AF305135

The Advanced Practitioner in Frailty and End-of-Life Care

The Advanced Practitioner in Frailty and End-of-Life Care

Hasan H. Alsararatee

Acute Medicine Advanced Practitioner
Northampton General Hospital
Northampton, United Kingdom

Senior Lecturer in Advanced Practice
Buckinghamshire New University
High Wycombe, United Kingdom

Series Editor

Ian Peate, OBE FRCN EN(G) RGN DipN(Lond) RNT
BEd(Hons) MA(Lond)LLM Hon DUniv (BNU)

WILEY

This edition first published 2026

© 2026 John Wiley & Sons Ltd

All rights reserved, including rights for text and data mining and training of artificial intelligence technologies or similar technologies. No part of this publication may be reproduced, stored in a retrieval system, or transmitted, in any form or by any means, electronic, mechanical, photocopying, recording or otherwise, except as permitted by law. Advice on how to obtain permission to reuse material from this title is available at http://www.wiley.com/go/permissions.

The right of Hasan H. Alsararatee to be identified as the author of this work has been asserted in accordance with law.

Registered Offices
John Wiley & Sons, Inc., 111 River Street, Hoboken, NJ 07030, USA
John Wiley & Sons Ltd, New Era House, 8 Oldlands Way, Bognor Regis, West Sussex, PO22 9NQ, UK

For details of our global editorial offices, customer services, and more information about Wiley products visit us at www.wiley.com.

The manufacturer's authorized representative according to the EU General Product Safety Regulation is Wiley-VCH GmbH, Boschstr. 12, 69469 Weinheim, Germany, e-mail: Product_Safety@wiley.com.

Wiley also publishes its books in a variety of electronic formats and by print-on-demand. Some content that appears in standard print versions of this book may not be available in other formats.

Trademarks: Wiley and the Wiley logo are trademarks or registered trademarks of John Wiley & Sons, Inc. and/or its affiliates in the United States and other countries and may not be used without written permission. All other trademarks are the property of their respective owners. John Wiley & Sons, Inc. is not associated with any product or vendor mentioned in this book.

Limit of Liability/Disclaimer of Warranty
The contents of this work are intended to further general scientific research, understanding, and discussion only and are not intended and should not be relied upon as recommending or promoting scientific method, diagnosis, or treatment by physicians for any particular patient. In view of ongoing research, equipment modifications, changes in governmental regulations, and the constant flow of information relating to the use of medicines, equipment, and devices, the reader is urged to review and evaluate the information provided in the package insert or instructions for each medicine, equipment, or device for, among other things, any changes in the instructions or indication of usage and for added warnings and precautions. While the publisher and the authors have used their best efforts in preparing this work, including a review of the content of the work, neither the publisher nor the authors make any representations or warranties with respect to the accuracy or completeness of the contents of this work and specifically disclaim all warranties, including without limitation any implied warranties of merchantability or fitness for a particular purpose. No warranty may be created or extended by sales representatives, written sales materials or promotional statements for this work. The fact that an organization, website, or product is referred to in this work as a citation and/or potential source of further information does not mean that the publisher and authors endorse the information or services the organization, website, or product may provide or recommendations it may make. This work is sold with the understanding that the publisher is not engaged in rendering professional services. The advice and strategies contained herein may not be suitable for your situation. You should consult with a specialist where appropriate. Further, readers should be aware that websites listed in this work may have changed or disappeared between when this work was written and when it is read. Neither the publisher nor authors shall be liable for any loss of profit or any other commercial damages, including but not limited to special, incidental, consequential, or other damages.

Library of Congress Cataloging-in-Publication Data
Names: Alsararatee, Hasan H. author | Peate, Ian series editor
Title: The advanced practitioner in frailty and end-of-life care / Hasan H.
  Alsararatee, Ian Peate.
Description: Hoboken, NJ : Wiley, [2026] | Includes bibliographical
  references and index.
Identifiers: LCCN 2026003772 (print) | LCCN 2026003773 (ebook) | ISBN
  9781394415823 hardback | ISBN 9781394415847 adobe pdf | ISBN
  9781394415830 epub
Subjects: LCSH: Terminal care–Great Britain | Palliative treatment–Great
  Britain | Geriatric nursing–Great Britain | Older people–Medical
  care–Great Britain | Geriatrics–Great Britain
Classification: LCC RT87.T45 A43 2026 (print) | LCC RT87.T45 (ebook)
LC record available at https://lccn.loc.gov/2026003772
LC ebook record available at https://lccn.loc.gov/2026003773

Cover Design: Wiley
Cover Image: © alfpoint/Shutterstock

Set in 10.5/13pt STIXTwoText by Straive, Pondicherry, India
Printed and bound by CPI Group (UK) Ltd, Croydon, CR0 4YY
C9781394415823_180526

Contents

About the Author vii

Preface viii

Acknowledgements ix

SECTION I   Foundations of Frailty and Advanced Practice **1**

CHAPTER 1   The Advanced Practitioner in Frailty and End-of-Life Medicine 3

CHAPTER 2   Conceptual Foundations of Frailty 15

CHAPTER 3   Frailty and Intrinsic Capacity: Frameworks for Healthy Ageing
and Advanced Practice 34

CHAPTER 4   Epidemiology of Frailty 46

CHAPTER 5   Frailty Risk Factors, Interventions, and Related Complications 56

SECTION II   Clinical Assessment and Frailty Assessment Tools **75**

CHAPTER 6   History-taken and Physical Examination Within the Context of Frailty 77

CHAPTER 7   Comprehensive Geriatric Assessment in Clinical Practice 98

CHAPTER 8   Frailty Assessment Tools 132

CHAPTER 9   Polypharmacy and Deprescribing 148

CHAPTER 10 Sarcopenia and Frailty 163

CHAPTER 11 Ageing and Physiological Changes 175

SECTION III   Geriatric Medicine   **195**

CHAPTER 12 Neurology System   201

CHAPTER 13 Psychiatry   217

CHAPTER 14 Cardiology   234

CHAPTER 15 Respiratory Medicine   253

CHAPTER 16 Gastroenterology   267

CHAPTER 17 Genitourinary System   279

CHAPTER 18 Renal System   289

CHAPTER 19 Endocrinology System   300

CHAPTER 20 Skin   315

CHAPTER 21 Musculoskeletal System   325

SECTION IV   End-of-Life Medicine and Ethical Dimensions   **345**

CHAPTER 22 Advance Care Planning and Difficult Conversations   347

CHAPTER 23 Managing the Most Common Symptoms in End-of-Life Medicine   357

CHAPTER 24 Ethical Consideration in Frailty and End-of-Life Medicine   369

SECTION V   Future Directions   **387**

CHAPTER 25 The Future of Frailty and End-of-Life Medicine   389

Index   398

About the Author

Hasan is a Senior Lecturer in Advanced Practice at Northampton General Hospital, England, and a Senior Lecturer in Advanced Practice at Buckinghamshire New University, London, England. He serves as a Committee Member of the Association of Advanced Practice Educators (AAPE), UK, and as an Editorial Board Member of the *International Journal of Advancing Practice*, as well as a peer reviewer across various peer-reviewed journals. He is also the winner of the UHN Research, Innovation and Improvement Excellence Award 2024.

Preface

Advanced practitioners (APs) are central to the delivery of safe, effective, and person-centred care for people living with frailty and approaching their end of life. This role requires clinical excellence, sound ethical judgement, and leadership across health and social care systems. This book is considered as part of the wider Advanced Practice series, providing an authoritative resource for APs who wish to evidence and extend their capabilities within these demanding fields.

Frailty and end-of-life medicine bring together the highest levels of clinical reasoning and compassionate care. Advanced practice in these areas is defined not by a job title but by a level of expertise and accountability, characterised by autonomy, complex decision-making and the ability to work across traditional professional boundaries. APs are expected to integrate the four pillars of advanced practice including clinical practice, leadership and management, education, and research while managing uncertainty, multimorbidity, and rapid change.

This volume builds on national developments including the Multi-Professional Framework for APs (NHS England, 2025) and the credentials for older people/frailty, palliative and end-of-life care, and acute medicine frameworks (NHS England, 2022; NHS England, 2023). It complements earlier titles in the *Advanced Practice* series, yet stands as a complete and independent guide. Each chapter combines evidence-based discussion with practical tools, reflective questions, and case studies, so that readers can map their learning to the competencies required for professional recognition and service improvement.

Our aim is to equip enhanced practitioners, APs, and those preparing for consultant-level practice with the knowledge, skills, and confidence to lead high-quality care for some of the most vulnerable patients. By integrating clinical science, ethical reflection, and system leadership, the book supports readers to demonstrate the standards of advanced practice and to shape services that are both responsive and sustainable.

Hasan H. Alsararatee

REFERENCES

NHS England (2022). Older people advanced practice area-specific capability and curriculum framework. Available at: `https://advanced-practice.hee.nhs.uk/wp-content/uploads/sites/28/2025/01/Older-people-advanced-practice-area-specific-capability-and-curriculum-framework-NHSE.pdf` (accessed 23 March 2026).

NHS England (2023). Palliative and end of life care advanced practice area-specific capability and curriculum framework. Available at: `https://advanced-practice.hee.nhs.uk/wp-content/uploads/sites/28/2025/01/Palliative-and-end-of-life-care-advanced-practice-area-specific-capability-and-curriculum-framework-NHSE.pdf` (accessed 23 March 2026).

NHS England (2025). *Multi-professional framework for advanced practice in England – Edition 2025*. NHS England. Available at: `https://advanced-practice.hee.nhs.uk/wp-content/uploads/sites/28/2025/05/Multi-professional-framework-for-advanced-practice-in-England---Edition-2025.pdf` (accessed 29 January 2026).

Acknowledgements

First, I wish to express my deepest thanks to my family especially my partner Raghad, my father Hazim and my beautiful son Abbas. They have stood by me, supported me, and courteously accepted the time that writing this book has taken from our lives. I remember many sleepless nights spent reviewing ideas, drafting and redrafting chapters, and seeking permissions from copyright holders. Writing and editing a book of this scope has been a massive achievement, and I am so proud of this achievement.

Second, I am especially grateful to my friend Professor Ian Peate, who consistently encouraged me to continue. I still recall his words when I doubted the structure of the book after reviewers' feedback: 'Are you getting cold feet?' a question that encouraged me to keep going.

Third, I extend sincere gratitude to the patients and families whose experiences have shaped my understanding of frailty and end-of-life care. Their courage and insights form the true foundation of this book.

Fourth, I warmly thank the editorial managers at Wiley, Tom and Christabel, whose guidance has been invaluable. I am particularly grateful to Christabel for her readiness to answer my many queries about permissions and publishing requirements.

Fifth, I thank the anonymous peer reviewers whose thoughtful comments shaped and strengthened the final content, even though their identities remain unknown to me.

Finally, I am grateful to my friends and colleagues at Northampton General Hospital and to the academic teams at Buckinghamshire New University for their continuing support and encouragement.

Hasan H. Alsararatee

FOUNDATIONS OF FRAILTY AND ADVANCED PRACTICE

The Advanced Practitioner in Frailty and End-of-Life Medicine

Aim

The aim of this chapter is to introduce the scope and capabilities of advanced practitioners (APs) in frailty and end-of-life medicine, to explain how the Centre for Advancing Practice structures credentials and curricula, and to map expectations to the multi-professional framework (MPF) 2025 and area-specific capability in older people/frailty and palliative and end-of-life care. The chapter sets the academic and professional context of the book and shows trainees and qualified APs how to evidence their capabilities across the four pillars using the chapters that follow.

LEARNING OUTCOMES

After reading this chapter, readers will be able to:

1. Describe the MPF (2025a), including the definition and scope of advanced practice and the four pillars, with specific reference to practice in contexts of complexity and uncertainty.
2. Summarise the role of the Centre for Advancing Practice in endorsing programmes, supporting credentials, and assuring quality via national standards and a directory.
3. Identify how area-specific frameworks for older people/frailty and palliative and end-of-life care complement the MPF and specify capabilities relevant to this book.
4. Use the structure of this book to evidence pillar-aligned competence (e.g. comprehensive geriatric assessment [CGA], frailty identification, advance care planning, ethical decision-making, and service improvement).

SELF-ASSESSMENT QUESTIONS

1. Explain how the MPF (2025a) defines advanced practice and describe how its four pillars underpin work with frailty and end-of-life care.
2. Discuss how the Centre for Advancing Practice's credentialing process supports governance, supervision, and evidencing of advanced practitioner capability in frailty and palliative care services.

> To practise at an advanced level is to lead within the grey zones of care, where evidence softens, ethics strengthen, and uncertainty guides professional judgement.

INTRODUCTION

Frailty and end-of-life care are shaped by the dynamic interaction between multimorbidity, functional decline, and ethical decision-making (Alsararatee et al., 2025). These areas necessitate autonomous and expert practice in contexts characterised by uncertainty, where information is often incomplete and clinical risk is high. The multi-professional framework (MPF) (NHS England, 2025a) highlights that advanced practice is a level of practice, rather than a job title, characterised by complex decision-making, accountability, and leadership, underpinned by four pillars: clinical practice, leadership and management, education, and research. Furthermore, the 2025 edition retains these pillar names but broadens their framing so that advanced practice is recognisable and applicable across professions and care contexts.

This book articulates this level of practice for advanced practitioners (APs) working with frailty and end-of-life needs. The early chapters define the key concepts, such as frailty models and intrinsic capacity. Later chapters address history-taking, physical examination, comprehensive geriatric assessment (CGA), and frailty assessment tools (e.g. the clinical frailty scale and the electronic frailty index [eFI]). Additional chapters explore geriatric medicine, communication, ethics, and future directions. Each of these topics is clearly linked to the four pillars of advanced practice and to the area-specific capabilities for older people and for palliative and end-of-life care. The chapters of the book are mapped to the MPF and other credentials, as outlined below.

Multi-Professional Framework (MPF) for APs (NHS England, 2025b)

This chapter is applicable to the MPF (NHS England, 2025b).

Accreditation Consideration

This chapter is applicable to the following specialist curriculum framework:

Curriculum framework for APs in the care of older people (NHS England, 2022a).
Curriculum framework for APs in the case of palliative and end-of-life care (NHS England, 2023a).
Curriculum for APs in acute medicine (NHS England, 2023b).

THE 2025 MPF: STABILITY AND ASSURANCE IN ADVANCED PRACTICE

The framework updates terminology ('advanced practice' and 'advanced practitioner'), clarifies that it is a distinct level exercised in complex contexts, and reaffirms the four pillars as the common backbone for capability development and assurance. There is a minor wording change to the CP1.5 and CP2.1 (Figure 1.1).

Why it matters for this book: The MPF 2025 is your baseline: wherever a chapter extends knowledge (for example, CGA or anticipatory prescribing), readers can map evidence to the relevant pillar descriptors and use that mapping in portfolios, supervision meetings, and appraisal. The MPF explicitly invites interpretation 'in light of the profession and context', which legitimises the way this book translates the four pillars into frailty and end-of-life contexts.

Capability number	2017 wording	2025 wording
Clinical practice: 1.5	Demonstrate effective communication skills, supporting people in making decisions, planning care or seeking to make positive changes, using Health Education England's Framework to promote person-centred approaches in health and care.	Demonstrate effective communication skills, supporting people in making decisions, planning care or seeking to make positive changes, using NHS England's Framework to promote person-centred approaches in health and care.
Leadership and management: 2.1	Pro-actively initiate and develop effective relationships, fostering clarity of roles within teams, to encourage productive working.	Demonstrate and role model inclusive attitudes and behaviours to pro-actively initiate and develop relationships, fostering clarity of roles within teams, to encourage productive working.

Terminology change: 'advanced practice' replaces 'advanced clinical practice'

FIGURE 1.1   Changes to the wording of the capabilities of MPF. *Source*: Adapted from NHS England (2025).

THE CENTRE FOR ADVANCING PRACTICE: GOVERNANCE, CREDENTIALS, AND DIRECTORY

The Centre for Advancing Practice oversees programme endorsement, area-specific capability frameworks ('credentials'), supervision standards, and quality management of advanced practice development. Its approach is laid out within the area-specific documents you provided (notably palliative and end-of-life care), which detail how learning outcomes, workplace supervision, and integrated academic/work-based assessment combine to evidence competence. These documents also reference governance standards and minimum supervision requirements published by the Centre for Advancing Practice, setting expectations for trainee and qualified APs and their organisations.

WHY APs SHOULD ENGAGE WITH AREA-SPECIFIC CAPABILITY FRAMEWORKS

APs should engage with the area-specific capability and curriculum frameworks because they provide a nationally recognised structure for evidencing advanced-level competence. Developed by the Centre for Advancing Practice, these frameworks, formerly known as credentials, define the precise skills, knowledge, and behaviours required to deliver safe, effective, and person-centred care within distinct clinical fields, such as frailty, palliative and end-of-life care, and acute medicine. They bring clarity by specifying what counts as credible evidence of capability, transferability through recognition across organisations and professional groups, and assurance by creating a shared national language for advanced practice. In addition, they support structured workplace supervision and assessment through portfolio tools such as logbooks, case-based discussions, and multi-source feedback. By aligning personal development and practice evidence with these frameworks, APs strengthen professional credibility, promote consistency in standards, and demonstrate leadership in shaping the future of advanced clinical care.

AREA-SPECIFIC FRAMEWORKS: OLDER PEOPLE/FRAILTY AND PALLIATIVE AND END-OF-LIFE CARE

Older People/Frailty

The Older People Advanced Practice Framework (NHS England, 2022b) provides a structured set of Capabilities in Practice (CiPs) that outline expectations for APs working with older adults. These are divided into three categories: core, generic clinical, and specialty clinical capabilities. Together, they establish a benchmark for the knowledge, skills, and behaviours required to deliver safe, person-centred care for older people, particularly in the context of frailty and end-of-life care.

At the core level, APs are expected to function within healthcare organisational and management systems, exercising autonomy within their scope of practice and sphere of influence. They should demonstrate the ability to manage complex ethical and legal challenges, employ advanced communication to support shared decision-making, and maintain professionalism and situational awareness. Core CiPs also emphasise leadership in service improvement, the capacity to critically appraise and contribute to research, and the responsibility to act as both learner and educator, modelling a culture of continuous development.

The generic clinical CiPs focus on the AP's ability to deliver care across a wide range of presentations and settings. These include undertaking advanced clinical assessments in the face of uncertainty, leading acute interventions for deteriorating patients, and managing the diagnosis and long-term care of individuals in outpatient, ambulatory, and community contexts. Practitioners must also demonstrate expertise in managing complex discharges, leading multi-professional teams, and applying palliative and end-of-life care skills where uncertainty and complexity are prominent. This positions APs as clinicians capable of responding flexibly to the varied and often unpredictable needs of older patients.

The specialty clinical CiPs reflect the unique expertise required in working specifically with older people. These include critically applying specialist knowledge of ageing and frailty, demonstrating advanced communication tailored to older adults and their families, and delivering comprehensive assessments that underpin anticipatory and advanced care planning. Collectively, these specialty expectations align closely with the delivery of CGA and the coordinated management of frailty syndromes, which remain central to high-quality care for older people.

Importantly, the framework not only explores the CiPs but also sets out entry criteria, learning content, assessment methods, and a decision aid that makes expectations transparent for learners, supervisors, and employers. By aligning CiPs to practice outcomes, the framework ensures that APs are supported to deliver holistic, evidence-informed care while driving service improvement across boundaries. Ultimately, these capabilities position APs to provide leadership in the care of older adults, bridging specialties and coordinating safe, effective, person-centred care in the context of complexity, multimorbidity, and frailty (Figure 1.2).

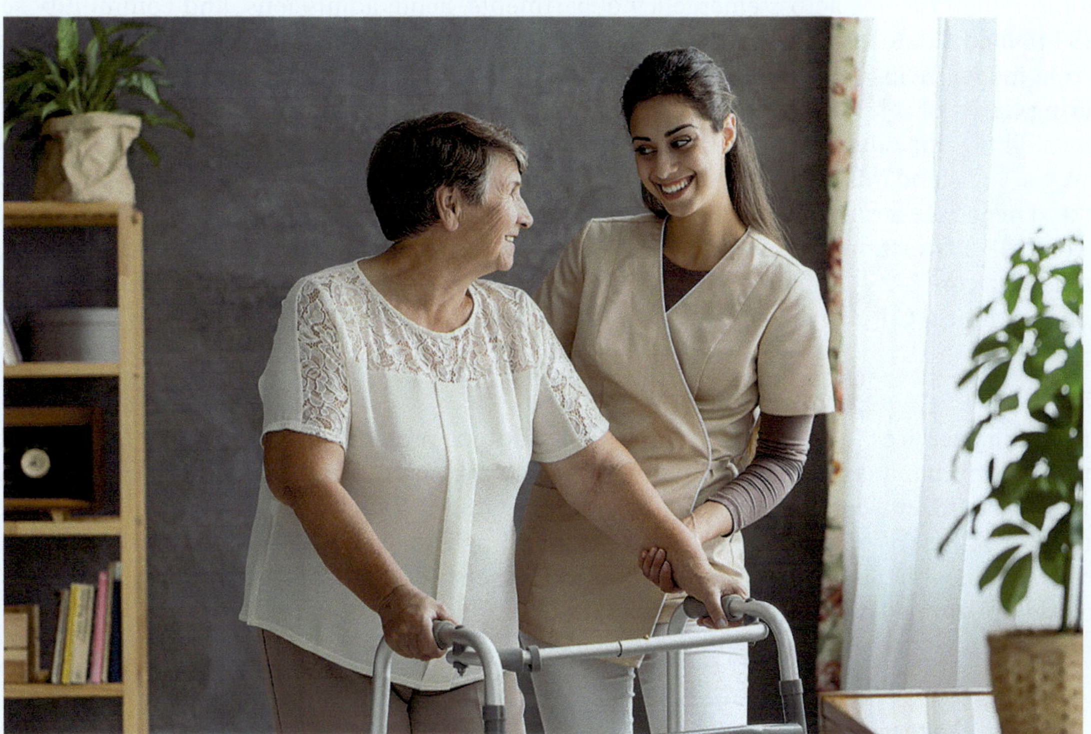

FIGURE 1.2   Person-centred care in frailty management. *Source*: Photographee.eu/Adobe Stock Photos.

What Does the Role of APs in Frailty Settings Look Like When Examined Across the Four Pillars of Advanced Practice?

Clinical Practice

In frailty services, APs bring advanced clinical assessment, diagnostic reasoning, and care-planning capabilities, enabling timely decision-making in complex presentations (NHS England, 2022a, 2025a). They synthesise multiple sources of data, including history, functional assessment, diagnostics, and risk stratification, and act under uncertainty, consistent with MPF core capability 1.6 to 'use expertise and decision-making ... synthesising information ... in complex situations' (NHS England, 2025b). Qualified and autonomous APs may manage patients screened for frailty in emergency departments, ambulatory care, or acute admissions, directing them into pathways such as admission, same-day discharge, or community management. These roles, increasingly used in 'front-door' frailty services, reduce length of stay and streamline care transitions. Practice also draws on generic clinical CiP 1 (advanced assessment in uncertainty) and CiP 3 (management of long-term conditions in complex settings). Because frailty is a syndrome of complexity and multimorbidity, APs should integrate specialty CiP 1 (critical use of advanced knowledge of older people and their contexts), CiP 2 (advanced communication with older people), and CiP 4 (expertise in advanced and anticipatory care planning). The evolving nature of these roles often blurs traditional boundaries with geriatricians and requires adaptability in role scope (Morley et al., 2022).

Leadership and Management

APs in frailty services frequently act as clinical leads and service-improvement catalysts, coordinating multidisciplinary teams across emergency departments, acute admissions, and community services (NHS England, 2025a). This reflects MPF leadership capability 2.1, which calls on APs to 'demonstrate and role model inclusive attitudes and behaviours to pro-actively initiate and develop relationships, fostering clarity of roles within teams, to encourage productive working' (NHS England, 2025b). Their responsibilities include developing and governing frailty screening protocols, admission-avoidance pathways, and standards of advanced practice. They may hold line-management duties for frailty team staff and negotiate service interfaces with social care and primary care providers. This work exemplifies core CiP 1 (functioning at an advanced level within healthcare organisational and management systems) and core CiP 4 (initiating and leading quality improvements focused on patient safety), as well as generic clinical CiP 5 (management of multi-professional teams and effective discharge planning).

Education

Within frailty services, APs act as educators and mentors, promoting best practice in CGA, falls prevention, delirium management, and frailty-syndrome principles. They design and deliver training for emergency, ward, and community teams, consistent with MPF capability 3.4 to 'advocate for and contribute to a culture of organisational learning' (NHS England, 2025a). This educational remit embodies core CiP 6, which expects APs to develop as learners, teachers, and supervisors, and it supports succession planning and the development of future leaders in frailty care.

Research

APs are expected to generate as well as apply evidence to strengthen frailty services. In line with MPF capability 4.2 to 'evaluate and audit own and others' clinical practice, quality improvement projects'

(NHS England, 2025a), they lead audits to measure outcomes such as length of stay, readmission rates, and functional recovery. They critically appraise emerging evidence on frailty phenotypes and multi-morbidity, integrate data from hospital and community services, and contribute to multicentre studies on new urgent-frailty care models. These responsibilities correspond to core CiP 5 (critical appraisal and research), generic clinical CiP 4 (management of complex or specialty problems), and specialty CiP 3 (assessing, planning, implementing, and evaluating specialist interventions). Dissemination through peer-reviewed publications and professional networks fulfils the MPF expectation that APs advance practice as researchers and educators (core CiP 6), ensuring that locally generated evidence informs national policy and future service design.

Reading this book through the lens of the Older People Advanced Practice Framework, the chapters on frailty concepts, intrinsic capacity, epidemiology, and assessment tools (such as Clinical Frailty Scale, Electronic Frailty Index, Edmonton Frail Scale, and Tilburg Frailty Indicator), together with those on polypharmacy, nutrition, and geriatric medicine, map directly onto the specialty CiPs. These areas equip APs to demonstrate clinical reasoning, optimise medicines management, mitigate risk, and coordinate multidisciplinary care.

PALLIATIVE AND END-OF-LIFE CARE FRAMEWORK

The capabilities and learning outcomes of APs working in palliative and end-of-life care can be understood through the four pillars of advanced clinical practice: clinical, leadership and management, education, and research. Within the clinical pillar, APs are expected to work autonomously within ethical and legal frameworks, taking responsibility for complex decisions in uncertain circumstances. Central to this role is the ability to establish therapeutic alliances through advanced communication skills, to undertake holistic assessments that integrate biological, psychological, social, and spiritual dimensions, and to co-produce care plans that support both current and future needs. APs must also manage continuity of care, responding to deterioration, supporting families, and coordinating bereavement care.

The leadership and management pillar highlights the AP's role in shaping services and creating supportive organisational cultures. This includes critical appraisal of health policy, leading service innovation, and promoting safety in the presence of complexity, risk, and unpredictability. APs are required to role-model collaborative teamworking across statutory and voluntary sectors, often in unfamiliar or challenging contexts.

The education pillar recognises the dual responsibility of APs as both learners and educators. APs must critically appraise and apply educational strategies to promote safe, evidence-based, and person-centred palliative care. They also facilitate interprofessional learning, contributing to a culture where teams, patients, and carers can engage in shared understanding.

The research pillar ensures that practice is grounded in evidence and continually advancing. APs in palliative care must be able to critically appraise research, contribute to governance systems, and apply quality improvement methodologies to strengthen care delivery. Working strategically across local, regional, and national systems, they influence policy and service development, thereby extending their impact beyond individual patient encounters. These four pillars provide a comprehensive framework for APs in palliative and end-of-life care. They ensure that APs are not only clinically competent, but also capable of leading change, supporting learning, and contributing to the evidence base, all while maintaining a strong focus on person-centred, ethically grounded care.

What Does the Role of APs in Frailty Settings Look Like When Examined Across the Four Pillars of Advanced Practice?

Clinical Practice

In palliative and end-of-life care, APs must deliver complex, holistic care, manage symptoms, participate in advanced care planning, and tailor care in uncertain prognostic contexts. The area-specific capability framework for palliative care builds on the core competencies while specifying additional expectations (e.g. care of dying, symptom control, and psychosocial and spiritual care) (NHS England, 2023). APs in palliative settings must interpret ambiguous presentations, manage complex pain and non-pain symptoms, lead deterioration decision-making, and support anticipatory care and end-of-life transitions. They must act as clinical leads in difficult conversations, capacity assessments, and shared decision-making.

Leadership and Management

APs in palliative care often lead or coordinate in multi-professional teams in hospice, hospital palliative units, or community services. They may shape service policies (for example, advance care planning protocols and framework for end-of-life pathways), liaise with hospital and community providers, and ensure governance of care standards. They may contribute to embedding palliative care strategies across wards or networks. This role demands capabilities in negotiation across boundaries, championing palliative culture, and system integration.

Education

Education is a critical pillar, particularly in palliative care: APs teach colleagues (physicians, nurses, and other allied healthcare professionals) in symptom management, communication skills, shared decision-making, and end-of-life care. They may deliver workshops on advanced care planning, breaking bad news skills, and capacity, and promote reflective practice. They also mentor trainees and act as supervisors, fostering a palliative mindset across disciplines. This meets capability 3.3 'work collaboratively to support health literacy ... for individuals, families and colleagues' (NHS England, 2025a).

Research

APs in palliative and end-of-life care are expected to engage in or lead research that advances practice and service delivery. They may evaluate interventions such as hospital-initiated palliative models for frail older people (Sharratt et al., 2024), explore the implementation of AP, or contribute to improvement science in symptom management and service models. In line with the NHS England palliative area-specific framework (2023), APs are required to use robust governance systems, apply appropriate research methodologies, and disseminate findings to build the specialty's evidence base. This includes leading implementation or service evaluation studies on integrated pathways and rapid discharge schemes, undertaking mixed-methods and participatory research with patients and carers, and managing large-scale data audits to monitor outcomes such as preferred place of death and hospital avoidance. Publication in peer-reviewed journals, presentation at professional conferences, and incorporation of findings into clinical guidelines complete the research cycle envisaged by the MPF.

FROM FRAMEWORK TO CURRICULUM: HOW APs BUILD AND PROVE CAPABILITY

The area-specific documents describe a joined-up model: academic learning (Higher Education Institution [HEI] modules at Level 7/8), workplace-based learning (supervised practice and reflective logs), and multi-method assessment (case-based discussions, Objective Structured Clinical Examination [OSCE]/ observed practice, multi-source feedback, and annual review). This is underpinned by governance, equality/inclusion commitments, and defined roles for coordinating and associate supervisors, ensuring educational quality and accountability while enabling flexibility for different professions and settings.

CORE PRACTICES THIS BOOK EXPECTS APs TO DEMONSTRATE

Comprehensive Geriatric Assessment (CGA) as a Method and Mindset

CGA is a team-delivered, person-centred process integrating medical, functional, psychological, and social assessments to guide coordinated plans. Your materials and references position CGA as the default lens for APs working with older adults, whether in community urgent response, same-day emergency care (SDEC), wards, or care homes linking directly to older-people CiPs and MPF Pillar-1 descriptors on holistic assessment and partnership working.

Frailty Identification and Grading, Sarcopenia

Chapters describe using CFS, eFI, and other validated tools to screen, stratify, and communicate risk. APs should record tool scores with context (baseline function, recent decline, cognition, and carers) and show how grading alters the plan (e.g. falls-prevention bundle, deprescribing, and Treatment Escalation Plan [TEP]/Do Not Attempt Cardiopulmonary Resuscitation [DNACPR] conversations). This is exemplary Pillar-1 and Pillar-2 evidence.

Polypharmacy and Deprescription, Undertaking a Comprehensive Frailty Assessment and Clinical Examination

Chapters outline how APs identify problematic polypharmacy and apply recognised deprescribing tools, highlighting key clinical considerations when withdrawing medicines. They describe performing a thorough history and advanced clinical examination within the frailty context, explicitly recognising sarcopenia and its functional impact. APs are expected to document findings with contextual details such as baseline function, recent decline, cognition, and carer support and to demonstrate how medicine optimisation changes management plans (e.g. falls-prevention measures, nutrition and exercise interventions, and TEP/DNACPR discussions). These are all related to the four pillars of MPF, the elderly medicine framework, and palliative care framework.

Advance Care Planning Process and Communication

The palliative framework's capabilities (e.g. CP1.8–CP1.10, CP2.1–CP2.5) align precisely with your ACP chapter: initiating goals-of-care dialogue, documenting preferences, and ensuring plans are visible across settings. APs can cite these capability codes when evidencing family meetings, treatment-escalation plans, and capacity/best-interests reasoning.

Ethics, Law, and Proportionality

Your ethics chapter aligns with CiPs on legal frameworks, capacity, best interests, confidentiality, and least-restrictive practices, and with MPF 2025 language on professional judgement and accountability. Portfolio entries should show transparent reasoning (risks/benefits, uncertainty, and burdens), especially when withholding/withdrawing therapies or using anticipatory medications under the doctrine of double effect.

Geriatric Medicine and Multidisciplinary Integration

Geriatric medicine underpins all aspects of frailty management, demanding advanced knowledge of age-related physiological changes, multimorbidity, and syndromic complexity. APs are expected to integrate diagnostic reasoning, therapeutics, and rehabilitation principles within multidisciplinary teams, ensuring evidence-based, person-centred care. Demonstration involves leadership in developing frailty pathways, implementing CGA outcomes, and contributing to service improvement through audit, education, and research.

HOW TO USE THIS BOOK

This textbook uses a consistent pedagogical structure to support effective learning and professional application. The following features appear throughout the chapters where relevant:

- Learning outcomes summarise the key topics addressed.
- Each chapter concludes with a wisdom phrase, inspiring APs to reflect, refine judgement, and translate knowledge into purposeful action.
- Self-assessment questions allow you to test and consolidate understanding.
- MPF for advanced clinical practice links content to professional development and accreditation standards.
- Centre for Advancing Practice accreditations including advanced clinical practitioners' framework in the care of the elderly, palliative and end-of-life care, and acute medicine.
- Examination scenarios encourage reflection on clinical reasoning and decision-making.
- Learning events prompt critical reflection on key issues.
- Pharmacological principles integrate pharmacology with clinical content.
- Case studies present practice-based scenarios to develop analytical and decision-making skills.
- Take-home points provide succinct summaries for quick review.

CONCLUSION

The MPF 2025 provides a stable spine for advanced practice; the older-people and palliative and end-of-life frameworks add the musculature specific to frailty and dying; and this book supplies the organs of daily practice methods, tools, cases, and reasoned positions you can present as evidence. Across settings (emergency department, urgent care, inpatient wards and care homes), APs are expected to assess holistically, decide under uncertainty, lead ethically, educate teams, and evaluate services. The chapters that follow are written to be lift-and-use evidence against the pillar statements (MPF 2025b) and the capability codes within area-specific frameworks, so that your growth as an AP is demonstrable, defensible, and transferable.

Take-Home Messages

1. Advanced practice is a defined level of practice characterised by complex decision-making, accountability, and leadership across four interdependent pillars: clinical, leadership and management, education, and research.

2. The Centre for Advancing Practice and its area-specific credentials (older people/frailty and palliative and end-of-life care) provide a national framework to evidence competence, support supervision, and ensure consistency and quality across diverse care settings.

3. APs should demonstrate transparent clinical reasoning and ethical judgement when managing frailty and end-of-life care, ensuring that decisions remain proportionate and person-centred.

4. Mapping the APs' activities to the MPF and relevant credentials strengthens professional credibility and supports appraisal, revalidation, and career progression.

REFERENCES

Alsararatee, H.H., Mukhtar, M., and Musawar, A. (2025). Ethical principles and challenges in end-of-life care for frail older adults. *British Journal of Nursing* 34 (11): 547–553.

Morley, D.A., Kilgore, C., Edwards, M. et al. (2022). The changing role of advanced clinical practitioners working with older people during the COVID-19 pandemic: a qualitative research study. *International Journal of Nursing Studies* 130: 104235.

NHS England (2022a). *Older people advanced practice area specific capability and curriculum framework.* NHS England. Available at: https://advanced-practice.hee.nhs.uk/wp-content/uploads/sites/28/2025/01/Older-people-advanced-practice-area-specific-capability-and-curriculum-framework-NHSE.pdf (accessed 30 January 2026).

NHS England (2022b). *Advanced Clinical Practice in Acute Medicine: Curriculum Framework.* London: Health Education England https://advanced-practice.hee.nhs.uk/wp-content/uploads/sites/28/2024/04/Advanced%20clinical%20practice%20in%20acute%20medicine%20curriculum%20framework.pdf (accessed 25 September 2025).

NHS England (2023a). *Palliative and end of life care advanced practice area specific capability and curriculum framework.* NHS England. Available at: https://advanced-practice.hee.nhs.uk/wp-content/uploads/sites/28/2025/01/Palliative-and-end-of-life-care-advanced-practice-area-specific-capability-and-curriculum-framework-NHSE.pdf (accessed 30 January 2026).

NHS England (2023b). *Acute medicine advanced practice area specific capability and curriculum framework.* NHS England. Available at: https://advanced-practice.hee.nhs.uk/wp-content/uploads/sites/28/2025/03/Acute-medicine-advanced-practice-area-specific-capability-and-curriculum-framework-NHSE.pdf (accessed 30 January 2026).

NHS England (2025a). *Multi-professional framework for advanced practice in England – Edition 2025.* NHS England. Available at: https://advanced-practice.hee.nhs.uk/wp-content/uploads/

sites/28/2025/05/Multi-professional-framework-for-advanced-practice-in-England---Edition-2025.pdf (accessed 29 January 2026).

NHS England (2025b). *Multi-professional framework (MPF) 2025: capabilities.* https://advanced-practice.hee.nhs.uk/mpf2025/capabilities (accessed 25 September 2025).

Sharratt, P., Zacharias, A., Nwosu, A.C., and Gadoud, A. (2024). Hospital-initiated palliative care interventions for adults with frailty: findings from a systematic review and narrative synthesis. *Age and Ageing* 53 (9): afae190.

CHAPTER 2

Conceptual Foundations of Frailty

Aim

The aim of this chapter is to provide a foundation for understanding frailty by exploring its conceptual development. It introduces the historical context in which frailty was described; explains the evolution of formal models such as the Fried frailty phenotype, the deficit accumulation model, and the frailty index; and explores the role of the electronic frailty index in current practice. This framework will support advanced practitioners to critically apply frailty concepts in clinical decision-making and service planning.

LEARNING OUTCOMES

After reading this chapter, readers will:

1. Understand the historical development of frailty and why formalised models were required.
2. Explain the key principles of the Fried frailty phenotype, deficit accumulation model, and frailty index.
3. Evaluate the advantages and disadvantages of the main frailty models in predicting outcomes and guiding care.
4. Describe the purpose and application of the electronic frailty index in general practice.
5. Apply knowledge of frailty concepts to inform personalised, multidisciplinary care planning.

SELF-ASSESSMENT QUESTIONS

1. How would you currently define frailty, and how does your understanding distinguish it from ageing, multimorbidity, and disability?
2. What formal models of frailty (e.g. phenotype, deficit accumulation, or electronic frailty index) are you already familiar with, and how might they influence your clinical decision-making?

Frailty is not the shadow of age but the mirror of accumulated burdens, biological, psychological, and social that gradually reduce resilience.

INTRODUCTION

Advanced practitioners (APs) require a critical understanding of frailty's conceptual development in order to assess, stratify, and plan care for older adults. The ability to apply models such as the frailty phenotype, deficit accumulation model, frailty index (FI), and electronic frailty index (eFI) supports advanced clinical reasoning, anticipatory care, and service design. This chapter situates these models within the multi-professional framework (MPF) for advanced practice (NHS England, 2025), which defines the four pillars of clinical practice, leadership and management, education, and research. By examining the historical origins of frailty, analysing key models and their predictive value, and highlighting their implications for personalised care, the chapter equips APs to embed robust conceptual foundations into everyday practice. It also maps to national advanced practice curricula for the care of older people, palliative and end-of-life care, and acute medicine, demonstrating how theoretical insight underpins the competencies and capabilities expected of APs across these domains.

Multi-Professional Framework (MPF) for Advanced Practitioners

(Adapted from NHS England, 2025)

This chapter maps to the following areas within the MPF:

- Clinical pillar: 1.1–1.11
- Leadership and management: 2.1, 2.2, 2.3, 2.5, 2.7, 2.8, 2.9
- Education: 3.1, 3.2, 3.3, 3.5, 3.7, 3.8
- Research: 4.1, 4.2, 4.3, 4.4, 4.5, 4.7, 4.8

Accreditation Consideration

This chapter maps to the statement with the following national accretional documents:

Curriculum framework for advanced practice in the care of older people (NHS England, 2022):

1. Core Capabilities in Practice (CiPs): 1–6
2. Generic Clinical CiPs: 1–6
3. Specialty Clinical CiPs: 1–4

Curriculum framework for APs in the case of palliative and end-of-life care (NHS England, 2023a):

1. Clinical pillar: 1.1–1.4
2. Leadership and research: 2.1–2.3
3. Education: 3.1–3.3
4. Research: 4.1–4.3

Curriculum for APs in acute medicine (NHS England, 2023b):

1. Core CiPs: 1, 2, 3, 5, 6
2. Generic Clinical CiPs: 1, 3, 5, 6
3. Specialty Clinical CiPs (Acute Medicine): 1–5 and acute medicine presentations.

THE CONCEPT OF FRAILTY PRIOR FRAILTY PHENOTYPE AND THE DEFICIT ACCUMULATION MODULE

The idea of frailty as a distinct condition in older adults predates the more formalised models of the frailty phenotype (Fried et al., 2001) and the deficit accumulation index (Rockwood and Mitnitski, 2007). Earlier understandings were descriptive and often inconsistent, with clinicians using the term to capture a general impression of vulnerability in later life. In seventeenth- and eighteenth-century medical writing, frailty was often equated with weakness, debility, or decrepitude and was closely linked with the ageing process itself (Bortz, 2002). These interpretations tended to conflate frailty with old age, disability, and comorbidity, meaning it was not conceptualised as a separate syndrome. By the mid-twentieth century, geriatric medicine began to frame frailty as more than chronological age alone. Observations in the 1950s and 1960s showed that individuals of similar ages could follow very different trajectories: some maintained independence despite multiple illnesses, while others experienced rapid decline despite fewer diagnoses (Gobbens et al., 2010). This recognition helped establish frailty as a multidimensional state characterised by reduced physiological reserve and increased susceptibility to stressors.

A policy innovation occurred in 1978 when the Federal Council on Aging in the United States introduced the term 'frail elderly'. This referred primarily to people over 75 years of age who were heavy users of health and social care services often because of overlapping medical, psychological, and functional problems (Kane et al., 1994). The phrase captured frailty as a combination of physical and cognitive decline, while emphasising that it was not an inevitable consequence of ageing but a state of vulnerability affecting a subgroup of older adults. During the 1980s and 1990s, frailty was increasingly understood as multidomain in nature. Researchers described it as the result of combined influences across physical, psychological, and social spheres, with issues such as isolation, withdrawal, and depression identified as accelerating decline (Strawbridge et al., 1998). At the same time, some authors proposed that frailty should be regarded as a pre-disability stage, occupying the space between healthy ageing and established functional dependence (Winograd et al., 1991). Others saw it as the cumulative impact of multiple physiological impairments that overlapped with geriatric syndromes such as falls, delirium, or incontinence (Campbell and Buchner, 1997). Despite these efforts, no agreed definition or measurement tool existed, and frailty remained a descriptive label applied variably in both research and clinical care.

Alongside these conceptual developments, comprehensive geriatric assessment emerged as a systematic way of evaluating older adults across medical, psychological, and social domains. Although not designed to define frailty specifically, this approach reflected the growing appreciation that the needs of vulnerable older people could not be understood through a single lens (Stuck et al., 1993). The multidomain framework of comprehensive geriatric assessment therefore helped pave the way for later operational models. In the years before Fried's phenotype and Rockwood's index, frailty was recognised as a state of vulnerability distinct from chronological age, multimorbidity, or disability, but without the precision required for clinical and research application. The limitations of this descriptive era underlined the need for reproducible tools, which emerged in the early 2000s and continue to shape practice today.

What Is Frailty?

It is a long-term condition characterised by loss of biological reserves across multiple systems and vulnerability to decompensation after a stressful event (Clegg et al., 2013). In addition, frailty is thought to arise from age-related decline in multiple organ systems, driven by oxidative stress, persistent inflammation, inadequate physical activity, and poor nutrition (2.2)

Figure 2.1 shows how frailty alters recovery from seemingly minor illness. Mrs. Margret, aged 79 years, recovered to baseline within two weeks after an lower respiratory tract infection (LRTI), supported by family and antibiotics. In contrast, Mrs. Cameron, also 79 years with LRTI, developed delirium and falls, was admitted to hospital, and discharged with carer support, having lost her previous independence.

For APs, this highlights that chronological age alone does not determine outcomes. Frailty amplifies vulnerability, leading to disproportionate decline after minor illness. Recognising frailty, conducting timely CGA, and planning anticipatory care are essential to supporting recovery and preventing avoidable dependence.

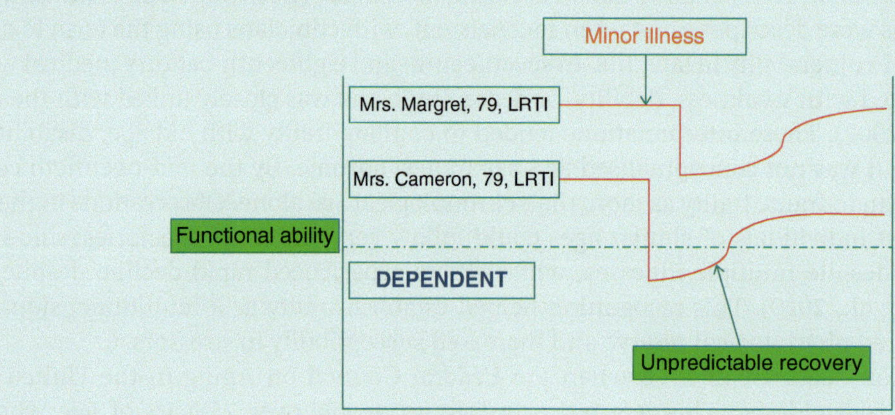

FIGURE 2.1   Variable recovery trajectories in frailty.

WHEN RESILIENCE FAILS: THE PATHWAY TO FRAILTY

Advancing age, multimorbidity, and disability interact to impair functional reserve, producing a cumulative loss of adaptability across multiple organ systems (Figure 2.3). This reduction in physiological reserve increases susceptibility to even minor stressors, such as infection or minor injury, which can precipitate acute illness, hospital admission, or functional decline. The model (Figure 2.3) highlights that frailty is not merely a by-product of ageing but a complex, dynamic process shaped by biological, psychological, and social factors. Once established, frailty creates a downward trajectory in which each episode of illness or decompensation further diminishes resilience, perpetuating a cycle that often culminates in dependency, institutionalisation, and death. Recognising frailty as a continuum rather than a fixed state allows APs to intervene early through comprehensive assessment, optimisation of comorbidities, and targeted rehabilitation to restore or preserve physiological reserve wherever possible. This conceptual understanding highlights the essence of geriatric medicine: care that prioritises function, independence, and quality of life over disease-specific outcomes. For APs, appreciating the mechanisms by which resilience fails is fundamental to anticipating deterioration, planning holistic care, and supporting patients and families through the progressive course of frailty (Figures 2.2–2.5).

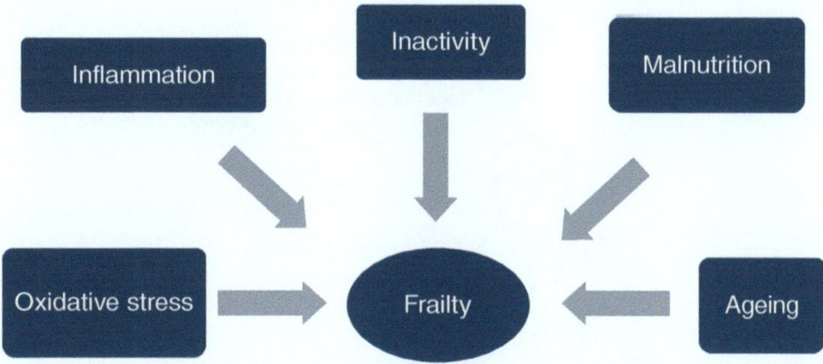

FIGURE 2.2 Mechanism of frailty development. *Source*: Umegaki (2025)/John Wiley & Sons.

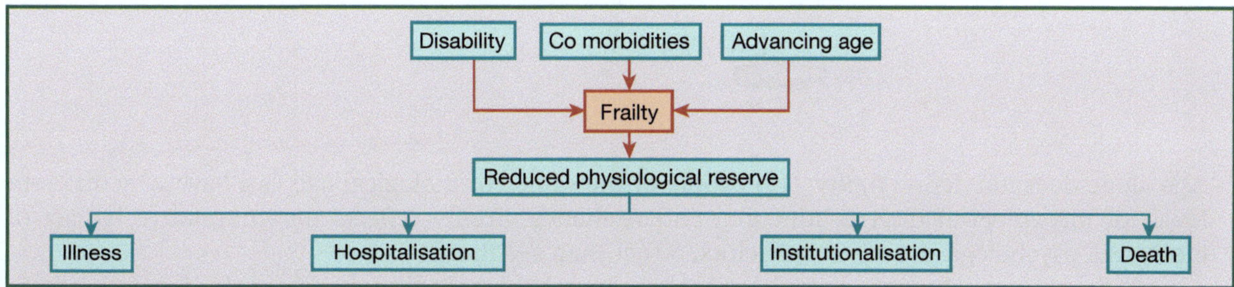

FIGURE 2.3 Frailty. *Source*: Adapted from Blundell and Gordon (2015) Wiley.

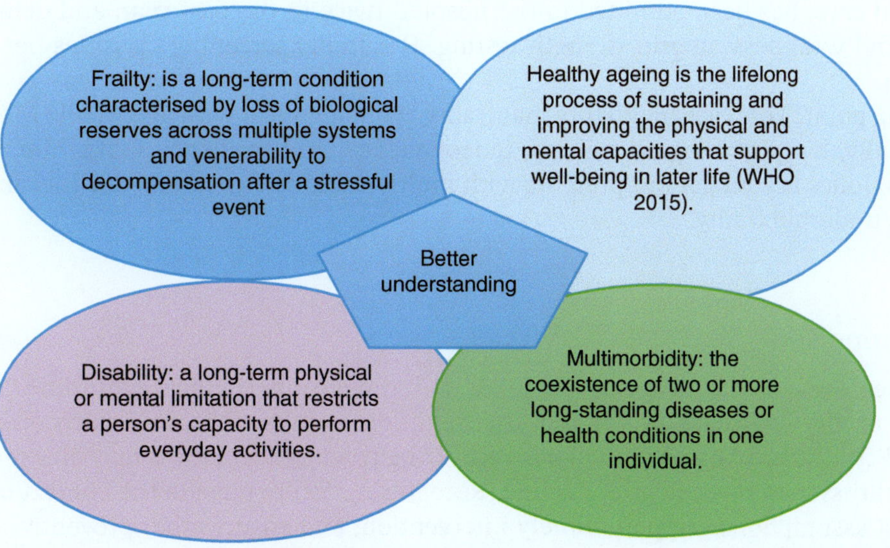

FIGURE 2.4 Frailty, healthy again, disability and multimorbidity.

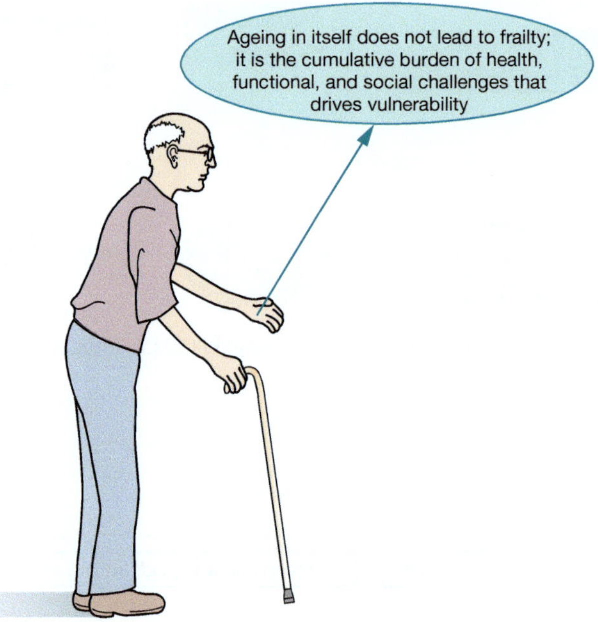

Age alone does not define frailty; two people of the same chronological age can have very different levels of physiological reserve, function, and resilience. Frailty reflects the cumulative impact of biological, psychological, and social factors, rather than age itself.

Mr. Smith is an 82-year-old retired schoolteacher who lives independently, walks two miles daily, and actively volunteers at his local library. He takes only one regular medication for mild hypertension and has no functional limitations. On screening, he scores as robust on the Clinical Frailty Scale (CFS 1–2).

In contrast, Mrs. Jones is a 70-year-old woman with poorly controlled type 2 diabetes, chronic obstructive pulmonary disease (COPD), obesity, and osteoarthritis. She requires help with shopping and personal care, has been admitted to the hospital twice in the past year, and demonstrates slow gait speed and weakness on grip strength testing. Her frailty screening classifies her as moderately frail (CFS 6).

Learning point: This case highlights that frailty is not identical with age. While Mr. Smith is older chronologically, his physiological reserve, independence, and resilience make him non-frail. Conversely, Mrs. Jones is younger but presents with multimorbidity, functional decline, and dependency, all of which underpin frailty.

Frailty Beyond Older Age

Frailty is often associated with ageing, yet it is a multidimensional clinical syndrome that can develop at any stage of life. Children with life-limiting conditions, adults with complex chronic diseases such as advanced cystic fibrosis, and individuals recovering from critical illness may all exhibit frailty arising from multi-system physiological decline. Recognising frailty outside the context of old age challenges ageist assumptions, supports timely intervention, and ensures that preventive, rehabilitative, and palliative strategies are applied equitably across the life course.

THE FIRST FRAILTY PHENOTYPE THROUGH THE CARDIOVASCULAR HEALTH STUDY

A decisive shift in the conceptualisation of frailty came with the work of Fried and colleagues in the Cardiovascular Health Study (CHS), a large, prospective, population-based cohort study of older adults in the United States. In 2001, Fried et al. published their landmark paper that operationalised frailty as a measurable clinical syndrome, now widely known as the frailty phenotype (Fried et al., 2001). This was the first attempt to create a reproducible definition of frailty that moved beyond descriptive language and clinical intuition, and instead provided a structured set of diagnostic criteria.

The CHS involved over 5,000 community-dwelling adults aged 65 years and older who were followed longitudinally to explore cardiovascular risk factors and outcomes. Within this cohort, frailty was characterised by a distinct cluster of features reflecting reduced physiological reserve. Through empirical analysis, Fried and colleagues identified five criteria that together defined the frailty phenotype: unintentional weight loss, self-reported exhaustion, weakness measured by grip strength, slow walking speed, and low levels of physical activity. An individual was classified as frail if three or more criteria were present, pre-frail if one or two criteria were met, and robust if none were identified. This gradation acknowledged that frailty exists on a continuum, rather than as an all-or-nothing condition. Importantly, the phenotype criteria were not chosen arbitrarily but reflected both theoretical constructs of diminished reserve and empirical associations with adverse outcomes.

The validation of this model within the CHS demonstrated that frailty, as defined by the phenotype, was strongly predictive of poor health outcomes. Individuals classified as frail had higher risks of falls, disability, hospitalisation, and mortality compared with robust or pre-frail counterparts. These findings provided the first large-scale evidence that frailty could be reliably measured and used to identify those at greatest risk of decline. The strength of the CHS approach lies in its ability to disentangle frailty from related but distinct concepts such as ageing, multimorbidity, and disability. Unlike disability, which describes established limitations in function, the frailty phenotype captured a state of vulnerability that preceded overt functional loss. Similarly, frailty was shown to predict adverse outcomes even after adjusting for the number of comorbidities, highlighting its independent contribution to risk.

The publication of the frailty phenotype marked a turning point in geriatric medicine. It provided clinicians and researchers with a practical tool to identify frail individuals in both research settings and, increasingly, in clinical practice. It also helped standardise terminology in a field that had previously been characterised by heterogeneity and imprecision. Subsequent studies have validated the phenotype across diverse populations and healthcare systems, though its limitations such as reliance on physical measures and less emphasis on psychosocial domains, have also been debated. Nonetheless, the CHS definition remains one of the most influential and widely cited models of frailty. It established the principle that frailty can be recognised as a distinct, measurable syndrome, paving the way for further refinements and the development of alternative approaches such as the deficit accumulation index.

FRAILTY PHENOTYPE CRITERIA

As explained previously in the CHS, Fried and colleagues proposed that frailty could be operationalised through five measurable criteria which together represent diminished physiological reserve and increased vulnerability. These criteria are unintentional weight loss, self-reported exhaustion, weakness, slowness, and low physical activity.

Unintentional weight loss was defined in the CHS as a reduction of 10 pounds (approximately 4.5 kg) or more in the previous year that was not attributable to dieting or intentional behaviour change. This parameter reflects declining nutritional status and metabolic reserve, often linked to sarcopenia, systemic inflammation, or underlying disease processes.

Exhaustion was measured through self-report using items from the Center for Epidemiologic Studies Depression Scale (CES-D). Participants who endorsed feelings of unusual tiredness or lack of energy on three or more days in the preceding week met the exhaustion criterion. This domain captures reduced endurance and subjective perceptions of poor physical resilience, often preceding measurable functional decline.

Weakness was assessed through grip strength, measured with a handheld dynamometer. Cut-off points were adjusted for sex and body mass index to account for natural variation. Grip strength was chosen as a simple yet powerful marker of global muscle strength and physical reserve, with low performance correlating strongly with risk of disability and mortality.

Slowness was evaluated using gait speed over a fixed distance. Thresholds were again stratified by sex and height, recognising the influence of anthropometry on walking velocity. Slow gait speed reflects deterioration in neuromuscular function and cardiorespiratory capacity and has consistently been associated with functional limitation and increased mortality in older populations.

Low physical activity was determined using a standardised questionnaire assessing weekly energy expenditure from leisure and household activities. Individuals whose reported activity fell in the lowest quintile, adjusted for sex, were classified as meeting this criterion. Low activity may both contribute to and result from frailty, reinforcing cycles of deconditioning and reduced resilience.

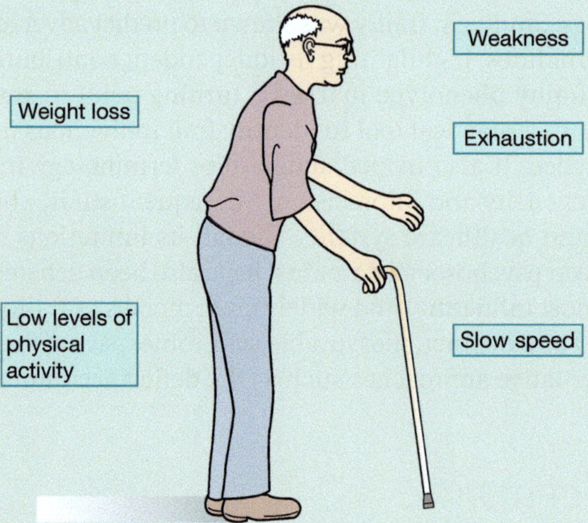

FIGURE 2.5   Frailty phenotype 3.4. *Source*: Adapted from Blundell and Gordon (2015) Wiley.

THE ADVANTAGES AND DISADVANTAGES OF FRAILTY PHENOTYPE (FRIED CRITERIA)

Advantages of the Fried Frailty Phenotype

Standardised and Reproducible Framework

The Fried frailty phenotype transformed a diffuse clinical intuition into a reproducible, five-item syndrome with clear staging: robust, pre-frail, and frail. In the original CHS, frailty independently predicted falls, disability, hospitalisation, and mortality over a three-year period. This established frailty as a distinct risk state, separate from multimorbidity and disability, and validated the concept of a pre-frail stage that is clinically actionable (Fried et al., 2001). In addition, clinical practice guidelines reinforce these strengths, recommending the frailty phenotype as a first-line tool for case finding in both community and primary care, with structured interventions such as exercise, nutritional optimisation, and medication review once frailty or pre-frailty is identified (Dent et al., 2019; Ruiz et al., 2020; Cesari et al., 2016).

Predictive Validity Across Populations

The predictive power of the frailty phenotype has been replicated globally. In the China Health and Retirement Longitudinal Study, which followed 5,874 adults aged 60 years and older, frailty at baseline predicted future adverse outcomes. The odds of falls increased by 54%, dependence in basic activities of daily living increased more than fourfold, and dependence in instrumental activities of daily living increased threefold. Even pre-frail individuals experienced elevated risks, underscoring the value of staging for early intervention (Zhang et al., 2020).

Early Identification of Progression

The Women's Health and Aging Study II demonstrated how frailty evolves over time. Exhaustion and unintentional weight loss conferred a threefold to fivefold increased risk of progression to frailty within follow-up, while weakness, slowness, and low activity often emerged earlier but were less predictive of full frailty. These findings justify monitoring single components, particularly exhaustion and weight loss, as early warning signals in older adults not yet frail (Xue et al., 2008).

Biological Plausibility and Epidemiology

Systematic reviews confirm the biological plausibility and widespread relevance of the phenotype. A meta-analysis of community cohorts estimated a weighted prevalence of 10.7%, though values ranged from 4.0% to 59.1%, reflecting both genuine variation and differences in operationalisation (Collard et al., 2012). The phenotype is therefore a useful framework for service planning, although heterogeneity in measurement requires careful interpretation.

Benefits of Standardisation

Research also shows that standardisation improves predictive ability. In the Toledo Study for Healthy Aging, harmonising cut-points and measurement protocols enhanced the ability of the phenotype to predict adverse outcomes (Bouzón et al., 2017). In contrast, a systematic review documented 262 modified versions of the phenotype, which produced prevalence estimates ranging from 12.7% to 28.2% when applied to European data. This highlights both the flexibility and the risk of inconsistency when the model is adapted without clear consensus (Theou et al., 2015). Subsequent studies have shown that standardisation not only improves frailty prediction but also enhances disease-specific risk discrimination, including cardiovascular outcomes (Boreskie et al., 2019). Together with the Toledo Study, these results highlight the necessity of harmonised protocols and population-specific cut-points to ensure both comparability and predictive accuracy (Alonso Bouzón et al., 2017).

Emerging Technological Applications

Recent innovations are exploring digital biomarkers and sensor-based tools to operationalise frailty phenotype components. For example, wearable sensors have been validated against traditional performance tests to approximate gait and cognitive-linked slowness (Zhou et al., 2019). Machine learning models built from daily activity data also show promise in detecting frailty phenotypes remotely, raising the prospect of scalable frailty monitoring beyond specialist clinics (Park et al., 2021).

Disadvantages of the Fried Frailty Phenotype

Feasibility Challenges in Clinical Settings

Although powerful in research, the phenotype is not always easy to implement in practice. In a study of 500 geriatric inpatients, only 65% could complete all five assessments (Bieniek et al., 2016). Overall, 35% were unassessable often because of cognitive impairment, inability to walk, or missing weight history. For example, 10% lacked weight data, 17.4% could not answer weight-loss questions, and 14% could not complete walking speed assessments. Prevalence exceeded 50% in this hospital cohort, increasing from 31.7% in the 60–69 age group to 67.6% among those aged 90 years and older. These findings illustrate the practical limitations of applying the full model in acute settings. Furthermore, similar concerns have been described in primary care, where time constraints, limited access to equipment, and uncertainty about responsibility for frailty assessment reduce uptake. Surveys of family physicians and practice nurses found that frailty screening often competes with other clinical demands and is inconsistently implemented across practices (Allison et al., 2021; Obbia et al., 2020; Abyad, 2021).

Barriers in Specialised Outpatient Care

Feasibility issues are not confined to hospital wards. In United States haemodialysis clinics, a 2023 feasibility study identified barriers such as limited time, lack of training, equipment requirements, and the absence of reimbursement (Wadhwa et al., 2023). These real-world constraints mean that precisely in the high-risk settings where frailty assessment would be valuable, implementation can be difficult without systemic support (Wadhwa et al., 2023).

Exclusion of Cognitive and Psychosocial Dimensions

The design of the phenotype deliberately focuses on physical criteria, but this can lead to under-recognition of individuals whose vulnerability arises primarily from cognitive or psychosocial deficits. Data from the French Three-City Study demonstrated that adding cognitive impairment to the phenotype improved its predictive power for disability in activities of daily living. Those who were both frail and cognitively impaired had the highest risk of functional decline, pointing to the value of integrating broader assessments into practice (Avila-Funes et al., 2009). A systematic review confirmed increasing incorporation of cognitive measures within frailty definitions, with evidence that cognition substantially improves predictive validity for adverse outcomes. Integrating cognitive testing into frailty assessment is now viewed as an essential step for comprehensive evaluation (Vella Azzopardi et al., 2018). Moreover, methodological analyses argue that focusing exclusively on predictive validity may lead to misclassification and advocate for concept-driven approaches to identification (Xue et al., 2020).

Variability in Operationalisation

Another challenge is the variability in how the phenotype has been applied across studies. Modifications in component definitions, cut-points, and instruments produce wide swings in prevalence and predictive accuracy, complicating meta-analysis and benchmarking. Without harmonised protocols, frailty prevalence estimates cannot be compared across populations with confidence (Theou et al., 2015).

Comparable Alternatives Exist

Finally, while the phenotype is validated, it is not universally superior. A systematic review published in 2022 concluded that both the Fried frailty phenotype and the deficit accumulation index had comparable ability to predict all-cause mortality in population studies. This suggests that instrument choice should be guided by context: the phenotype for simple case finding and the index for more detailed monitoring (Kim et al., 2022).

The Deficit Accumulation Module

The deficit accumulation model, developed by Kenneth Rockwood and Arnold Mitnitski in the early 2000s, conceptualises frailty as the result of a lifelong process in which damage progressively builds at molecular, cellular, and physiological levels until it becomes clinically visible (Mitnitski et al., 2001). Evidence shows that while the specific deficits may vary between individuals, the overall number of deficits is more predictive of survival than which deficits are present (Mitnitski and Rockwood, 2015). This perspective differs from traditional disease risk models that emphasise single causative factors, instead framing frailty as an actuarial marker of biological ageing and heterogeneity in mortality risk across people of the same chronological age (Vaupel et al., 1979). Large-scale pooled analyses involving over 150,000 participants demonstrate that the accumulation of health deficits is strongly associated with cardiovascular morbidity and mortality (Farooqi et al., 2020). Deficit accumulation also amplifies the expression of late-life conditions such as dementia. Biomarkers and neuropathological changes are more likely to manifest clinically when individuals have high frailty scores, suggesting that frailty itself can act as a gateway for disease expression (Howlett et al., 2021; Ward et al., 2022; Canevelli et al., 2024). At the biological level, mechanisms such as DNA methylation changes, telomere shortening, protein misfolding, inflammation, and impaired DNA repair have all been linked to the accumulation of deficits (López-Otín et al., 2023; Goh et al., 2023). Longitudinal research indicates that clinical deficits double approximately every 12–15 years in older adults, reinforcing the progressive nature of frailty (Hoogendijk et al., 2018). Animal models and computational simulations further support the validity of this framework, showing that frailty emerges from interacting systems and can be modelled mathematically to predict trajectories of decline (Farrell et al., 2021). The deficit accumulation model therefore provides a flexible and biologically grounded lens for understanding frailty, accommodating diverse determinants from genetics to social and environmental exposures, while retaining strong predictive value for adverse outcomes (Mitnitski et al., 2001).

Frailty Index

The FI was first proposed by Mitnitski, Mogilner, and Rockwood in 2001 as part of the deficit accumulation model, using data from the Canadian Study of Health and Aging (Mitnitski et al., 2001). This framework defines frailty not by single conditions, but by the cumulative effect of multiple health problems across the life course. The FI is calculated by dividing the number of health deficits present by the total number considered, producing a score between 0 and 1. Although a score of 1 would indicate the presence of every possible deficit, in practice, values rarely exceed 0.7 because survival is highly unlikely at such high levels of frailty (Rockwood and Mitnitski, 2007). Thresholds around 0.25 have been shown to consistently identify individuals at increased risk of adverse outcomes, making the FI a powerful predictor of mortality, hospitalisation, institutionalisation, and functional decline (Clegg et al., 2013).

The strength of the FI lies in its flexibility. A wide range of health variables spanning comorbidities, disabilities, functional measures, and clinical signs can be incorporated. To ensure validity, however, certain principles guide construction: deficits should increase with age, be associated with poor outcomes, and not be universally present or absent within the study population. Typically, at least 30 variables are recommended for a robust index (Searle et al., 2008). More recent methodological updates have emphasised standardised approaches to variable selection and scoring, including the exclusion of overly rare or common deficits, coding partial deficits where appropriate, and ensuring longitudinal consistency in repeated assessments (Theou et al., 2023).

Because of this adaptable design, the FI has been applied across diverse contexts. Large-scale cohort studies, randomised controlled trial datasets, and routine electronic health records have all been used to construct valid indices (Clegg et al., 2016; Kim et al., 2018, 2020). The tool has also been adapted to measure frailty within specific disease populations. For example, FIs have been developed for systemic sclerosis, HIV, and systemic lupus erythematosus, where they predict survival and multimorbidity independently of disease severity markers (Rockwood et al., 2014; Guaraldi et al., 2015; Legge et al., 2020). Laboratory and biomarker-based frailty indices provide another dimension, capturing subclinical vulnerability that may precede functional decline (Sapp et al., 2023). The same principles have been extended to social determinants of health, leading to the creation of a social vulnerability index that quantifies the impact of social and environmental exposures on frailty and mortality risk (Andrew et al., 2008).

Preclinical studies further support the model's generalisability. Versions of the FI have been successfully applied to animal populations, including mice, dogs, and non-human primates, confirming that frailty emerges from multi-system deficit accumulation rather than disease-specific mechanisms (Kane and Howlett, 2021). This translational evidence has strengthened the biological plausibility of the index and its use in experimental gerontology.

Despite its strengths, some limitations remain. A single FI measurement may not capture fluctuations in health, particularly in acutely ill patients or those undergoing recovery. Questions also persist about whether certain deficits, such as controlled hypertension, should continue to be scored once treated. Furthermore, electronic frailty indices developed from administrative or primary care data may inadvertently include 'immortal time' variables, where a condition once recorded is never updated, potentially inflating frailty scores (Hatheway et al., 2017). Nonetheless, the FI continues to be one of the most widely validated and applied frailty measures globally, providing a robust, scalable, and biologically grounded means of quantifying vulnerability in older adults.

The Electronic Frailty Index

The eFI is a digital adaptation of the deficit accumulation model, designed to enable the routine identification of frailty in primary care using data already recorded in electronic health records. It was developed in the United Kingdom by Clegg and colleagues in collaboration with the University of Leeds, the University of Southampton, and NHS England, and first validated in 2016 using data from over 900,000 patients in the ResearchOne and THIN databases (Clegg et al., 2016).

The eFI is based on the principles of the FI introduced by Mitnitski et al. (2001), which quantifies frailty as the proportion of health deficits present out of a total set of possible deficits. In the electronic version, 36 deficits are used, covering a wide range of domains including:

- Functional impairments
- Clinical signs and symptoms
- Diseases and long-term conditions
- Disabilities and social vulnerability markers

Each deficit is scored as present or absent, and the total number of deficits is divided by 36 to create a score between 0 and 1. This continuous score is then categorised into four frailty strata:

- Fit (0–0.12)
- Mild frailty (0.13–0.24)
- Moderate frailty (0.25–0.36)
- Severe frailty ($\geq$0.36)

The eFI has been widely adapted because it can be automated within primary care systems, providing a consistent, scalable approach to case finding without requiring additional data collection. Its predictive validity has been demonstrated across multiple outcomes. In the original validation, higher eFI scores were strongly associated with increased risk of hospitalisation, nursing home admission, and mortality (Clegg et al., 2016).

Importantly, the 2017/2018 GP contract in England introduced a requirement for practices to use an evidence-based tool such as the eFI to identify patients aged 65 years and over living with moderate or severe frailty (NHS England, 2017). For those identified with severe frailty, practices must provide a structured medication review, undertake a falls risk assessment where appropriate, and ensure an enriched Summary Care Record is in place.

The eFI has also been extended and validated in different populations and datasets, including secondary care and international cohorts. Studies have demonstrated its utility in predicting adverse outcomes among hospitalised patients, those with multimorbidity, and disease-specific groups such as people living with dementia or cardiovascular disease (Kim et al., 2018; Hollinghurst et al., 2021). However, limitations of the eFI mirror those of the broader deficit accumulation approach. As a record-based tool, its accuracy depends on the quality and completeness of coded data, and it does not directly capture dynamic changes in a person's health. Concerns have also been raised about potential over- or under-identification if deficits are miscoded or not updated regularly (Hollinghurst et al., 2021). Despite these challenges, the eFI represents a major step in embedding frailty assessment into routine primary care and has become a cornerstone of the NHS policy for supporting older people living with frailty.

Case Study 2.1   Using the FI in Clinical Practice

Background

Mrs. Jones, an 82-year-old woman, attends a primary care clinic after two episodes of dizziness and a recent fall at home. She has hypertension, osteoarthritis, mild cognitive impairment, urinary incontinence, and takes eight regular medications. She lives alone but receives occasional help from her daughter.

Assessment by an AP

The AP undertakes a CGA, covering physical, functional, psychological, social and future wishes domains. Alongside this, the FI is applied using 40 health variables recorded in her clinical notes and through direct questioning. Mrs. Jones is identified as having 14 deficits, including polypharmacy, falls, impaired mobility, urinary incontinence, memory difficulties, and mood disturbance.
FI Calculation

$$14 \text{ deficits} \div 40 \text{ items} = 0.35 \left(\text{moderate frailty} \right)$$

Clinical Reasoning

- The FI confirms Mrs. Jones is at increased risk of hospitalisation and functional decline.
- The CGA provides context, highlighting that medication burden, cognitive impairment, and environmental risks are key contributors to her vulnerability.

Management Plan

1. Medication review: The AP works with a pharmacist to reduce polypharmacy and deprescribe medications contributing to dizziness.
2. Falls prevention: Referral to physiotherapy for balance and strength training, and an occupational therapy home visit to minimise environmental hazards.
3. Continence support: Bladder assessment and conservative management plan, including pelvic floor exercises.
4. Cognitive and psychological support: Memory clinic referral and signposting to local dementia support groups.
5. Social care liaison: Contact with social services to explore additional home support and respite options for her daughter.

Follow-Up

At four months, Mrs Jones has not experienced further falls, reports improved mood, and is managing daily activities with greater independence. A repeat FI shows a small reduction to 0.32, reflecting stabilisation. Importantly, the FI facilitated structured communication of her risk level to the wider MDT and helped prioritise tailored interventions within the CGA framework.

Key Learning Points

The FI provides a practical, numerical measure of frailty that complements CGA. For the AP, it supports risk stratification, monitoring of change over time, and targeted, person-centred interventions across the GCA domains.

Frailty Following Critical Illness

Frailty may emerge as a late consequence of critical illness, especially in survivors of sepsis or prolonged intensive care. Many patients develop ICU-acquired weakness (ICU-AW), a condition of diffuse muscle wasting and neuromuscular dysfunction affecting limb and respiratory muscles, which is associated with long-term morbidity and increased mortality (Vanhorebeek et al., 2020). Post-sepsis syndrome similarly contributes to a frailty phenotype by inducing chronic inflammation, neurocognitive impairment, fatigue and functional decline: sepsis survivors commonly acquire new limitations in activities of daily living after hospital discharge (Prescott and Angus, 2018). Together, these processes erode multi-system physiological reserve independent of chronological age and may accelerate or mimic classical frailty, reinforcing the need to include post-critical illness states in any comprehensive frailty framework.

Frailty in paediatrics can be described as a state of heightened susceptibility to health decline and mortality, most evident in children with severe, progressive, or life-limiting illness (Brenner et al., 2018; Gallo et al., 2021). It arises from multi-system dysfunction involving neurological, endocrine, immune, and musculoskeletal compromise, resulting in complex care requirements and diminished quality of life (Feng et al., 2017; Calcaterra et al., 2021).

Frail children often present with a wide range of underlying conditions, including neurological, respiratory, metabolic, and congenital disorders, with malignancy accounting for only a minority of cases. Their care is further complicated by developmental delay, meaning many remain dependent on caregivers for basic functions such as feeding and hygiene. Families require sensitive, timely communication about prognosis and management, with decision-making framed as a shared process. Multidisciplinary, family-centred care is widely regarded as best practice, particularly when provided at home, where familiar surroundings can reduce distress and support both the medical and psychosocial needs of children and their families.

CONCLUSION

Frailty has moved from being a vague descriptor of age-related vulnerability to a measurable and clinically meaningful construct. The transition from early descriptive accounts to formal models such as the Fried frailty phenotype and the deficit accumulation model has provided robust tools for identifying, staging, and managing frailty across settings. The FI has extended these principles into flexible, data-driven applications, while the eFI has embedded frailty assessment within routine primary care, reflecting its importance in policy and practice. Each model has strengths and limitations, yet together they demonstrate that frailty is distinct from chronological ageing, disability, or multimorbidity, and is a powerful predictor of adverse outcomes. For APs, understanding these conceptual foundations is essential for critical appraisal, appropriate application, and integration of frailty assessment into holistic, person-centred care.

Take-Home Messages

1. Frailty is a distinct, multidimensional condition, separate from ageing, disability, and multimorbidity, defined by loss of physiological reserve and heightened vulnerability to stressors.

2. Historical shifts from descriptive use of 'frailty' to formal models such as the Fried phenotype and the deficit accumulation model provide measurable tools to predict adverse outcomes.

3. The FI and its electronic adaptation enable systematic risk stratification, integrating frailty assessment into everyday clinical and primary care practice.

4. Each model offers different strengths such as simplicity, biological grounding, or scalability, so APs should select and combine approaches according to clinical context.

5. Embedding these conceptual foundations supports anticipatory, person-centred, and multidisciplinary care planning, aligning with national advanced practice frameworks and policy expectations.

REFERENCES

Abyad, A. (2021). Is primary health care capable of addressing frailty? *European Geriatric Medicine* 12 (5): 899–902.

Allison, R., Assadzandi, S., and Adelman, M. (2021). Frailty: evaluation and management. *American Family Physician* 103 (4): 219–226.

Andrew, M.K., Mitnitski, A.B., and Rockwood, K. (2008). Social vulnerability, frailty and mortality in elderly people. *PLoS One* 3 (5): e2232.

Avila-Funes, J.A., Amieva, H., Barberger-Gateau, P. et al. (2009). Cognitive impairment improves the predictive validity of the phenotype of frailty for adverse health outcomes: the three-city study. *Journal of the American Geriatrics Society* 57: 453–461.

Bieniek, J., Wilczyński, K., and Szewieczek, J. (2016). Fried frailty phenotype assessment components as applied to geriatric inpatients. *Clinical Interventions in Aging* 11: 453–459.

Blundell, A. and Gordon, A. (2015). *Geriatric Medicine at a Glance*, 1e. Chichester: Wiley Blackwell.

Boreskie, K.F., Kehler, D.S., Costa, E.C. et al. (2019). Standardization of the Fried frailty phenotype improves cardiovascular disease risk discrimination. *Experimental Gerontology* 119: 40–44.

Bortz, W.M. (2002). A conceptual framework of frailty: a review. *The Journals of Gerontology. Series A, Biological Sciences and Medical Sciences* 57 (5): M283–M288.

Bouzón, C.A., Carnicero, J.A., Turin, J.G. et al. (2017). The standardization of frailty phenotype criteria improves its predictive ability: The Toledo Study for Healthy Aging. *Journal of the American Medical Directors Association* 18 (5): 402–408.

Brenner, M., Kidston, C., Hilliard, C. et al. (2018). Children's complex care needs: a systematic concept analysis of multidisciplinary language. *European Journal of Pediatrics* 177 (11): 1641–1652.

Calcaterra, V., Cena, H., Ruggieri, A. et al. (2021). Metabolically unhealthy phenotype: a key factor in determining paediatric frailty. *Pediatric Reports* 13 (3): 340–346.

Campbell, A.J. and Buchner, D.M. (1997). Unstable disability and the fluctuations of frailty. *Age and Ageing* 26 (4): 315–318.

Canevelli, M., Wallace, L.M., Bruno, G. et al. (2024). Frailty is associated with the clinical expression of neuropsychological deficits in older adults. *European Journal of Neurology* 31 (1): e16072.

Cesari, M., Prince, M., Thiyagarajan, J.A. et al. (2016). Frailty: an emerging public health priority. *Journal of the American Medical Directors Association* 17 (3): 188–192.

Clegg, A., Young, J., Iliffe, S. et al. (2013). Frailty in elderly people. *The Lancet* 381 (9868): 752–762.

Clegg, A., Bates, C., Young, J. et al. (2016). Development and validation of an electronic frailty index using routine primary care electronic health record data. *Age and Ageing* 45 (3): 353–360.

Collard, R.M., Boter, H., Schoevers, R.A., and Oude Voshaar, R.C. (2012). Prevalence of frailty in community-dwelling older persons: a systematic review. *Journal of the American Geriatrics Society* 60 (8): 1487–1492.

Dent, E., Morley, J.E., Cruz-Jentoft, A.J. et al. (2019). Physical frailty: ICFSR International Clinical Practice Guidelines for identification and management. *Journal of Nutrition, Health & Aging* 23 (9): 771–787.

Farooqi, M.A.M., Gerstein, H., Yusuf, S., and Leong, D.P. (2020). Accumulation of deficits as a key risk factor for cardiovascular morbidity and mortality: a pooled analysis of 154, 000 individuals. *Journal of the American Heart Association* 9 (3): e014686.

Farrell, S., Stubbings, G., Rockwood, K. et al. (2021). The potential for complex computational models of aging. *Mechanisms of Ageing and Development* 193: 111403.

Feng, Z., Lugtenberg, M., Franse, C. et al. (2017). Risk factors and protective factors associated with incident or increase of frailty among community-dwelling older adults: a systematic review of longitudinal studies. *PLoS One* 12 (6): e0178383.

Fried, L.P., Tangen, C.M., Walston, J. et al. (2001). Frailty in older adults: evidence for a phenotype. *The Journals of Gerontology. Series A, Biological Sciences and Medical Sciences* 56 (3): M146–M156.

Gallo, M., Agostiniani, R., Pintus, R., and Fanos, V. (2021). The child with medical complexity. *Italian Journal of Pediatrics* 47 (1): 1–7.

Gobbens, R.J., Luijkx, K.G., Wijnen-Sponselee, M.T., and Schols, J.M. (2010). Toward a conceptual definition of frailty: a review of the literature. *Nursing Outlook* 58 (2): 76–86.

Goh, J., Wong, E., Soh, J. et al. (2023). Targeting the molecular and cellular pillars of human aging with exercise. *FEBS Journal* 290 (3): 649–668.

Guaraldi, G., Brothers, T.D., Zona, S. et al. (2015). A frailty index predicts survival and incident multimorbidity independent of markers of HIV disease severity. *AIDS* 29 (13): 1633–1641.

Hatheway, O.L., Mitnitski, A., and Rockwood, K. (2017). Frailty affects the initial treatment response and time to recovery of mobility in acutely ill older adults admitted to hospital. *Age and Ageing* 46 (6): 920–925.

Hollinghurst, J., Housley, G., Watkins, A. et al. (2021). A comparison of two national frailty scoring systems. *Age and Ageing* 50 (4): 1208–1214.

Hoogendijk, E.O., Rockwood, K., Theou, O. et al. (2018). Tracking changes in frailty throughout later life: results from a 17-year longitudinal study in the Netherlands. *Age and Ageing* 47 (5): 727–733.

Howlett, S.E., Rutenberg, A.D., and Rockwood, K. (2021). The degree of frailty as a translational measure of health in aging. *Nature Aging* 1 (8): 651–665.

Kane, A.E. and Howlett, S.E. (2021). Sex differences in frailty: comparisons between humans and preclinical models. *Mechanisms of Ageing and Development* 198: 111546.

Kane, R.A., Kane, R.L., and Ladd, R.C. (1994). *The Heart of Long-Term Care*. New York: Oxford University Press.

Kim, D.H., Schneeweiss, S., Glynn, R.J. et al. (2018). Measuring frailty in Medicare data: development and validation of a claims-based frailty index. *The Journals of Gerontology. Series A, Biological Sciences and Medical Sciences* 73 (7): 980–987.

Kim, D.H., Patorno, E., Pawar, A. et al. (2020). Measuring frailty in administrative claims data: comparative performance of four claims-based frailty measures in the US Medicare data. *The Journals of Gerontology. Series A, Biological Sciences and Medical Sciences* 75 (6): 1120–1125.

Kim, D.J., Massa, M.S., Potter, C.M. et al. (2022). Systematic review of the utility of the frailty index and frailty phenotype to predict all-cause mortality in older people. *Systematic Reviews* 11 (1): 187.

Legge, A., Kirkland, S., Rockwood, K. et al. (2020). Construction of a frailty index as a novel health measure in systemic lupus erythematosus. *The Journal of Rheumatology* 47 (1): 72–81.

López-Otín, C., Blasco, M.A., Partridge, L. et al. (2023). Hallmarks of aging: an expanding universe. *Cell* 186 (2): 243–278.

Mitnitski, A. and Rockwood, K. (2015). Aging as a process of deficit accumulation: its utility and origin. *Interdisciplinary Topics in Gerontology* 40 (1): 85–98.

Mitnitski, A.B., Mogilner, A.J., and Rockwood, K. (2001). Accumulation of deficits as a proxy measure of aging. *The Scientific World Journal* 1 (2): 323–336.

NHS England (2017). Electronic frailty index (eFI). `https://www.england.nhs.uk/ourwork/clinical-policy/older-people/frailty/efi` (accessed 9 July 2025).

NHS England (2022). *Older people advanced practice area specific capability and curriculum framework*. NHS England. Available at: `https://advanced-practice.hee.nhs.uk/wp-content/uploads/sites/28/2025/01/Older-people-advanced-practice-area-specific-capability-and-curriculum-framework-NHSE.pdf` (accessed: 30 January 2026).

NHS England (2023a). *Palliative and end of life care advanced practice area specific capability and curriculum framework*. NHS England. Available at: `https://advanced-practice.hee.nhs.uk/wp-content/uploads/sites/28/2025/01/Palliative-and-end-of-life-care-advanced-practice-area-specific-capability-and-curriculum-framework-NHSE.pdf` (accessed 30 January 2026).

NHS England (2023b). *Acute medicine advanced practice area specific capability and curriculum framework*. NHS England. Available at: `https://advanced-practice.hee.nhs.uk/wp-content/uploads/sites/28/2025/03/Acute-medicine-advanced-practice-area-specific-capability-and-curriculum-framework-NHSE.pdf` (accessed: 30 January 2026).

NHS England (2025). *Multi-professional framework for advanced practice in England – Edition 2025*. NHS England. Available at: `https://advanced-practice.hee.nhs.uk/wp-content/uploads/sites/28/2025/05/Multi-professional-framework-for-advanced-practice-in-England---Edition-2025.pdf` (accessed 29 January 2026).

Obbia, P., Graham, C., Duffy, F.J.R., and Gobbens, R.J.J. (2020). Preventing frailty in older people: an exploration of primary care professionals' experiences. *International Journal of Older People Nursing* 15 (2): e12297.

Park, C., Mishra, R., and Najafi, B. (2021). Digital biomarkers of physical frailty and frailty phenotypes using sensor-based physical activity and machine learning. *Sensors* 21 (16): 5289.

Prescott, H.C. and Angus, D.C. (2018). Enhancing recovery from sepsis: a review. *JAMA* 319 (1): 62–75.

Rockwood, K. and Mitnitski, A. (2007). Frailty in relation to the accumulation of deficits. *The Journals of Gerontology. Series A, Biological Sciences and Medical Sciences* 62 (7): 722–727.

Rockwood, M.R., MacDonald, E., Sutton, E. et al. (2014). Frailty index to measure health status in people with systemic sclerosis. *The Journal of Rheumatology* 41 (4): 698–705.

Ruiz, J.G., Dent, E., Morley, J.E. et al. (2020). Screening for and managing the person with frailty in primary care: ICFSR consensus guidelines. *Journal of Nutrition, Health & Aging* 24 (9): 920–927.

Sapp, D.G., Cormier, B.M., Rockwood, K. et al. (2023). The frailty index based on laboratory test data as a tool to investigate the impact of frailty on health outcomes: a systematic review and meta-analysis. *Age and Ageing* 52 (1): afac309.

Searle, S.D., Mitnitski, A., Gahbauer, E.A. et al. (2008). A standard procedure for creating a frailty index. *BMC Geriatrics* 8: 24.

Strawbridge, W.J., Shema, S.J., Balfour, J.L. et al. (1998). Antecedents of frailty over three decades in an older cohort. *Journal of Gerontology. Social Sciences* 53B (1): S9–S16.

Stuck, A.E., Siu, A.L., Wieland, G.D. et al. (1993). Comprehensive geriatric assessment: a meta-analysis of controlled trials. *The Lancet* 342 (8878): 1032–1036.

Theou, O., Cann, L., Blodgett, J. et al. (2015). Modifications to the frailty phenotype criteria: systematic review of the current literature and investigation of 262 frailty phenotypes in the Survey of Health, Ageing, and Retirement in Europe. *Ageing Research Reviews* 21: 78–94.

Theou, O., Haviva, C., Wallace, L. et al. (2023). How to construct a frailty index from an existing dataset in 10 steps. *Age and Ageing* 52 (12): afad221.

Umegaki, H. (2025). Frailty, multimorbidity, and polypharmacy: proposal of the new concept of the geriatric triangle. *Geriatrics & Gerontology International* 25 (5): 657–662.

Vanhorebeek, I., Latronico, N., and Van den Berghe, G. (2020). ICU-acquired weakness. *Intensive Care Medicine* 46 (4): 637–653.

Vaupel, J.W., Manton, K.G., and Stallard, E. (1979). The impact of heterogeneity in individual frailty on the dynamics of mortality. *Demography* 16 (3): 439–454.

Vella Azzopardi, R., Beyer, I., Vermeiren, S. et al. (2018). Increasing use of cognitive measures in the operational definition of frailty: a systematic review. *Ageing Research Reviews* 43: 10–16.

Wadhwa, A., Balbale, S.N., Palleti, S.K. et al. (2023). Prevalence and feasibility of assessing the frailty phenotype among hemodialysis patients in a dialysis unit. *BMC Nephrology* 24 (1): 371.

Ward, D.D., Ranson, J.M., Wallace, L.M. et al. (2022). Frailty, lifestyle, genetics and dementia risk. *Journal of Neurology, Neurosurgery & Psychiatry* 93 (4): 343–350.

Winograd, C.H., Gerety, M.B., Chung, M. et al. (1991). Screening for frailty: criteria and predictors of outcomes. *Journal of the American Geriatrics Society* 39 (8): 778–784.

Xue, Q.L., Bandeen-Roche, K., Varadhan, R. et al. (2008). Initial manifestations of frailty criteria and the development of frailty phenotype in the Women's Health and Aging Study II. *The Journals of Gerontology Series A: Biological Sciences and Medical Sciences* 63 (9): 984–990.

Xue, Q.-L., Tian, J., Walston, J.D. et al. (2020). Discrepancy in frailty identification: move beyond predictive validity. *The Journals of Gerontology. Series A, Biological Sciences and Medical Sciences* 75 (2): 387–393.

Zhang, Q., Zhao, X., Liu, H., and Ding, H. (2020). Frailty as a predictor of future falls and disability: a four-year follow-up study of Chinese older adults. *BMC Geriatrics* 20 (1): 388.

Zhou, H., Razjouyan, J., Halder, D. et al. (2019). Instrumented trail-making task: application of wearable sensor to determine physical frailty phenotypes. *Gerontology* 65 (2): 186–197.

Frailty and Intrinsic Capacity: Frameworks for Healthy Ageing and Advanced Practice

Aim

The aim of this chapter is to critically explore the concepts of frailty and intrinsic capacity (IC), examining their theoretical foundations, measurement approaches, and implications for clinical practice. It demonstrates how these frameworks inform assessment, care planning, and person-centred interventions, with a particular focus on the role of advanced practitioners (APs) in promoting healthy ageing.

LEARNING OUTCOMES

On completion of this chapter, readers will be able to:

1. Differentiate between frailty and intrinsic capacity (IC), explaining their conceptual bases, orientations, and clinical significance.
2. Critically appraise the tools and methods used to assess frailty and IC, including the WHO Integrated Care for Older People (ICOPE) framework.
3. Analyse how frailty and IC complement one another in guiding proactive, person-centred interventions to support older adults.
4. Apply the principles of frailty and IC to advanced practice, demonstrating their relevance across the four pillars of the multi-professional framework.
5. Evaluate the implications of frailty and IC for national and international healthy-ageing policies, and how these shape advanced practice roles.

SELF-ASSESSMENT QUESTIONS

1. How do you presently distinguish frailty from intrinsic capacity in concept, measurement, and purpose, and what would this mean for anticipatory care in your setting?
2. Which components of the WHO ICOPE framework could you implement immediately, and what resources or service changes across the MPF pillars would be required to do so safely and effectively?

> Frailty is not about how old you are, but how strong your reserves remain.

INTRODUCTION

Intrinsic capacity (IC) is a key concept in contemporary healthy-ageing policy and practice, emphasising the preservation of physical and mental reserves rather than focusing only on disease. Originating from the World Health Organization's World Report on Ageing and Health and developed in the Integrated Care for Older People (ICOPE) guidelines (WHO, 2024), IC provides a functional, life-course perspective that complements frailty models. For advanced practitioners (APs), understanding IC is essential for early risk identification, proactive intervention, and integration of preventive strategies across community and acute settings. This chapter explores the conceptual basis and evidence for IC, examines its six domains, and demonstrates how IC assessment and the ICOPE pathway align with the multi-professional framework (MPF) for advanced clinical practice (NHS England, 2025) and national curricula for older people and palliative care. By linking these frameworks, the chapter supports APs to embed IC into everyday decision-making, service design, and person-centred care.

Multi-Professional Framework (MPF) for Advanced Practitioners

(Adapted from NHS England, 2025)

This chapter maps to the following areas within the multi-professional framework (MPF):

1. Clinical practice: 1.1–1.11
2. Leadership and management: 2.1, 2.2, 2.3, 2.5, 2.6, 2.7, 2.8
3. Education: 3.3, 3.5, 3.8
4. Research: 4.2, 4.3, 4.6

Accreditation Consideration

This chapter maps to the statement with the following national accretional document:

Curriculum framework for advanced practice in the care of older people (NHS England, 2022)

1. Core Capabilities in Practice (CiPs): 1–6
2. Generic Clinical CiPs: 1, 3, 5, 6
3. Specialty Clinical CiPs (older People): 1, 2, 3, 4

Curriculum framework for APs in the case of palliative and end-of-life care (NHS England, 2023a):

1. Clinical pillar: 1.1–1.4
2. Leadership and management: 2.1, 2.2, 2.3
3. Education: 3.1, 3.2, 3.3
4. Research: 4.1, 4.2, 4.3

Curriculum for APs in acute medicine (NHS England, 2023b):

1. Core CiPs: 1–6
2. Generic Clinical CiPs: 1, 3, 5, 6
3. Specialty Clinical CiPs (Acute Medicine): 1, 2, 3, 5, and acute medicine presentations

INTRINSIC CAPACITY: CONCEPT, EVIDENCE, AND IMPLICATIONS FOR ADVANCED PRACTITIONERS

The concept of IC originated in the WHO World report on ageing and health, which laid the foundation for the ICOPE guidelines (WHO, 2024). Unlike disease-based models of ageing, IC provides a more holistic measure of functional reserve and resilience. The decline in these capacities underpins the development of frailty. These documents shifted global thinking away from a disease-focused view of ageing towards a functional model that emphasises maintaining independence, resilience, and quality of life. IC is now recognised as the biological core of frailty and a key focus of ageing research, public health policy, and clinical practice worldwide. For APs, understanding and monitoring IC allows earlier identification of at-risk individuals and more proactive, person-centred interventions across community and acute settings.

WHY IC MATTERS?

A recent systematic review and meta-analysis by Sánchez-Sánchez et al. (2024) found that lower IC is associated with increased risks of functional decline and all-cause mortality, independent of age and comorbidity. The authors argue that IC performs as a prognostic marker of healthy ageing and recommend consistent operationalisation across settings in order to realise its value for care planning and outcome prediction. From a population perspective, a systematic review and meta-analysis by Cao et al. (2024) reported that approximately two-thirds of community-dwelling older adults exhibit a measurable decline in at least one IC domain, with a pooled prevalence of 67.8% (95% CI 57.0–78.5%). Their analysis highlights both the scale of potentially modifiable deficits and the importance of structured assessment. Identified risk factors encompass cardiometabolic disease, low education, living alone, smoking, physical inactivity, and osteoarthritis, all of which are clinically recognisable and, at least in part, amenable to intervention.

Newer modelling work is also clarifying IC trajectories. A recent study by Bernal et al. (2025) applied functional data approaches to demonstrate domain-specific ageing paths and showed that trajectories are associated with modifiable lifestyle factors, including physical activity, body mass index, alcohol use, and smoking. The study also found that residence outside nursing homes was linked to higher vitality, cognition, and locomotion scores. These findings strengthen the case for proactive, domain-targeted interventions that are anchored in both behaviour change and environmental support. Emerging cohort studies provide further insights. Zhang et al. (2025) reported that engagement in social and intellectual activities is associated with more favourable IC trajectories. This observation resonates with the wider literature on cognitive reserve and social participation in later life. Although the evidence base is still developing, these messages suggest practical levers that extend beyond biomedical treatment and underline the importance of psychosocial engagement.

Longitudinal analyses from large population studies also reinforce the prognostic value of IC. Evidence from the English Longitudinal Study of Ageing and the China Health and Retirement Longitudinal Study confirms that IC and its subdomains robustly predict subsequent care dependence, dementia, and mortality, even when adjusted for age and comorbidities. The functional framing provided by IC therefore offers a sharper and more actionable marker than traditional frailty indices, supporting its integration into clinical and public health strategies. Furthermore, studies using nationally representative cohort data demonstrate the social patterning of IC. Salinas-Rodríguez et al. (2024), drawing on data from Mexico's WHO SAGE study, showed that IC decline trajectories are strongly influenced by wealth, education, gender, and ethnicity. Their findings highlight that IC is not only clinically valuable but also provides a lens for identifying and targeting health inequalities, which is critical for the development of effective national healthy-ageing strategies.

THE SIX DOMAINS OF INTRINSIC CAPACITY

WHO identifies six core domains of IC, each of which declines with age at different rates and contributes to frailty:

Locomotor Capacity

Locomotor capacity represents the musculoskeletal system and can be defined as the ability to move in one's environment. Walking speed, chair-stand tests, and balance tasks are validated measures (WHO, 2024). Reduced gait speed over 12 months significantly increased the likelihood of falls among community-dwelling older adults, independent of cognitive status (Adam et al., 2023). A multi-country analysis showed that poor chair-stand performance independently predicted cardiovascular and all-cause mortality in older adults with hypertension (Polo-López et al., 2025). Handgrip strength, recently updated with international reference values, is also a strong predictor of functional limitations and disability (Tomkinson et al., 2025). Identifying sedentary and low-performance individuals allows timely interventions to maintain locomotor capacity.

Vitality/Nutrition

Vitality refers to energy balance and metabolic activity and is closely linked to nutritional status (WHO, 2024). Ageing reduces basal energy expenditure (Zampino et al., 2020) and alters body composition, with muscle replaced by fat even in the absence of weight loss (Briand et al., 2025). A 2025 systematic review and meta-analysis by Salari et al. (2025) pooled data from 98 studies ($n = 79{,}976$) and estimated a global malnutrition prevalence of 18.6% (95% CI 16.4–21.1%) in older adults, with the highest rates in Africa (35.7%) and Americas (20.3%) and the highest by the assessment tool (NRS-2002) reaching 39.9%.

The GLIM criteria, validated across multiple settings, link malnutrition to sarcopenia, frailty, and increased mortality (Yeung et al., 2021). Risk factors include poverty, isolation, dysphagia, depression, and anorexigenic drugs, all of which should be screened to prevent nutritional decline.

Cognitive Capacity

Cognitive capacity covers memory, attention, and executive function. The WHO ICOPE tool includes subjective cognitive decline and brief cognitive screens (WHO, 2024). The motoric cognitive risk (MCR) syndrome—defined by subjective complaint plus slow gait—predicts dementia, disability, and falls in meta-analysis (Xiang et al., 2022). A prospective cohort study found that combined slow gait and poor processing speed increase mortality risk compared with either deficit alone (Yang et al., 2025). Early identification is important because even mild cognitive impairment accelerates decline in other IC domains (Merchant et al., 2024).

Psychological Capacity

Psychological capacity relates to mood, coping, and emotional well-being (WHO, 2024). Late-life depression is prevalent and predicts functional decline, increased falls, and mortality. Depression and anxiety also interact with cognitive impairment to accelerate dependence (Lindert et al., 2021). The 2024 *Lancet Commission on Dementia* identified depression as a modifiable risk factor for dementia, underscoring the need for proactive detection (Livingston et al., 2024). Simple mood screens embedded in ICOPE have high sensitivity, while formal tools improve specificity in complex cases (de Oliveira et al., 2023).

Sensory Capacity (Hearing and Vision)

Sensory capacity covers hearing and vision. Impairments reduce quality of life and functional ability (Tseng et al., 2018). Hearing loss is strongly linked with dementia risk (Alzheimer's Society, 2024), while vision impairment is associated with cognitive decline and dementia incidence (Shang et al., 2021). Dual sensory impairment confers the highest risk of disability and dementia (Yoshida et al., 2025). The 2024 Lancet Commission includes untreated vision and hearing loss as modifiable dementia risk factors (Livingston et al., 2024).

Continence

Continence refers to bladder and bowel control, often compromised by age-related changes, mobility decline, and medication use. Urinary incontinence (UI) is common, linked with falls, institutionalisation, and mortality (Moon et al., 2021). UI is common in frailty, affecting over 39% of frail older adults (a rate approximately twice that observed in their non-frail peers). Moreover, in older women, UI—particularly urgency type—doubles the risk of falls, and the 12-month incidence of falls among women with even one episode per week may be as high as 54%. Conservative measures such as pelvic floor muscle training and timed voiding improve continence outcomes (Cho and Kim, 2021). Despite this, continence remains under-reported, requiring proactive enquiry (WHO, 2024).

IC and Frailty

Frailty and IC are closely related concepts, but they describe ageing in different ways and guide care planning differently. Frailty has traditionally been defined as a state of vulnerability arising from cumulative physiological decline, whereas IC represents the reserves and capacities that can be harnessed and maintained across the life course (Clegg et al., 2013; WHO, 2024). Table 3.1 provides a structured comparison between the two frameworks, highlighting differences in orientation, measurement, and clinical application.

TABLE 3.1   Comparison between frailty and IC.

Aspect	Frailty	IC
Definition	Progressive decline of physiological systems, leading to increased vulnerability to stressors and risk of adverse health outcomes (Clegg et al., 2013).	Composite of all mental and physical capacities, reflecting reserves and residual function across multiple domains (WHO, 2015, 2024).
When observed	Geriatric condition, usually identified in later life.	Relevant across the life course, but operationalised particularly after midlife to track decline against healthy-ageing goals.
Time dimension	Typically, cross-sectional assessment identifying a vulnerable state at a point in time.	Longitudinal construct designed for tracking capacity trajectories over time.
Characteristics	Defined by deficits and abnormalities (e.g. Fried's criteria including weakness, slowness, weight loss, low activity, and exhaustion).	Defined by reserves and capacities across six domains: locomotion, vitality, cognition, psychological, sensory, and continence (WHO, 2024).
Original purpose	Developed to address unmet clinical needs of older adults, primarily in geriatric medicine and risk stratification.	Developed to inform public health strategies for promoting healthy ageing, prevention, and early intervention.
Measurement tools	Frailty phenotype (Fried et al., 2001), frailty index (Rockwood and Mitnitski, 2007), and clinical frailty scale.	WHO ICOPE screening and assessment tools, based on domain-specific measures such as gait speed, grip strength, cognition, mood, sensory checks, and nutrition.
Orientation	Deficit-based, focusing on loss of reserve and resilience.	Asset-based, focusing on capacities that can be preserved or enhanced.
Clinical implications	Used to stratify high-risk patients for comprehensive geriatric assessment and targeted interventions.	Used to design proactive, domain-targeted interventions before frailty and dependency develop.
Policy implications	Incorporated into national strategies on frailty management (e.g. NHS England FRAIL framework).	Central to WHO healthy-ageing framework and ICOPE guidelines, influencing global and national ageing policy.
Interventions	Comprehensive geriatric assessment, often within integrated care models; rehabilitation and secondary prevention.	Comprehensive, person-centred interventions integrating healthcare, behavioural change, and social services, with emphasis on prevention and capacity maintenance.

Source: Adapted from Fried et al. (2001), WHO (2024), Clegg et al. (2013), and Rockwood and Mitnitski (2007).

As shown in the table, frailty is deficit-based, typically observed in later life, and often measured cross-sectionally to identify those at immediate risk of adverse outcomes. By contrast, IC is asset-based, designed for longitudinal tracking of functional domains, and aims to inform preventive strategies that maintain independence. Both constructs have value: frailty is well established in geriatric medicine for risk stratification and care planning, while IC has been promoted by the WHO as a foundation of the healthy-ageing agenda. For APs, recognising the differences and complementarities between frailty and IC is essential for delivering proactive, person-centred care that both mitigates vulnerability and enhances resilience.

THE ICOPE ASSESSMENT PATHWAY: A PRACTICAL APPROACH FOR APs

The WHO developed the ICOPE framework as a structured method to evaluate IC in adults aged 65 years and older (WHO, 2024). The approach emphasises early detection, holistic assessment, and person-centred care planning, all of which align closely with the scope of practice for APs. The following pathway illustrates (Figure 3.1) how APs can operationalise IC assessment in both primary and secondary settings.

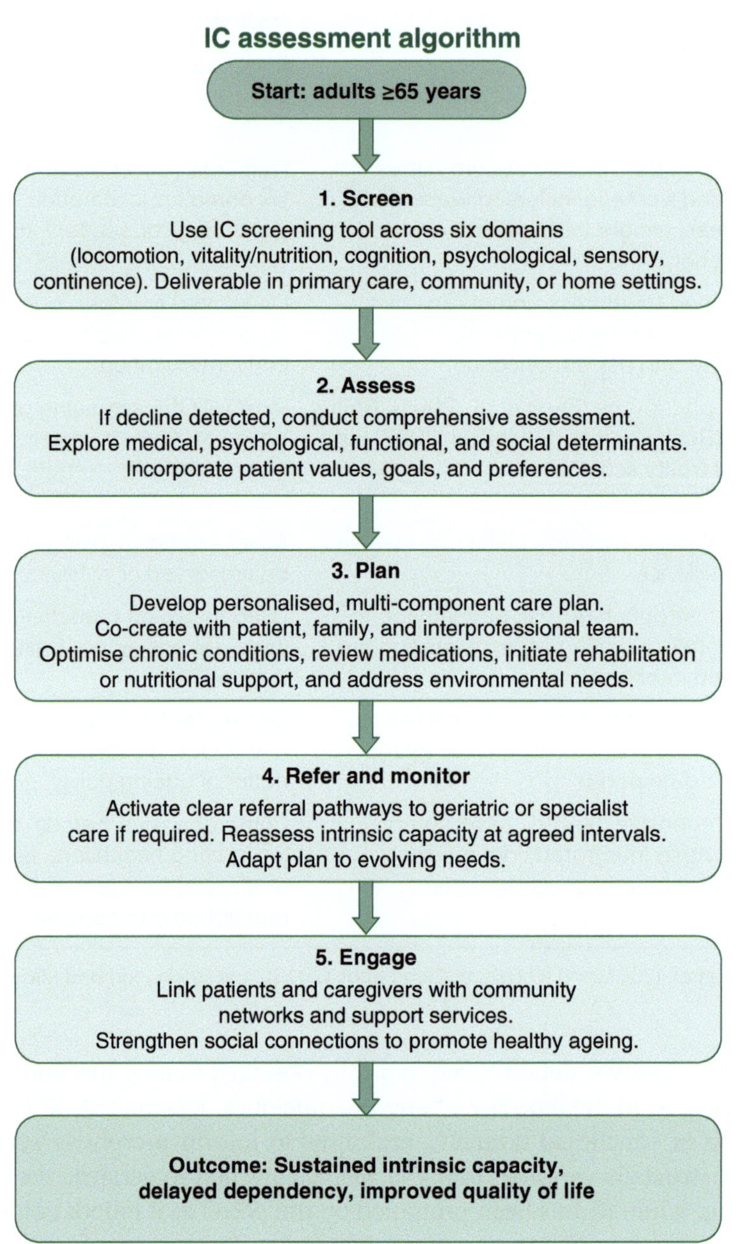

FIGURE 3.1   IC assessment methods.

Step 1: Initial IC Screening

Assessment begins with a brief screening tool designed to detect early changes in six IC domains: locomotion, vitality and nutrition, cognition, psychological well-being, sensory function, and continence. The screening consists of simple questions and short tasks that can be administered in primary care clinics, same-day emergency care, or the patient's home. For APs, this first step offers an efficient way to identify those at risk of decline, particularly in environments where time and resources are limited.

Step 2: Comprehensive Person-centred Assessment

When deficits are identified at screening, a more detailed assessment follows. This involves a structured exploration of potential causes such as acute illness, chronic disease, medication side effects, or social factors including isolation and poverty. APs are well placed to perform this stage, drawing upon their advanced history-taking and diagnostic skills while integrating social and functional perspectives. Importantly, this assessment also involves exploring the patient's goals, values, and preferences, ensuring that the process is genuinely person-centred.

Step 3: Development of a Personalised Care Plan

Based on the findings, a tailored care plan is co-created by the AP, the patient, family members, and, where appropriate, other members of the inter-professional team. The plan may involve optimising chronic disease management, reviewing medications where polypharmacy is evident, initiating rehabilitation or nutrition support, and connecting the patient with community resources. APs, with their ability to work across professional boundaries, are ideally positioned to coordinate this plan.

Step 4: Referral, Monitoring, and Review

Care planning does not end with formulation. Ongoing monitoring is essential, and APs play a pivotal role in reassessing IC trajectories at agreed intervals. Clear referral pathways to specialist geriatric services should be activated when complex needs arise, but APs remain central to continuity of care, ensuring that interventions remain relevant and responsive to changes in health status or social circumstances.

Step 5: Community and Caregiver Engagement

IC cannot be preserved through healthcare interventions alone. APs are instrumental in linking patients and families with local community groups, voluntary organisations, and caregiver support networks. By doing so, they extend the reach of ICOPE beyond the clinic, addressing the environmental and social enablers of healthy ageing.

This structured approach highlights the unique contribution that APs can make. Their advanced diagnostic capability, combined with a holistic appreciation of social and functional health, places them at the centre of IC assessment and management. By embedding ICOPE into routine practice, health services can shift from reactive responses to frailty and dependency towards proactive maintenance of capacity and independence (Table 3.2).

TABLE 3.2   Mapping the ICOPE assessment pathway for APs to the MPF capabilities.

ICOPE step	MPF pillar(s)	Precisely relevant capability numbers
1. Initial IC screening	1. Clinical practice	1.4 work in partnership using a range of assessment methods; 1.5 effective communication to support decisions and planning; 1.6 apply clinical reasoning to differentiated and undifferentiated presentations.
2. Comprehensive person-centred assessment	1. Clinical practice	1.4 holistic and diagnostic assessment; 1.6 synthesise information to make evidence-based judgements and diagnoses; 1.8 manage risk in complex or unpredictable situations; 1.3 exercise judgement about when to seek help.
	2. Leadership and management	2.1 role model inclusive behaviours to build effective relationships when coordinating complex assessment.
3. Personalised care plan	1. Clinical practice	1.7 initiate, evaluate, and modify interventions including medicines, therapies, lifestyle advice, and care; 1.9 work collaboratively with multi-agency and inter-professional resources; 1.10 act as a clinical role model and advocate for responsive care.
	2. Leadership and management	2.2 role model person-centred service delivery; 2.5 lead new practice and service redesign across boundaries.
	3. Education	3.3 support health literacy and empower individuals to participate in care decisions.
4. Referral, monitoring, and review	1. Clinical practice	1.7 modify interventions over time; 1.8 manage risk during trajectory monitoring; 1.9 maintain links across organisations for safe referral.
	2. Leadership and management	2.3 participate in service and team evaluation to demonstrate impact; 2.7 provide consultancy across boundaries to enhance quality and reduce unwarranted variation; 2.8 demonstrate team leadership and resilience.
	4. Research	4.2 evaluate and audit practice and act on findings; 4.3 appraise and synthesise evidence to inform ongoing care; 4.6 implement robust governance and documentation processes.
5. Community and caregiver engagement	1. Clinical practice	1.9 develop, maintain, and evaluate links with multi-agency resources to manage risk and issues across settings.
	2. Leadership and management	2.6 co-produce service improvements with individuals, families, carers, and communities; 2.1 inclusive relationship building to foster productive working.
	3. Education	3.3 empower individuals and carers through education; 3.5 facilitate collaboration and peer learning; 3.8 act as educator, supervisor, coach, and mentor.

CONCLUSION

Frailty and IC represent two conceptually aligned frameworks for understanding ageing. Frailty highlights vulnerability and the need for targeted support once reserve is diminished, while IC emphasises strengths and the potential for prevention across the life course. For APs, applying both perspectives offers a balanced approach that supports timely risk identification while promoting interventions to preserve independence and quality of life.

> **Take-Home Messages**
>
> 1. Frailty and IC are different in orientation: frailty is deficit-based, whereas IC is asset-based and focuses on capacities that can be maintained or enhanced.
> 2. Frailty is usually identified later in life, while IC can be measured and tracked earlier, making it a proactive tool for prevention.
> 3. Measurement approaches are different in frailty tools that assess vulnerability, while IC uses the WHO ICOPE framework to track six functional domains.
> 4. Both models are complementary for practice: frailty helps to stratify risk, whereas IC supports person-centred, preventive care aligned with healthy-ageing strategies.

REFERENCES

Adam, C.E., Fitzpatrick, A.L., Leary, C.S. et al. (2023). Change in gait speed and fall risk among community-dwelling older adults with and without mild cognitive impairment: a retrospective cohort analysis. *BMC Geriatrics* 23 (1): 328.

Alzheimer's Society (2024). Hearing loss and the risk of dementia. www.alzheimers.org.uk/about-dementia/managing-the-risk-of-dementia/reduce-your-risk-of-dementia/hearing-loss (accessed 10 September 2025).

Bernal, M.C., Batista, E., Martínez-Ballesté, A., and Solanas, A. (2025). A functional approach to model intrinsic capacity in ageing trajectories. *Scientific Reports* 15 (1): 7878.

Briand, M., Raffin, J., Gonzalez-Bautista, E. et al. (2025). Body composition and aging: cross-sectional results from the INSPIRE study in people 20 to 93 years old. *GeroScience* 47 (1): 863–875.

Cao, X., Yi, X., Chen, H. et al. (2024). Prevalence of intrinsic capacity decline among community-dwelling older adults: a systematic review and meta-analysis. *Aging Clinical and Experimental Research* 36 (1): 157.

Cho, S.T. and Kim, K.H. (2021). Pelvic floor muscle exercise and training for coping with urinary incontinence. *Journal of Exercise Rehabilitation* 17 (6): 379–387.

Clegg, A., Young, J., Iliffe, S. et al. (2013). *Frailty in elderly people. The lancet 381* (9868): 752–762.

Fried, L.P., Tangen, C.M., Walston, J. et al. (2001). Frailty in older adults: evidence for a phenotype. *The Journals of Gerontology Series A: Biological Sciences and Medical Sciences* 56 (3): M146–M157.

Lindert, J., Paul, K.C., Lachman, M.E. et al. (2021). Depression-, anxiety-, and anger and cognitive functions: findings from a longitudinal prospective study. *Frontiers in Psychiatry* 12: 665742.

Livingston, G., Huntley, J., Liu, K.Y. et al. (2024). Dementia prevention, intervention, and care: 2024 report of the Lancet standing Commission. *The Lancet* 404 (10452): 572–628.

Merchant, R.A., Chan, Y.H., Anbarasan, D., and Vellas, B. (2024). Association of intrinsic capacity with functional ability, sarcopenia and systemic inflammation in pre-frail older adults. *Frontiers in Medicine* 11: 1374197.

Moon, S., Chung, H.S., Kim, Y.J. et al. (2021). The impact of urinary incontinence on falls: a systematic review and meta-analysis. *PLoS One* 16 (5): e0251711.

NHS England (2022). *Older people advanced practice area specific capability and curriculum framework.* NHS England. Available at: `https://advanced-practice.hee.nhs.uk/wp-content/uploads/sites/28/2025/01/Older-people-advanced-practice-area-specific-capability-and-curriculum-framework-NHSE.pdf` (accessed 30 January 2026).

NHS England (2023a). *Palliative and end of life care advanced practice area specific capability and curriculum framework.* NHS England. Available at: `https://advanced-practice.hee.nhs.uk/wp-content/uploads/sites/28/2025/01/Palliative-and-end-of-life-care-advanced-practice-area-specific-capability-and-curriculum-framework-NHSE.pdf` (accessed 30 January 2026).

NHS England (2023b). *Acute medicine advanced practice area specific capability and curriculum framework.* NHS England. Available at: `https://advanced-practice.hee.nhs.uk/wp-content/uploads/sites/28/2025/03/Acute-medicine-advanced-practice-area-specific-capability-and-curriculum-framework-NHSE.pdf` (accessed 30 January 2026).

NHS England (2025). *Multi-professional framework for advanced practice in England – Edition 2025.* NHS England. Available at: `https://advanced-practice.hee.nhs.uk/wp-content/uploads/sites/28/2025/05/Multi-professional-framework-for-advanced-practice-in-England---Edition-2025.pdf` (accessed 29 January 2026).

de Oliveira, V.P., Ferriolli, E., Lourenço, R.A. et al. (2023). The sensitivity and specificity of the WHO's ICOPE screening tool, and the prevalence of loss of intrinsic capacity in older adults: a scoping review. *Maturitas* 177: 107818.

Polo-López, A., López-Bueno, R., Calatayud, J. et al. (2025). Association of chair stand performance with all-cause and cardiovascular mortality in older adults with hypertension: a 28-country study. *Maturitas* 196: 108248.

Rockwood, K. and Mitnitski, A. (2007). Frailty in relation to the accumulation of deficits. *The Journals of Gerontology Series A: Biological Sciences and Medical Sciences* 62 (7): 722–727.

Salari, N., Darvishi, N., Bartina, Y. et al. (2025). Global prevalence of malnutrition in older adults: a comprehensive systematic review and meta-analysis. *Public Health in Practice* 9: 100583.

Salinas-Rodríguez, A., Fernández-Niño, J.A., Rivera-Almaraz, A., and Manrique-Espinoza, B. (2024). Intrinsic capacity trajectories and socioeconomic inequalities in health: the contributions of wealth, education, gender, and ethnicity. *International Journal for Equity in Health* 23 (1): 48.

Sánchez-Sánchez, J.L., Lu, W.H., Gallardo-Gómez, D. et al. (2024). Association of intrinsic capacity with functional decline and mortality in older adults: a systematic review and meta-analysis of longitudinal studies. *The Lancet Healthy Longevity* 5 (7): e480–e492.

Shang, X., Zhu, Z., Wang, W. et al. (2021). The association between vision impairment and incidence of dementia and cognitive impairment: a systematic review and meta-analysis. *Ophthalmology* 128 (8): 1135–1149.

Tomkinson, G.R., Lang, J.J., Rubín, L. et al. (2025). International norms for adult handgrip strength: a systematic review of data on 2.4 million adults aged 20 to 100+ years from 69 countries and regions. *Journal of Sport and Health Science* 14: 101014.

Tseng, Y.C., Liu, S.H.Y., Lou, M.F., and Huang, G.S. (2018). Quality of life in older adults with sensory impairments: a systematic review. *Quality of Life Research* 27 (8): 1957–1971.

World Health Organization (2015). *World report on ageing and health.* Geneva: World Health Organization. Available at:`https://www.who.int/publications/i/item/9789241565042`(accessed 30 January 2026).

World Health Organization (2024). *Integrated Care for Older People (ICOPE): Guidance for Person-Centred Assessment and Pathways in Primary Care,* 2e. Geneva: World Health Organization `https://www.who.int/publications/i/item/9789240103726` (accessed 9 September 2025).

Xiang, K., Liu, Y., and Sun, L. (2022). Motoric cognitive risk syndrome: symptoms, pathology, diagnosis, and recovery. *Frontiers in Aging Neuroscience* 13: 728799.

Yang, H., Zhou, Y., Wang, X., and Xu, X. (2025). Combined association of gait speed and processing speed on cardiometabolic disease mortality risk in the US older adults: a prospective cohort study from NHANES. *Frontiers in Aging Neuroscience* 17: 1537413.

Yeung, S.S.Y., Leung, J., Woo, J. et al. (2021). Malnutrition according to the Global Leadership Initiative on Malnutrition (GLIM) criteria predicts sarcopenia, frailty and long-term mortality in community-dwelling older Chinese adults: a 14-year follow-up study. *Journal of the Academy of Nutrition and Dietetics* 121 (12): 2567–2576. `https://www.sciencedirect.com/science/article/abs/pii/S152586102030829X` (accessed 10 September 2025).

Yoshida, Y., Hiratsuka, Y., Umeya, R. et al. (2025). The association between dual sensory impairment and dementia: a systematic review and meta-analysis. *Journal of Alzheimer's Disease* 103 (3): 637–648.

Zampino, M., AlGhatrif, M., Kuo, P.L. et al. (2020). Longitudinal changes in resting metabolic rates with aging are accelerated by diseases. *Nutrients* 12 (10): 3061.

Zhang, X., Zheng, X., Zheng, T. et al. (2025). Associations between leisure activities with trajectories of intrinsic capacity among Chinese older adults: the China health and retirement longitudinal study. *Archives of Public Health* 83 (1): 162.

CHAPTER 4

Epidemiology of Frailty

Aim

The aim of this chapter is to provide advanced practitioners (APs) with a critical understanding of the global and regional epidemiology of frailty, highlighting how prevalence patterns are shaped by methodological choices, demographic variation, and social determinants. It seeks to equip APs with the ability to interpret prevalence data critically and apply these insights to inform clinical practice, service design, and policy implementation across community, acute, and end-of-life settings.

LEARNING OUTCOMES

By the end of this chapter, learners will be able to:

1. Explain the epidemiological patterns of frailty across global, regional, and national contexts, with attention to age, sex, and social gradients.
2. Critically appraise the strengths and limitations of epidemiological research, including systematic reviews, meta-analyses, national surveys, and electronic health record (EHR)-based studies.
3. Analyse how methodological variability (e.g. frailty phenotype versus deficit accumulation index) influences prevalence estimates and their interpretation.
4. Discuss the implications of frailty epidemiology for health inequalities, service planning, and anticipatory care.
5. Apply epidemiological insights to clinical decision-making, including case finding, comprehensive geriatric assessment (CGA), medicines optimisation, and end-of-life care planning within advanced practice roles.

SELF-ASSESSMENT QUESTIONS

1. How would you interpret different frailty prevalence estimates when derived from phenotype versus deficit accumulation approaches, and what biases or sampling issues would you anticipate in each?
2. Given your local population's age, sex, and deprivation profile, what proportion of older adults would you prioritise for case finding and CGA, and how would this inform medicines optimisation and anticipatory care planning?

> Frailty is not a fixed number in a chart, but a reflection of how biology, life course, and society combine.

INTRODUCTION

Frailty has become a defining concept in gerontological medicine and policy, but its epidemiology remains complex and challenging to characterise (Dlima et al., 2024). Unlike conditions defined by single biomarkers or disease codes, frailty represents a syndrome of diminished physiological reserve, often operationalised through models such as the Fried frailty phenotype or the deficit accumulation index. For advanced practitioners (APs) working across community, acute, and end-of-life care, the prevalence of frailty within populations has direct implications for service design, proactive case finding, and anticipatory care planning. However, the literature reveals wide variation in prevalence estimates depending on the measurement tool, the demographic context, and the healthcare system in which data are collected. For APs, engaging with this evidence requires not only attention to pooled prevalence estimates but also critical appraisal of research design, awareness of the limitations inherent in systematic reviews and meta-analyses, and consideration of how such data are operationalised within national guidance and translated into frontline practice.

Multi-Professional Framework (MPF) for Advanced Practitioners

(Adapted from NHS England, 2025a)

This chapter maps to the following areas within the MPF:

1. Clinical: 1.4, 1.6, 1.7, 1.9
2. Leadership and management: 2.3, 2.5, 2.6, 2.7, 2.9, 2.10
3. Education: 3.4, 3.5, 3.7
4. Research: 4.1, 4.2, 4.3, 4.4, 4.6, 4.7

Accreditation Consideration

This chapter maps to the statement with the following national accretional documents:

Curriculum framework for advanced practice in the care of older people (NHS England, 2022):

1. Core Capabilities in Practice (CiPs): 1, 2, 3, 4, 5
2. Generic Clinical CiPs: 1, 3, 5, 6
3. Specialty Clinical CiPs (Older People): 1, 3, 4

Curriculum framework for APs in the case of palliative and end-of-life care (NHS England, 2023a):

1. Clinical: 1.2, 1.3
2. Leadership and management: 2.1, 2.2, 2.3
3. Education: 3.1, 3.2
4. Research: 4.1, 4.2, 4.3

Curriculum for APs in acute medicine (NHS England, 2023b):

1. Coe CiPs: 1, 2, 3, 5
2. Generic Clinical CiPs: 1, 3, 5, 6
3. Specialty Clinical CiPs (Acute Medicine): 1, 2, 3, 5

EPIDEMIOLOGY OF FRAILTY

One of the earliest attempts to synthesise frailty prevalence globally was the systematic review and meta-analysis by Collard and colleagues, who analysed 21 studies across high-income countries (Collard et al., 2012). Their meta-analysis reported an overall prevalence of 10.7% in community-dwelling older adults, but with individual studies ranging from 4% to nearly 60%. The methodological strength of this review lies in its systematic approach and pooled weighting, but limitations included heterogeneity between instruments and the under-representation of non-Western countries. Importantly, Collard et al. demonstrated that prevalence increases steeply with age, from less than 5% at ages 65–69 years to over 25% in those aged 85 years and older, and that women consistently exhibit higher frailty prevalence than men.

Subsequent reviews expanded the scope to Europe and low- and middle-income countries (LMICs). The ADVANTAGE Joint Action, which drew together data from European community samples, reported a pooled prevalence of around 12%, highlighting the variation between northern and southern Europe (O'Caoimh et al., 2018). By contrast, Siriwardhana et al. (2018) synthesised evidence from LMICs and found higher prevalence rates of approximately 17.4%, suggesting that socioeconomic determinants, multimorbidity, and health system constraints magnify frailty burden. A separate meta-analysis focused on Latin America and the Caribbean, incorporating 29 studies and 43,083 participants, reported a prevalence of approximately 19.6% (Da Mata et al., 2016). These findings highlight that frailty is both a biological phenomenon and a reflection of structural disadvantage, reinforcing the importance for APs to consider local context when applying epidemiological data. The most comprehensive synthesis to date is the global meta-analysis of 240 studies across 62 countries, involving nearly 1.8 million participants (O'Caoimh et al., 2021). This review is methodologically robust, drawing on a vast evidence base, but its limitations include residual heterogeneity and variation in age cut-offs. It confirmed that prevalence differs depending on the definition: 12% with physical phenotype criteria and 24% with a frailty index, while pre-frailty affected nearly half of the older adults. The consistency across reviews, phenotype yielding lower prevalence and deficit accumulation yielding higher prevalence, highlights the importance of specifying measurement methods. Without this, comparisons across studies or countries are misleading.

Theou et al. (2013) demonstrated this strongly by applying eight different frailty tools to the same cohort, yielding prevalence estimates ranging from 6% to 44%. This demonstrates that epidemiology is partly a function of conceptualisation, which has direct implications for policy. For instance, a national health system adopting a multidimensional tool may report higher prevalence than one relying on physical criteria, even within demographically similar populations.

Regional variation is also evident. In Asia, Japanese pooled estimates suggest frailty prevalence of around 7% in those aged 65 years and older, but rates rise to more than 35% in those over 85 years (Kojima et al., 2017). Chinese surveys, particularly the CHARLS cohort, reveal that approximately 7.0% of community-dwelling adults aged 60 years or older are frail. Prevalence varies geographically, ranging from about 3.3% in the Southeast and Northeast to 9.1% in the Northwest, and is higher in rural areas (about 1.5-fold greater) than in urban centres (Kojima et al., 2017). In India, national data from the Longitudinal Ageing Study of India (LASI) indicate a frailty prevalence of 29.2%, with pre-frailty at 58.8%, alongside substantial variation between states, ranging from 14.5% in Uttarakhand to 41.3% in Arunachal Pradesh (Nagarkar and Kulkarni, 2024). These findings highlight the association of demographic ageing, socioeconomic disadvantage, and healthcare infrastructure. For APs working in increasingly diverse populations, such variation cautions against assuming uniform risk across ethnic or cultural groups.

European data demonstrate considerable heterogeneity, with analyses from the Survey of Health, Ageing and Retirement in Europe (SHARE), indicating frailty prevalence as low as 3% in Switzerland and rising to over 15% in Portugal (Manfredi et al., 2019). A pooled analysis of 18 countries found an average prevalence of 7.7% for frailty and 42.9% for pre-frailty (Manfredi et al., 2019). These figures reflect not only methodological inconsistency but also a genuine north–south and east–west gradient, with higher rates in southern and eastern countries. In acute settings, the prevalence is markedly higher. The FEED study, conducted in 14 European countries, found that around 40% of adults aged 65 years and older presenting to emergency departments were frail, with national figures ranging from 26% to 51%. For APs, this has direct relevance: frailty should be expected in at least one in three older patients attending acute care (Coats et al., 2024).

The United Kingdom (UK) presents a unique case in epidemiology because frailty is embedded within national policy through the electronic frailty index (eFI). This tool, based on cumulative deficits coded in primary care records, stratifies people aged 65+ years into mild, moderate, and severe categories (NHS England, 2025b). Around 12% of older adults are classified as moderately frail, with a smaller proportion severely frail (NHS England, 2025a). Longitudinal primary care data from a cohort of more than two million adults in England show that the average age of frailty onset is around 69 years, although a notable minority (over 10% of those aged 50–64 years) were already frail at baseline. Prevalence rises steeply with age, exceeding 50% by age 85 years, reflecting both biological ageing and the cumulative impact of social determinants. These findings highlight the importance of early identification in midlife to slow progression and inform anticipatory care planning. This trajectory is further reinforced by demographic projections. Population estimates from the Office for National Statistics indicate that by 2045, there will be approximately 73% more individuals aged 85 years and over in England compared with 2025

Population projections for people aged 65 or over in England, 2025 to 2045

It is projected that in 20 years there will be 73% more people aged 85 or over in England

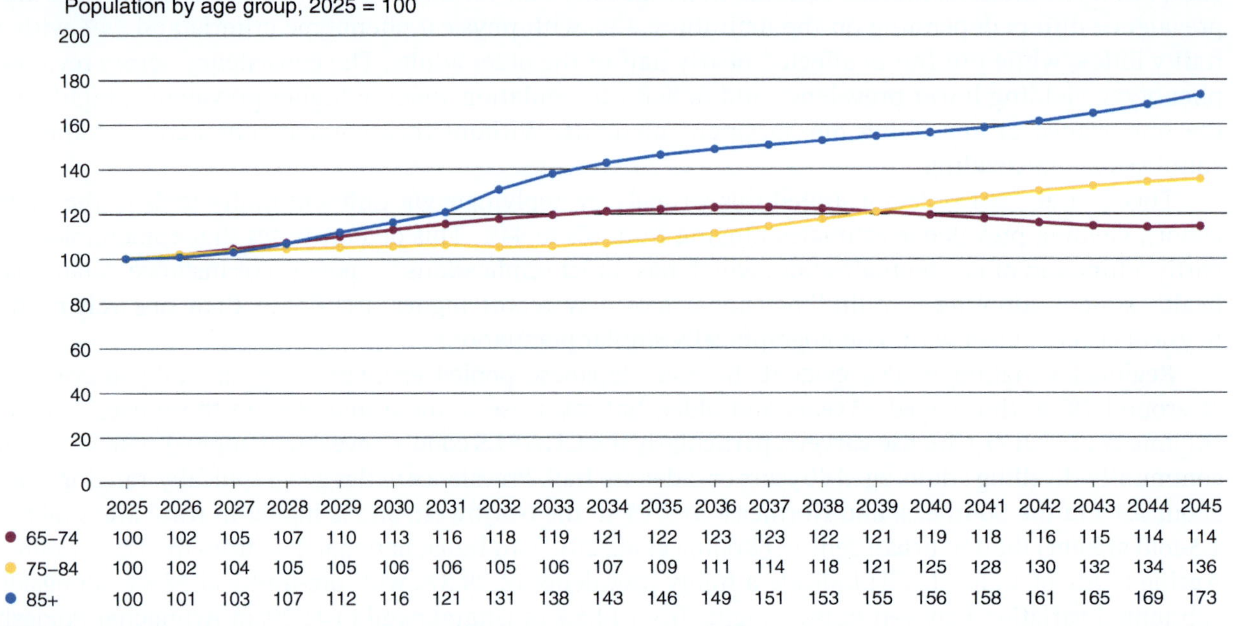

	2025	2026	2027	2028	2029	2030	2031	2032	2033	2034	2035	2036	2037	2038	2039	2040	2041	2042	2043	2044	2045
65–74	100	102	105	107	110	113	116	118	119	121	122	123	123	122	121	119	118	116	115	114	114
75–84	100	102	104	105	105	106	106	105	106	107	109	111	114	118	121	125	128	130	132	134	136
85+	100	101	103	107	112	116	121	131	138	143	146	149	151	153	155	156	158	161	165	169	173

Note

1   The Office for National Statistics' population projections are based upon combining the latest mid-year population estimate with long run assumptions about life expectancy, fertility and migration, and are typically published every two years. The projections reported here were published in 2025 and are based upon mid-2022 population estimates.

FIGURE 4.1   Population projections for people aged 65 years and over in England, 2025 to 2045. Adapted from National Audit Office (2025).

(Figure 4.1) (National Audit Office, 2025). Given that frailty prevalence exceeds 50% in this age group, this demographic shift is likely to lead to a substantial increase in the overall burden of frailty, strengthening the case for proactive, system-level approaches to prevention and management.

Strong social gradients exist: prevalence is roughly twice as high in the most deprived areas compared with the least deprived. The strength of electronic health record (EHR) surveillance lies in its population coverage and predictive utility for planning, but limitations include reliance on coded data quality and conceptual divergence from phenotype measures. This inequality is further illustrated in Figure 4.2, which demonstrates significant differences in healthy life expectancy across deprivation groups. Women aged 50 years and over living in the most deprived areas experience substantially fewer years in good health compared with those in the least deprived areas, with the gap evident from midlife and persisting into older age. For example, at ages 50 to 54 years, those in the least deprived decile can expect around 26 years of healthy life compared with approximately 14 years in the most deprived decile, with this disparity narrowing but remaining evident in later life. These findings highlight the cumulative impact of deprivation across the life course and its contribution to earlier onset and increased burden of frailty (National Audit Office, 2025).

National guidance has operationalised these epidemiological insights. The British Geriatrics Society's Fit for Frailty consensus outlines best practice for community management (BGS, 2014), while NHS England's Proactive Care Framework requires identification and proactive support for people with moderate or severe frailty (NHS England, 2023). NICE guidance on multimorbidity

Years of healthy life expectancy for women aged 50 or over in England by age and deprivation, 2018 to 2020

Women aged 50 or over from the most deprived areas of England have around half the years of healthy life expectancy compared to those from the least deprived areas

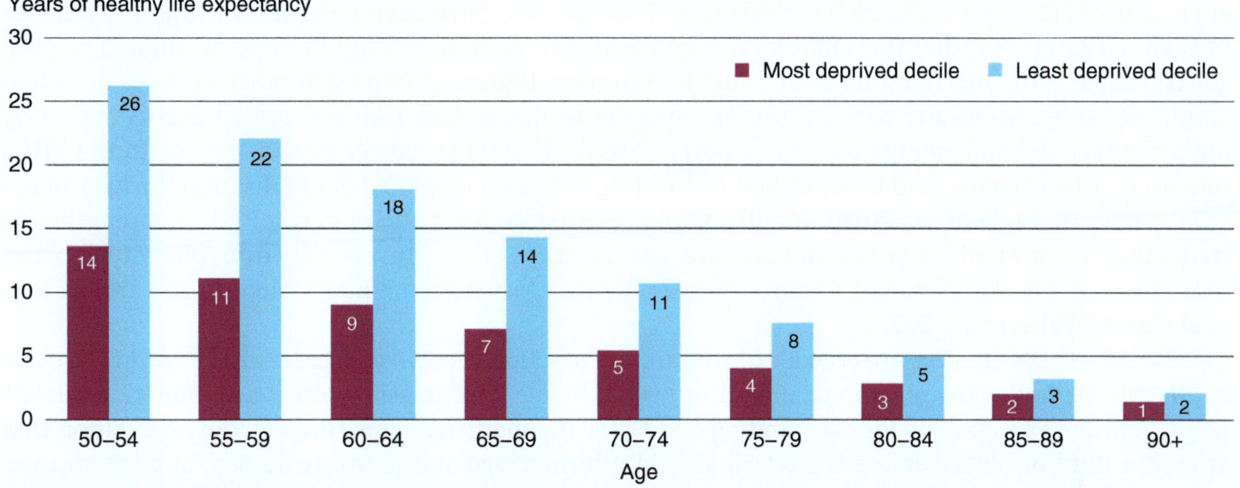

FIGURE 4.2 Years of healthy life expectancy for women aged 50 or over in England by age and deprivation, 2018 to 2020. Adapted from the National Audit Office (2025).

incorporates frailty assessment into prescribing and deprescribing decisions (NICE, 2016), while the Centre for Perioperative Care (Centre for Perioperative Care and British Geriatrics Society, 2021) mandates frailty assessment in surgical pathways. Front Door Frailty guidance supports emergency departments in embedding frailty-attuned models of care, acknowledging the high prevalence in acute settings (BGS, 2023).

At an international level, the World Health Organization (WHO) (2017) situates frailty within its Healthy Ageing and Integrated Care for Older People frameworks. Rather than prescribing fixed prevalence figures, WHO emphasises the concept of intrinsic capacity and functional ability. Implementation studies, such as Integrated Care for Older People Screening and Prevention of Care Dependency (INSPIRE) and Integrated Care for Older People – Care Pathways (ICOPE-CARE), demonstrate that early identification and intervention can be embedded within primary care systems (Tavassoli et al., 2022). This represents a shift from merely counting frailty cases to designing systems that preserve independence and dignity.

IMPLICATIONS FOR PRACTICE

The epidemiological evidence base offers both strengths and limitations. Its strengths lie in the consistency of key patterns: frailty prevalence increases progressively with age, is more common among women, and shows strong social patterning (Collard et al., 2012; O'Caoimh et al., 2018, 2021). Systematic reviews and meta-analyses contribute valuable *aggregate prevalence estimates*, enabling service planners to forecast caseloads and inform workforce strategies. The growing use of nationally representative surveys and large-scale EHR data provides an increasingly reliable basis for longitudinal monitoring of frailty trajectories across populations (Clegg et al., 2016; Collard et al., 2012).

Nonetheless, the limitations are substantial. Variability in measurement instruments undermines comparability, with prevalence estimates differing widely depending on whether frailty is operationalised through a physical phenotype or a multidimensional deficit accumulation model (Theou et al., 2015; O'Caoimh et al., 2021). Many prevalence studies have been conducted using convenience or regional samples rather than nationally representative designs, raising the risk of inflated or non-generalisable estimates (Kojima et al., 2018). Moreover, figures drawn from acute settings are often conflated with community-based estimates, despite evidence that frailty prevalence is consistently higher in hospital and emergency care cohorts (Ellis et al., 2011) Coats et al., 2024). Data from LMICs remain relatively sparse and heterogeneous, limiting the scope of global generalisation (Siriwardhana et al., 2018; Da Mata et al., 2016). Finally, while EHR-based tools such as the eFI have strengthened frailty identification in UK policy and practice, these indices differ conceptually from phenotype-based measures and are therefore not directly comparable in international epidemiological research (Clegg et al., 2016; Walsh et al., 2023).

For APs, these nuances are crucial. In community practice, recognising that around one in ten older adults may be frail using phenotype measures but up to one in four using deficit accumulation models helps calibrate expectations for case-finding and CGA. In emergency departments, the expectation that at least a third of older attendees are frail should inform triage and pathway design. In primary care, using eFI data to stratify patients enables proactive care planning, but APs must interpret scores critically, acknowledging coding variability and the risk of over-labelling.

At a policy level, the translation of epidemiology into national frameworks demonstrates how data can shape services. The UK's Proactive Care Framework and Fit for Frailty guidance provide APs with structured approaches to identifying and supporting frail individuals at home. Perioperative guidance ensures frailty is considered in surgical decision-making, while NICE multimorbidity guidance reinforces the link between frailty, prescribing, and shared decision-making. These frameworks encourage APs to move beyond viewing prevalence as abstract numbers and instead apply it to practical decisions about medicines optimisation, anticipatory care, and end-of-life planning.

Therefore, frailty epidemiology shows that prevalence figures are not static truths but reflections of measurement choices, demographic context, and social determinants. For APs, the key is not to memorise a prevalence rate but to critically appraise how figures were produced and apply them judiciously in clinical decision-making. Doing so ensures that epidemiological data becomes a tool for improving care, rather than a contested statistic.

CONCLUSION

Frailty epidemiology is complex, with prevalence shaped by methodology, demographics, and social determinants. Despite variation across studies, consistent patterns emerge: frailty increases with age, is more common in women, and reflects health inequalities. National and international frameworks—such as the eFI, BGS guidance, NICE recommendations, and WHO Healthy Ageing—show how epidemiological data drive policy and service design. For APs, the key is not to rely on a single prevalence figure but to critically interpret the evidence and apply it to practice, supporting case finding, CGA, medicines optimisation, and anticipatory care across diverse settings.

Take-Home Messages

1. Frailty epidemiology is variable but patterned. While prevalence figures differ depending on measurement tools and study designs, consistent trends show that frailty rises with age, is more common in women, and is socially patterned.

2. Methodological choices shape prevalence estimates. Systematic reviews, meta-analyses, and EHR data provide valuable insights, but differences between phenotype and multidimensional models, as well as sample representativeness, limit direct comparisons across studies and regions.

3. Policy and practice are informed by epidemiology. National and international frameworks (e.g. NHS England's eFI, BGS guidance, NICE multimorbidity, and WHO Healthy Ageing) translate prevalence data into service models, shaping case finding, care planning, and resource allocation.

4. Implications for APs are practical and critical. APs must not memorise single prevalence figures but instead critically appraise how data are produced and apply them to clinical practice, from CGA and medicines optimisation to anticipatory and end-of-life care planning.

REFERENCES

British Geriatrics Society (2014). *Fit for Frailty: Consensus Best Practice Guidance for the Care of Older People Living in Community and Outpatient Settings*. London: British Geriatrics Society www.bgs.org.uk/resources/resource-series/fit-for-frailty (accessed 9 September 2025).

British Geriatrics Society (2023). Front door frailty: advice on setting up services. www.bgs.org.uk/front-door-frailty-advice-on-setting-up-services (accessed 9 September 2025).

Centre for Perioperative Care and British Geriatrics Society (2021). Guideline for perioperative care for people living with frailty undergoing elective and emergency surgery. www.cpoc.org.uk/guidelines-and-resources/guidelines/perioperative-care-people-living-frailty (accessed 9 September 2025).

Clegg, A., Bates, C., Young, J. et al. (2016). Development and validation of an electronic frailty index using routine primary care data. *Age and Ageing* 45 (3): 353–360.

Coats, T., Nickel, C.H., Conroy, S.P. et al. (2024). Prevalence of frailty in European emergency departments: the FEED study. *European Geriatric Medicine* 15 (2): 463–470.

Collard, R.M., Boter, H., Schoevers, R.A., and Oude Voshaar, R.C. (2012). Prevalence of frailty in community-dwelling older persons: a systematic review. *Journal of the American Geriatrics Society* 60 (8): 1487–1492.

Da Mata, F.A.F., Pereira, P.P.D.S., Andrade, K.R.C.D. et al. (2016). Prevalence of frailty in Latin America and the Caribbean: a systematic review and meta-analysis. *PLoS One* 11 (8): e0160019.

Dlima, S.D., Hall, A., Aminu, A.Q. et al. (2024). Frailty: a global health challenge in need of local action. *BMJ Global Health* 9 (8): e015173.

Ellis, G., Whitehead, M.A., Robinson, D. et al. (2011). Comprehensive geriatric assessment for older adults admitted to hospital: meta-analysis of randomised controlled trials. *Bmj* 343: d6553.

Kojima, G., Iliffe, S., Taniguchi, Y. et al. (2017). Prevalence of frailty in Japan: a systematic review and meta-analysis. *Journal of Epidemiology* 27 (8): 347–353.

Kojima, G., Iliffe, S., and Walters, K. (2018). Frailty index as a predictor of mortality: a systematic review and meta-analysis. *Age and Ageing* 47 (2): 193–200.

Manfredi, G., Midão, L., Paúl, C. et al. (2019). Prevalence of frailty status among the European elderly population: findings from the Survey of Health, Aging and Retirement in Europe. *Geriatrics & Gerontology International* 19 (8): 723–729.

Nagarkar, A. and Kulkarni, A.S. (2024). Regional variation in prevalence of frailty in India: evidence from longitudinal ageing study in India (LASI) wave-1. *The Indian Journal of Medical Research* 159 (5): 441–448.

National Audit Office (2025). Primary and community healthcare support for people living with frailty. London: National Audit Office. Available at: https://www.nao.org.uk/wp-content/uploads/2025/12/Primary-and-community-healthcare-support-for-people-living-with-frailty.pdf (accessed 29 March 2026).

NHS England (2022). *Older people advanced practice area specific capability and curriculum framework.* NHS England. Available at: https://advanced-practice.hee.nhs.uk/wp-content/uploads/sites/28/2025/01/Older-people-advanced-practice-area-specific-capability-and-curriculum-framework-NHSE.pdf accessed 30 January 2026.

NHS England (2023). Proactive care: providing care and support for people living at home with moderate or severe frailty. https://www.england.nhs.uk/long-read/proactive-care-providing-care-and-support-for-people-living-at-home-with-moderate-or-severe-frailty (accessed 9 September 2025).

NHS England (2023a). *Palliative and end of life care advanced practice area specific capability and curriculum framework.* NHS England. Available at: https://advanced-practice.hee.nhs.uk/wp-content/uploads/sites/28/2025/01/Palliative-and-end-of-life-care-advanced-practice-area-specific-capability-and-curriculum-framework-NHSE.pdf .

NHS England (2023b) *Acute medicine advanced practice area specific capability and curriculum framework.* NHS England. Available at: https://advanced-practice.hee.nhs.uk/wp-content/uploads/sites/28/2025/03/Acute-medicine-advanced-practice-area-specific-capability-and-curriculum-framework-NHSE.pdf (accessed 30 January 2026).

NHS England (2025a). Electronic frailty index (eFI). https://www.england.nhs.uk/ourwork/clinical-policy/older-people/frailty/efi (accessed 9 September 2025).

NHS England (2025b). *Multi-professional framework for advanced practice in England – Edition 2025.* NHS England. Available at: https://advanced-practice.hee.nhs.uk/wp-content/uploads/sites/28/2025/05/Multi-professional-framework-for-advanced-practice-in-England---Edition-2025.pdf (accessed 29 January 2026).

NICE (2016). *Multimorbidity: Clinical Assessment and Management (NG56).* National Institute for Health and Care Excellence www.nice.org.uk/guidance/ng56 (accessed 9 September 2025).

O'Caoimh, R., Galluzzo, L., Rodríguez-Laso, Á. et al. (2018). Prevalence of frailty at population level in European ADVANTAGE Joint Action Member States: a systematic review and meta-analysis. *Annali dell'Istituto Superiore di Sanità* 54 (3): 226–238.

O'Caoimh, R., Sezgin, D., O'Donovan, M.R. et al. (2021). Prevalence of frailty in 62 countries across the world: a systematic review and meta-analysis of population-level studies. *Age and Ageing* 50 (1): 96–104.

Siriwardhana, D.D., Hardoon, S., Rait, G. et al. (2018). Prevalence of frailty and prefrailty among community-dwelling older adults in low-income and middle-income countries: a systematic review and meta-analysis. *BMJ Open* 8 (3): e018195.

Tavassoli, N., de Souto Barreto, P., Berbon, C. et al. (2022). Framework implementation of the INSPIRE ICOPE-CARE programme in collaboration with the World Health Organization in the Occitania region. *The Lancet Healthy Longevity* 3 (6): e394–e404. https://doi.org/10.1016/S2666-7568(22)00097-6 (accessed 9 September 2025).

Theou, O., Brothers, T.D., Mitnitski, A., and Rockwood, K. (2013). Operationalization of frailty using eight commonly used scales and comparison of their ability to predict all-cause mortality. *Journal of the American Geriatrics Society* 61 (9): 1537–1551.

Theou, O., Cann, L., Blodgett, J. et al. (2015). Modifications to the frailty phenotype criteria: Systematic review of the current literature and investigation of 262 frailty phenotypes in the Survey of Health, Ageing, and Retirement in Europe. *Ageing Research Reviews* 21: 78–94.

World Health Organization (2017). *Integrated Care for Older People: Guidelines on Community-Level Interventions to Manage Declines in Intrinsic Capacity.* Geneva: WHO https://www.who.int/publications/i/item/9789241550109 (accessed 9 September 2025).

CHAPTER 5

Frailty Risk Factors, Interventions, and Related Complications

Aim

The aim of this chapter is to critically explores the multidimensional risk factors that drive the development and progression of frailty and to analyse the complications that arise as a consequence of this syndrome. The chapter also evaluates evidence-based interventions and policy implications to inform clinical practice, service delivery, and future research.

LEARNING OUTCOMES

By the end of this chapter, readers will be able to:

1. Identify the biological, psychological, social, and lifestyle risk factors contributing to the onset and progression of frailty and evaluate intervention strategies aimed at slowing or preventing its development.
2. Analyse the major complications associated with frailty, including disability, falls, hospitalisation, institutionalisation, mortality, cognitive decline, malnutrition, infection, and reduced quality of life.
3. Evaluate the association between frailty, multimorbidity, and polypharmacy, and their collective impact on the complexity of care, health outcomes, and health system burden.
4. Critically appraise the effectiveness of multidomain interventions such as comprehensive geriatric assessment, exercise and nutrition support, psychosocial approaches, and medication optimisation in mitigating frailty risks and complications.
5. Apply insights from emerging constructs such as intrinsic capacity and resilience to enhance prognostication, prevention, and personalised approaches to frailty management.

SELF-ASSESSMENT QUESTIONS

1. Which modifiable risk factors for frailty are most prevalent in your patient cohort, and how would you prioritise evidence-based interventions (exercise, nutrition, psychosocial support, and medication optimisation) to address them safely?
2. How will you identify and mitigate the key complications you anticipate such as falls, delirium, malnutrition, readmission, and treatment burden from polypharmacy while aligning actions with patient goals and available services?

> Frailty is not destiny. It emerges from risks that can be reduced and from strengths that can be rebuilt.

INTRODUCTION

Advanced practitioners (APs) play an essential role in identifying frailty risk factors, preventing progression, and managing related complications through evidence-based, multidomain interventions. This chapter examines the biological, psychological, social, and lifestyle determinants of frailty; the complications they precipitate; and the interventions that mitigate these risks. It links this evidence to the multi-professional framework (MPF) for advanced clinical practice (NHS England, 2025) and national curricula, enabling APs to integrate advanced clinical reasoning, leadership, education, and research in person-centred frailty care.

Multi-Professional Framework (MPF) for Advanced Practitioners

(Adapted from NHS England, 2025)

This chapter maps to the following statements within the MPF:

1. Clinical practice: 1.6, 1.7, 1.8, 1.9
2. Leadership and management: 2.3, 2.5, 2.7, 2.8
3. Education: 3.3, 3.5, 3.7
4. Research: 4.1, 4.2, 4.3

Accreditation Consideration

This chapter maps to the statement with the following national accretional documents:

Curriculum framework for advanced practice in the care of older people (NHS England, 2022):

1. Core Capabilities in Practice (CiPs): 4, 5
2. Generic Clinical CiPs: 1, 3, 5
3. Specialty Clinical CiPs (Older People): 1, 3, 4

Curriculum framework for APs in the case of palliative and end-of-life care (NHS England, 2023a):

1. Clinical pillar: 1.2, 1.4
2. Research: 4.1, 4.2, 4.3

Curriculum for APs in acute medicine (NHS England, 2023b):

1. Core CiPs: 3, 5
2. Generic Clinical CiPs: 1, 5
3. Specialty Clinical CiPs (Acute Medicine): 1, 2, 3, 5 and acute medicine presentations

FRAILTY RISK FACTORS

Biological and Clinical Factors

Sarcopenia, chronic inflammation, and multimorbidity are tightly linked with frailty progression; recent consensus and reviews reaffirm sarcopenia as a driver of adverse outcomes, while multimorbidity and frailty show bidirectional amplification over time (Beaudart et al., 2025). Multimorbidity also accelerates progression, with frailty and multiple chronic conditions reinforcing one another in a cyclical relationship. A meta-analysis shows that 72% of frail individuals also have multimorbidity, with a two-way association between the conditions (Vetrano et al., 2019).

Psychological and Cognitive Factors

Mental health plays a crucial role in frailty progression. Depression and anxiety are independently linked with worsening frailty, and their co-occurrence amplifies vulnerability (Mutz et al., 2022). Cognitive impairment, including mild cognitive impairment, often accelerates frailty progression and predicts poorer outcomes; for example, older adults with both frailty and mild cognitive impairment have significantly higher mortality (more than threefold increased risk), highlighting shared pathways of neurodegeneration and loss of physiological reserve (Liu et al., 2025a,b).

Social and Environmental Determinants

Frailty is influenced not only by biological health but also by social context. Evidence from a 14-year longitudinal study of English older adults (English Longitudinal Study of Ageing [ELSA]) shows that loneliness substantially increases the risk of frailty, with medium levels raising risk by 57% (HR 1.57) and high levels by 162% (HR 2.62) compared with low levels. Social isolation exerts a similar, though smaller, effect, increasing frailty risk by 12% at medium levels and 32% at high levels, even after adjusting for age, sex, wealth, and smoking status (Davies et al., 2021). In parallel, socioeconomic disadvantage including poverty, low education, and poor housing has been consistently linked with earlier onset and faster progression of frailty, highlighting the role of structural inequalities in shaping health trajectories (Sinclair et al., 2025).

Lifestyle Factors

Low physical activity markedly increases the odds of incident frailty. A recent meta-analysis found that higher levels of physical activity were associated with 37% lower odds of physical frailty, 49% lower odds of multidimensional frailty, and 30% less likelihood of deficit accumulation frailty, compared to lower activity levels (Zhao et al., 2022). In addition, malnutrition, particularly when associated with sarcopenia, significantly elevates frailty risk, and this effect is mediated by muscle loss and moderated by activity levels, especially in those achieving moderate physical activity (Celik et al., 2024). Furthermore, smoking is a causal risk factor for frailty. A Mendelian randomisation study confirmed that smoking is associated with increased frailty, while traditional observational studies show that current smokers have 61% higher odds of frailty compared to non-smokers (Crane et al., 2022; Liu et al., 2023). Alcohol consumption has less consistent evidence, with some studies suggesting no clear causal relationship with frailty. These lifestyle factors, which also drive non-communicable diseases, interact with ageing to promote systemic inflammation and accelerate both the onset and progression of frailty, while chronic diseases in turn hasten frailty, creating a bidirectional relationship (Figure 5.1).

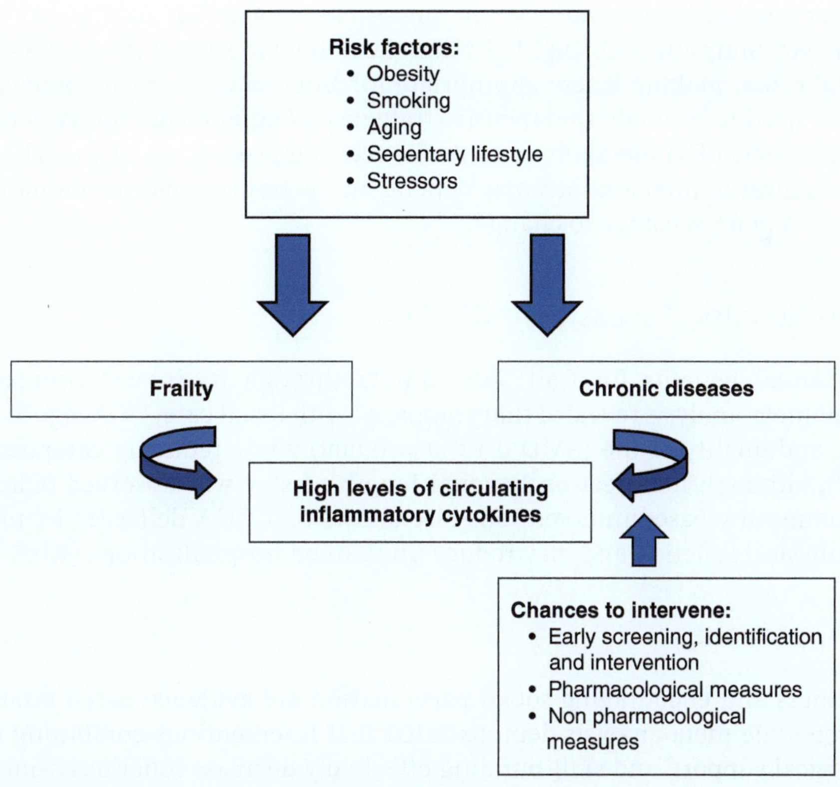

FIGURE 5.1 Graphical representation of the bidirectional relationship between frailty and chronic diseases. *Source*: Adapted from Bhattarai et al. (2024), distributed under the terms of the Creative Commons Attribution 4.0 International License (CC BY 4.0).

INTERVENTIONS TO PREVENT OR SLOW PROGRESSION

Multicomponent Interventions

Multicomponent interventions are highly effective in managing frailty. A 24-week trial found that combined resistance and balance training markedly improved walking speed, balance, and strength compared to resistance training alone (Jiang et al., 2025). Systematic review evidence further shows that multimodal exercise, including low-intensity programmes such as yoga and tai chi, can reduce frailty risk and improve physical function (Loewenthal et al., 2023). Exercise may also interact with underlying health conditions; in patients with chronic heart failure, frailty status significantly modified the benefits of training, with frail participants experiencing the greatest gains (Pandey et al., 2021).

A systematic review in 2024 confirmed that such programmes enhance cognitive performance, muscle strength, lower frailty scores, and reduce depressive symptoms (Luo et al., 2024). When exercise is paired with protein supplementation, the benefits are amplified, with randomised controlled trials showing significant improvements in muscle mass and handgrip strength (Yoshimura et al., 2025). A 12-week body-weight resistance programme also improved lower-limb strength and balance among older women, underlining the importance of functional training in frailty prevention (Liu et al., 2025a,b).

Findings from the Look AHEAD trial and its extension reinforce the role of lifestyle-based approaches. While intensive lifestyle interventions did not alter phenotypic frailty, they were associated with long-term reductions in frailty when measured using deficit accumulation models (Espinoza, 2021). Moreover, Simpson et al., highlight that the phenotype approach places disproportionate emphasis on weight loss, making it less appropriate for interventions involving caloric restriction. This highlights the need to evaluate therapeutic strategies using multiple frailty constructs, as each captures different aspects of vulnerability and resilience (Simpson et al., 2020). These data emphasise that the effectiveness of interventions may depend on the frailty construct employed, with deficit accumulation models more sensitive to change.

Comprehensive Geriatric Assessment (CGA)

CGA offers substantial benefits for frail older adults through its interdisciplinary and holistic approach. A recent meta-analysis revealed that compared with usual care, CGA significantly improves functional ability and quality of life (SMD 0.12, $p = 0.009$) while reducing caregiver burden (SMD -0.56, $p = 0.007$), although no effect on hospital length of stay was observed (Chen et al., 2021). Evidence from community-based interventions also shows that CGA delivered by multidisciplinary teams enhances physical function and may reduce unplanned hospitalisations (Kim, 2024).

Psychosocial Approaches

Addressing loneliness and encouraging social participation are evidence-based strategies to reduce frailty risk. A large-scale meta-analysis demonstrated that interventions combining animal-assisted therapy, psychological support, and skill-building effectively decrease loneliness among older adults in long-term care settings, with medium to large effect sizes (Patil et al., 2024). In a longitudinal study from China, older adults engaging more frequently in leisure-based social and intellectual activities were significantly less likely to follow a persistently low intrinsic capacity (IC) trajectory (OR 0.36 for social activities; OR 0.37 for intellectual activities) (Zhang et al., 2025). These findings suggest that enhancing social connectedness, whether through structured interventions or regular engagement in meaningful group activities, can bolster both psychological and functional resilience. For older people, particularly those experiencing frailty or IC decline, integrating such approaches into care plans holds promise for maintaining capacity and preventing decline.

Medication Optimisation

Effective management of medication burden is essential in frailty prevention. A systematic review confirms that deprescribing in frail older people is not only feasible and well tolerated but also reduces inappropriate medication use (Ibrahim et al., 2021). Real-world interventions, including pharmacist-led reviews using STOPP/START criteria, have already demonstrated reductions in potentially inappropriate prescriptions in primary care from 1.15 to 0.90 medications per person (Khera et al., 2019). A multidisciplinary medication review and deprescribing programme has also been developed using rigorous, theory-informed design, tailored to frail older adults with polypharmacy (Radcliffe et al., 2025).

Future Directions

Future research on frailty should prioritise a more precise understanding of how biological, psychological, social, and lifestyle risk factors interact to drive progression. Longitudinal studies that integrate biomarkers of inflammation, sarcopenia, and multimorbidity with social determinants such as poverty, housing, and isolation would clarify cumulative and synergistic effects. Advances in digital health, including wearable technology, may allow earlier detection of functional decline and more responsive monitoring of modifiable risk factors in community settings.

In terms of intervention, greater attention is needed on multimodal strategies that combine exercise, nutrition, psychosocial support, and medication optimisation, rather than focusing on single components in isolation. Large-scale trials should investigate how tailoring interventions to individual frailty trajectories and risk profiles might improve outcomes, and whether integrating such programmes into primary care and community services can deliver sustainable benefit. In addition, policy-level strategies also require evaluation, particularly those addressing structural inequalities that accelerate frailty onset. Embedding frailty risk assessment into routine health checks, supported by validated tools sensitive to change, could provide a platform for prevention. Future work should also explore how interventions can be adapted for diverse populations, ensuring equity in access and impact.

COMPLICATIONS OF FRAILTY

Introduction

Frailty is a multidomain state of diminished physiological reserve and impaired homeostatic recovery that renders older people disproportionately vulnerable to stressors. The two most widely used operationalisations: the frailty phenotype and the frailty index (FI) (Fried et al., 2001; Mitnitski et al., 2002). Substantial evidence base demonstrates that frailty is associated with disability, falls and fractures, unplanned hospital use, institutionalisation, and premature death, with effect sizes that are both statistically and clinically meaningful across contexts and time frames (Vermeiren et al., 2016; Peng et al., 2022). Beyond biology, psychosocial determinants including social capital, resilience, and cognitive reserve modulate these risks and their trajectories.

Functional Decline and Disability

Functional decline is at the centre of frailty and represents a major determinant of loss of independence in older adults. A systematic review and meta-analysis of longitudinal studies found that frailty approximately trebles the odds of subsequent disability in instrumental activities of daily living (IADLs) and more than doubles the odds of basic activities of daily living (ADLs), notwithstanding heterogeneity due to definitions and settings (Kojima, 2017). Evidence from meta-analyses also indicates that the FI, by quantifying accumulated health deficits, has strong predictive validity for adverse outcomes including disability and mortality, with each incremental increase in the index conferring a significantly higher risk of death (Kojima et al., 2018). Mechanistically, sarcopenia, chronic low-grade inflammation, malnutrition, impaired balance and gait, and executive dysfunction converge to reduce performance capacity and limit recovery after intercurrent illness. Disability then functions as both a consequence and a mediator, amplifying subsequent risks of hospitalisation, institutional care, and mortality through deconditioning, immobility-related harms, and caregiver strain.

Falls, Fractures, and Injury

Evidence from the Lifestyle Interventions and Independence for Elders (LIFE) study shows that a deficit accumulation FI predicts mobility decline: each one-unit increase in FI raised the hazard for major mobility disability by about 4%, with the highest quintile displaying nearly double the risk compared with the lowest (Brown et al., 2020). In another cohort free of major disability or dementia at baseline, higher FI scores were associated with dramatically increased hazard of the composite outcome of persistent disability or dementia (HR 21.3) (Ryan et al., 2022). Moreover, systematic reviews indicate that using the FI as a continuous score enhances prediction accuracy for adverse outcomes (Kim et al., 2022).

Complications of frailty include a markedly higher propensity to falls, fractures, and injury. Meta-analyses show frailty (and cognitive frailty) predicts future falls, with a graded risk that begins in pre-frailty; large cohorts demonstrate dose–response increases in fall- and fracture-related outcomes with increasing frailty severity (Yang et al., 2023; Guo et al., 2023; Dent et al., 2024; Jing et al., 2025). In hospital, frailty is linked with patient-safety incidents including falls, underscoring the need for targeted, multidomain prevention and rehabilitation (Alotaibi et al., 2025).

Healthcare Utilisation: Hospitalisation and Readmission

Frailty is a strong predictor of unscheduled care, acute hospital admission, prolonged length of stay, and early readmission. A systematic review and meta-analysis of prospective cohorts demonstrated that physical frailty significantly increases the risk of hospitalisation among community-dwelling older adults (Kojima, 2016a,b). Within hospitals, frailty identifies patients at high risk of in-hospital complications (delirium, infections, and pressure injuries) and functional loss; incorporation of frailty scores into emergency and acute pathways improves prognostic discrimination beyond physiological early warning scores and supports anticipatory care planning and timely discharge support (Boucher et al., 2023).

A recent systematic review of multidisciplinary home-based interventions found no convincing evidence that such programmes reduced mortality, emergency visits, or hospital readmissions among frail older people, and their effect on quality of life was minimal (Ruiz-Grao et al., 2024). These findings underline the need for interventions that are directly linked to frailty assessment and targeted at modifiable risks. In the acute care setting, the Clinical Frailty Scale (CFS) has been shown to be both feasible and acceptable in emergency departments, with most staff perceiving it as relevant and easy to use, though workload pressures and unclear follow-up actions remain barriers (Hörlin et al., 2023). These studies highlight that while frailty tools such as the CFS can support case-finding and prognostication, their utility depends on integration with CGA and robust transitional care planning to translate prediction into prevention.

Institutionalisation and Loss of Autonomy

Institutional care represents a sentinel transition for many frail individuals and carries profound personal and economic implications. A systematic review and meta-analysis found that both frailty and pre-frailty significantly increase the risk of nursing home placement among community-dwelling older adults, independent of sociodemographic factors and baseline function (Kojima, 2018). Repeated falls, progressive disability, cognitive impairment, carer burnout, and environmental barriers in housing and transport cumulatively drive the move to institutional settings. Proactive community-based approaches such as reablement, continence management, falls services, carer support and respite, nutrition and oral health programmes, and timely advance care planning can delay or prevent institutionalisation where home circumstances permit (Kojima et al., 2018).

Mortality and Prognosis

Mortality is the best recognised adverse outcome linked to frailty, with a graded relationship across severity levels and consistent findings across tools. A recent systematic review and meta-analysis concluded that frailty is associated with increased all-cause mortality and is a strong predictor of cause-specific mortality from cardiovascular, cancer, and respiratory disease in community cohorts (Peng et al., 2022). Emerging analyses reinforce that the FI, by capturing cumulative multi-system deficit burden, often shows particularly strong discrimination for death at medium-term follow-up, though both index and phenotype are prognostic (Kojima et al., 2018; Stolz et al., 2024). Clinically, these data inform shared decision-making about the goals and proportionality of interventions, trigger early conversations about preferences, and support timely involvement of palliative and supportive care in trajectories marked by recurrent complications and functional decline.

Cognitive Decline, Delirium, and Mental Health

Frailty and neurocognitive vulnerability frequently co-occur and interact. Meta-analytic syntheses indicate that 'cognitive frailty', defined as the coexistence of physical frailty and cognitive impairment in the absence of dementia, is associated with increased risks of mortality, disability, and incident dementia, exceeding the risks associated with either condition alone (Zhang et al., 2022; Grande et al., 2019). In hospital, frailty is an independent risk factor for delirium; a 2022 meta-analysis reported a 66% higher risk of delirium among frail inpatients compared with non-frail peers, with pooled frailty and delirium prevalences of 34% and 21%, respectively (Cechinel et al., 2022). These relationships likely operate through shared mechanisms of systemic inflammation, cerebral small vessel disease, reduced synaptic plasticity, sensory impairment, and medication burden, and they have practical significance: combining frailty assessment with brief cognitive screening improves prognostic accuracy and identifies modifiable targets for delirium prevention (hydration, mobilisation, sleep preservation, sensory aids) and for community cognitive health promotion.

Multimorbidity, Polypharmacy, and Complexity of Care

Frailty commonly co-occurs with multimorbidity and polypharmacy, creating a constellation of complexity that magnifies vulnerability to adverse outcomes. Longitudinal evidence demonstrates that polypharmacy itself is not merely an indicator but a driver of frailty progression: among older inpatients, it significantly increased the risk of frailty aggravation over two years (OR 1.43, 95% CI 1.26–1.63), mortality (OR 1.37, 95% CI 1.17–1.59), and falls (OR 1.36, 95% CI 1.06–1.72), with the association between polypharmacy and falls partly explained by multimorbidity (Liu et al., 2024). At the population level, an umbrella review reported that nearly 60% of frail older adults live with polypharmacy and confirmed a bidirectional relationship: polypharmacy contributes to frailty, while frailty increases the likelihood of multiple prescribing (Kim et al., 2024).

The clinical consequences of this association are wide-ranging. In outpatient cohorts, high anticholinergic burden, often a by-product of polypharmacy, has been shown to compromise safety through increased risks of falls and cognitive impairment (De Zoysa et al., 2025). In disease-specific populations such as chronic kidney disease, the co-occurrence of frailty, multimorbidity, and polypharmacy amplifies hospitalisation and mortality risk. Yet, appropriate pharmacological therapy, including SGLT2 inhibitors, remains effective and may even deliver greater absolute benefit among frail subgroups (Mayne et al., 2024). Beyond functional decline, polypharmacy independently represents a modifiable risk factor for fractures in older adults (Gagnon et al., 2024). Furthermore, interventions that target prescribing quality demonstrate tangible benefits: reducing inappropriate medication use in frail inpatients was associated with a 37% reduction in mortality (Inglis et al., 2024).

Although frailty is distinct from multimorbidity, the two syndromes cluster and reinforce one another. Frail individuals accumulate long-term conditions that are more treatment refractory and interact adversely under stress. Polypharmacy, frequently used as a proxy for clinical complexity, adds a further layer of risk by increasing the likelihood of falls, delirium, bleeding, hypotension, and acute kidney injury. Harmful prescribing patterns such as anticholinergics and long-acting benzodiazepines have been specifically associated with increased readmission and mortality in frail populations (Inglis et al., 2024). Thus, frailty-informed medication review and deprescribing, anchored in patient goals and functional priorities, is an essential complication-mitigation strategy across care settings.

Measurement and Setting: How Prediction Varies

Predictive strength depends on the instrument and the clinical environment. The FRAILTOOLS project compared eight commonly used instruments across geriatric wards, outpatient clinics, primary care, and nursing homes (Oviedo-Briones et al., 2021, 2022). Inter-test agreement was low, implying that instruments approach the construct from different perspectives; sensitivity and specificity profiles were setting-dependent, with several tools showing good sensitivity for inpatient outcomes (mortality and ADL worsening) but limited specificity, the reverse pattern in geriatric clinics, and weak performance in primary care (Oviedo-Briones et al., 2021, 2022). These findings argue against a universal gold standard and for purposive selection: brief screens for case-finding and workflow triggers; more detailed measures for prognosis, care planning, or research phenotyping. They also highlight that measurement must be linked to action; for instance, a positive screen in the emergency department should trigger CGA, not sit in isolation.

Malnutrition and Sarcopenia

Malnutrition often coexists with frailty and acts both as a driver and a complication of declining physiological resilience. Community-based longitudinal studies using GLIM criteria have shown that malnourished older adults face dramatically increased risks of developing frailty (OR = 4.4) and frailty progression (OR = 6.25) over approximately three years, particularly in those with musculoskeletal pain (Rodríguez-Sánchez et al., 2025). Systematic reviews further highlight that malnutrition is associated with a fourfold to fivefold greater prevalence of sarcopenia and frailty, reinforcing its key role in their pathogenesis (Beaudart et al., 2019; Norazman et al., 2020).

Infections and Compromised Immunity

Frailty markedly increases susceptibility to infections—a clinically significant but underappreciated complication. A large prospective cohort in China demonstrated that frail older adults experienced a 50% higher rate of infectious disease incidence (HR 1.50, 95% CI 1.14–1.97), particularly for respiratory (IRR 1.97) and gastrointestinal infections (IRR 3.67) (Yang et al., 2024). These findings align with broader immunosenescence frameworks: chronic low-grade inflammation and weakened immune response (so-called inflamm-ageing) render frail individuals more vulnerable to infection and less responsive to vaccination (Quiros-Roldán et al., 2024).

Decline in Quality of Life and Well-being

Frailty and its associated physiological burdens are allied with profound reductions in life quality, mental well-being, and social engagement. A bibliometric synthesis of frailty and sarcopenia trends highlights the intrinsic link between muscle loss, functional impairment, and poor patient-reported outcomes, including diminished independence and mood (Ye et al., 2023). Moreover, in-hospital studies show that the co-presence of frailty, sarcopenia, or malnutrition markedly increases the risk of post-operative delirium, with odds ratios of approximately 5.3 for frailty and 5.6 for sarcopenia, underscoring the interaction between physical vulnerability, nutritional status, and neurocognitive outcomes (Moellmann et al., 2024).

Economic and Caregiver Burden

Frailty imposes substantial economic strain on healthcare systems and exacts a profound toll on caregivers. A registry-based study found that over three years, frail individuals ($n = 39,363$) incurred healthcare costs totalling US $1.28 billion, approximately US $457 per month per individual, with 75% of excess spending driven by hospital admissions (incidence rate ratio for frailty status versus expected non-frail: IRR 1.76) (Toson et al., 2024). In community-dwelling older adults, transitions to frailty are associated with increased inpatient days, frequency, and costs. Converting from pre-frail to frail yielded an average US $2,339 rise in healthcare costs over two years compared with stable, robust individuals (Kim et al., 2023). Similarly, a Spanish population-based cohort study ($n = 9,315$) demonstrated that frailty was associated with a graded rise in healthcare costs, from €1,420 per year in robust older adults to over €5,600 in those classified as very frail; independent of age and sex, frailty incurred an additional €1,171 per person annually, equivalent to more than double the costs of non-frail individuals (Lavado et al., 2023). These observations are reinforced by prospective Medicare-linked analyses showing that phenotypic frailty increases incremental annual healthcare costs by US $6,172–8,532, depending on sex, even after adjusting for existing comorbidity patterns (Ensrud et al., 2023). Beyond direct care costs, frailty also burdens caregivers qualitatively and financially. Prior reviews confirm that caregivers of frail older adults experience elevated stress, depressive symptoms, and out-of-pocket expenses, though comprehensive quantitative estimates remain limited, highlighting a critical gap (Ringer et al., 2017).

Intrinsic Capacity and Resilience as Modifiers of Risk

Intrinsic capacity (IC), the World Health Organization construct encompassing an individual's physical and mental capacities, offers a complementary lens that may identify decline before the emergence of overt frailty. Longitudinal validation in a nationally representative cohort showed that lower IC predicts subsequent decline in ADLs and IADLs (Beard et al., 2022). Prospective studies suggest that IC decline is associated with later frailty onset, implying a potential window for earlier intervention in community settings (Tay et al., 2023). Existing work continues to explore the predictive validity of composite IC scores for falls, disability, and mortality in clinical populations (Yong et al., 2024).

Resilience (the capacity to resist, absorb, and recover from stress) modulates trajectories; analyses across animal and human datasets indicate that both robustness (damage resistance) and resilience (repair capacity) diminish with age and influence survival, helping explain heterogeneous outcomes among individuals with similar frailty severity (Farrell et al., 2022). Incorporating IC and resilience into assessment may therefore refine risk estimation, prioritise reversible domains (e.g. mobility, mood, and sensory function), and support stepped-care interventions.

Clinical and Public Health Implications

First, anticipate complications by embedding rapid, validated frailty screening tools in ambulatory, emergency, and pre-operative pathways, with clear thresholds for CGA and rehabilitation referrals. Second, target modifiable risks: multicomponent exercise (progressive resistance, balance, and gait), adequate protein and energy intake with micronutrient repletion where indicated, osteoporosis assessment and secondary fracture prevention, medication optimisation with deprescribing of high-risk agents, and adherence to evidence-based delirium prevention bundles. Third, integrate cognition and mental health into care plans; combined frailty and cognitive impairment is associated with additive risk, and addressing depression, loneliness, and sleep disturbance can improve adherence, participation in activity, and functional outcomes. Fourth, plan transitions: early discharge planning, carer education, and home-based reablement help to mitigate readmissions and avoid institutional transitions when consistent with patient values (Boucher et al., 2023; Ruiz-Grao et al., 2024). Finally, use frailty for shared decisions: prognosis communicated with sensitivity can align treatments with what matters to the person, including timely palliative involvement where appropriate.

Future Directions

Priorities for research and implementation include: (1) robust comparisons of instruments linked to actionable care bundles in primary care and community settings, where current performance is weakest; (2) trials testing scalable, multidomain interventions that target specific complication pathways (falls, sarcopenia, cognitive decline, and delirium) and report patient-centred outcomes; (3) integration of IC trajectories and resilience metrics alongside frailty phenotypes to personalise prevention; (4) development and external validation of parsimonious prediction models that combine frailty with routinely collected clinical data to guide resource allocation without entrenching inequities; and (5) evaluation of policy-level strategies such as frailty-attuned pathways in emergency care and reablement funding that demonstrably reduce institutionalisation and preserve independence.

Case Study 5.1   AP-Led Multidomain Management of Frailty

Background

Mrs. A, a 78-year-old woman, lives alone in a deprived urban area. She has type 2 diabetes, osteoarthritis, mild cognitive impairment, and takes nine regular medicines, including two with anticholinergic effects. She attends a same day emergency care (SDEC) unit following a fall at home. Triage notes indicate a previous fall three months ago and recent unintentional weight loss.

Assessment by the AP

- Frailty screening: Clinical Frailty Scale score of 6 (moderately frail); positive electronic frailty index (eFI) record from primary care.
- CGA: Identifies sarcopenia (reduced grip strength), low mood, polypharmacy, vitamin D deficiency, and poor nutritional intake.
- Risk factors: Chronic inflammation from diabetes, multimorbidity, loneliness, and physical inactivity.
- Complications: Recurrent falls, malnutrition, and risk of delirium during acute illness.

AP-led Interventions

1. Exercise and nutrition: Referral to a community strength-and-balance exercise programme and prescription of oral protein–energy supplements with dietitian support.
2. Medication optimisation: Deprescribing of a sedative antihistamine and review of antihypertensive therapy to reduce postural hypotension, in line with STOPP/START criteria.
3. Psychosocial support: Connection to a local befriending service and group activities to address loneliness and mood.
4. Integrated care planning: Advance care discussion to align treatment goals with Mrs. A's priorities, ensuring involvement of her daughter and primary care team.
5. Follow-up: Monthly review of weight, strength, and falls risk, with digital monitoring via a wearable gait sensor.

Learning Points for APs

Demonstrates how early recognition of multidimensional risk factors (sarcopenia, malnutrition, social isolation, and polypharmacy) can guide targeted, evidence-based interventions.

- Illustrates the value of linking frailty assessment to action: CGA, deprescribing, and strength-and-balance training.
- Highlights leadership and coordination roles within the MPF, including interagency working and patient-centred care planning.

CONCLUSION

Frailty is a multidimensional syndrome that substantially increases vulnerability to a wide range of complications, including disability, falls, hospitalisation, institutionalisation, mortality, cognitive decline, malnutrition, infection, and reduced quality of life. Its impact extends beyond the individual, generating significant economic burden and caregiver strain. The predictive validity of frailty varies across tools and settings, underscoring the importance of purposive measurement linked to timely, multidomain interventions such as CGA, exercise and nutrition programmes, psychosocial support, and medication optimisation. Emerging constructs, including IC and resilience, may enhance prognostication and prevention strategies by capturing earlier stages of decline. Addressing frailty requires coordinated action across clinical, community, and policy levels to prevent progression, mitigate complications, and preserve independence and well-being in older adults.

Take-Home Messages

1. Frailty is a multidomain syndrome of reduced physiological reserve that increases vulnerability to complications such as functional decline, falls, fractures, hospitalisation, institutionalisation, cognitive deterioration, infection, malnutrition, and premature death.

2. These complications often interact in cyclical ways: disability amplifies the risk of admission and institutionalisation; multimorbidity and polypharmacy reinforce frailty progression; and malnutrition, sarcopenia, and cognitive impairment heighten delirium and mortality risk.

3. The impact of frailty extends beyond clinical outcomes, driving substantial healthcare costs and placing significant strain on caregivers, with evidence showing more than a doubling of healthcare expenditure and measurable increases in psychological and financial burden among carers.

4. Effective responses require early identification and integrated interventions, including CGA, exercise and nutrition support, medication review, psychosocial strategies, and policy-level approaches that address structural inequalities and embed frailty-informed care across health systems.

REFERENCES

Alotaibi, F., Alshibani, A., Banerjee, J., and Manktelow, B. (2025). The association between frailty and hospital-related adverse events in older hospitalised patients: a systematic literature review. *European Geriatric Medicine* 6 (4): 1303–1318.

Beard, J.R., Si, Y., Liu, Z. et al. (2022). Intrinsic capacity: validation of a new WHO concept for healthy aging in a longitudinal Chinese study. *The Journals of Gerontology. Series A, Biological Sciences and Medical Sciences* 77 (1): 94–100.

Beaudart, C., Sanchez-Rodriguez, D., Locquet, M. et al. (2019). Malnutrition as a strong predictor of the onset of sarcopenia. *Nutrients* 11 (12): 2883.

Beaudart, C., Alcazar, J., Aprahamian, I. et al. (2025). Health outcomes of sarcopenia: a consensus report by the outcome working group of the Global Leadership Initiative in Sarcopenia (GLIS). *Aging Clinical and Experimental Research* 37 (1): 100.

Bhattarai, U., Bashyal, B., Shrestha, A. et al. (2024). Frailty and chronic diseases: a bi-directional relationship. *Aging Medicine* 7 (4): 510–515.

Boucher, E.L., Gan, J.M., Rothwell, P.M. et al. (2023). Prevalence and outcomes of frailty in unplanned hospital admissions: a systematic review and meta-analysis of hospital-wide and general (internal) medicine cohorts. *EClinicalMedicine* 59: 101973.

Brown, J.D., Alipour-Haris, G., Pahor, M., and Manini, T.M. (2020). Association between a deficit accumulation frailty index and mobility outcomes in older adults: secondary analysis of the lifestyle interventions and independence for elders (LIFE) study. *Journal of Clinical Medicine* 9 (11): 3757.

Cechinel, C., Lenardt, M.H., Rodrigues, J.A.M. et al. (2022). Frailty and delirium in hospitalized older adults: a systematic review with meta-analysis. *Revista Latino-Americana de Enfermagem* 30: e3687.

Celik, H.I., Koc, F., Siyasal, K. et al. (2024). Exploring the complex associations among risks of malnutrition, sarcopenia, and frailty in community-dwelling older adults. *European Review of Aging and Physical Activity* 21 (1): 18.

Chen, Z., Ding, Z., Chen, C. et al. (2021). Effectiveness of comprehensive geriatric assessment intervention on quality of life, caregiver burden and length of hospital stay: a systematic review and meta-analysis of randomised controlled trials. *BMC Geriatrics* 21 (1): 377.

Crane, H.M., Ruderman, S.A., Whitney, B.M. et al. (2022). Associations between drug and alcohol use, smoking, and frailty among people with HIV across the United States in the current era of antiretroviral treatment. *Drug and Alcohol Dependence* 240: 109649.

Davies, K., Maharani, A., Chandola, T. et al. (2021). The longitudinal relationship between loneliness, social isolation and frailty in older adults in England: a prospective analysis. *The Lancet Healthy Longevity* 2 (9): e628–e636.

De Zoysa, W., Mendis, S.A., Rathnayake, N. et al. (2025). Multimorbidity, medications, and their association with falls, physical activity, and cognitive functions in older adults: multicenter study in Sri Lanka. *Scientific Reports* 15 (1): 6233.

Dent, E., Dalla Via, J., Bozanich, T. et al. (2024). Frailty increases the long-term risk for fall and fracture-related hospitalizations and all-cause mortality in community-dwelling older women. *Journal of Bone and Mineral Research* 39 (3): 222–230.

Ensrud, K.E., Schousboe, J.T., Kats, A.M. et al. (2023). Incremental health care costs of self-reported functional impairments and phenotypic frailty in community-dwelling older adults: a prospective cohort study. *Annals of Internal Medicine* 176 (4): 463–471.

Espinoza, S.E. (2021). The association of prior intensive lifestyle intervention and diabetes support and education with frailty prevalence at long-term follow-up in the Action for Health in Diabetes Extension Study. *The Journals of Gerontology. Series A, Biological Sciences and Medical Sciences* 76 (12): 2195–2201.

Farrell, S., Kane, A.E., Bisset, E. et al. (2022). Measurements of damage and repair of binary health attributes in aging mice and humans reveal that robustness and resilience decrease with age, operate over broad timescales, and are affected differently by interventions. *eLife* 11: e77632.

Fried, L.P., Tangen, C.M., Walston, J. et al. (2001). *Frailty in older adults: evidence for a phenotype. The Journals of Gerontology: Series A, Biological Sciences and Medical Sciences* 56 (3): M146–M156.

Gagnon, M.E., Talbot, D., Tremblay, F. et al. (2024). Polypharmacy and risk of fractures in older adults: a systematic review. *Journal of Evidence-Based Medicine* 17 (1): 145–171.

Grande, G., Haaksma, M.L., Rizzuto, D. et al. (2019). Co-occurrence of cognitive impairment and physical frailty, and incidence of dementia: systematic review and meta-analysis. *Neuroscience & Biobehavioral Reviews* 107: 96–103.

Guo, X., Pei, J., Ma, Y. et al. (2023). Cognitive frailty as a predictor of future falls in older adults: a systematic review and meta-analysis. *Journal of the American Medical Directors Association* 24 (1): 38–47.

Hörlin, E., Ehrlington, S.M., John, R.T. et al. (2023). Is the Clinical Frailty Scale feasible to use in an emergency department setting? A mixed methods study. *BMC Emergency Medicine* 23: 124. https://doi.org/10.1186/s12873-023-00850-2.

Ibrahim, K., Cox, N.J., Stevenson, J.M. et al. (2021). A systematic review of the evidence for deprescribing interventions among older people living with frailty. *BMC Geriatrics* 21 (1): 258.

Inglis, J.M., Caughey, G., Thynne, T. et al. (2024). Inappropriate prescribing and association with readmission or mortality in hospitalised older adults with frailty: a systematic review and meta-analysis. *BMC Geriatrics* 24 (1): 718.

Jiang, G., Tan, X., Zou, J., and Wu, X. (2025). A 24-week combined resistance and balance training program improves physical function in older adults: A randomized controlled trial. *The Journal of Strength & Conditioning Research* 39 (1): e62–e69.

Jing, H., Chen, Y., Liang, B. et al. (2025). Risk factors for falls in older people with pre-frailty: a systematic review and meta-analysis. *Geriatric Nursing* 62: 272–279.

Khera, S., Abbasi, M., Dabravolskaj, J. et al. (2019). Appropriateness of medications in older adults living with frailty: impact of a pharmacist-led structured medication review process in primary care. *Journal of Primary Care & Community Health* 10: 2150132719890227.

Kim, D.H. (2024). CGA and multidisciplinary intervention improve fried frailty phenotype (high certainty) and may reduce unplanned hospitalisation (low certainty). *Frailty in Older Adults.* Available at: PubMed Central (accessed 10 September 2025).

Kim, D.J., Massa, M.S., Potter, C.M. et al. (2022). Systematic review of the utility of the frailty index and frailty phenotype to predict all-cause mortality in older people. *Systematic Reviews* 11 (1): 187.

Kim, M.J., Lee, S., Cheong, H.K. et al. (2023). Healthcare utilization and costs according to frailty transitions after two years: a Korean frailty and aging cohort study. *Journal of Korean Medical Science* 38 (24): e191.

Kim, S., Lee, H., Park, J. et al. (2024). Global and regional prevalence of polypharmacy and related factors, 1997–2022: an umbrella review. *Archives of Gerontology and Geriatrics* 124: 105465.

Kojima, G. (2016a). Frailty as a predictor of fractures among community-dwelling older people: a systematic review and meta-analysis. *Bone* 90: 116–122.

Kojima, G. (2016b). Frailty as a predictor of hospitalisation among community-dwelling older people: a systematic review and meta-analysis. *Journal of Epidemiology and Community Health* 70 (7): 722–729. https://doi.org/10.1136/jech-2015-206978.

Kojima, G. (2017). Frailty as a predictor of disabilities among community-dwelling older people: a systematic review and meta-analysis. *Disability and Rehabilitation* 39 (19): 1897–1908.

Kojima, G. (2018). Frailty as a predictor of nursing home placement among community-dwelling older adults: a systematic review and meta-analysis. *Journal of geriatric physical therapy* 41 (1): 42–48.

Kojima, G., Iliffe, S., and Walters, K. (2018). Frailty index as a predictor of mortality: a systematic review and meta-analysis. *Age and Ageing* 47 (2): 193–200.

Lavado, À., Serra-Colomer, J., Serra-Prat, M. et al. (2023). Relationship of frailty status with health resource use and healthcare costs in the population aged 65 and over in Catalonia. *European Journal of Ageing* 20 (1): 20.

Liu, W., Yang, H., Lv, L. et al. (2023). Genetic predisposition to smoking in relation to the risk of frailty in ageing. *Scientific Reports* 13 (1): 2405.

Liu, X., Zhao, R., Zhou, X. et al. (2024). Association between polypharmacy and 2-year outcomes among Chinese older inpatients: a multi-center cohort study. *BMC Geriatrics* 24 (1): 748.

Liu, A.B., Lin, Y.X., Li, G.Y. et al. (2025a). Associations of frailty and cognitive impairment with all-cause and cardiovascular mortality in older adults: a prospective cohort study from NHANES 2011–2014. *BMC Geriatrics* 25 (1): 124.

Liu, Z., Sawada, S., Deng, P. et al. (2025b). Effect of body-weight-based resistance training on balance ability and fear of falling in community-dwelling older Japanese women. *Sports* 13 (1): 8.

Loewenthal, J.I.K., Mitzner, M., Mita, C., and Orkaby, A.R. (2023). The effect of yoga on frailty in older adults: a systematic review. *Annals of Internal Medicine* 176 (4): 524–535. (accessed 10 September 2025).

Luo, H., Zheng, Z., Yuan, Z. et al. (2024). The effectiveness of multicomponent exercise in older adults with cognitive frailty: a systematic review and meta-analysis. *Archives of Public Health* 82 (1): 229.

Mayne, K.J., Sardell, R.J., Staplin, N. et al. (2024). Frailty, multimorbidity, and polypharmacy: exploratory analyses of the effects of empagliflozin from the EMPA-KIDNEY Trial. *Clinical Journal of the American Society of Nephrology* 19 (9): 1119–1129.

Mitnitski, A.B., Mogilner, A.J., and Rockwood, K. (2002). *Accumulation of deficits as a proxy measure of aging. The Scientific World Journal* 2: 323–336.

Moellmann, H.L., Alhammadi, E., Boulghoudan, S. et al. (2024). Risk of sarcopenia, frailty and malnutrition as predictors of postoperative delirium in surgery. *BMC Geriatrics* 24 (1): 971.

Mutz, J., Choudhury, U., Zhao, J., and Dregan, A. (2022). Frailty in individuals with depression, bipolar disorder and anxiety disorders: longitudinal analyses of all-cause mortality. *BMC Medicine* 20 (1): 274.

NHS England (2022). *Older people advanced practice area specific capability and curriculum framework.* NHS England. Available at: https://advanced-practice.hee.nhs.uk/wp-content/uploads/sites/28/2025/01/Older-people-advanced-practice-area-specific-capability-and-curriculum-framework-NHSE.pdf (accessed 30 January 2026).

NHS England (2023a). *Palliative and end of life care advanced practice area specific capability and curriculum framework.* NHS England. Available at: https://advanced-practice.hee.nhs.uk/wp-content/uploads/sites/28/2025/01/Palliative-and-end-of-life-care-advanced-practice-area-specific-capability-and-curriculum-framework-NHSE.pdf (accessed 30 January 2026).

NHS England (2023b). *Acute medicine advanced practice area specific capability and curriculum framework.* NHS England. Available at: https://advanced-practice.hee.nhs.uk/wp-content/uploads/sites/28/2025/03/Acute-medicine-advanced-practice-area-specific-capability-and-curriculum-framework-NHSE.pdf (accessed 30 January 2026).

NHS England (2025). *Multi-professional framework for advanced practice in England – Edition 2025.* NHS England. Available at: https://advanced-practice.hee.nhs.uk/wp-content/uploads/sites/28/2025/05/Multi-professional-framework-for-advanced-practice-in-England---Edition-2025.pdf (accessed 29 January 2026).

Norazman, C.W., Adznam, S.N.A., and Jamaluddin, R. (2020). Malnutrition as key predictor of physical frailty among Malaysian older adults. *Nutrients* 12 (6): 1713.

Oviedo-Briones, M., Laso, Á.R., Carnicero, J.A. et al. (2021). A comparison of frailty assessment instruments in different clinical and social care settings: the FRAILTOOLS project. *Journal of the American Medical Directors Association* 22 (3): 607.e7–607.e12.

Oviedo-Briones, M., Rodríguez-Laso, Á., Carnicero, J.A. et al. (2022). The ability of eight frailty instruments to identify adverse outcomes across different settings: the FRAILTOOLS project. *Journal of Cachexia, Sarcopenia and Muscle* 13 (3): 1487–1501.

Pandey, A., Segar, M.W., Singh, S. et al. (2022). Frailty status modifies the efficacy of exercise training among patients with chronic heart failure and reduced ejection fraction: an analysis from the HF-ACTION trial. *Circulation* [Online ahead of print at time of citation] 146: 80–90.

Patil, U., Williamson, J., Deixler, J. et al. (2024). Interventions for loneliness in older adults: effectiveness of animal, psychological, and skill-based approaches. *Frontiers in Public Health* 12: Article 1427605.

Peng, Y., Zhong, G.C., Zhou, X. et al. (2022). Frailty and risks of all-cause and cause-specific death in community-dwelling adults: a systematic review and meta-analysis. *BMC Geriatrics* 22 (1): 725.

Quiros-Roldán, E., Sottini, A., Natali, P.G., and Imberti, L. (2024). The impact of immune system aging on infectious diseases. *Microorganisms* 12 (4): 775.

Radcliffe, E., Saucedo, A.R., Howard, C. et al. (2025). Development of a complex multidisciplinary medication review and deprescribing intervention in primary care for older people living with frailty and polypharmacy. *PLoS One* 20 (4): e0319615.

Ringer, T., Hazzan, A.A., Agarwal, A. et al. (2017). Relationship between family caregiver burden and physical frailty in older adults without dementia: a systematic review. *Systematic Reviews* 6 (1): 55.

Rodríguez-Sánchez, I., Carnicero-Carreño, J.A., Álvarez-Bustos, A. et al. (2025). Effects of malnutrition on the incidence and worsening of frailty in community-dwelling older adults with pain. *Nutrients* 17 (9): 1400.

Ruiz-Grao, M.C., Álvarez-Bueno, C., Garrido-Miguel, M. et al. (2024). Multidisciplinary home-based interventions in adverse events and quality of life among frail older people: a systematic review and meta-analysis. *Heliyon* 10 (21): e40015. PMID: 39583819; PMCID: PMC11582431.

Ryan, J., Espinoza, S., Ernst, M.E. et al. (2022). Validation of a deficit-accumulation frailty index in the ASPirin in reducing events in the elderly study and its predictive capacity for disability-free survival. *The Journals of Gerontology. Series A, Biological Sciences and Medical Sciences* 77 (1): 19–26.

Simpson, F.R., Pajewski, N.M., Nicklas, B.J. et al. (2020). Impact of multidomain lifestyle intervention on frailty through the lens of deficit accumulation in adults with type 2 diabetes mellitus. *The Journals of Gerontology. Series A, Biological Sciences and Medical Sciences* 75 (10): 1921–1927.

Sinclair, D.R., Maharani, A., Kingston, A. et al. (2025). Frailty-free life expectancy and its association with socio-economic characteristics: an analysis of the English Longitudinal Study of Ageing cohort study. *BMC Medicine* 23 (1): 276.

Stolz, E., Schultz, A., Schüssler, S. et al. (2024). Frailty predicts all-cause and cause-specific mortality among older adults in Austria: 8-year mortality follow-up of the Austrian Health Interview Survey (ATHIS 2014). *BMC Geriatrics* 24 (1): 13.

Tay, L., Tay, E.L., Mah, S.M. et al. (2023). Association of intrinsic capacity with frailty, physical fitness and adverse health outcomes in community-dwelling older adults. *The Journal of Frailty & Aging* 12 (1): 7–15.

Toson, B., Edney, L.C., Haji Ali Afzali, H. et al. (2024). Economic burden of frailty in older adults accessing community-based aged care services in Australia. *Geriatrics & Gerontology International* 24 (9): 939–947.

Vermeiren, S., Vella-Azzopardi, R., Beckwee, D. et al. (2016). Frailty and the prediction of negative health outcomes: a meta-analysis. *Journal of the American Medical Directors Association* 17 (12): 1163. e1–1163.e17.

Vetrano, D.L., Palmer, K., Marengoni, A. et al. (2019). Frailty and multimorbidity: a systematic review and meta-analysis. *The Journals of Gerontology. Series A, Biological Sciences and Medical Sciences* 74 (5): 659–666.

Yang, Z.C., Lin, H., Jiang, G.H. et al. (2023). Frailty is a risk factor for falls in the older adults: a systematic review and meta-analysis. *The Journal of Nutrition, Health & Aging* 27 (6): 487–495.

Yang, Y., Che, K., Deng, J. et al. (2024). Assessing the impact of frailty on infection risk in older adults: prospective observational cohort study. *JMIR Public Health and Surveillance* 10 (1): e59762.

Ye, L., Liang, R., Liu, X. et al. (2023). Frailty and sarcopenia: a bibliometric analysis of their association and potential targets for intervention. *Ageing Research Reviews* 92: 102111.

Yong, K., Chew, J., Low, K. et al. (2024). Predictive validity of intrinsic capacity composite scores for risk of frailty at 2 years: a comparison of 4 scales. *Journal of the American Medical Directors Association* 25 (9): 105146.

Yoshimura, Y., Matsumoto, A., Inoue, T. et al. (2025). Protein supplementation alone or combined with exercise for sarcopenia and physical frailty: a systematic review and meta-analysis of randomised controlled trials. *Archives of Gerontology and Geriatrics* 131: 105783.

Zhang, X.M., Wu, X.J., Cao, J. et al. (2022). Association between cognitive frailty and adverse outcomes among older adults: a meta-analysis. *The Journal of Nutrition, Health & Aging* 26 (9): 817–825.

Zhang, X., Zheng, X., Zheng, T. et al. (2025). Associations between leisure activities with trajectories of intrinsic capacity among Chinese older adults: the China Health and Retirement Longitudinal Study. *Archives of Public Health* 83 (1): Article 162.

Zhao, W., Hu, P., Sun, W. et al. (2022). Effect of physical activity on the risk of frailty: a systematic review and meta-analysis. *PLoS One* 17 (12): e0278226.

SECTION **II**

CLINICAL ASSESSMENT AND FRAILTY ASSESSMENT TOOLS

CHAPTER 6

History-taken and Physical Examination Within the Context of Frailty

Aim

To develop and strengthen advanced practitioners' (APs) competence and capability in person-centred history-taking and physical examination of frail adults, supporting accurate assessment and safe, holistic care planning.

LEARNING OUTCOMES

By the end of this chapter, readers will be able to:

1. Apply a structured approach to history-taking in frail adults, identifying changes from baseline, eliciting collateral information, and recognising the impact of multimorbidity and polypharmacy.
2. Identify and explore common frailty presentations, including decreased mobility, new confusion, falls, reduced eating and drinking, and continence problems, linking these to likely underlying causes.
3. Demonstrate an adapted physical examination that is safe, dignified, and tailored to the tolerance of frail adults, while capturing key signs across cardiovascular, respiratory, abdominal, neurological, and functional domains.
4. Integrate findings from history and examination to form an initial clinical impression, justify further investigations, and contribute to person-centred care planning within a comprehensive geriatric assessment (CGA) framework.

SELF-ASSESSMENT QUESTIONS

1. How would you adapt your history-taking and physical examination when a frail adult presents with vague/atypical functional decline rather than a clear organ-specific symptom?
2. Which frailty assessment tools (e.g. Clinical Frailty Scale and electronic frailty index) would you select in your clinical setting, and how would their findings guide immediate management and longer-term care planning?

> In frailty, the smallest changes speak the loudest; it is the careful history and gentle examination that discover the truth.

> The giants of geriatrics are immobility, instability, incontinence, and intellectual impairment. They have in common multiple causation, chronic course, deprivation of independence and no simple cure.
>
> Bernard Isaacs, *The Challenge of Geriatric Medicine*. Oxford University Press, 1997.

INTRODUCTION

Frailty is now recognised as a central concept in adult health and social care, particularly as populations age and people live longer with multiple conditions. It is best understood as a state of reduced physiological reserve that leaves the individual more vulnerable to even minor stressors. For advanced practitioners (APs), this reality means that the approach to history-taking and physical examination requires adaptation. Unlike in younger or fitter patients, the frail adult rarely presents with a single, neatly defined symptom that points directly to a diagnosis. More often, there are vague complaints such as 'feeling weaker', 'not being quite themselves', or 'slowing down'. These symptoms may reflect underlying infections, medication side effects, metabolic imbalance, or simply the consequences of cumulative decline. The task of the AP is therefore to straighten out these overlapping threads with both skill and sensitivity. A central principle is that history-taking and examination should be person-centred. The values, preferences, and usual baseline of the patient must remain at the heart of the consultation. The CGA provides a gold standard model, bringing together medical, psychological, functional, and social aspects of health. While not every clinical setting allows a full CGA, APs can adopt its principles by thinking broadly and holistically (see Chapter 7, CGA).

Multi-Professional Framework (MPF) for Advanced Practitioners

(Adapted from NHS England, 2025)

This chapter maps to the following areas within the MPF:

1. Clinical practice: 1.1–1.11
2. Leadership and management: 2.3, 2.5, 2.7, 2.8, 2.10
3. Education: 3.3, 3.4, 3.5, 3.7, 3.8
4. Research: 4.1, 4.2, 4.3

Accreditation Consideration

This chapter maps to the statement with the following national accretional document:

Curriculum framework for advanced practice in the care of older people (NHS England, 2022):

1. Core Capabilities in Practice (CiPs): 1–6
2. Generic Clinical CiPs: 1, 3, 5, 6
3. Specialty Clinical CiPs (Older People): 2, 3

Curriculum framework for APs in the case of palliative and end-of-life care (NHS England, 2023a):

1. Clinical Pillar: 1.2, 1.4, 1.5

Curriculum for APs in acute medicine (NHS England, 2023b):

1. Core CiPs: 1–6
2. Generic Clinical CiPs: 1–6
3. Specialty Clinical CiPs (Acute Medicine): Generic: 1–4 and acute medicine presentations

FACTORS INFLUENCING HISTORY-TAKING

Functional Decline and Decompensation

Frailty means that illness often presents through functional deterioration rather than textbook symptoms. A urinary tract infection, for instance, may cause sudden immobility or delirium rather than dysuria. Pneumonia may manifest as a fall or a refusal to eat rather than cough and fever. APs should be alert to these atypical pathways and frame their questions carefully. It is often more revealing to ask, 'What has changed from your usual pattern?' than 'Do you have pain on passing urine?' The emphasis should be on exploring shifts in baseline function. Because physiological reserve is limited, small challenges can trigger major deterioration. Something as seemingly trivial as a change in medication timing or a day of poor oral intake can lead to significant decompensation. History-taking therefore requires a focus on subtle changes and triggers.

Communication Challenges

Communication is a frequent barrier in history-taking with frail adults. Problems may arise from hearing loss, speech impairment, or cognitive decline. A useful framework is the 'seven Ds' as outlined in Box 6.1.

Box 6.1   Communication Challenges, The 7 Ds

Deafness: hearing impairment can make even simple questioning difficult.
Dysarthria: slurred or unclear speech, often seen after a stroke or in Parkinson's disease.
Dysphasia: difficulty finding words or forming sentences.

Dementia: gradual cognitive decline affecting memory and orientation.

Delirium: acute confusion, fluctuating in severity over hours or days.

Depression: low mood or apathy that reduces engagement.

Dependence: reliance on carers may influence the accuracy of history or create reluctance to disclose difficulties.

Source: Adapted from Innes et al. (2018).

Being aware of these challenges helps APs to adapt their approach. Strategies include sitting face to face, speaking slowly and clearly, avoiding medical jargon, and checking understanding regularly. Collateral history from relatives, carers, or residential staff is invaluable and often essential.

Multimorbidity and Overlapping Symptoms

Most frail adults live with multiple long-term conditions. Heart failure, diabetes, chronic kidney disease, arthritis, and cognitive impairment often coexist, creating complex and overlapping symptom profiles. For example, breathlessness might be due to anaemia, heart failure, lung disease, or general deconditioning. Pain may be the result of arthritis, peripheral neuropathy, or both.

For APs, it is important to avoid the tendency to focus on a single explanation too quickly. Symptoms of frailty are often the result of several conditions acting together, so keeping an open mind and considering multiple possible causes will lead to a more accurate assessment. A broad and systematic approach is necessary to ensure that important contributors are not overlooked. Multimorbidity also complicates management, making it vital to capture a complete picture during history-taking.

Under-reporting of Symptoms

Older adults often do not report symptoms for several reasons: attributing changes to normal ageing, fear of hospital admission or institutional care, or a wish to avoid worrying relatives. Some express ('What do you expect at my age?') or ('My son will worry if he knows I fell twice this week'). Cognitive impairment may limit recall, and negative attitudes such as hopelessness can further reduce disclosure. Awareness of these factors helps APs probe gently and validate concerns, ensuring important problems are not missed.

KEY COMPONENTS OF THE HISTORY

Presenting Complaint (PC)

In frailty, the PC is often vague, generalised, or reported by a carer rather than the patient themselves. For example, a neighbour might say, 'She just seems different', or a care worker may report that the patient has been less mobile than usual. For APs, the challenge is to frame the PC in a way that guides further exploration. Rather than expecting a clear symptom such as 'chest pain', it is often more helpful to describe the concern in functional terms, such as 'new confusion' or 'loss of independence with walking'.

There is no single correct order for history-taking in older adults. If dementia is suspected, it can be less threatening to begin with the social or family history, using an opening such as, 'I would like to get to know you first, could you tell me a little about yourself before we talk about any memory concerns'. Early questions about key personal facts, for example the number of children or educational background, can give an initial impression of cognitive function. Even a simple enquiry such as 'How did you travel here today?' may provide valuable insights into orientation, memory, and executive ability.

History of Presenting Complaints (HPCs)

Older adults often present with multiple health problems and several overlapping complaints. A single symptom may arise from more than one underlying cause, and it is rarely possible to address every issue in a single consultation. It is therefore helpful to invite the patient and family to identify the most pressing concerns and agree on priorities for that visit. Where feasible, collecting background information in advance can make the encounter more focused and effective. Clinical heterogeneity is the rule in later life, so the approach should remain flexible and individualised.

Exploring the HPC involves understanding what is normal for the patient and identifying changes from that baseline. Questions should focus on the timing, progression, and associated features of the problem.

For example:

- Has mobility always been limited, or is this a new deterioration?
- Did confusion appear gradually over months, or suddenly over days?
- Is pain continuous or intermittent?

Understanding the speed and pattern of change is crucial. Rapid changes often indicate an acute and potentially reversible problem, whereas slow, gradual changes usually point to long-term decline or progression of a chronic illness. Box 6.2 demonstrates the most common PCs.

Box 6.2   The Most Common Presenting Complaints in Older Adults

Decreased Mobility

- Establish baseline level: walking independently, using a stick, or requiring a frame.
- Identify recent deterioration: new need for support, reduced walking distance, and difficulty standing from a chair.
- Explore associated symptoms: pain, weakness, joint stiffness, and dizziness.
- Consider contributing systems: neurological (stroke and Parkinson's), musculoskeletal (arthritis and fracture), and cardiovascular (postural hypotension and heart failure).

Confusion

It may represent delirium, dementia, or both. Key distinctions include:

- Delirium: sudden onset, fluctuating course, often reversible with treatment of the underlying cause.
- Dementia: slow and progressive decline, not usually reversible.

APs should enquire about recent illness, medication changes, hydration, and nutrition, as these are common triggers of delirium.

Falls

They are highly significant in frail adults and may reflect underlying pathology. History should cover:

- Frequency and number of falls (National Institute for Health and Care Excellence, 2013).
- Circumstances: location, time, and activity.
- Preceding symptoms: dizziness, chest pain, palpitations, and loss of consciousness.
- Consequences: injuries, fractures, and fear of falling.
- Use of mobility aids and their effectiveness.

Reduced Eating and Drinking

Risk factors:

- Cognitive impairment (dementia, delirium, and depression).
- Physical difficulties such as dysphagia, poor dentition, or Parkinsonism.
- Social factors including isolation, lack of carer support, or difficulty preparing meals.
- Medication side effects (for example, opioids, antibiotics, or chemotherapy).

Ask about:

- Appetite changes, food preferences, and meal patterns.
- Swallowing difficulties, coughing or choking during meals.
- Weight loss, fatigue, or recurrent infections.
- Carer observations about intake.
- Practical barriers such as poor mobility, limited finances, or inadequate kitchen facilities.

Assess for contributing factors:

- Neurological: dysphagia following stroke and Parkinson's disease.
- Gastrointestinal: reflux, oesophageal disease, constipation, and malignancies.
- Psychological: depression and social withdrawal.
- Medication-related: altered taste, nausea, and dry mouth.

Urinary Incontinence

Risk factors:

- Age-related changes such as reduced bladder capacity and detrusor instability.
- Neurological disease (stroke, Parkinson's disease, and dementia).
- Medication side effects (diuretics and sedatives).
- Mobility problems that delay reaching the toilet.
- Constipation, which can worsen bladder symptoms.

Ask about:

- Onset, frequency, and type (urgency, stress, overflow, and functional).
- Associated symptoms such as pain, haematuria, or recurrent infections.
- Fluid intake and use of caffeine or alcohol.

- Night-time symptoms including nocturia.
- Impact on dignity, quality of life, and carer burden.

Assess for contributing factors:

- Neurological: multiple sclerosis and spinal cord pathology.
- Urological: prostate enlargement and urinary tract infection.
- Functional: reduced mobility and cognitive impairment.
- Medication-related: diuretics, sedatives, and anticholinergics.

Bowel Incontinence

Risk factors:

- Chronic constipation with overflow.
- Neurological impairment (stroke, dementia, spinal disease).
- Medication effects (laxatives, antibiotics, chemotherapy).
- Reduced mobility and functional dependence.
- Poor diet, dehydration, or inadequate fibre intake.

Ask about:

- Frequency and pattern of incontinence.
- Stool consistency (use Bristol Stool Chart if appropriate).
- Associated symptoms such as abdominal pain, rectal bleeding, or urgency.
- Recent changes in diet, mobility, or medications.
- Impact on daily activities, skin integrity, and psychological well-being.

Assess for contributing factors:

- Gastrointestinal: colorectal cancer, inflammatory bowel disease, and diverticular disease.
- Neurological: dementia, Parkinson's disease, and spinal cord pathology.
- Medication-related: laxatives, metformin, and antibiotics.
- Functional: immobility, poor carer support, and environmental barriers to toilet access.

PAST MEDICAL AND SURGICAL HISTORY

Past Medical History (PMH) provides context for current symptoms and helps to shape management. Many frail adults have multiple chronic conditions, and these may limit treatment choices or affect prognosis (Figure 6.1).

Examples include:

- Chronic kidney disease influencing safe use of antibiotics.
- Advanced chronic obstructive pulmonary disease limiting tolerance of procedures.
- Dementia shaping discussions about goals of care.

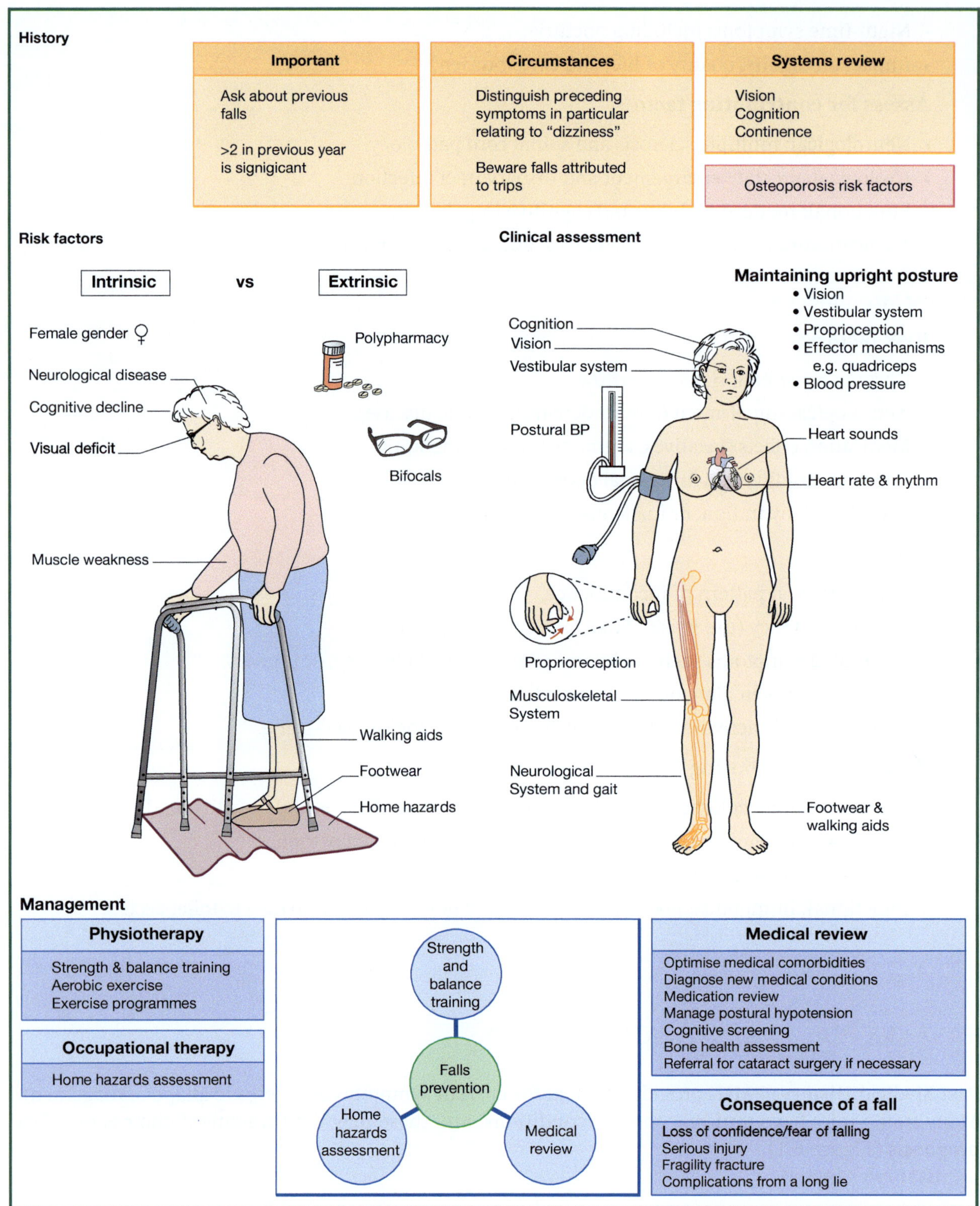

FIGURE 6.1 Falls. *Source*: Adapted from Blundell and Gordon (2015) Wiley.

Information should be gathered from multiple sources, including medical records, discharge summaries, and carers, as patients may not recall their full history accurately.

DRUG HISTORY AND POLYPHARMACY

Polypharmacy is a defining feature of frailty. Most frail adults take multiple medications, increasing the risks of drug interactions, side effects, and adherence problems (see Chapter 10 of polypharmacy and deprescribing).

A good drug history involves:

- Documenting all prescribed, over-the-counter, and herbal medications (Figure 6.2).
- Identifying recent changes.
- Exploring possible links between symptoms and drugs.
- Assessing the patient's ability to manage their regimen.
- Checking for omitted doses, such as diuretics skipped to avoid incontinence.
- Confirming allergies and adverse reactions.

Because frail adults have reduced physiological reserve, they are more sensitive to medication effects. For example, sedatives can trigger delirium, and anticoagulants increase risk after falls. Regular review and deprescribing are essential.

FAMILY HISTORY

Family history may reveal genetic predispositions such as dementia, diabetes, or cardiovascular disease. It can also highlight the availability of family support, which is vital when planning care. In younger frail patients, inherited conditions such as muscular dystrophy may be particularly relevant.

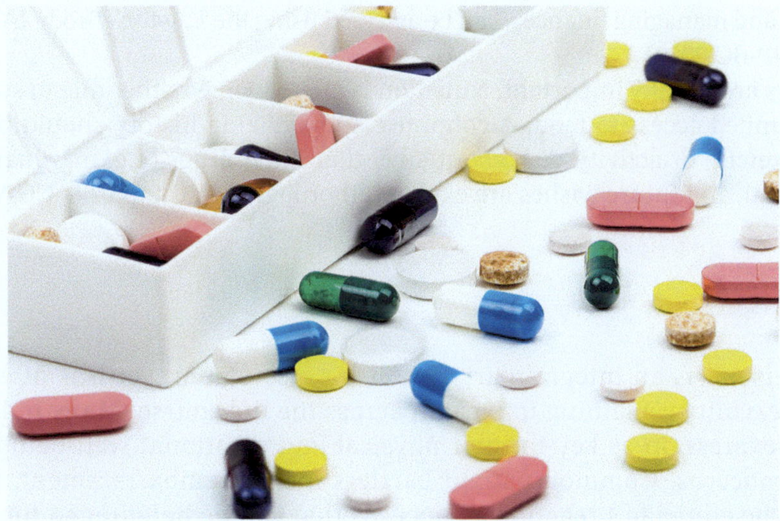

FIGURE 6.2   Polypharmacy. *Source*: viperfzk/Adobe Stock Photos.

SOCIAL AND FUNCTIONAL HISTORY

Frailty cannot be fully understood without exploring the patient's social and functional circumstances. APs should ask about:

- Living arrangements: alone, with spouse, in residential, or nursing care.
- Home environment: stairs, adaptations, and accessibility.
- Carer support: family involvement, frequency of visits, and reliability.
- Social networks: friends, community links, and risk of isolation.

Functional status is best assessed using activities of daily living (ADLs) such as bathing, dressing, and feeding. The Katz Index of Independence in Activities of Daily Living (Katz-ADL) is a widely used tool that evaluates basic ADLs and assesses mobility specifically through the ability to transfer (e.g. move from bed to chair) (Figure 6.3; Wallace and Shelkey, 2007). Instrumental activities of daily living (IADLs), including shopping, cooking, and managing finances, can be assessed using the Lawton–Brody IADL scale (Figure 6.2; Coyne and AGACNP-BC 2019).

Lifestyle factors are equally important. Nutrition is often poor, whether due to swallowing problems, dental issues, or limited access to food. Alcohol use and smoking history should be considered, along with patterns of exercise or activity. Ask about any other illicit drugs (e.g. marijuana). The functional, social, environmental, and future wishes are explored thoroughly in Chapter 8, CGA.

SEXUAL HISTORY

For APs, sexual history is an integral part of holistic assessment, yet it is often omitted in older patients despite sexuality remaining important across the life course. Many individuals value intimacy and sexual expression as key to their physical and emotional well-being, but may hesitate to discuss these concerns. Common patient barriers include embarrassment, fear of judgement, or worries about the clinician's reaction—concerns that can be heightened for sexual and gender minorities. Clinician barriers include insufficient training, time pressures, and discomfort with sensitive topics.

Patient Name:______________________ **Date:**______________

Patient ID #______________________

Katz Index of Independence in Activities of Daily Living

Activities Points (1 or 0)	Independence (1 Point)	Dependence (0 Points)
	NO supervision, direction or personal assistance.	WITH supervision, direction, personal assistance or total care.
BATHING Points: __________	**(1 POINT)** Bathes self completely or needs help in bathing only a single part of the body such as the back, genital area or disabled extremity.	**(0 POINTS)** Need help with bathing more than one part of the body, getting in or out of the tub or shower. Requires total bathing
DRESSING Points: __________	**(1 POINT)** Get clothes from closets and drawers and puts on clothes and outer garments complete with fasteners. May have help tying shoes.	**(0 POINTS)** Needs help with dressing self or needs to be completely dressed.
TOILETING Points: __________	**(1 POINT)** Goes to toilet, gets on and off, arranges clothes, cleans genital area without help.	**(0 POINTS)** Needs help transferring to the toilet, cleaning self or uses bedpan or commode.
TRANSFERRING Points: __________	**(1 POINT)** Moves in and out of bed or chair unassisted. Mechanical transfer aids are acceptable	**(0 POINTS)** Needs help in moving from bed to chair or requires a complete transfer.
CONTINENCE Points:	**(1 POINT)** Exercises complete self control over urination and defecation.	**(0 POINTS)** Is partially or totally incontinent of bowel or bladder
FEEDING Points: __________	**(1 POINT)** Gets food from plate into mouth without help. Preparation of food may be done by another person.	**(0 POINTS)** Needs partial or total help with feeding or requires parenteral feeding.

TOTAL POINTS: ________   **SCORING:** 6 = High (*patient independent*) 0 = Low (*patient very dependent*

FIGURE 6.3 The Katz Index of Independence in Activities of Daily Living. *Source*: Wallace and Shelkey (2007)/ Hartford Institute for Geriatric Nursing.

A patient-centred approach helps to overcome these challenges. Introduce the subject by normalising it within routine care, for example: 'Sexual health is an important part of overall wellbeing. May we talk about this together?' Use open questions that invite discussion, such as: 'Have you been sexually active in the past year, and with how many partners?'; 'Do you have sex with men, women, or both?'; or 'Have you noticed any changes in sexual function as you have got older?' Explore any specific concerns physical, psychological, or relationship-related and offer evidence-based information or referral if appropriate (Box 6.3).

Box 6.3   Systematic Enquiry

A systematic enquiry is essential when assessing frail adults because symptoms are often subtle, vague, or masked by comorbidities. Rather than relying on a focused history alone, APs should undertake a structured review of systems to uncover problems that may otherwise go unnoticed.

Cardiovascular system: Ask about chest pain, palpitations, breathlessness, orthopnoea, ankle swelling, or dizziness. Even mild complaints may reflect significant underlying pathology such as heart failure or arrhythmia.

Respiratory system: Explore cough, sputum, wheeze, or breathlessness. In frail adults, pneumonia may present with reduced mobility or confusion rather than typical respiratory symptoms.

Gastrointestinal system: Enquire about swallowing difficulties, reflux, abdominal pain, changes in bowel habit, rectal bleeding, or weight loss. Constipation is common and can worsen confusion, urinary symptoms, and mobility.

Genitourinary system: Ask about frequency, urgency, nocturia, haematuria, incontinence, or retention. Urinary Tract Infection (UTIs) are common precipitants of delirium in frail adults.

Neurological system: Explore history of stroke, seizures, tremor, gait disturbance, memory loss, and functional decline. Pay attention to any acute changes in speech, vision, or limb power.

Musculoskeletal system: Ask about pain, stiffness, reduced range of movement, and falls. Arthritis and osteoporosis increase the risk of immobility and fractures.

Psychological health: Enquire about mood, interest in activities, sleep, and feelings of loneliness or hopelessness. Depression is common yet often under-recognised in frail adults.

A systematic enquiry not only reveals hidden pathology but also supports the holistic ethos of frailty care by capturing physical, psychological, and functional issues in parallel.

PHYSICAL EXAMINATION IN THE FRAIL ADULT

General Principles

The physical examination of a frail adult requires sensitivity, patience, and flexibility. APs should approach the examination at a slower pace, allowing time for rest and explanation. The emphasis should be on comfort, dignity, and prioritising the areas most relevant to the presenting problem. Frail adults often tire quickly, so the examination may need to be adapted or performed in stages. Observation begins the moment the AP meets the patient: their posture, facial expression, clothing, and interaction provide valuable clues about function, mood, and general health.

Core Elements of Examination

See Boxes 6.4 and 6.5.

Box 6.4   Core Elements of Physical Examinations

General Assessment

- Look for weight loss, muscle wasting, dehydration, or poor hygiene.
- Assess skin integrity, noting bruises, pressure areas, or signs of neglect.
- Check for signs of frailty syndromes such as immobility, incontinence, and cognitive impairment.

Vital Signs

- Record blood pressure, pulse, respiratory rate, oxygen saturation, temperature, and pain.
- Measure lying and standing blood pressure to identify postural hypotension.
- Note that 'normal' readings may still indicate illness in frail adults, who often mount a blunted physiological response.

Cardiovascular System

- Inspect for peripheral oedema, cyanosis, or pallor.
- Palpate the pulse for rate, rhythm, and volume.
- Auscultate the heart for murmurs, extra sounds, or irregular rhythms.
- Pay attention to signs of heart failure such as raised jugular venous pressure.

Respiratory System

- Observe breathing pattern, effort, and use of accessory muscles.
- Percuss and auscultate the lung fields for crackles, wheeze, or reduced air entry.
- Subtle findings, such as fine basal crackles, may signal early infection (Figure 6.3) or pulmonary oedema.

Abdominal Examination

- Look for scars, distension, or visible peristalsis.
- Palpate gently for tenderness, masses, or organomegaly.
- Assess for constipation, which is common and often overlooked.

Neurological Examination

- Screen cognition using simple tools such as the Abbreviated Mental Test Score (AMTS) or 4AT for delirium.
- Assess cranial nerves where indicated, limb tone, power, reflexes, and coordination.
- Observe gait and balance if safe to do so (Figure 6.4).

Musculoskeletal Examination

- Inspect for deformity, joint swelling, or restricted movement.
- Assess muscle strength and tone.
- Pay close attention to pain, which may limit cooperation with examination.

ADDITIONAL CONSIDERATIONS

- Atypical presentations: Frail adults often fail to display 'classic' signs. For instance, infection may present without fever, and myocardial infarction without chest pain.
- Functional assessment: Observing the patient stand, transfer, or walk a few steps can be as informative as formal neurological testing.

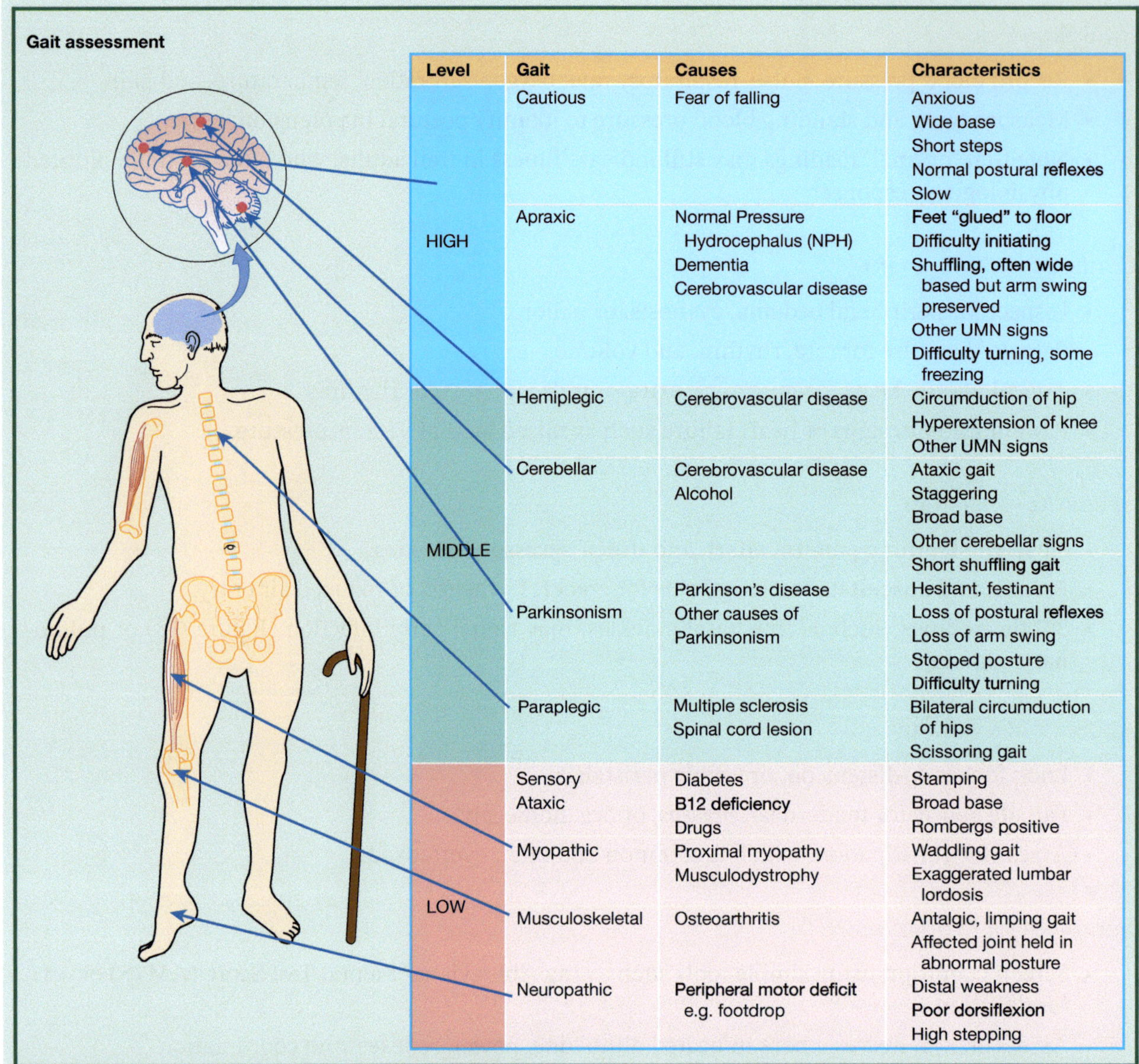

Level	Gait	Causes	Characteristics
HIGH	Cautious	Fear of falling	Anxious Wide base Short steps Normal postural reflexes Slow
	Apraxic	Normal Pressure Hydrocephalus (NPH) Dementia Cerebrovascular disease	Feet "glued" to floor Difficulty initiating Shuffling, often wide based but arm swing preserved Other UMN signs Difficulty turning, some freezing
MIDDLE	Hemiplegic	Cerebrovascular disease	Circumduction of hip Hyperextension of knee Other UMN signs
	Cerebellar	Cerebrovascular disease Alcohol	Ataxic gait Staggering Broad base Other cerebellar signs
	Parkinsonism	Parkinson's disease Other causes of Parkinsonism	Short shuffling gait Hesitant, festinant Loss of postural reflexes Loss of arm swing Stooped posture Difficulty turning
	Paraplegic	Multiple sclerosis Spinal cord lesion	Bilateral circumduction of hips Scissoring gait
LOW	Sensory Ataxic	Diabetes B12 deficiency Drugs	Stamping Broad base Rombergs positive
	Myopathic	Proximal myopathy Musculodystrophy	Waddling gait Exaggerated lumbar lordosis
	Musculoskeletal	Osteoarthritis	Antalgic, limping gait Affected joint held in abnormal posture
	Neuropathic	Peripheral motor deficit e.g. footdrop	Distal weakness Poor dorsiflexion High stepping

FIGURE 6.4   Gait assessment. *Source*: Adapted from Blundell and Gordon (2015).

- Cognitive and mood assessment: Screening tools should be used alongside collateral history from carers.
- Safety: Examinations must be conducted with awareness of falls risk, fatigue, and discomfort.

Box 6.5   Interpretation of Common Investigations in Frailty

Routine laboratory and imaging tests often have different implications in frail older adults compared to younger populations. For example, middle-range urea values may mask severe dehydration, while low creatinine may falsely reassure due to reduced muscle mass. Electrolyte disturbances such as hyponatraemia are frequent and may present with confusion rather than classic neurological symptoms. Similarly, asymptomatic bacteriuria on urinalysis should not be treated without clinical signs.

Key points for APs include:

- Always interpret results against the background of physiological ageing, reduced reserve, and multimorbidity.
- Subtle abnormalities can represent significant pathology in frail adults.
- 'Normal' values may still be clinically significant depending on the trajectory of change.
- Collateral clinical information and CGA remain essential for accurate interpretation.

Test/investigation	Clinical considerations in frailty	Cautions and interpretation notes
Urea	May reflect dehydration, renal function, or catabolic state.	Mid-range urea can indicate severe dehydration in frail adults; interpret alongside clinical context and fluid balance.
Creatinine	Assesses renal function and muscle mass.	Low muscle bulk can mask renal impairment; Cockcroft–Gault may overestimate eGFR, leading to overdiagnosis of CKD.
Electrolytes (Na+, K+)	Reflect hydration, renal, and endocrine balance.	Sodium <125 mmol/L → confusion/tiredness; <115 mmol/L → seizure s/coma/death. Consider rate of change; some frail adults tolerate chronic mild hyponatraemia.
Glucose	Screens for diabetes, hypoglycaemia, or stress response.	Frail adults have blunted autonomic response → higher hypoglycaemia risk; interpret in light of nutrition and medication (e.g. insulin and sulphonylureas).
Liver function tests (LFTs)	Assess hepatobiliary function and bone turnover.	Elevated alkaline phosphatase (ALP) with other normal LFTs may indicate Paget's disease or a recent fracture.
Calcium	Indicates metabolic bone disease or malignancy.	Abnormalities common with vitamin D deficiency, parathyroid disease, or metastases; interpret with phosphate and ALP.
C-reactive protein (CRP)	Marker of inflammation or infection.	Mildly raised CRP may be non-specific in frail patients; trends more meaningful than single results.
Thyroid function tests (TFTs)	Screens for thyroid dysfunction.	'Sick euthyroid' common in acute illness; if symptoms persist despite normalisation, consider autoimmune comorbidity (e.g. Addison's and pernicious anaemia).
Full blood count (FBC)	Evaluates anaemia, infection, and marrow health.	Hb declines with age; anaemia is common in elderly adults. Assess rate of decline, MCV, and haematinics. Fluid overload may lower Hb; dimorphic picture may mask dual deficiencies.

Test/investigation	Clinical considerations in frailty	Cautions and interpretation notes
Erythrocyte sedimentation rate (ESR)	Screening/monitoring inflammation.	ESR >90 mm/h may indicate *comprehensive geriatric assessment*. malignancy, chronic infection, or paraproteinaemia. Normal up to 35 mm/h (female) or 30 mm/h (male) in ≥70 years.
Urinalysis	Detects infection, glucose, protein, or blood.	Asymptomatic bacteriuria common; treat only if symptomatic. New incontinence → investigate with culture.
Chest X-ray (CXR)	Identifies infection, heart failure, or malignancy.	Interpret cautiously: dehydration, kyphosis, and poor inspiration can obscure signs.
Electrocardiograph (ECG)	Detects arrhythmia, ischaemia, and electrolyte imbalance.	Frail adults may have silent ischaemia or atypical symptoms; monitor QT interval in polypharmacy.
Bone profile	Evaluates fracture risk and metabolic bone disorders	Raised ALP or low calcium may reflect bone disease or vitamin D deficiency.
Urine sodium/osmolality	Helps differentiate causes of hyponatraemia.	Useful in syndrome of inappropriate antidiuretic hormone secretion; interpret alongside serum osmolality and fluid status.
Arterial or venous blood gas (Arterial blood gas (ABG) /Venous blood gas (VBG))	Assesses acid–base balance, CO_2 retention, and oxygenation.	Use VBG if less invasive; interpret in context of chronic respiratory disease.
Inflammatory markers, Ferritin and Lactate dehydrogenase)	Identify underlying infection, malignancy, or inflammation.	Ferritin may be elevated in inflammation even with iron deficiency.

Case Study 6.1   Frail Adult with New Confusion and Cough

Mrs. J, an 87-year-old woman, lives alone in her own home. Her daughter visits twice weekly and provides collateral information. Until recently, she was independent in basic activities of daily living, requiring only a stick for mobility indoors. She has now developed new confusion and a persistent cough.

Presenting Complaint

The patient's daughter reports that her mother 'is not herself' and appears confused. This began within the last 48 hours. She has also developed a productive cough.

History of Presenting Complaint

Two days ago, Mrs. J was orientated and conversational, managing her meals and personal care. Today she is disorientated, lethargic, and forgetful. She appears to have difficulty recalling recent events and is unable to provide a coherent history herself.

The daughter notes that Mrs. J has had a moist cough for three days, worse at night, associated with reduced appetite and oral intake. She denies haemoptysis. There is no reported chest pain or pleuritic pain. The daughter has not noticed a fever, but Mrs. J has been unusually sleepy during the day and restless at night.

There is no history of recent falls, head injury, seizures, or new medications. No vomiting or diarrhoea reported.

Past Medical History

- Hypertension.
- Osteoarthritis affecting knees and hips.
- No known respiratory disease.
- No previous diagnosis of cognitive impairment.

Drug History

- Amlodipine 5 mg once daily.
- Paracetamol as needed for joint pain.
- No recent changes.
- No known drug allergies.

Family History

- Mother had dementia.
- No strong family history of respiratory disease or cancer.

Social and Functional History

Mrs. J lives alone. Daughter provides meals for the week during her visits. Normally independent in personal care and light household tasks. Uses a walking stick indoors. Previously enjoyed gardening but has been less active in recent months.

No alcohol use. Non-smoker. Adequate support from neighbours who check in daily. Her Clinical Frailty Scale (CFS) before admission was 5 (Mildly frail).

Systematic Enquiry

- Cardiovascular: No chest pain or palpitations. Mild ankle swelling is long-standing.
- Respiratory: Productive cough, increased breathlessness, and reduced exercise tolerance.
- Gastrointestinal: Poor appetite, no nausea, vomiting, or abdominal pain. No constipation.
- Genitourinary: Urine darker and no dysuria.
- Neurological: Confusion, fluctuating attention. No focal weakness or slurred speech reported.
- Musculoskeletal: Generalised weakness and reduced mobility.
- Psychological: No previous diagnosis of depression or anxiety.

EXAMINATION

General Appearance

An elderly woman sitting in a chair appears confused and disorientated. Looks frail, with reduced muscle bulk and evidence of poor oral intake.

Vital Signs

- Temperature: 37.8 °C (low-grade pyrexia).
- Blood pressure: 108/60 mmHg (mildly low for baseline).
- Pulse: 104 beats per minute, regular.
- Respiratory rate: 24 per minute.
- Oxygen saturation: 90% on air.

Cardiovascular System

Pulse regular. Heart sounds normal, no murmurs. No peripheral cyanosis. Mild ankle oedema present.

Respiratory System

Inspection: Tachypnoea with mild use of accessory muscles.
Palpation: Reduced chest expansion on the right side.
Percussion: Dullness over the right lower zone.
Auscultation: Crackles and bronchial breathing over the right base. Left lung clear.

Abdomen

Soft, non-tender. No organomegaly. Bowel sounds present.

Neurological Examination

Alert but disorientated to time and place. Attention impaired. No cranial nerve deficits. Power in all limbs normal for age but reduced effort due to fatigue. Reflexes symmetrical. Gait not assessed due to unsteadiness.

Cognitive Assessment

Unable to complete AMTS due to inattention. Fluctuating awareness consistent with delirium.

Musculoskeletal System

Evidence of sarcopenia and reduced grip strength. No acute joint swelling.

Skin

Dry, reduced turgor. No pressure sores.

Clinical Impression

Mrs. J presents with acute confusion and cough, likely delirium secondary to community-acquired pneumonia. The history points to a sudden onset of cognitive change, poor oral intake, and functional decline. Examination findings of pyrexia, hypoxia, tachypnoea, and right basal consolidation support pneumonia as the trigger.

Contributory factors include frailty, dehydration, and reduced reserve, which heighten her vulnerability to infection and delirium.

NEXT STEPS

- Immediate investigations: blood tests, chest X-ray, urine dip and culture, and ECG.
- Oxygen therapy to maintain saturations >94% (adjust for frailty goals).
- Initiate empirical antibiotics guided by local policy.
- Intravenous fluids if dehydrated.
- Monitor for complications: sepsis, worsening delirium, and reduced mobility.
- Early discussion with the patient's daughter about goals of care and escalation planning (Figure 6.5).

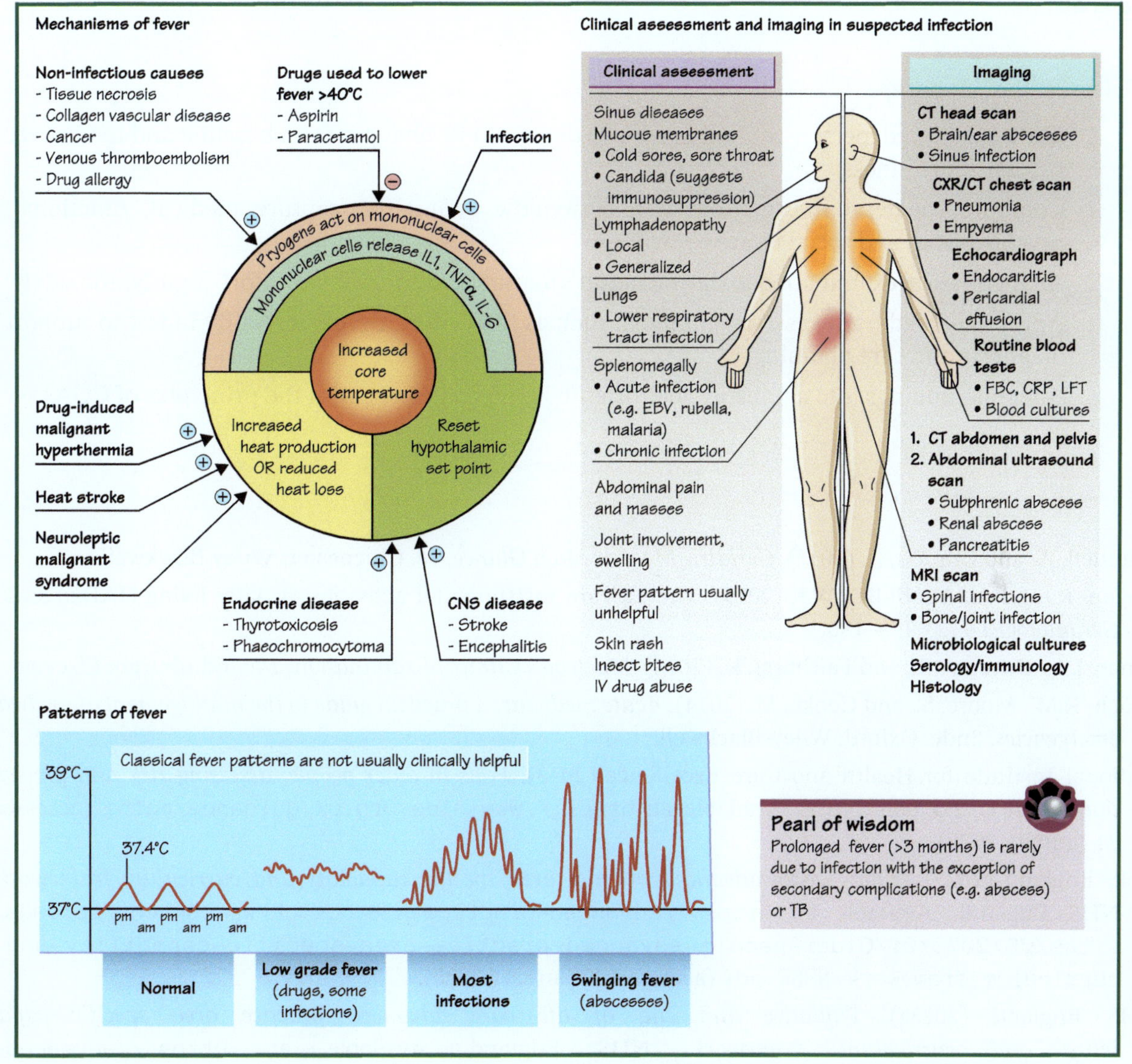

FIGURE 6.5 Assessment of the suspect infection. *Source*: Adapted from Leach et al. (2014) published by John Wiley & Sons, Ltd.

CONCLUSION

History-taking and physical examination in the frail adult require APs to adapt their clinical skills with patience, sensitivity, and breadth of vision. Presentations are rarely straightforward, often involving subtle functional changes or non-specific symptoms. Collateral history, systematic enquiry, and awareness of frailty syndromes are essential in reaching accurate conclusions. Physical examination should be focused on the patient's tolerance, prioritising comfort and dignity. The AP should look not only for organ-specific disease but also for wider indicators such as hydration, nutrition, cognition, and function. The goal is not simply to identify pathology but to place the patient within their broader context of comorbidities, functional capacity, and social support. This person-centred approach, guided by the ethos of CGA, ensures that frail adults receive care that is both clinically effective and aligned with their values and goals.

Take-Home Message

1. Use a structured, person-centred history to detect subtle changes from baseline and to uncover hidden acute illness.

2. Combine collateral information with systematic enquiry to capture medical, functional, psychological, and social issues.

3. Adapt physical examination to the frail adult's tolerance, prioritising comfort, dignity, and safety.

4. Apply validated frailty assessment tools, such as the CFS or electronic frailty index, to support diagnosis and care planning.

5. Integrate findings into a holistic, goal-oriented plan consistent with the principles of CGA.

REFERENCES

Blundell, A. and Gordon, A. (2015). *Geriatric Medicine at a Glance*, 1e. Chichester: Wiley Blackwell.

Coyne, R. and AGACNP-BC, W.K (2019). The Lawton instrumental activities of daily living (IADL) scale. *Gerontologist* 9 (3): 179–186.

Innes, J.A., Dover, A.R., and Fairhurst, K. (2018). *Macleod's Clinical Examination*, 14e. Edinburgh: Elsevier.

Leach, R.M., Moore, S., and Cooke, M. (2014). *Acute medicine: a practical guide to the management of medical emergencies*, 2nde. Oxford: Wiley-Blackwell.

National Institute for Health and Care Excellence (2013). *Falls in older people: assessing risk and prevention (CG161)*. London: NICE. Available at: https://www.nice.org.uk/guidance/cg161 (accessed 31 January 2026).

NHS England (2022). *Older people advanced practice area specific capability and curriculum framework*. NHS England. Available at: https://advanced-practice.hee.nhs.uk/wp-content/uploads/sites/28/2025/01/Older-people-advanced-practice-area-specific-capability-and-curriculum-framework-NHSE.pdf (accessed 30 January 2026).

NHS England (2023a). *Palliative and end of life care advanced practice area specific capability and curriculum framework*. NHS England. Available at: https://advanced-practice.hee.nhs.uk/wp-content/uploads/sites/28/2025/01/Palliative-and-end-of-life-care-advanced-practice-area-specific-capability-and-curriculum-framework-NHSE.pdf (accessed 30 January 2026).

NHS England (2023b). *Acute medicine advanced practice area specific capability and curriculum framework.* NHS England. Available at: https://advanced-practice.hee.nhs.uk/wp-content/uploads/sites/28/2025/03/Acute-medicine-advanced-practice-area-specific-capability-and-curriculum-framework-NHSE.pdf (accessed 30 January 2026).

NHS England (2025). *Multi-professional framework for advanced practice in England – Edition 2025.* NHS England. Available at: https://advanced-practice.hee.nhs.uk/wp-content/uploads/sites/28/2025/05/Multi-professional-framework-for-advanced-practice-in-England---Edition-2025.pdf (accessed 29 January 2026).

Wallace, M. and Shelkey, M. (2007). Katz index of independence in activities of daily living (ADL). *Urologic Nursing* 27 (1): 93–94.

CHAPTER 7

Comprehensive Geriatric Assessment in Clinical Practice

Aim

This chapter aims to provide advanced practitioners (APs) and the wider multidisciplinary team (MDT) with a comprehensive understanding of comprehensive geriatric assessment (CGA) in clinical practice. It outlines its rationale, evidence base, domains, and implementation, equipping healthcare professionals with the knowledge and skills to conduct and apply CGA systematically to improve outcomes for older adults living with frailty.

LEARNING OUTCOMES

By the end of this chapter, readers will be able to:

1. Define CGA and explain its role as a multidimensional, multidisciplinary process rather than a task confined to geriatricians.
2. Justify the rationale for using CGA, drawing on its robust clinical and economic evidence base.
3. Systematically conduct CGA using the six domains outlined by the British Geriatrics Society (BGS): physical, functional, psychological, social, environmental, and future wishes.
4. Describe the steps involved in conducting CGA, from initial assessment to care planning, documentation, and multidisciplinary implementation.

SELF-ASSESSMENT QUESTIONS

1. How will you operationalise the six CGA domains in your setting (including tool selection and MDT roles), and what triggers will you use to escalate from screening to full CGA?
2. Which outcome and cost measures will you track to demonstrate CGA impact (e.g. ADL change, readmissions, length of stay, or institutionalisation), and how will the results inform service redesign?

INTRODUCTION

Comprehensive geriatric assessment (CGA) is a structured, multidisciplinary process that enables APs to convert complex presentations of frailty into coordinated person-centred care plans. Grounded in the four pillars of the multi-professional framework (MPF), APs lead advanced clinical assessment, medicines optimisation, and shared decision-making; they coordinate teams and pathways, educate colleagues, and evaluate outcomes to sustain quality improvement. This chapter defines CGA, summarises its evidence base and cost-effectiveness, and sets out practical steps for implementation across settings including acute, community, and end-of-life care, so APs can deliver consistent, measurable benefits for older people living with frailty (Figure 7.1).

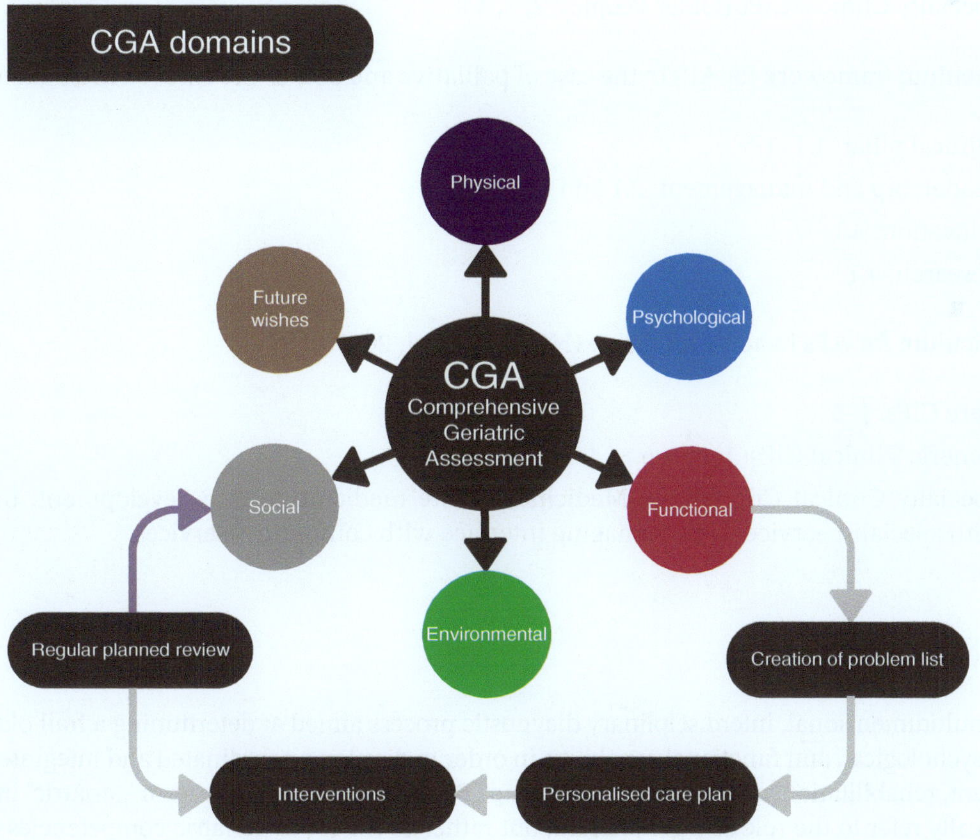

FIGURE 7.1   Comprehensive geriatric assessment. *Source*: The British Geriatrics Society (2025e)/British Geriatrics Society.

Multi-Professional Framework (MPF) for Advanced Practitioners

(Adapted from NHS England, 2025)

This chapter maps to the following areas within the MPF:

1. Clinical practice: 1.1–1.11
2. Leadership and management: 2.2
3. Education: 3.3, 3.8
4. Research: 4.1, 4.2, 4.3

Accreditation Consideration

This chapter maps to the statement with the following national accretional document:

Curriculum framework for advanced practice in the care of older people (NHS England, 2022):

1. Core Capabilities in Practice (CiPs): 1–4
2. Generic Clinical CiPs: 1, 3, 5, 6
3. Specialty Clinical CiPs (Older People): 2, 3, 4

Curriculum framework for APs in the case of palliative and end-of-life care (NHS England, 2023a):

1. Clinical pillar: 1.1–1.5
2. Leadership and management: 2.1 and 2.2
3. Education: 3.1
4. Research: 4.1

Curriculum for APs in acute medicine (NHS England, 2023b):

1. Core CiPs: 1–5
2. Generic Clinical CiPs: 1, 3, 5, 6
3. Specialty Clinical CiPs (Acute Medicine): Acute medicine service development, integration with specialist services, and managing interface with community services.

CGA DEFINITION

CGA is a multidimensional, interdisciplinary diagnostic process aimed at determining a frail older person's medical, psychological, and functional capability, in order to develop a coordinated and integrated care plan for treatment, rehabilitation, and long-term follow-up (Briggs et al., 2022). The term 'geriatric' in CGA does not specifically refer to the role of a geriatrician, but rather to the set of geriatric competencies required to meet the complex needs of older people. Contributions from a wide range of professionals may address one or more components of CGA, even if these are not initially recognised as part of the formal process.

Note: CGA cannot be undertaken by a single professional. It is fundamentally a multi-agency, multidisciplinary process, drawing on the expertise of different team members. While APs may be primarily involved in the physical domain, other members of the multidisciplinary team (MDT) contribute across the remaining domains to ensure a truly holistic assessment.

WHO CAN DO CGA?

See Table 7.1.

TABLE 7.1   Who can conduct CGA.

Team members
Medical experts (consultant geriatricians, associate specialists; GPs with a specialist interest in older people and frailty).
Advanced nurse practitioners
Advanced clinical practitioner/advanced practitioners
Nursing teams
Allied health professionals (physiotherapists, occupational therapists, speech and language therapists, and dietitians)
Pharmacists and pharmacy technicians
Paramedics
Social workers, social prescribers, and care coordinators

WHEN TO CONSIDER CONDUCTING CGA

See Figure 7.2.

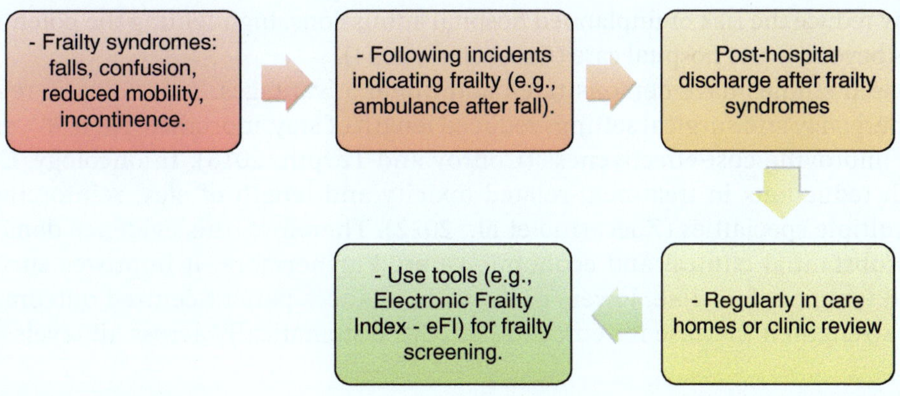

FIGURE 7.2   How to perform CGA.

WHY CGA MATTERS IN EVERYDAY CARE

CGA has a robust evidence base demonstrating its value in improving outcomes for older people living with frailty and complex needs. An influential meta-analysis of 22 randomised controlled trials ($n = 10{,}315$) found that CGA significantly increased the likelihood of older adults being alive and living at home at 12 months (OR 1.16, NNT 33), while also reducing the risk of institutionalisation (OR 0.78) (Ellis et al., 2011). More recently, a systematic review and meta-analysis of 18 randomised controlled trials ($n = 3{,}254$, hospital-based setting) reported that CGA reduced decline in activities of daily living (ADLs) (RR 0.55, 95% CI 0.33–0.92; $p = 0.021$) and decreased mortality (RR 0.85, 95% CI 0.73–0.99), with strong certainty of evidence (Xu et al., 2024).

In the United Kingdom, CGA is embedded within national policy and professional standards. The National Institute for Health and Care Excellence (NICE) recommends that older people with complex needs, including frailty, should receive a CGA at the point of admission, with the aim of shortening hospital stay and supporting faster recovery of independence (NICE, 2016). Similarly, professional bodies emphasise CGA as a marker of high-quality care. The Royal College of Emergency Medicine (RCEM) advises that hospitals should establish acute frailty services, incorporating early frailty identification and access to CGA as part of a multidisciplinary pathway (RCEM, 2025). Similarly, the Royal College of Physicians (RCP) and the British Geriatrics Society (BGS) have developed toolkits promoting the use of CGA from admission through to the later stages of care (RCP/BGS, 2015).

CGA has also been shown to be cost-effective across a range of care settings. An evaluation of hospital-at-home services incorporating CGA found them to be less costly than traditional admission, with mean savings of between £2,265 and £2,840 per patient, without compromising quality-adjusted survival (Singh et al., 2022). Similarly, a Swedish study of outpatient CGA for multimorbid older adults reported an additional cost of €25,000 per patient but a gain of 0.54 quality-adjusted life years (QALYs), resulting in an incremental cost-effectiveness ratio (ICER) of €46,000 per QALY (a figure considered acceptable within European health economics thresholds) (Lundqvist et al., 2018).

The integration of CGA into primary care has further demonstrated system-wide benefits. A large-scale intervention in Swedish primary care, combining CGA with digital risk prediction among 1,604 patients aged 75 years and above, reduced hospital days by 22%, admissions by 17%, and overall costs by 17% (€4,324 per patient) over two years (Nord et al., 2021). Evidence from the Community Epidemiology of Ageing (CEpiA) cluster randomised trial in France also suggests that GP- and nurse-led CGA in the community may reduce the risk of unplanned hospital admissions, highlighting the potential for CGA to deliver benefits beyond acute hospital care (Orcel et al., 2024).

Hospital-based studies have demonstrated additional advantages. A systematic review reported that CGA in emergency and surgical settings reduced length of stay, mortality (RR 0.78), and functional decline, while improving cost-effectiveness (Conroy and Turpin, 2016). In oncology, CGA has been associated with reductions in treatment-related toxicity and length of stay, reinforcing its applicability across multiple specialties (Zuccarino et al., 2022). Therefore, this evidence demonstrates that CGA delivers substantial clinical and economic value. Furthermore, it improves survival, reduces admissions and functional decline, lowers costs, and enhances patient-centred outcomes. Moreover, these findings strengthen the case for embedding CGA systematically across all levels of health and social care.

HOW TO CONDUCT CGA IN CLINICAL PRACTICE

The six steps of CGA provide a clear framework for APs working within the MDT to deliver coordinated, person-centred care. The process begins with data gathering, where APs contribute by undertaking thorough physical assessments, reviewing medications, and identifying risks across the domains of frailty. This information is then taken to the team discussion, where APs share their findings and integrate them with insights from other professionals, ensuring a balanced view of the person's needs. Together, the MDT and APs generate a problem list, clarifying the priority areas that require intervention. In the next step, APs play a key role in developing a plan with the person, ensuring that clinical priorities are balanced with the individual's goals and values. Once agreed, APs help lead on implementing and sharing the plan, coordinating actions across services, and communicating clearly with the person, carers, and professionals involved. The process is sustained through regular planned review, where APs monitor progress, reassess needs, and adapt the plan as the person's condition changes, ensuring care remains proactive and responsive.

THE SIXTH ELEMENTS OF CGA

The CGA is built around six key domains, each addressing a vital aspect of an older person's health and well-being (Royal College of Physicians, 2015). All these domains provide a holistic foundation for developing a personalised and coordinated care plan (Figure 7.3).

PHYSICAL DOMAIN

The physical domain of CGA forms the foundation of holistic assessment, focusing on the medical, functional, and biological aspects of ageing and frailty (BGS, 2025a). It encompasses detailed exploration of past medical and surgical history, long-term condition management, and recognition of frailty syndromes. Key components include structured medication reviews, assessment of nutrition and hydration, evaluation of pain and joint health, and falls risk identification. This domain also addresses the challenges of multimorbidity and polypharmacy, recognising how these interact to influence health outcomes. By systematically reviewing these elements, APs can identify modifiable risks and create person-centred care plans that maintain function and independence.

Frailty Status

Frailty status is a vital component of the physical domain in CGA, as it identifies individuals at greatest risk of falls, hospitalisation, disability, and mortality. For APs, recognising frailty involves more than observation; it requires advanced clinical reasoning, integration of comorbidities, medication burden, cognition, and function, and use of validated tools such as the Clinical Frailty Scale (CFS), Fried Frailty Phenotype, or Edmonton Frail Scale (Chapter 8). Importantly, APs must establish baseline function at least two weeks prior to acute illness to avoid misclassification. Frailty assessment guides personalised interventions such as exercise programmes, nutritional optimisation, and structured deprescribing that can slow progression and reduce admissions. It also informs prognostic

Capital Health

Comprehensive Geriatric Assessment Form

WNL = Within Normal Limits   ASST = Assisted   IND = Independent   DEP = Dependent

○ **Cognition** ☐ WNL   ☐ CIND   ☐ MCI   ☐ Dementia   ☐ Delirium   MMSE: _________   FAST: _________
Chief lifelong occupation: _________________________________   Education (years): _______________

● **Action Required**
○ **Monitor**

○ **Emotional** ☐ WNL   ☐ ↓ Mood ☐ Depression ☐ Anxiety ☐ Fatigue ☐ Halluncination ☐ Delusion ☐ Other

○ **Motivation** ☐ High ☐ Usual ☐ Low   **Health Attitude** ☐ Excellent ☐ Good ☐ Fair ☐ Poor ☐ Couldn't say

○ **Communication**   **Speech** ☐ WNL ☐ Impaired   **Hearing** ☐ WNL ☐ Impaired   **Vision** ☐ WNL ☐ Impaired

○ **Strength**   ☐ WNL   ☐ Weak   Upper: PROXIMAL DISTAL   Lower: PROXIMAL DISTAL

○ **Exercise** ☐ Frequent   ☐ Occassional   ☐ Not

Patient contact:
☐ Inpatient
☐ Clinic
☐ GDH
☐ NH
☐ Outreach
☐ Home
☐ Assisted Living
☐ ER
☐ Other
PT = PATIENT
CG = CAREGIVER

Current Frailty Score:

	BASELINE (two weeks ago)				CURRENT (today)				NOTES
Balance Balance / Falls	WNL N Y	Impaired Number ____			WNL N Y	Impaired Number ____			
Mobility Walk Outside	IND		ASST Can't		IND		ASST Can't		
Walking	IND SLOW	ASST	DEP		IND SLOW	ASST	DEP		
Transfers	IND Stand by	ASST	DEP		IND Stand by	ASST	DEP		
Bed	IND PULL	ASST	DEP		IND PULL	ASST	DEP		
Aid	None Cane	Walker	Chair		None Cane	Walker	Chair		
Nutrition Weight / Appetite	GOOD UNDER OVER OBESE / WNL FAIR POOR				STABLE LOSS GAIN / WNL FAIR POOR				
Elimination Bowel / Bladder	CONT CONSTIP INCONT / CONT CATHETER INCONT				CONT CONSTIP INCONT / CONT CATHETER INCONT				
ADLs Feeding	IND	ASST	DEP		IND	ASST	DEP		
Bathing	IND	ASST	DEP		IND	ASST	DEP		
Dressing	IND	ASST	DEP		IND	ASST	DEP		
Toileting	IND	ASST	DEP		IND	ASST	DEP		
IADLs Cooking	IND	ASST	DEP		IND	ASST	DEP		
Cleaning	IND	ASST	DEP		IND	ASST	DEP		
Shopping	IND	ASST	DEP		IND	ASST	DEP		
Medications	IND	ASST	DEP		IND	ASST	DEP		
Driving	IND	ASST	DEP		IND	ASST	DEP		
Banking	IND	ASST	DEP		IND	ASST	DEP		

Scale | PT | CG
1. Very fit
2. Well
3. Well with Rx'd co-morbid disease
4. Apparently vulnerable
5. Mildly frail
6. Moderately frail
7. Severely frail
8. Very severely frail
9a. Terminally ill - walker
9b. Terminally ill - bed

○ **Sleep** ☐ Normal ☐ Disrupted ☐ Daytime drowsiness   **Socially Engaged** ☐ Frequent ☐ Occasional ☐ Not

○ **Social**   ☐ Married   ☐ Divorced   ☐ Widowed   ☐ Single

Lives   ☐ Alone   ☐ Spouse   ☐ Other

Home   ☐ House (Levels___)   ☐ Steps (Number ___)   ☐ Apartment   ☐ Assisted Living   ☐ Nursing home   ☐ Other

Supports   ☐ Informal   ☐ HCNS   ☐ Other   ☐ Req. more support   ☐ None   ○ **Code Status** ☐ Do not resuscitate ☐ Rescuscitate

Caregiver Relationship   ☐ Spouse   ☐ Sibling   ☐ Offspring   ☐ Other

Caregiver Stress   ☐ None   ☐ Low   ☐ Moderate   ☐ High

Caregiver occupation (CG): _________________

○ **Advance directive in place?** ☐ Yes ☐ No

ACTION REQUIRED (check appropriate circles)

Problems: Med adjust req.   Associated Medication: (*mark meds started in hospital with an asterisk)
1. _______________________________   ○ _________________________________
2. _______________________________   ○ _________________________________
3. _______________________________   ○ _________________________________
4. _______________________________   ○ _________________________________
5. _______________________________   ○ _________________________________
6. _______________________________   ○ _________________________________
7. _______________________________   ○ _________________________________
8. _______________________________   ○ _________________________________
9. _______________________________   ○ _________________________________
10. ______________________________   ○ _________________________________
11. ______________________________   ○ _________________________________
12. ______________________________   ○ _________________________________

Assessor/Physician: _________________________________   Date: _________________
(YYYY/MM/DD)

Assessment Forms
CD0184MR_06_09

© 2007-2016 v1.2.2 All rights reserved. Kenneth Rockwood Inc.
Permission granted to copy for research and education use only.

Page 1 of 1

FIGURE 7.3   CGA (Dalhousie University, 2025) copy write was taken for reuse/reprint.

discussions, advance care planning, and decisions around escalation of treatment. By embedding frailty assessment into CGA, APs ensure care is proactive, person-centred, and focused on maintaining quality of life and independence.

Past Medical and Surgical History

A thorough exploration of an older person's past medical and surgical history is a cornerstone of CGA, as it provides essential context for understanding the interplay between comorbidity, frailty, and disability. Multimorbidity, defined as the coexistence of two or more long-term health conditions, is highly prevalent in older adults and often coexists with frailty, though the two are distinct constructs (NICE, 2023). With ageing comes the accumulation of diagnoses and interventions, increasing the potential for interactions between conditions and their treatments, which in turn creates a complexity that necessitates holistic assessment. A structured review of past and current diagnoses, together with details of previous surgical or interventional procedures, ensures that clinicians can identify which conditions are active, which are historical, and which professionals or services are currently involved in ongoing care. This is particularly relevant in the surgical context, where a robust body of evidence demonstrates that frailty is associated with poorer long-term outcomes, including higher rates of post-operative complications, longer hospital stays, and increased mortality (Ambler et al., 2020; Panayi et al., 2019). However, the risks associated with frailty are not immutable: the integration of CGA into perioperative pathways has been shown to mitigate adverse outcomes, optimise recovery, and even deliver cost-effective improvements in patient care (Dhesi et al., 2019; Eamer et al., 2017). Consequently, careful documentation and critical interpretation of a patient's medical and surgical history are not only diagnostic but also prognostic, informing both personalised treatment planning and broader multidisciplinary coordination.

Medication History and Review

Polypharmacy is common among older adults with frailty, and its safe management is a critical component of CGA (see Chapter 9). APs have a central role in undertaking comprehensive medication reviews and exploring prior medication use to ensure prescribing is appropriate, person-centred, and aligned with current best practice. A thorough medication history should include prescribed, over-the-counter, complementary and alternative medicines, as well as lifestyle factors such as alcohol, smoking, and recreational drug use, which may otherwise be overlooked in older adults due to assumptions about age-related behaviour (NICE, 2015). Importantly, APs should also check immunisation status to identify any missed opportunities for preventive care.

The risks of inappropriate polypharmacy are well established. As the number of medicines increases, so does the risk of adverse outcomes, including falls, cognitive impairment, and hospitalisation (Davies et al., 2020). Evidence demonstrates that people prescribed 10 or more medicines are 300 times more likely to require hospital admission due to medication-related problems (Payne et al., 2014), and up to 1 in 5 unplanned hospital admissions in older adults are attributable to adverse drug reactions (Pirmohamed et al., 2004). Frailty and polypharmacy are closely linked, with multimorbidity driving higher prescribing rates, and polypharmacy itself associated with an increased prevalence of frailty (Veronese et al., 2017). Prescribing cascades, where one drug is added to treat the side effects of another, are particularly common and must be identified and addressed by APs to prevent harm and improve quality of life (McCarthy et al., 2022).

The scale of polypharmacy in England highlights the urgency of this issue: in January 2025, more than 1.1 million people were prescribed 10 or more medicines, of whom 457,285 were aged 75 or older (NHSBSA, 2025). Beyond clinical consequences, the Department of Health and Social Care's National Overprescribing Review reported that 10% of prescriptions in primary care are inappropriate, representing both harm to patients and waste of NHS resources (DHSC, 2021). For APs, this reinforces the importance of embedding structured, systematic approaches into practice.

Structured Medication Reviews (SMRs), as defined by NICE, are a central tool within CGA for older adults with frailty. They involve a person-centred, critical evaluation of all prescribed and non-prescribed medicines, with the aim of optimising therapeutic benefit while reducing risks and waste (NICE, 2015; NICE QS120, 2017). Reviews should prioritise high-risk drug classes, including those contributing to a high anticholinergic burden (ACB), which has been strongly linked to cognitive decline, dementia, falls, and mortality (bpacnz, 2024). Evidence indicates that two-thirds of unplanned admissions due to adverse drug reactions are preventable (Howard et al., 2006), underscoring the value of proactive, AP-led medication optimisation.

By combining advanced pharmacological knowledge with clinical leadership, APs can bridge gaps in prescribing guidance, much of which is derived from trials that excluded frail older adults or those with multimorbidity (Davies et al., 2020). In doing so, APs not only reduce the dangers of inappropriate polypharmacy but also deliver care that aligns with patient values, improves outcomes, and safeguards NHS resources.

Falls History

Falls are a critical component of CGA because they are common in older adults and strongly associated with morbidity, mortality, and loss of independence. Falls are often sentinel events signalling functional loss (Ellmers et al., 2023). They may mark the beginning of a 'downward spiral' of hospitalisation, deconditioning, and dependency. For APs, a focused falls history provides vital insight into frailty progression, identifies modifiable risk factors, and guides evidence-based interventions. NICE guidance highlights the importance of structured falls assessment in older adults and those aged 50 and over at higher risk (NICE, 2025).

Frailty significantly increases falls risk due to sarcopenia, impaired balance, slower reaction times, and polypharmacy. Evidence shows that people with frailty not only fall more frequently but are more likely to sustain serious consequences, such as fractures, head injuries, hospitalisation, and subsequent functional decline (Montero-Odasso et al., 2022). For APs, identifying these risks proactively enables timely prevention strategies that reduce admissions and maintain independence.

A comprehensive falls history should include:

- **History of falls**: number, frequency, timing, location, circumstances, associated injuries, and fear of falling.
- **Stability**: gait and balance assessment using tools such as the Timed Up and Go Test (TUGT), postural blood pressure measurement for orthostatic hypotension (Asai et al., 2018). A comprehensive systematic review and meta-analysis of 50 longitudinal and cross-sectional studies, including over 49,000 individuals aged $\geq$65 years, reported a pooled odds ratio of 1.73 (95% CI 1.50–1.99), indicating a significant positive association between orthostatic hypotension and falls (Mol et al., 2019).
- **Feet and footwear**: pain, deformities, peripheral neuropathy, or unsafe footwear.
- **Medications**: review of sedatives, antihypertensives, anticholinergics, and psychotropics.

> - **Other risk factors**: vision, cognition, continence, and environmental hazards.
> - **Bone protection**: fracture risk using Fracture Risk Assessment Tool (FRAX) or QFracture, adjusting FRAX if the patient reports ≥2 falls per year (NOGG, 2021).

The AP's role is to integrate this information, distinguishing between modifiable and non-modifiable risks, and to provide practical guidance. For example, where falls risk cannot be fully eliminated, patients and carers should be advised on safe strategies for managing falls, such as how to get up safely.

Multifactorial interventions are the most effective approach, combining exercise (strength and balance training), medication review, vision correction, and home hazard modification. APs are central to coordinating these interventions, ensuring that falls history is translated into actionable, personalised care plans. Falls are often the first marker of declining health in frailty. Addressing them proactively is therefore not only preventive but also diagnostic, signalling when a broader CGA or escalation of support is required.

Pain and Joint Problems

Pain assessment is a vital component of CGA, yet it is frequently under-recognised and under-treated in older adults. APs have a crucial role in identifying and managing pain, not only as a symptom but also as a driver of frailty, reduced mobility, and functional decline. Misconceptions that pain is a 'normal' part of ageing, along with concerns about the adverse effects of analgesics, often contribute to undertreatment (Ali et al., 2018). Untreated pain is linked to poor sleep, low mood, impaired cognition, social isolation, and loss of independence, all of which can significantly reduce quality of life (Chan and Chan, 2022).

A holistic approach is required, recognising the biological, psychological, and social dimensions of pain. For patients with cognitive impairment or communication difficulties, APs should apply validated observational tools such as the Abbey Pain Scale (Abbey et al., 2004) or the Pain Assessment in Advanced Dementia (PAINAD) scale (Warden et al., 2003). These tools are endorsed in UK national guidelines, which emphasise structured pain assessment as part of routine practice (Schofield, 2018). A recent COSMIN-based systematic review examined the psychometric properties of nine such tools used in people living with dementia ($n = 5,924$) (Smith and Harvey, 2022). The review identified strong to moderate evidence supporting the Pain Assessment Checklist for Seniors with Limited Ability to Communicate—Revised (PACSLAC-II), the Checklist of Nonverbal Pain Indicators (CNPI), the DOLOPLUS-2 Scale, the Mobilisation–Observation–Behaviour–Intensity–Dementia Pain Scale (MOBID), and the Face, Legs, Activity, Cry, Consolability Scale (FLACC/FACs). In contrast, the Abbey Pain Scale, though widely used in UK settings, was found to have only limited evidence of reliability and validity due to concerns regarding its structural and criterion validity (Smith and Harvey, 2022).

Effective management should address underlying causes wherever possible, complemented by careful pharmacological strategies and non-pharmacological approaches such as physiotherapy, occupational therapy, and social support. APs are ideally placed to coordinate multidisciplinary input and ensure that treatment is person-centred, balancing analgesic benefits with the risks of adverse effects, falls, or drug interactions.

Joint problems are among the most common sources of pain in older adults, with osteoarthritis being a major contributor to mobility loss, functional impairment, and falls risk. APs should perform systematic joint examinations, looking for swelling, tenderness, deformity, and reduced range of movement. Functional impact must also be assessed, including the ability to dress, prepare meals, and handle medications. Where joint injury is suspected following a fall, a low threshold for radiological investigation is warranted to avoid missed diagnoses. Referral to physiotherapy or specialist services may be needed for detailed assessment and management planning.

Through early recognition and holistic management of pain and joint problems, APs can significantly improve well-being, independence, and quality of life in frail older adults.

Nutrition and Hydration

Nutrition and hydration are fundamental to CGA, underpinning physical, psychological, and social well-being. Poor nutritional status can accelerate frailty progression, impair recovery, and increase the risk of adverse outcomes, while dehydration contributes to delirium, falls, and hospitalisation. For APs, early recognition and intervention are critical, as they often act as coordinators across MDTs.

Malnutrition and frailty are strongly interlinked, with evidence showing that malnourished individuals are four times more likely to develop frailty (Laur et al., 2017). The diagnostic criteria for frailty overlap with those for malnutrition and sarcopenia, including weight loss, exhaustion, and muscle weakness. This overlap highlights the importance of integrated management approaches targeting nutrition, muscle health, and functional capacity (Khor et al., 2022). Screening should include validated tools such as the Malnutrition Universal Screening Tool (MUST), with attention also paid to obesity and sarcopenia. Although muscle mass is difficult to measure directly, muscle strength offers a practical and reliable proxy.

APs should consider a wide range of factors when assessing nutrition and hydration: appetite, oral health, gastrointestinal symptoms, polypharmacy, and the impact of socio-economic deprivation or psychological distress. Older people are more likely to have B12 or folate deficiency due to diet or malabsorption, which may be difficult to detect clinically (Ni Lochlainn et al., 2021). Sensory impairments, functional decline, and dysphagia are also key contributors to reduced intake and should not be overlooked. Importantly, there is no validated screening tool for dehydration, making careful clinical judgement and collateral history essential (Parkinson et al., 2023).

Interventions should be holistic and person-centred. Food-based strategies remain the cornerstone of management and may include tailored healthy eating advice, fortified meals, and practical support for shopping or cooking. Oral nutritional supplements (ONS) are widely prescribed; however, recent systematic review evidence demonstrates limited effectiveness in frail older adults, raising questions about their routine use (Thomson et al., 2022).

International frameworks such as the Global Leadership Initiative on Malnutrition (GLIM) criteria provide consensus standards for diagnosing malnutrition (Cederholm et al., 2019), while UK-specific reviews highlight nutritional requirements for adults over 65, particularly regarding protein, vitamin D, and hydration (Dorrington et al., 2020). The European Society for Clinical Nutrition and Metabolism (ESPEN) guidelines further recommend structured, multidisciplinary approaches to nutrition and hydration in older people (Volkert et al., 2019).

For APs, the priority is to embed nutrition and hydration into every CGA, recognising their cross-cutting influence on all domains of health. By coordinating early screening, initiating food-first interventions, and aligning management with individual values, APs can prevent decline, improve outcomes, and support independence in frail older adults.

Sensory Impairment

Sensory impairment is a frequently overlooked but highly significant domain of CGA. The prevalence of sensory dysfunction rises sharply with age: around 40% of people aged 70–79 experience impairment in at least one sense, and over a quarter report dysfunction in multiple senses (Völter et al., 2021). For APs, recognising and managing sensory impairment is critical because it has wide-ranging impacts on physical function, communication, mental health, nutrition, and independence.

Hearing loss is especially common, affecting an estimated 80% of people aged 80 years and over (Erwin and Chen, 2025). Despite this, it remains under-recognised and under-treated. Consequences include reduced communication, social isolation, depression, anxiety, and an increased risk of cognitive decline (Dalton et al., 2003). Encouragingly, treatment of hearing loss such as the use of hearing aids or cochlear implants is associated with improved physical, mental, emotional, and social well-being. For APs undertaking CGA, assessment may begin with simple bedside methods, including enquiry about hearing aid use, direct questioning, and the whisper test. Where impairment is suspected, referral to audiology services for formal testing, such as pure tone audiometry, should be facilitated.

Visual impairment is similarly prevalent, with over 2 million people in the United Kingdom living with sight loss, the vast majority of whom are aged over 65 (Royal National Institute of Blind People [RNIB], 2025). Visual impairment affects daily functioning, contributing to difficulties with reading, cooking, and medication management, and is strongly linked with depression, anxiety, and social isolation (Brown and Barrett, 2011). Importantly, vision loss increases the risk of falls and related injuries, compounding frailty-related vulnerabilities. CGA should therefore include an enquiry about glasses use, any history of sight loss, and where appropriate, an objective assessment of visual acuity. Early detection enables timely referral to ophthalmology or low-vision services, with interventions such as corrective lenses, cataract surgery, or environmental adaptations.

Beyond hearing and vision, other senses also warrant consideration. Changes in smell and taste can reduce appetite and compromise dietary intake, exacerbating malnutrition and frailty. Impairments in touch and spatial awareness may further increase falls risk and hinder safe mobility. APs should remain vigilant for these subtle but impactful deficits, incorporating collateral history from carers or family members where self-report is unreliable.

Ultimately, addressing sensory impairment within CGA allows APs to mitigate risks, optimise communication, and support holistic well-being. Integrating screening, appropriate referrals, and practical interventions into frailty care can significantly enhance independence and quality of life for older adults.

Bowel and Bladder Health

Bladder and bowel dysfunction are highly prevalent in older adults and represent important domains of CGA. While common, these issues are not an inevitable part of ageing. Their impact on quality of life, independence, dignity, and mental health is profound, and they also impose substantial economic and health system burdens. For APs conducting CGA, early recognition and sensitive management are essential, particularly given the close association of continence problems with frailty, falls, and institutionalisation.

Bladder health problems in older adults typically present as incontinence, retention, or urinary tract infection (UTI). Urinary incontinence can be urge, stress, or mixed in nature and is frequently under-reported due to embarrassment. It can limit social participation and contribute to depression and carer strain. Retention is also common, particularly in older men, with around one in three over the age of 65 years experiencing incomplete emptying, often related to benign prostatic enlargement (BAUS, 2024). Retention can also result from constipation or medications, particularly opiates and anticholinergics.

UTIs are another frequent concern, with incidence increasing with age (Ahmed et al., 2018). Importantly, APs should recognise that asymptomatic bacteriuria is highly prevalent in older adults, especially in those with catheters. Reliance on urine dipsticks should be avoided due to their poor predictive value in this group. Diagnosis should instead be based on clinical features such as dysuria, urgency, frequency, suprapubic pain, or systemic signs, ensuring that antibiotics are prescribed appropriately to avoid resistance.

Bowel health problems are similarly multifactorial. Constipation is widespread, driven by reduced mobility, low-fibre diets, inadequate hydration, polypharmacy, and conditions such as Parkinson's disease. Conversely, diarrhoea may reflect medication side effects (e.g. laxatives and metformin), infection, or underlying gastrointestinal pathology. Faecal incontinence, which may be functional (due to mobility or cognitive impairment) or passive (due to sphincter dysfunction), is particularly common, with prevalence rising sharply in care home settings where up to 60% of residents are affected (NICE, 2022).

For APs, the management of bladder and bowel dysfunction requires a holistic, person-centred approach. A comprehensive medication review is essential, both to identify drugs contributing to dysfunction and to weigh the risks of medications used for incontinence, which may increase falls risk. Consideration should also be given to environmental and functional factors (as explained in the environmental and functional domains below): Is the toilet accessible and safe? Is urgency increasing falls risk? Does nocturia disrupt sleep and affect both patient and carer well-being? These practical questions enable APs to tailor interventions that extend beyond clinical management to address safety and quality of life.

Equally important is the psychosocial dimension. Incontinence often leads to embarrassment, social withdrawal, and reduced confidence, with downstream effects on mood and physical activity. APs should explicitly explore how continence issues affect daily life, relationships, and mental health, and work collaboratively with patients and carers to establish realistic goals. Shared decision-making ensures that management aligns with what matters most to the individual, whether this is reducing nocturia, enabling social participation, or minimising carer burden.

Interventions may include bladder training, pelvic floor exercises, dietary modification, laxative optimisation, and referral to continence services or physiotherapy. In some cases, urological or gastroenterological input may be necessary. However, the emphasis in CGA is always on multifactorial, coordinated management rather than isolated symptom treatment.

Skin Integrity

The maintenance of skin integrity is a critical domain of CGA, given the vulnerability of older adults with frailty to skin breakdown and chronic wounds. Ageing naturally results in thinning of the dermis, reduced collagen, diminished vascularity, and impaired immune response, all of which reduce resilience and healing capacity. These physiological changes are further compounded by multimorbidity, polypharmacy, and functional decline, meaning that APs must always approach skin health as both a stand-alone concern and an indicator of wider systemic vulnerability. Chronic wounds, including pressure injuries, moisture lesions, venous leg ulcers, and diabetic foot complications, are increasingly prevalent in older people with frailty (Ferris and Harding, 2020). They not only cause pain and functional restriction but also carry a substantial risk of infection, sepsis, and hospitalisation. The financial and social costs are equally significant, with tissue viability services representing a major area of healthcare expenditure (Wounds International, 2020). For APs, the challenge lies in recognising early signs of deterioration, implementing preventive strategies, and embedding skin assessment into the holistic CGA process.

Early identification and intervention are essential. The NICE (2024) recommends the use of validated risk assessment tools, such as the Braden Scale, Waterlow Score, or Norton Risk Assessment Scale, when evaluating an individual's vulnerability to pressure damage. Small changes such as altering positioning, adjusting equipment to redistribute pressure, or applying emollients to maintain hydration can prevent escalation into chronic wounds (Figure 7.4). Regular structured inspection, particularly of pressure-prone

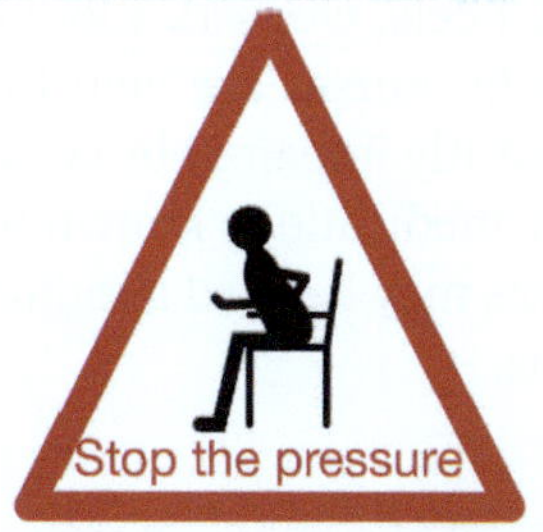

Stage 1: Non-blanching erythema

Intact skin with non-blanchable redness of a localised area over a bony prominence. Darkly pigmented skin may not have visible blanching but the local area may be painful or have a bluish tinge and feel warmer. Stage 1 may be difficult to detect in individuals with dark skin tones

Stage 2: Partial thickness

Partial thickness with loss of dermis presenting as a shallow open ulcer with a red pink wound bed, without slough. May also present as an intact or open/ruptured serum-filled or sero-sanginous filled blister. This stage should not be confused with moisture lesions

Stage 3: Full thickness

Full thickness tissue loss with loss of subcutaneous fat, some of which may still be visible but bone, tendon or muscle is not visible or directly palpable. Slough or eschar may be present and may include undermining and tunnelling. *Wounds covered with 100% eschar or slough are at least stage 3*

Stage 4: Full thickness

Full thickness tissue loss with exposed bone, tendon or muscle visible or palpable. Slough or eschar may be present and there may be undermining and tunnelling. The depth of stage 3 and 4 pressure ulcers vary by anatomical location depending on where subcutaneous tissue is naturally stored. Stage 4 ulcers extend into muscle and/or fascia, tendon or joint capsule, making osteomyelitis a high risk factor

Suspected deep tissue injury: Skin intact

Purple localised area of discoloured intact skin or blood-filled blister due to damage of underlying soft tissue from pressure and/or *shear*. The area may be preceded by tissue that is painful or warmer than adjacent tissue. Deep tissue injury may be difficult to detect in individuals with dark skin tones. A thin blister may develop over a dark wound bed. Changes may be rapid exposing additional layers of tissue despite optimal treatment

Moisture lesion: NOT a pressure ulcer

Redness or partial thickness skin loss involving the epidermis, upper dermis or both. Caused by excessive moisture to the skin from urine, faeces or sweat. This is not a pressure ulcer and must not be confused with one

FIGURE 7.4   Pressure ulcer. Adapted from Blundell and Gordon (2015) Wiley.

areas (sacrum, heels, elbows), should be routine within CGA. Routine inspection and documentation of pressure areas by nurses are vital to ensure early recognition of tissue compromise. Healing outcomes may be significantly impaired by coexisting factors such as vascular disease, poor glycaemic control, or the prescription of medications known to exacerbate ulceration risk, for example nicorandil. Therefore, risk assessment tools may be used as adjuncts, but APs must exercise clinical judgement and not rely solely on scoring systems.

Assessment of skin integrity within CGA also requires consideration of wider contributory factors such as:

- **Incontinence:** Moisture from urine or faeces increases the risk of dermatitis, infection, and delayed wound healing. This highlights the need for bladder and bowel assessment, timely continence management, and use of appropriate barrier products.
- **Polypharmacy and medication side effects:** Frail older adults are often prescribed complex regimens, some of which impair skin healing. Nicorandil, for example, has been linked with ulceration, while medicines affecting vascular perfusion can exacerbate ischaemia (Wounds International, 2020). APs should incorporate skin health into structured medication reviews, balancing risks and benefits.
- **Nutrition and hydration:** Malnutrition and dehydration reduce tissue repair, muscle mass, and mobility, increasing the risk of pressure damage. As highlighted in the nutrition domains of CGA, ensuring adequate protein, micronutrient intake, and fluid balance is central to maintaining skin health.
- **Mobility and functional status:** Limited movement or prolonged immobility increases susceptibility to pressure damage. Assessing how long patients remain in one position, whether they can reposition independently, and the suitability of support surfaces is essential. Linking with physiotherapists and occupational therapists can help develop strategies to optimise positioning and activity.

The care plan emerging from CGA must therefore adopt a holistic, person-centred approach to skin integrity. For APs, this involves integrating skin assessment with continence, medication, nutritional, and functional reviews, and then co-producing management plans with patients and carers. Shared decision-making is particularly important where interventions require lifestyle adjustments, equipment use, or adherence to regular repositioning schedules. Ultimately, skin integrity is both a marker and mediator of frailty: deterioration often signals wider decline, while proactive management can improve comfort, reduce complications, and preserve independence. By embedding tissue viability into CGA, APs can deliver care that not only treats wounds but also actively prevents them, aligning with best practice recommendations for maintaining skin health in older adults with frailty (Wound International, 2020).

FUNCTIONAL DOMAIN

The functional domain of CGA refers to an older person's ability to undertake everyday activities essential for independent living. It includes both ADLs, such as feeding, dressing, toileting, and mobility, and instrumental activities of daily living (IADLs), such as managing finances, using transport, shopping, and medication adherence (Kendall and Wiltjer, 2019). Decline in functional capacity is often the first visible sign of deterioration, making functional assessment fundamental to anticipatory and person-centred care. For APs, this provides essential insights into independence and care needs.

Assessing ADLs and IADLs

Validated tools support structured assessment. The Barthel Index measures independence across 10 domains, including mobility, grooming, and continence (Martinsson and Eksborg, 2006). The Lawton and Brody IADL Scale is particularly useful in community and outpatient settings (Ward et al., 1998). A recent study of 264 older adults demonstrated that IADL scores declined significantly with frailty, showing the tool's utility in identifying early decline (Özdemir and Telli, 2024). For APs, these tools support monitoring and targeted interventions.

Influences on Function

Ageing brings physiological and cognitive changes that influence function. Reduced muscle mass, joint stiffness, sensory loss, and balance problems can limit ADLs. Cognitive impairment, including mild cognitive impairment and dementia, affects the ability to perform more complex tasks (Preston and Biddell, 2021). Functional decline is often gradual, manifesting as difficulty with stairs before walking or transferring. Acute illness or injury may accelerate this decline. For APs, recognising underlying drivers is key to proactive care.

Structured Functional Assessment

APs should begin with a detailed history of what the person can currently do, tasks requiring support, and activities recently given up (BGS, 2018). Functional assessment includes evaluating transfers (e.g. bed to chair), use of aids, and barriers such as tremors, pain, postural hypotension, or environmental limitations. Where deficits are identified, referral to physiotherapy or occupational therapy may be required for gait assessment, provision of aids, or environmental modifications. For APs, structured assessment informs multidisciplinary planning.

Cognition, Nutrition, and Continence

Cognition is integral to function. Loss of ability may result from impaired executive function or judgement. Forgetting to eat or neglecting hygiene may reflect cognitive decline rather than choice. Screening tools such as the Mini-Cog, Abbreviated Mental Test (10-item version) (AMT-10) (Borson et al., 2000), or Abbreviated Mental Test Score (AMTS) (Hodkinson, 1972) should be used to inform interpretation of functional findings. Nutrition and continence are also closely linked: malnutrition or constipation can cause fatigue and immobility, while fear of incontinence may lead to restricted activity. APs should explore these interdependencies during CGA. For APs, this highlights the need for holistic assessment.

Continuity and Care Planning

Functional assessment must be dynamic and continuous rather than a one-off exercise (Kendall and Wiltjer, 2019). Changes should be documented against baseline to guide interventions, whether decline is transient (e.g. following hospitalisation) or progressive (e.g. neurodegenerative disease). Care plans should be person-centred, reflecting the individual's goals and meaningful activities (BGS, 2018, 2023). The aim is not necessarily full independence but supported independence through aids, adaptations, or assistance. For APs, continuity ensures meaningful and sustainable care plans.

Interventions and Reablement

APs play a central role in preventing or slowing functional decline by encouraging safe activity, setting goals, and educating patients on mobility and safety. Hospital-associated deconditioning can be reduced through mobilisation strategies such as the #EndPJparalysis campaign (Swinnerton and Price, 2023). Reablement, a short-term intensive intervention delivered at home, has strong evidence of improving functional ability. A systematic review and meta-analysis confirmed significant benefits for older adults, though the extent varied by context (Chen et al., 2022). Embedding reablement into care pathways supports independence while reducing demand for long-term care. For APs, these interventions highlight their leadership role in supporting function.

The functional domain provides a lens through which to assess an older adult's ability to live safely and well. It links closely with physical, psychological, and social domains, requiring a holistic approach. APs and nurses, as frontline assessors and advocates, are essential to identifying functional decline early, coordinating interventions, and ensuring care plans uphold independence, dignity, and quality of life.

PSYCHOLOGICAL DOMAIN

The psychological domain of CGA is essential to understanding the interplay between mental health, cognition, and frailty. Psychological well-being affects adherence to treatment, engagement in rehabilitation, and overall quality of life. For APs, recognising and addressing psychological issues early is critical, as they frequently coexist with physical frailty and exacerbate its impact. This domain covers mood disorders such as depression and anxiety, cognitive decline, and the identification and management of delirium. Refer to Chapter 12, where the psychiatry assessment and management within geriatric medicine is explored.

Depression

Depression is more common in people with frailty, with prevalence increasing as frailty severity worsens (Hamada et al., 2024). Evidence suggests a bidirectional relationship: depression accelerates frailty and cognitive decline, while frailty increases susceptibility to depression (Sang et al., 2024). Clinical features in older adults may resemble those seen in younger populations, but somatic presentations such as fatigue, gastrointestinal complaints, poor sleep, and weight loss are more prominent. Anxiety, agitation, and slowing of emotional responses are also common (Triolo et al., 2023). Social withdrawal and loss of interest in once-meaningful activities such as disengaging from family or hobbies should alert APs to possible depression. For APs, recognising these atypical presentations is essential to avoid under-diagnosis.

Depression in older people is often chronic and relapsing, with serious consequences: around 20% of suicides occur in later life, and lethality of attempts is higher in older people than in younger groups (Conwell et al., 2011). Risk factors include male gender, bereavement, physical illness, chronic pain, substance misuse, and previous suicidal behaviour. Screening tools are vital for early recognition.

The two-question screener ('Have you felt down, depressed, or hopeless in the last month?' and 'Have you had little interest or pleasure in doing things?') is simple and sensitive. If positive, further assessment may be undertaken using validated instruments such as the Geriatric Depression Score, PHQ-9, or the Cornell Scale for Depression in Dementia. For APs, using these tools within CGA supports early identification, timely intervention, and appropriate referral.

COGNITION

Cognitive impairment is highly prevalent in frail populations. Early signs of dementia—such as forgetting conversations, repeating questions, or misplacing items are often dismissed as 'normal ageing'. More complex functional impairments, including managing finances or planning journeys, may also be over-looked. Routine screening is therefore recommended, even if conversational skills appear intact. Useful approaches include the Single Question in Dementia ('Has the person been more forgetful in the last 12 months to the extent that it has affected their daily life?'), collateral histories, and structured questionnaires such as the Informant Questionnaire on Cognitive Decline in the Elderly (IQCODE). For APs, combining collateral history with screening tools ensures that subtle cognitive decline is not missed.

Validated cognitive tests, such as the 6-CIT, can support assessment but should not be used in isolation. More detailed tools, such as the Addenbrooke's Cognitive Examination, are typically reserved for memory clinics. Before dementia is diagnosed, reversible causes such as thyroid dysfunction, vitamin deficiencies, or infection must be excluded through targeted investigations. For APs, this highlights their role in ordering, interpreting, or escalating investigations to exclude reversible causes.

DELIRIUM

Delirium is an acute, fluctuating disturbance of attention and cognition that is distressing and carries long-term consequences. Frailty is an independent risk factor, increasing the likelihood of delirium by 66% compared to non-frail peers (Cechinel et al., 2022). Detection requires proactive screening, as subtle cases are easily missed. The Single Question in Delirium ('Has this person been more confused lately?') and the 4AT tool are recommended for their speed, accuracy, and ease of use. When delirium is identified, APs should systematically address contributory factors (Figure 7.5). For APs, embedding these screening approaches within routine CGA ensures delirium is recognised early and treated promptly.

The psychological domain of CGA allows APs to identify and address depression, cognitive impairment, and delirium conditions that profoundly shape outcomes in frailty. By embedding routine screening, utilising validated tools, and adopting proactive, person-centred strategies, APs can reduce suffering, promote independence, and integrate psychological well-being into holistic care planning. For APs, this domain is central to safeguarding mental health, supporting autonomy, and coordinating care across services.

THE SOCIAL DOMAIN

The social domain of CGA examines the interpersonal, economic, and environmental aspects of older people's lives. It encompasses relationships, social support, financial resources, living arrangements, and risks such as neglect and abuse. Although sometimes perceived as 'non-clinical', these factors profoundly

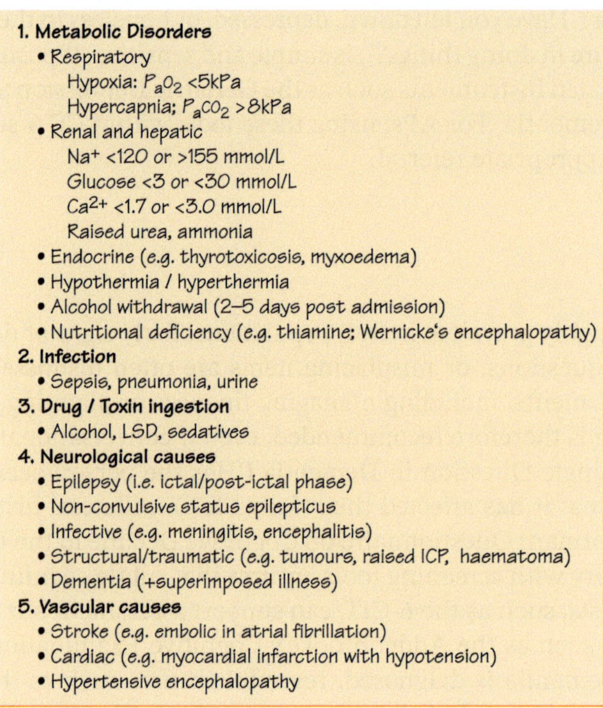

FIGURE 7.5   Causes of confusion states and coma. *Source*: Adapted from Leach et al. (2014) published by John Wiley & Sons, Ltd.

shape health outcomes, care utilisation, and well-being. For older adults living with frailty, the social environment can act as a safeguard that preserves independence or as a driver of decline where support is absent. For APs, this domain is central to holistic care, ensuring that treatment plans are aligned with the person's social reality.

Social Support, Isolation, and Loneliness

Social isolation and loneliness are recognised public health concerns. Age UK (2024) reports that almost one million older adults over 65 are often lonely, with projections suggesting that this will rise to 1.2 million by 2034. Loneliness is linked with depression, cognitive decline, malnutrition, and increased mortality (Cardona and Andrés, 2023; Kantilafti et al., 2024; Barnes et al., 2022). While isolation is an objective lack of social contact, and loneliness is the subjective perception of being alone, they frequently overlap.

Validated tools such as the UCLA Loneliness Scale (Russell et al., 1978) or the De Jong Gierveld Loneliness Scale (de Jong-Gierveld and Kamphuis, 1985) can support structured assessment, though APs may also use targeted, conversational questions such as 'Do you have someone you can call in a crisis?' or 'How often do you have meaningful contact with others?'. Observation is equally important, as indicators such as poor hygiene, withdrawn affect, or hesitancy to share information may suggest social vulnerability. For APs, assessing loneliness and isolation requires sensitivity, empathy, and the ability to link findings with personalised interventions.

Carer Needs and Burden

Where older people rely on informal carers such as spouses or adult children, the health and well-being of carers must also be considered. The Zarit Burden Interview (Zarit et al., 1980) is a widely used tool for measuring caregiver strain. High levels of burden can precipitate breakdown of home care arrangements, leading to unplanned admissions. Carers also have legal rights to assessment and support under the Care Act (2014), which APs should uphold. Carers may require access to respite services, emotional support, and benefits advice. APs are often best placed to signpost or refer carers to appropriate services and to incorporate carer well-being into care planning.

Financial Concerns

Financial well-being directly influences diet, heating, social engagement, and access to care. Many older adults are reluctant to disclose financial difficulties, but neutrally framed questions such as 'Are you managing to pay for everything you need?' or 'Would you like help checking your benefits entitlement?' can enable disclosure. Referrals to Age UK, Citizens Advice, or welfare rights organisations provide practical support, while official resources (Gov.uk, 2025) can assist with planning, including power of attorney. For APs, incorporating financial concerns into CGA is essential, as financial insecurity is often hidden yet closely linked to poorer health.

Spiritual and Cultural Well-being

The cultural and spiritual significance of social roles cannot be underestimated. For many older adults, family structures, religious practice, and community engagement form the core of identity and belonging (BGS, 2025b). Loss of these roles due to illness, bereavement, or relocation may lead to spiritual distress and diminished self-worth. APs should explore these dimensions sensitively, acknowledging their importance and identifying opportunities for reconnection through social prescribing, voluntary groups, or culturally specific networks. Supporting spiritual needs enhances resilience and ensures that care planning respects personal values.

Safeguarding and Modern Risks

Older adults with frailty are at greater risk of abuse, whether physical, emotional, financial, or neglect. Social isolation, dependency, and cognitive impairment all increase vulnerability. Signs may include unexplained injuries, fearfulness, controlling family dynamics, or repeated missed appointments. APs must be alert to these indicators and follow local safeguarding procedures rigorously, including referral to adult safeguarding services and capacity assessments where needed.

Digital exclusion is an emerging social risk. As healthcare increasingly relies on digital access for appointments and prescriptions, older adults without internet access or digital literacy may be disadvantaged. This can deepen isolation and exacerbate health inequalities (Mohan et al., 2024). APs should assess digital capability and, where necessary, refer patients to services offering basic training or access to devices.

Protective Factors

The social domain also highlights protective elements that can buffer against frailty. Social capital—the value of networks, trust, and reciprocity—supports well-being and resilience. Strong friendship networks, purposeful activities such as volunteering, and hobbies contribute to maintaining independence.

Frameworks such as the Five Ways to Well-being and initiatives from the National Academy for Social Prescribing (2025) provide evidence-based approaches to building resilience. APs can help older adults access interventions such as befriending schemes, day centres, Men's Sheds, or intergenerational projects. In end-of-life care, protective social interventions may involve facilitating reconciliation, enabling family visits, or supporting legacy-building.

The social domain shapes how older adults interact with the world, influences health behaviours, and mediates resilience or vulnerability. For APs, engaging with this domain demands empathy, cultural competence, and awareness of structural inequalities. By systematically addressing support networks, carer needs, financial security, spiritual well-being, and safeguarding, APs ensure that CGA is not only clinically robust but also personally meaningful.

THE ENVIRONMENTAL DOMAIN

The environmental domain of CGA explores the interaction between older adults and the spaces in which they live, move, and receive care. It encompasses home safety, accessibility, the availability of community services, and the use of assistive technology (BGS, 2025c). These elements are fundamental to supporting independence, minimising falls risk, and enhancing quality of life in people living with frailty. Frailty increases vulnerability to environmental hazards because diminished physiological reserves reduce adaptability to stressors (Hemadeh et al., 2025). For APs, a thorough environmental assessment is therefore not simply about risk identification but about creating enabling conditions that support dignity, safety, and continued participation in everyday life.

Home Safety

Older adults with frailty face significantly increased risks of domestic accidents, including falls, burns, and fractures. These are often linked to reduced mobility, slower reaction times, polypharmacy, and cognitive impairment (Montero-Odasso et al., 2022). Seemingly minor features such as inadequate lighting, uneven flooring, or cluttered spaces can present substantial hazards. Home safety assessments therefore play a central role within CGA, enabling the identification of modifiable risks.

Evidence supports the role of targeted home modifications in reducing accidents and promoting independence. Cha's systematic review found that approximately 65% of studies reported positive outcomes from environmental adaptations, including fall prevention, improved functional independence, and cost savings. Similarly, Goddard et al. (2025) highlighted that measures such as improved lighting and installable devices reduced strain and increased safety in domiciliary care settings. For APs, such findings emphasise the value of early and proactive intervention. Interventions such as grab rails, stair rails, and non-slip flooring may appear small, but they can transform confidence and prevent injury.

Equally important is the psychological impact of the environment. Perceptions of an unsafe home can foster fear of falling, leading to reduced mobility, avoidance of activity, and deconditioning. This highlights the bidirectional relationship between environment and physical capacity. APs should recognise that the role of home safety interventions extends beyond risk reduction, contributing also to confidence and engagement in daily life.

Accessibility

Accessibility extends the scope of environmental assessment beyond discrete safety hazards to consider the overall design and usability of the home. Many older people live in houses that were not designed for ageing populations, with steep stairs, narrow corridors, or inaccessible bathrooms. For individuals with frailty, such features can become major barriers to independence. A thorough CGA should therefore evaluate the physical layout and functionality of essential rooms, the adequacy of lighting, and environmental controls such as heating and ventilation. Poor temperature regulation, for example, places frail individuals at heightened risk of hypothermia in winter and heat-related illness in summer. APs should also evaluate environmental barriers to continence management, nutrition, and personal care, since these domains interact closely with functional capacity.

Accessibility interventions range from simple adaptations, such as raising toilet seats or widening doorways, to more significant modifications, such as stair lifts or bathroom reconfiguration. These can substantially reduce care needs and delay or prevent admission to long-term care facilities. However, APs must also take into account the financial context of the patient and family, as resources determine whether such changes are realistic. Collaborative discussions with occupational therapists, local authorities, and housing services are often required to facilitate sustainable adaptations.

Community Services and Support

Environmental factors cannot be separated from the broader social environment. Even the most carefully adapted homes may fail to support independence if the individual lacks access to community services or support networks. Social isolation and lack of engagement are themselves hazards associated with depression, cognitive decline, and malnutrition. APs play a vital role in bridging the gap between clinical care and community provision. This includes referral to falls prevention programmes, domiciliary care services, and voluntary sector initiatives. Involving link workers or community connectors can help embed older adults within local resources, such as lunch clubs, day centres, or social prescribing schemes. Access to these services not only addresses practical needs but also sustains social capital and promotes psychological resilience. In cases where living independently is no longer safe, APs may also support decision-making around alternative living arrangements, including sheltered housing, supported living, or residential care. These decisions should always be guided by the patient's values and future wishes, ensuring that dignity and autonomy remain central.

Technology Aids

Technology plays an increasingly important role in environmental assessment, providing tools that enhance safety, communication, and monitoring. Pendant alarms and telecare devices ensure rapid access to help in emergencies, reducing the consequences of falls or acute illness. Environmental sensors can detect hazards such as gas leaks or unsafe stove use, which are particularly relevant for those with cognitive impairment. Assistive devices such as properly fitted canes, walkers, or powered mobility aids are essential to safe movement within and beyond the home. Smart home technologies, including motion-activated lighting, remote monitoring systems, and automated reminders, offer additional layers of support. Research has demonstrated that these interventions can improve independence, reduce hospitalisation, and generate cost savings for health systems (Cha, 2025; Goddard et al., 2025). For APs, the challenge lies in balancing technological solutions with individual capacity and preferences. Digital literacy, willingness to use devices, and affordability all affect uptake. APs should therefore assess readiness and provide education, while also linking patients with community services that can offer training or financial support for technology adoption.

The environmental domain of CGA highlights how the physical and social surroundings of older adults influence safety, independence, and quality of life. For APs, systematic assessment of home safety, accessibility, community support, and technology use enables interventions that reduce risk and promote autonomy. Addressing environmental issues is not only about preventing harm but also about fostering confidence, dignity, and continued participation in community life. By making targeted adjustments and mobilising community resources, APs can transform the living environment from a source of vulnerability into a foundation for resilience.

THE FUTURE WISHES DOMAIN

'The best way to predict the future, is to predict it.'

The future wishes domain of CGA is central to person-centred care, ensuring that decisions about treatment, care planning, and living arrangements are aligned with an individual's preferences, values, and level of frailty (BGS, 2025d). Unlike end-of-life care, discussions around future wishes are not confined to those who are imminently dying. Instead, they anticipate the likely progression of frailty across multiple domains and help pre-empt decisions that may arise during periods of deterioration. This process supports autonomy, reduces uncertainty, and allows patients and their families to feel prepared for future changes in health or functional ability.

Conversations and Communication

Conversations about future wishes should be approached with sensitivity, recognising that people differ in the extent to which they have considered or expressed their thoughts about illness, dying, and medical interventions (NHS England, 2022). While some older adults may already have communicated their preferences to family or made legal arrangements, many have not. APs should therefore create a compassionate and safe environment for these conversations, aware of the emotional significance they carry (Fujimoto et al., 2025).

Treatment Preferences

Future wishes may relate to relatively simple decisions, such as whether a person would consent to routine blood tests, but decline more invasive investigations such as endoscopy. Equally, they can involve complex choices about hospital admission, long-term residential care, or artificial nutrition and hydration. Documenting such preferences is essential so that they are visible to all relevant professionals and carers, and can be enacted promptly and appropriately when required. Many healthcare systems have developed templates or shared records to capture these decisions, such as electronic care planning tools accessible to paramedics and community staff during emergencies.

Legal Tools

Several legal and clinical instruments can support the documentation of future wishes. A Lasting Power of Attorney (LPA) allows a trusted person to make decisions about health, welfare, or finances if capacity is lost (UK Government, 2014; UK Government, 2025). This process must be completed when the individual has capacity and is legally binding across England and Wales, with equivalent systems in Scotland and Northern Ireland. An Advance Decision to Refuse Treatment (ADRT), sometimes referred to as a living will, is another formal mechanism through which a person can specify treatments they do not wish to receive under certain circumstances (Age UK, 2025; NHS England, 2022). ADRTs are legally enforceable, provided they are completed while the person has capacity and apply to the clinical situation at hand.

Elder abuse is a significant contributor to illness and premature death in later life. The Elder Abuse Suspicion Index is a validated screening instrument that supports clinicians, including family physicians, in recognising and addressing suspected abuse (Box 7.1).

Box 7.1   Elder Abuse Suspicion Index: Questions 1 Through 5 are Asked of the Patient, and Question 6 Is Answered by the Physician; 1 or More Positive Responses on Questions 2–6 Could Suggest Elder Abuse

Question: over the past 12 months…	Answer (circle one)	
1. Have you relied on people for any of the following: bathing, dressing, shopping, banking, or meals?	Yes	No
2. Has anyone prevented you from getting food, clothes, medication, glasses, hearing aids, or medical care, or from being with people you wanted to be with?	Yes	No
3. Have you been upset because someone talked to you in a way that made you feel shamed or threatened?	Yes	No
4. Has anyone tried to force you to sign papers or to use your money against your will?	Yes	No
5. Has anyone made you afraid, touched you in ways that you did not want, or hurt you physically?	Yes	No
6. Doctor: Elder abuse might be associated with findings such as poor eye contact, withdrawn nature, malnourishment, hygiene issues, cuts, bruises, inappropriate clothing, or medication compliance issues. Did you notice any of these today or in the past 12 months?	Yes	No

Source: Adapted from Yaffe and Tazkarji (2012).

Emergency Care and Escalation Planning

The Recommended Summary Plan for Emergency Care and Treatment (ReSPECT) has increasingly replaced traditional 'Do Not Attempt Cardiopulmonary Resuscitation' (DNACPR) forms in the UK (Resuscitation Council UK, 2025). Unlike the older one-dimensional documentation, the ReSPECT form provides a broader framework for recording treatment preferences, escalation limits, and legally binding directives. It is designed to be a concise yet comprehensive record accessible in emergencies, ensuring that decisions reflect the patient's values rather than being driven solely by clinical assumptions.

In addition, treatment escalation plans and local initiatives, such as future planning resources and e-learning modules on advanced care planning (`https://portal.e-lfh.org.uk/Component/Details/391377`), help APs embed structured approaches into routine practice. The inclusion of family members and carers in these discussions is vital, both to ensure understanding of the patient's wishes and to reduce the burden of uncertainty on relatives during crises.

The future wishes domain therefore plays a vital role in CGA by ensuring that older adults with frailty remain central to decisions about their care. It is not only a matter of medical planning but also an ethical commitment to uphold dignity, autonomy, and personhood in later life. When well implemented, this domain fosters coordinated care across community, primary, and hospital settings, preventing unnecessary interventions and supporting older people to live and ultimately die in accordance with their values.

NEXT STEPS: IMPLEMENTATION

The true value of CGA lies in its practical application. While the principles and domains provide a structured framework, it is through real-world implementation that its benefits for older people are realised. Embedding CGA into routine care requires commitment, flexibility, and collaboration across MDTs. It is not a one-off assessment but a dynamic process that must adapt to the individual's changing needs and circumstances. Successful implementation often depends on leadership, staff training, and clear pathways to ensure that information from CGA translates into meaningful, coordinated care plans. Lessons learned from practice highlight the importance of early involvement of patients and carers, effective use of shared documentation, and integration of CGA findings into existing services such as frailty pathways, community nursing, and hospital admission avoidance schemes. The author encourages colleagues to view CGA not simply as an additional task, but as a way of working that supports person-centred, holistic care. Sharing practical experiences and innovations can help refine approaches and overcome barriers such as workforce pressures, time constraints, or digital exclusion.

Case Study 7.1   An AP-LED CGA in General Practice Surgery

Mrs. D, a 79-year-old woman, attended her general practice surgery for a review with the AP. She had a history of hypertension, type 2 diabetes, osteoarthritis, urinary incontinence, and depression. Her daughter, who accompanied her, expressed concerns about two recent falls, increasing forgetfulness, and reduced confidence in daily activities. At the time of review, Mrs. D was prescribed amlodipine 10 mg once daily, Bendroflumethiazide 2.5 mg once daily, metformin 500 mg three times daily, gliclazide 80 mg twice daily, simvastatin 40 mg at night, amitriptyline 25 mg at night, citalopram 20 mg once daily, oxybutynin 5 mg three times daily, omeprazole 20 mg once daily, paracetamol 1 g four times daily as required, and ibuprofen 400 mg three times daily as required. Using the ACB calculator, the AP identified that amitriptyline scored 3, oxybutynin scored 3, and citalopram scored 1, giving a cumulative score of 7 (King and Rabino, 2024), which is strongly associated with falls, constipation, confusion, and delirium in frail older adults. Mrs. D's blood pressure was recorded at 128/68 mmHg, which raised concern that tight control, in combination with thiazide therapy, was contributing to her instability and recent falls.

The AP applied the CGA across all six domains. Within the physical domain, the focus was on multimorbidity and medication risk, with frailty screening using the CFS confirming a score of 5 (Rockwood et al., 2005). Functionally, Mrs. D was independent in her personal care but increasingly dependent on her daughter for shopping, finances, and cooking. She described difficulty climbing stairs because of knee pain and a fear of falling, with her daughter reporting that she was reluctant to leave the house alone. Psychologically, Mrs. D admitted to fluctuating mood and worsening forgetfulness. Her Abbreviated Mental Test (AMT-10) score was 7/10, suggesting possible mild cognitive impairment in addition to longstanding depression. Her sleep was disturbed by nocturia, raising further concerns about fatigue and reduced resilience. From a social perspective, she lived alone in a two-storey house, with her daughter visiting twice weekly. She had become increasingly socially isolated and had disengaged from community groups that she previously attended. Environmental assessment revealed hazards within the home, including loose rugs and the absence of stair rails, while the location of her bathroom upstairs exacerbated continence difficulties and increased falls risk. In terms of future wishes, Mrs. D stated clearly that she wanted to remain at home for as long as possible and avoid hospital admission if safe to do so, with her daughter agreeing but requesting reassurance that additional support would be put in place.

The AP led a structured polypharmacy review, guided by the Scottish 7-Step Approach and STOPP/START criteria (O'Mahony et al., 2015), and framed around shared decision-making (Scottish Government Polypharmacy Model of Care Group, 2018). Using the Ask 3 Questions model, the AP encouraged Mrs. D and her daughter to consider their options: whether to continue her current medicines or reduce treatment burden, the benefits and risks of deprescribing, and what support would be available to help them decide. Together, they agreed on a plan to taper amitriptyline over two weeks and switch to duloxetine 30 mg once daily for neuropathic pain, providing a lower anticholinergic risk. Oxybutynin was discontinued, with bladder retraining and referral to a continence nurse arranged. Citalopram was switched to sertraline 50 mg daily, a safer option with reduced risk of hyponatraemia. Bendroflumethiazide was deprescribed, as it posed a significant risk for hyponatraemia and hypotension, with blood pressure to be monitored against frailty-adjusted targets of <150/90 mmHg. Simvastatin was also stopped, as the marginal long-term benefit in the context of frailty did not outweigh the burden of polypharmacy and aligned with Mrs. D's preferences. After these changes, her revised ACB score was 0, reflecting a substantial reduction in her risk of anticholinergic adverse effects.

The AP coordinated with the community pharmacist to optimise medicines and ensure safe withdrawal, referred Mrs. D to the memory clinic for further cognitive assessment, and requested an occupational therapy home visit for falls prevention and safety modifications. Anticipatory care planning was introduced, with her preferences documented to ensure care aligned with her goals. At the six-week follow-up, Mrs. D reported fewer dizzy spells, improved bowel function, and better confidence leaving the house, with no further falls. Her daughter observed that she appeared brighter and more engaged. This case demonstrates how an AP in general practice applied CGA as a multidimensional process, integrating frailty assessment, functional review, medication optimisation, psychological screening, social and environmental evaluation, and future care planning. By applying validated tools, using prescribing authority, and embedding shared decision-making, the AP ensured that deprescribing reduced harm and promoted independence, aligning care with what mattered most to the patient.

CGA in End-of-Life Medicine

CGA remains important even at the end of life (EoL), as it helps distinguish when deterioration reflects a palliative rather than restorative trajectory. In this context, CGA shifts focus from aggressive treatment and rehabilitation to careful symptom management, advanced care planning, and alignment of care with the person's values and goals. For APs, the role lies not only in identifying the physical burden of frailty but also in addressing psychological, social, environmental, and future wishes domains in order to ensure dignity, comfort, and person-centred care. Early involvement of patients and families in these discussions is essential, and when individuals lack capacity, previous wishes or best interests must guide decisions.

Case Study 7.2   CGA in EoL

Mr. F, an 86-year-old man with advanced heart failure, chronic kidney disease, and severe frailty (CFS score 8), was reviewed by an AP in his own home after increasing episodes of breathlessness and reduced oral intake. His daughter reported that he was sleeping most of the day, eating very little, and struggling with fatigue. A physical review revealed bilateral ankle oedema, oxygen saturation of 89% on air, and a markedly reduced exercise tolerance. Functionally, Mr. F was largely bedbound and reliant on carers for all ADLs. Psychologically, he expressed feelings of exhaustion and acknowledged that repeated hospital admissions had become 'too much'. Socially, his daughter provided round-the-clock care but admitted she was struggling, and environmental assessment highlighted that his small, terraced home was poorly suited to further medical interventions. When discussing future wishes, Mr. F stated clearly that he wanted no further hospital admissions, preferring to remain at home with his family.

The AP used CGA to frame care planning, ensuring a holistic approach. The physical domain highlighted the symptom burden of heart failure and renal disease, while the functional and psychological domains captured his loss of independence and emotional fatigue. The social and environmental domains confirmed carer strain and practical limitations, while the future wishes domain established his preference for home-based palliative care. This multidimensional assessment guided decision-making away from hospital-based interventions towards anticipatory care planning. The AP organised community palliative care input, initiated anticipatory medications for breathlessness and anxiety, and supported the daughter with information about carer support services. The outcome was a coordinated plan that prioritised Mr. F's comfort, reduced unnecessary hospital transfers, and ensured that care was aligned with his expressed values. This scenario demonstrates that CGA at the EoL is not redundant but transformative, reframing the goals of care around what matters most to the person. For APs, applying CGA in this way ensures that clinical expertise, prescribing authority, and leadership skills are used to promote dignified, person-centred care at life's final stage.

CONCLUSION

CGA provides APs and the wider MDT with a structured, evidence-based way to address the multidimensional needs of older adults living with frailty. By working systematically across the physical, functional, psychological, social, environmental, and future wishes domains, CGA delivers coordinated, person-centred care that adapts to change over time. The evidence base shows that CGA improves survival and function, reduces admissions, and is cost-effective across community and hospital settings. APs contribute advanced assessment, medication optimisation, and leadership for shared decision-making that reflects what matters to the person. CGA remains equally valuable at EoL, when priorities shift from restoration to comfort, dignity, and alignment with the person's goals.

Take-Home Messages

1. CGA is a multidimensional, multidisciplinary process spanning six domains that together guide a coordinated care plan.
2. CGA requires collaboration across the MDT; APs often lead on advanced assessment, medication optimisation, and care coordination.
3. Strong evidence supports CGA for improving outcomes and reducing costs across settings.
4. Validated tools such as CFS, STOPP/START, ACB calculators, Barthel Index, and AMT-10 enable consistent, evidence-informed practice.
5. CGA is dynamic and should be reviewed regularly to reflect changes in health, function, and personal priorities.

6. At EoL, CGA reframes goals towards symptom relief, anticipatory planning, and respect for values and preferences.
7. APs use clinical reasoning, prescribing authority, and service leadership to translate CGA findings into practical, person-centred action.

SELF-ASSESSMENT QUESTIONS

1. How do the six domains of CGA interact to create a holistic picture that informs decision-making?
2. Which tools would you select to assess physical and functional domains in your setting, and what trade-offs do they involve?
3. How can APs use CGA to identify and address polypharmacy risks while aligning with the person's goals?
4. In what ways does the focus of CGA change at EoL, and how do you ensure that this shift is reflected in care plans and conversations?
5. What local barriers limit routine use of CGA, and what actions can APs take to embed CGA reliably in everyday workflows?

REFERENCES

Abbey, J., Piller, N., De Bellis, A. et al. (2004). The Abbey Pain Scale: a 1-minute numerical indicator for people with end-stage dementia. *International Journal of Palliative Nursing* 10 (1): 6–13.

Age UK (2024). *Age UK's New Report Shows 'You Are Not Alone in Feeling Lonely'*. Age UK [Online]. Published 02 December 2024 www.ageuk.org.uk/latest-press/articles/age-uks-new-report-shows-you-are-not-alone-in-feeling-lonely (accessed 30 August 2025).

Age UK (2025). *What Is a Living Will (Advance Decision)?* Age UK [Online]. Last updated 10 February 2025 www.ageuk.org.uk/information-advice/money-legal/legal-issues/advance-decisions (accessed 31 August 2025).

Ahmed, H., Farewell, D., Jones, H.M. et al. (2018). Incidence and antibiotic prescribing for clinically diagnosed urinary tract infection in older adults in UK primary care. *PLoS One* 13 (1): e0190521.

Ali, A., Arif, A.W., Bhan, C. et al. (2018). Managing chronic pain in the elderly: an overview of the recent therapeutic advancements. *Cureus* 10 (9): e3293.

Ambler, G.K., Kotta, P.A., Zielinski, L. et al. (2020). The effect of frailty on long term outcomes in vascular surgical patients. *European Journal of Vascular and Endovascular Surgery* 60 (2): 264–272. https://doi.org/10.1016/j.ejvs.2020.04.009.

Asai, T., Oshima, K., Fukumoto, Y. et al. (2018). *Association of fall history with the timed up and go test among independent community-dwelling older adults. Geriatrics & Gerontology International* 18 (6): 1189–1193.

Barnes, T.L., Ahuja, M., MacLeod, S. et al. (2022). Loneliness, social isolation, and all-cause mortality in a large sample of older adults. *Journal of Aging and Health* 34 (6–8): 883–892.

Best Practice Advocacy Centre New Zealand (bpacnz) (2024). Anticholinergic burden: reducing the risk of adverse effects in older people. Published 15 March. https://bpac.org.nz/2024/anticholinergic.aspx (accessed 5 September 2025).

Blundell, A. and Gordon, A. (2015). *Geriatric Medicine at a glance*. John Wiley & Sons.

Borson, S., Scanlan, J.M., Brush, M. et al. (2000). The Mini-Cog: a cognitive "vital signs" measure for dementia screening in multi-lingual elderly. *International Journal of Geriatric Psychiatry* 15 (11): 1021–1027.

Briggs, R., McDonough, A., Ellis, G. et al. (2022). Comprehensive geriatric assessment for community-dwelling, high-risk, frail, older people. *Cochrane Database of Systematic Reviews* 5 (5): CD012705.

British Association of Urological Surgeons (BAUS) (2024). Prostate symptoms (bladder outlet obstruction). `www.baus.org.uk/patients/conditions/9/prostate_symptoms_bladder_outlet_obstruction` (accessed 5 September 2025).

British Geriatrics Society (2018). CGA in primary care settings: functional and social assessment. `www.bgs.org.uk/4-cga-in-primary-care-settings-functional-and-social-assessment` (accessed 27 August 2025).

British Geriatrics Society (2023). *Be Proactive: Delivering Proactive Care for Older People with Frailty*. London: BGS `www.bgs.org.uk/sites/default/files/content/attachment/2024-11-13/Be%20proactive%20-%20Delivering%20proactive%20care%20for%20older%20people%20with%20frailty.pdf` (accessed 27 August 2025).

British Geriatrics Society (2025a). *BGS Key Messages: Older People's Healthcare*. London: British Geriatrics Society `www.bgs.org.uk/keymsgs` (accessed 30 August 2025).

British Geriatrics Society (2025b). *Comprehensive Geriatric Assessment (CGA): Social Domain*. London: British Geriatrics Society `www.bgs.org.uk/cga-social-domain` (accessed 30 August 2025).

British Geriatrics Society (2025c). *Comprehensive Geriatric Assessment (CGA): Environmental Domain*. London: British Geriatrics Society `www.bgs.org.uk/cga-environmental-domain` (accessed 30 August 2025).

British Geriatrics Society (2025d). *Comprehensive Geriatric Assessment (CGA): Future Wishes*. London: British Geriatrics Society. Published 18 June 2025 `www.bgs.org.uk/cga-future-wishes` (accessed 30 August 2025).

British Geriatrics Society (2025e). *Comprehensive Geriatric Assessment (CGA) Hub* [Online]. `www.bgs.org.uk/CGA` (accessed 25 September 2025).

Brown, R.L. and Barrett, A.E. (2011). Visual impairment and quality of life among older adults: an examination of explanations for the relationship. *The Journals of Gerontology: Series B, Psychological Sciences and Social Sciences*. 66B (3): 364–373.

Cardona, M. and Andrés, P. (2023). Are social isolation and loneliness associated with cognitive decline in ageing? *Frontiers in Aging Neuroscience* 15: 1075563.

Cechinel, C., Lenardt, M.H., Rodrigues, J.A.M. et al. (2022). Frailty and delirium in hospitalized older adults: a systematic review with meta-analysis. *Revista Latino-Americana de Enfermagem* 30: e3687.

Cederholm, T., Jensen, G.L., Correia, M.I.T.D. et al. (2019). Glim criteria for the diagnosis of malnutrition—a consensus report from the global clinical nutrition community. *Journal of Cachexia, Sarcopenia and Muscle* 10 (1): 207–217.

Cha, S.M. (2025). A systematic review of home modifications for aging in place in older adults. *Healthcare* 13 (7): 752. `https://doi.org/10.3390/healthcare13070752`.

Chan, H.K.I. and Chan, C.P.I. (2022). Managing chronic pain in older people. *Clinical Medicine* 22 (4): 292–294. `https://doi.org/10.7861/clinmed.2022-0274`.

Chen, S.M., Wu, C.J.J., Devin, R., and Atherton, J.J. (2022). Effects of reablement programs for older people: a systematic review and meta-analysis. *Collegian 29* (6): 894–903.

Conroy, S.P. and Turpin, S. (2016). New horizons: urgent care for older people with frailty. *Age and Ageing* 45 (5): 577–584.

Conwell, Y., Van Orden, K., Caine, E.D., and Druss, B.G. (2011). Suicide in older adults. *Psychiatric Clinics of North America* 34 (2): 451–68, ix.

Dalhousie University (2025) *Comprehensive Geriatric Assessment.* Available at: `https://www.dal.ca/sites/gmr/our-tools/comprehensive-geriatric-assessment.html` (accessed 30 January 2026).

Dalton, D.S., Cruickshanks, K.J., Klein, B.E. et al. (2003). The impact of hearing loss on quality of life in older adults. *Gerontologist* 43 (5): 661–668.

Davies, L.E., Spiers, G., Kingston, A. et al. (2020). Adverse outcomes of polypharmacy in older people: systematic review of reviews. *Journal of the American Medical Directors Association* 21 (2): 181–187.

Department of Health and Social Care (DHSC) (2021). *Good for You, Good for Us, Good for Everybody: A Plan to Reduce Overprescribing to Make Patient Care Better and Safer, Support the NHS, and Reduce Carbon Emissions.* London: DHSC `https://assets.publishing.service.gov.uk/media/614a10fed3bf7f05ab786551/good-for-you-good-for-us-good-for-everybody.pdf` (accessed 5 September 2025).

Dhesi, J.K., Lees, N.P., and Partridge, J.S. (2019). Frailty in the perioperative setting. *Clinical Medicine* 19 (6): 485–489. `https://doi.org/10.7861/clinmed.2019-0283`.

Dorrington, N., Fallaize, R., Hobbs, D.A. et al. (2020). A review of nutritional requirements of adults aged $\geq$ 65 years in the UK. *The Journal of Nutrition* 150 (9): 2245–2256.

Eamer, G., Saravana-Bawan, B., van der Westhuizen, B. et al. (2017). Economic evaluations of comprehensive geriatric assessment in surgical patients: a systematic review. *Journal of Surgical Research* 218: 9–17. `https://doi.org/10.1016/j.jss.2017.03.041`.

Ellis, G., Whitehead, M.A., Robinson, D. et al. (2011). Comprehensive geriatric assessment for older adults admitted to hospital: meta-analysis of randomised controlled trials. *BMJ* 343: d6553.

Ellmers, T.J., Delbaere, K., and Kal, E.C. (2023). Frailty, falls and poor functional mobility predict new onset of activity restriction due to concerns about falling in older adults: a prospective 12-month cohort study. *European Geriatric Medicine* 14 (2): 345–351.

Erwin, D.Z. and Chen, P. (2025). Hearing loss in the elderly. In: *StatPearls.* Treasure Island, FL: StatPearls Publishing.[Internet]`https://www.ncbi.nlm.nih.gov/books/NBK580566`(accessed 5 September 2025).

Ferris, A.E. and Harding, K.G. (2020). Are chronic wounds a feature of frailty? *British Journal of General Practice* 70 (694): 256–257. `https://doi.org/10.3399/bjgp20X709829`.

Fujimoto, M., Evans, C.J., Zhou, Y. et al. (2025). Enhancing readiness for advance care planning among community-dwelling older adults with frailty: a mixed-method systematic review. *International Journal of Nursing Studies* 168: 105111.

Goddard, K.S., Hall, J.P., Greiman, L. et al. (2025). Examining the effects of home modifications on perceptions of exertion and safety among people with mobility disabilities. *Disability and Health Journal* 18 (3): 101590. `https://doi.org/10.1016/j.dhjo.2024.101590`.

Hamada, S., Sasaki, Y., Son, B.K. et al. (2024). Association of coexistence of frailty and depressive symptoms with mortality in community-dwelling older adults: Kashiwa Cohort Study. *Archives of Gerontology and Geriatrics* 119: 105322.

Hemadeh, A., Lema-Arranz, C., Bonassi, S. et al. (2025). Lifestyle, environment and other major determinants of frailty in older adults: a population-based study from the UK biobank. *Biogerontology* 26 (3): 1–23. `https://doi.org/10.1007/s10522-025-10152-8`.

Hodkinson, H.M. (1972). Evaluation of a mental test score for assessment of mental impairment in the elderly. *Age and Ageing* 1 (4): 233–238.

Howard, R.L., Avery, A.J., Slavenburg, S. et al. (2006). Which drugs cause preventable admissions to hospital? A systematic review. *British Journal of Clinical Pharmacology* 63 (2): 512–526. https://doi.org/10.1111/j.1365-2125.2006.02794.x.

de Jong-Gierveld, J. and Kamphuis, F. (1985). The development of a Rasch-type loneliness scale. *Journal of Psychology: Interdisciplinary and Applied* 119 (3): 335–341.

Kantilafti, M., Hadjikou, A., and Chrysostomou, S. (2024). The association between malnutrition, depression and cognitive decline in free-living elderly people in Cyprus: a cross-sectional study. *BMC Public Health* 24 (1): 3556. https://doi.org/10.1186/s12889-024-13556-5.

Kendall, N. and Wiltjer, H. (2019). Assessment of older people 3: assessing the functional domain. *Nursing Times* 115 (7): 52–55.

Khor, P.Y., Vearing, R.M., and Charlton, K.E. (2022). The effectiveness of nutrition interventions in improving frailty and its associated constructs related to malnutrition and functional decline among community-dwelling older adults: a systematic review. *Journal of Human Nutrition and Dietetics* 35 (3): 566–582.

King, R. and Rabino, S. (2024). ACB calculator. A tool for Calculating Anticholinergic Cognitive Burden (ACB) scores. https://www.acbcalc.com (accessed 6 September 2025).

Laur, C., McNicholl, T., Valaitis, R., and Keller, H. (2017). Malnutrition or frailty? Overlap and evidence gaps in the diagnosis and treatment of frailty and malnutrition. *Applied Physiology, Nutrition, and Metabolism* 42 (5): 449–458.

Leach, R.M., Moore, S., and Cooke, M. (2014). *Acute medicine: a practical guide to the management of medical emergencies*, 2nde. Oxford: Wiley-Blackwell.

Lundqvist, M., Alwin, J., Henriksson, M. et al. (2018). Cost-effectiveness of comprehensive geriatric assessment at an ambulatory geriatric unit based on the AGe-FIT trial. *BMC Geriatrics* 18 (1): 32.

Martinsson, L. and Eksborg, S. (2006). Activity index: a complementary ADL scale to the Barthel Index in the acute stage in patients with severe stroke. *Cerebrovascular Diseases* 22 (4): 231–239.

McCarthy, L.M., Savage, R.D., Dalton, K. et al. (2022). ThinkCascades: a tool for identifying clinically important prescribing cascades affecting older people. *Drugs & Aging* 39 (10): 829–840. https://doi.org/10.1007/s40266-022-00964-9.

Mohan, R., Saleem, F., Voderhobli, K., and Sheikh-Akbari, A. (2024). Ensuring sustainable digital inclusion among the elderly: a comprehensive analysis. *Sustainability* 16 (17): 7485.

Mol, A., Bui Hoang, P.T.S., Sharmin, S. et al. (2019). *Orthostatic hypotension and falls in older adults: a systematic review and meta-analysis. Journal of the American Medical Directors Association* 20 (5): 589–597.e5.

Montero-Odasso, M., van der Velde, N., Martin, F.C. et al. (2022). World guidelines for falls prevention and management for older adults: a global initiative. *Age and Ageing* 51 (9): afac205. https://doi.org/10.1093/ageing/afac205.

National Academy for Social Prescribing (2025) National Academy for Social Prescribing. https://socialprescribingacademy.org.uk (accessed 30 August 2025).

National Institute for Health and Care Excellence (2024). How should I assess a person's risk of developing a pressure ulcer? https://cks.nice.org.uk/topics/pressure-ulcers/diagnosis/risk-assessment (accessed 27 August 2025).

National Institute for Health and Care Excellence (NICE) (2015). Medicines optimisation: the safe and effective use of medicines to enable the best possible outcomes (NG5). www.nice.org.uk/guidance/ng5 (accessed 5 September 2025).

National Institute for Health and Care Excellence (NICE) (2016). *Multimorbidity: Quality Standard [QS136]. Quality Statement 2: Comprehensive Geriatric Assessment*. London: NICE www.nice.org.uk/guidance/qs136/chapter/Quality-statement-2-Comprehensive-geriatric-assessment (accessed 27 August 2025).

National Institute for Health and Care Excellence (NICE) (2017). Medicines optimisation: structured medication review (QS120). www.nice.org.uk/guidance/qs120 (accessed 5 September 2025).

National Institute for Health and Care Excellence (NICE) (2022). Faecal incontinence in adults: clinical knowledge summary. Last revised September 2022. https://cks.nice.org.uk/topics/faecal-incontinence-in-adults (accessed 5 September 2025).

National Institute for Health and Care Excellence (NICE) (2023). Multimorbidity: clinical knowledge summary. https://cks.nice.org.uk/topics/multimorbidity (accessed 5 September 2025).

National Institute for Health and Care Excellence (NICE) (2025). Falls: assessment and prevention in older people and in people 50 and over at higher risk (NG249). www.nice.org.uk/guidance/ng249 (accessed 5 September 2025).

National Osteoporosis Guideline Group (NOGG) (2021). Clinical guideline for the prevention and treatment of osteoporosis. www.nogg.org.uk/full-guideline (accessed 5 September 2025).

NHS Business Services Authority (NHSBSA) (2025). Polypharmacy prescribing comparators. https://www.nhsbsa.nhs.uk/prescription-data/analysis/medicines-optimisation/polypharmacy-prescribing-comparators (accessed 5 September 2025).

NHS England (2022). *Universal Principles for Advance Care Planning*. NHS England [Online]. https://www.england.nhs.uk/wp-content/uploads/2022/03/universal-principles-for-advance-care-planning.pdf (accessed 30 August 2025).

NHS England (2025). Five steps to mental wellbeing. https://www.nhs.uk/mental-health/self-help/guides-tools-and-activities/five-steps-to-mental-wellbeing (accessed 30 August 2025).

Ni Lochlainn, M., Cox, N.J., Wilson, T. et al. (2021). Nutrition and frailty: opportunities for prevention and treatment. *Nutrients* 13 (7): 2349.

Nord, M., Lyth, J., Alwin, J., and Marcusson, J. (2021). Costs and effects of comprehensive geriatric assessment in primary care for older adults with high risk for hospitalisation. *BMC Geriatrics* 21 (1): 263.

O'Mahony, D., O'Sullivan, D., Byrne, S. et al. (2015). STOPP/START criteria for potentially inappropriate prescribing in older people: version 2. *Age and Ageing* 44 (2): 213–218. https://doi.org/10.1093/ageing/afu145.

Orcel, V., Banh, L., Bastuji-Garin, S. et al. (2024). Effectiveness of comprehensive geriatric assessment adapted to primary care when provided by a nurse or a general practitioner: the CEpiA cluster-randomised trial. *BMC Medicine* 22 (1): 414.

Özdemir, Ç. and Telli, H. (2024). Evaluation of pain, activities of daily living, mood changes, and stress levels in frail individuals. *Turkish Journal of Osteoporosis*. 30: 157–163.

Panayi, A.C., Orkaby, A.R., Sakthivel, D. et al. (2019). Impact of frailty on outcomes in surgical patients: a systematic review and meta-analysis. *American Journal of Surgery* 218 (2): 393–400. https://doi.org/10.1016/j.amjsurg.2018.11.020.

Parkinson, E., Hooper, L., Fynn, J. et al. (2023). Low-intake dehydration prevalence in non-hospitalised older adults: systematic review and meta-analysis. *Clinical Nutrition* 42 (8): 1510–1520.

Payne, R.A., Avery, A.J., Duerden, M. et al. (2014). Is polypharmacy always hazardous? A retrospective cohort analysis using linked electronic health records from primary and secondary care. *British Journal of Clinical Pharmacology* 77 (6): 1073–1082.

Pirmohamed, M., James, S., Meakin, S. et al. (2004). Adverse drug reactions as cause of admission to hospital: prospective analysis of 18,820 patients. *BMJ* 329 (7456): 15–19.

Preston, J. and Biddell, B. (2021). The physiology of ageing and how these changes affect older people. *Medicine* 49 (1): 1–5.

Resuscitation Council UK (2025). *ReSPECT: Recommended Summary Plan for Emergency Care and Treatment.* Resuscitation Council UK [Online]. www.resus.org.uk/respect (accessed 31 August 2025).

Rockwood, K., Song, X., MacKnight, C. et al. (2005). A global clinical measure of fitness and frailty in elderly people. *CMAJ* 173 (5): 489–495. https://doi.org/10.1503/cmaj.050051.

Royal College of Emergency Medicine (RCEM) (2025). *Care of Older People in the Emergency Department.* London: RCEM https://rcem.ac.uk/wp-content/uploads/2025/04/Care-of-Older-People-in-the-Emergency-Department.pdf (accessed 27 August 2025).

Royal College of Physicians (RCP) (2015). *New Toolkit Aims to Improve Care for Frail Older People.* London: RCP www.rcp.ac.uk/news-and-media/news-and-opinion/new-toolkit-aims-to-improve-care-for-frail-older-people (accessed 27 August 2025).

Royal College of Physicians and British Geriatrics Society (2015). *Comprehensive geriatric assessment toolkit for hospitals.* London: Royal College of Physicians. Available at: https://www.rcp.ac.uk/news-and-media/news-and-opinion/new-toolkit-aims-to-improve-care-for-frail-older-people/ (accessed 31 January 2026).

Royal National Institute of Blind People (2025). Key information and statistics on sight loss in the UK. www.rnib.org.uk/professionals/research-and-data/key-information-and-statistics-on-sight-loss-in-the-uk (accessed 5 September 2025).

Russell, D., Peplau, L.A., and Ferguson, M.L. (1978). Developing a measure of loneliness. *Journal of Personality Assessment* 42 (3): 290–294.

Sang, N., Liu, R.C., Zhang, M.H. et al. (2024). Changes in frailty and depressive symptoms among middle-aged and older Chinese people: a nationwide cohort study. *BMC Public Health* 24 (1): 301.

Schofield, P. (2018). The assessment of pain in older people: UK national guidelines. *Age and Ageing* 47 (Suppl. 1): i1–i22.

Scottish Government Polypharmacy Model of Care Group (2018). *Polypharmacy Guidance, Realistic Prescribing,* 3e. Scottish Government [Online]. http://therapeutics.scot.nhs.uk/wp-content/uploads/2018/04/Polypharmacy-Guidance-2018.pdf.

Singh, S., Gray, A., Shepperd, S. et al. (2022). Is comprehensive geriatric assessment hospital at home a cost-effective alternative to hospital admission for older people? *Age and Ageing* 51 (1): afab220.

Smith, T.O. and Harvey, K. (2022). Psychometric properties of pain measurements for people living with dementia: a COSMIN systematic review. *European Geriatric Medicine* 13 (5): 1029–1045.

Swinnerton, E. and Price, A. (2023). Recognising, reducing and preventing deconditioning in hospitalised older people. *Nursing Older People* 35 (2): 34–41.

Thomson, K.H., Rice, S., Arisa, O. et al. (2022). Effectiveness and cost-effectiveness of oral nutritional supplements in frail older people who are malnourished or at risk of malnutrition: a systematic review and meta-analysis. *The Lancet Healthy Longevity* 3 (10): e654–e666.

Triolo, F., Sjöberg, L., Calderón-Larrañaga, A. et al. (2023). Late-life depression and multimorbidity trajectories: the role of symptom complexity and severity. *Age and Ageing* 52 (2): afac315.

UK Government (2014). *Care Act 2014.* London: The Stationery Office www.legislation.gov.uk/ukpga/2014/23/contents/enacted (accessed 30 August 2025).

UK Government (2025). *Make, Register or End a Lasting Power of Attorney: Overview.* GOV.UK [Online]. `https://www.gov.uk/power-of-attorney` (accessed 30 August 2025).

Veronese, N., Stubbs, B., Noale, M. et al. (2017). Polypharmacy is associated with higher frailty risk in older people: an 8-year longitudinal cohort study. *Journal of the American Medical Directors Association* 18 (7): 624–628.

Volkert, D., Beck, A.M., Cederholm, T. et al. (2019). ESPEN guideline on clinical nutrition and hydration in geriatrics. *Clinical Nutrition* 38 (1): 10–47.

Völter, C., Thomas, J.P., Maetzler, W. et al. (2021). Sensory dysfunction in old age. *Deutsches Ärzteblatt International* 118 (29–30): 512–520.

Ward, G., Jagger, C., and Harper, W. (1998). A review of instrumental ADL assessments for use with elderly people. *Reviews in Clinical Gerontology* 8 (1): 65–71.

Warden, V., Hurley, A.C., and Volicer, L. (2003). Development and psychometric evaluation of the Pain Assessment in Advanced Dementia (PAINAD) scale. *Journal of the American Medical Directors Association* 4 (1): 9–15.

Wounds International (2020). *Wound balance: achieving wound healing with confidence.* London. Available at: `https://woundsinternational.com/wp-content/uploads/2023/02/3030301f766e16fe15684829ac4f20e4.pdf`: Wounds International (accessed 31 January 2026).

Xu, Y., Ji, T., Li, X. et al. (2024). The effectiveness of the comprehensive geriatric assessment for older adults with frailty in hospital settings: a systematic review and meta-analysis. *International Journal of Nursing Studies* 159: 104849.

Yaffe, M.J. and Tazkarji, B. (2012). Understanding elder abuse in family practice. *Canadian Family Physician* 58 (12): 1336–1340.

Zarit, S.H., Reever, K.E., and Bach-Peterson, J. (1980). Relatives of the impaired elderly: correlates of feelings of burden. *The Gerontologist* 20 (6): 649–655.

Zuccarino, S., Monacelli, F., Antognoli, R. et al. (2022). Exploring cost-effectiveness of the comprehensive geriatric assessment in geriatric oncology: a narrative review. *Cancers* 14 (13): 3235.

CHAPTER 8

Frailty Assessment Tools

Aim

The aim of this chapter is to provide advanced practitioners (APs) with a critical understanding of key frailty measurement tools, including the Clinical Frailty Scale (CFS), Pictorial Fit-Frail Scale (PFFS), FRAIL Scale, Edmonton Frail Scale (EFS), and Tilburg Frailty Indicator (TFI), and to demonstrate how their use supports the four pillars of the multi-professional framework (MPF) for advanced clinical practice (NHS England, 2025). The chapter equips readers to select, apply, and evaluate these tools in diverse clinical settings to improve person-centred care, safety, and service quality.

LEARNING OUTCOMES

On completion of this chapter, readers will be able to:

1. Critically appraise the conceptual basis, structure, strengths, and limitations of the CFS, PFFS, FRAIL Scale, EFS, and TFI.
2. Demonstrate how the application of these tools fulfils the MPF clinical practice capabilities across the four pillars.
3. Reflect on their own practice to identify further learning and service-development needs in the assessment and management of frailty.

SELF-ASSESSMENT QUESTIONS

1. How would you decide which frailty assessment tool is most appropriate for an older adult with complex multimorbidity in your clinical setting?
2. After completing a frailty assessment, what key indicators would prompt you to escalate care or involve a wider multidisciplinary team?

Frailty assessment tools empower every healthcare professional to recognise vulnerability early, guide interventions, and restore dignity through informed, collaborative care.

INTRODUCTION

Frailty is a multidimensional syndrome that increases vulnerability to adverse health outcomes and is now recognised as a key determinant of care planning for older adults across acute, primary, and community settings. Accurate identification and grading of frailty are essential for timely interventions, shared decision-making, and the prevention of avoidable hospital admissions. Advanced practitioners (APs) require robust, evidence-based tools that allow them to assess frailty comprehensively and consistently, while demonstrating the competencies expected at master's level clinical practice. This chapter presents five widely validated instruments for frailty assessment: Clinical Frailty Scale (CFS), Pictorial Fit-Frail Scale (PFFS), Fatigue, Resistance, Ambulation, Illnesses, Loss of weight (FRAIL) Scale, Edmonton Frail Scale (EFS), and Tilburg Frailty Indicator (TFI).

Using validated frailty assessment tools such as the CFS, PFFS, FRAIL Scale, EFS, and TFI exemplifies the breadth of knowledge, skills, and behaviours expected of APs. Through expert, holistic assessment, these tools support autonomous decision-making, critical reasoning, and evidence-based care planning, while ensuring professional accountability and recognition of personal scope and limits. They foster partnerships with individuals, families, and carers and encourage clear, person-centred communication in situations of complexity, risk, and uncertainty. Their implementation provides opportunities to lead service redesign, improve quality and safety, and build effective interprofessional relationships across organisational boundaries. By introducing and supervising their use, practitioners act as educators and mentors, strengthening team capability and supporting a culture of shared learning. Engagement in audit, evaluation, and research using frailty data drives continuous improvement, contributes to the evidence base and facilitates the dissemination of best practice. In this way, the consistent and reflective use of these instruments demonstrates advanced practice across clinical care, leadership, education and research, and evidences the high level of professional judgement and accountability required for contemporary healthcare. APs integrate these tools into routine pathways and governance structures, ensuring frailty assessment informs every stage of planning, intervention, and review.

Multi-Professional Framework (MPF) For Advanced Practitioners

(Adapted from NHS England, 2025)

This chapter maps to the following areas within the MPF:

1. Clinical practice: 1.1, 1.4, 1.6, 1.9
2. Leadership and management: 2.2, 2.4, 2.6
3. Education: 3.1, 3.3, 3.5
4. Research: 4.1, 4.3, 4.5

Accreditation Consideration

This chapter maps to the statement with the following national accretional document:

Curriculum framework for advanced practice in the care of older people (NHS England, 2022):

1. Core Capabilities (CiPs): 1.1, 1.2, 1.3, 1.4, 1.5, 1.6
2. Generic Clinical CiPs: 2.1, 2.2, 2.3, 2.4, 2.5, 2.6
3. Specialty Clinical CiPs (Older People): 3.1, 3.2, 3.3, 3.4, 3.5

Curriculum framework for APs in the case of palliative and end-of-life care (NHS England, 2023a):

1. Clinical pillar: 1.1, 1.2, 1.3, 1.4
2. Leadership and management: 2.1
3. Education: 3.1
4. Research: 4.1

Curriculum for APs in acute medicine (NHS England, 2023b):

1. Core CiPs: 1.1, 1.2, 1.3, 1.4, 1.5, 1.6
2. Generic Clinical CiPs: 2.1, 2.2, 2.3, 2.4, 2.5, 2.6
3. Specialty Clinical CiPs (Acute Medicine): 3.1, 3.2, 3.3, 3.4, 3.5 and acute medicine presentations

FRAILTY ASSESSMENT TOOLS

The Clinical Frailty Scale (CFS) was first developed in Halifax, Nova Scotia, during the Canadian Study of Health and Ageing as a means of summarising comprehensive geriatric assessments (CGAs) carried out by clinicians with varied expertise in gerontology (Rockwood et al., 2005). Initially designed as a research tool to provide an integrated view of older adults' health and to predict adverse outcomes, it soon became widely adopted in clinical practice to guide care planning (Granata et al., 2022; Church et al., 2020). The CFS is not a questionnaire but a judgement-based tool that synthesises information on comorbidities, functional status, mobility, symptoms, and cognition to categorise an individual's overall level of fitness or frailty (Rockwood and Theou, 2020). Since its introduction, the tool has been expanded from an original 7-point scale to a 9-point scale, now ranging from 'very fit' (level 1) to 'terminally ill' (level 9), thereby offering greater clinical granularity, particularly in acute-care contexts (Theou et al., 2021).

The CFS has demonstrated strong predictive validity for a range of outcomes including mortality, hospitalisation, institutionalisation, and length of stay (Wallis et al., 2015; Lee et al., 2022). A study by Zwawi et al. (2025) found that using the simplified version of the CFS (SCFS) was shown to predict 90-day mortality among emergency patients with acute dyspnoea, outperforming traditional triage systems when used in combination. Furthermore, a recent systematic review and meta-analysis reported CFS $\geq$ 5 yields sensitivity 81% (62–91), specificity 71% (54–83), LR+ 2.80 (1.96–3.82), LR– 0.29 (0.15–0.48), and AUC 0.82 (0.77–0.85) for adverse outcomes, supporting clinically meaningful rule-in/rule-out utility (Ku et al., 2025).

Its appeal lies in its simplicity, rapid applicability, and international validation across multiple settings, with use reported in more than 20 countries and translation into numerous languages (Church

CLINICAL FRAILTY SCALE

	1	**VERY FIT**	People who are robust, active, energetic and motivated. They tend to exercise regularly and are among the fittest for their age.
	2	**FIT**	People who have **no active disease symptoms** but are less fit than category 1. Often, they exercise or are very **active occasionally**, e.g., seasonally.
	3	**MANAGING WELL**	People whose **medical problems are well controlled**, even if occasionally symptomatic, but often are **not regularly active** beyond routine walking.
	4	**LIVING WITH VERY MILD FRAILTY**	Previously "vulnerable," this category marks early transition from complete independence. While **not dependent** on others for daily help, often **symptoms limit activities**. A common complaint is being "slowed up" and/or being tired during the day.
	5	**LIVING WITH MILD FRAILTY**	People who often have **more evident slowing**, and need help with **high order instrumental activities of daily living** (finances, transportation, heavy housework). Typically, mild frailty progressively impairs shopping and walking outside alone, meal preparation, medications and begins to restrict light housework.
	6	**LIVING WITH MODERATE FRAILTY**	People who need help with **all outside activities** and with **keeping house**. Inside, they often have problems with stairs and need **help with bathing** and might need minimal assistance (cuing, standby) with dressing.
	7	**LIVING WITH SEVERE FRAILTY**	**Completely dependent for personal care**, from whatever cause (physical or cognitive). Even so, they seem stable and not at high risk of dying (within ~6 months).
	8	**LIVING WITH VERY SEVERE FRAILTY**	Completely dependent for personal care and approaching end of life. Typically, they could not recover even from a minor illness.
	9	**TERMINALLY ILL**	Approaching the end of life. This category applies to people with a **life expectancy <6 months**, who are **not otherwise living with severe frailty**. (Many terminally ill people can still exercise until very close to death.)

SCORING FRAILTY IN PEOPLE WITH DEMENTIA

The degree of frailty generally corresponds to the degree of dementia. Common **symptoms in mild dementia** include forgetting the details of a recent event, though still remembering the event itself, repeating the same question/story and social withdrawal.

In **moderate dementia**, recent memory is very impaired, even though they seemingly can remember their past life events well. They can do personal care with prompting.

In **severe dementia**, they cannot do personal care without help.

In **very severe dementia** they are often bedfast. Many are virtually mute.

FIGURE 8.1   CFS. *Source*: Permission has been taken to reuse this tool.

et al., 2020). Nonetheless, important limitations exist. The CFS relies heavily on clinical judgement, which may introduce inter-rater variability, particularly among less experienced assessors (Theou et al., 2021; Ellis et al., 2025). Furthermore, while highly useful in older populations, its validity in younger adults remains underexplored (Granata et al., 2022). Importantly, the scale reflects an individual's baseline health status, typically defined as two weeks prior to an acute illness rather than their immediate clinical presentation, which is crucial when applying it in emergency or critical care (Hubbard et al., 2020). Despite these limitations, the CFS remains one of the most widely applied frailty measures in geriatric and acute medicine, supporting prognostication, risk stratification, and shared decision-making (Figure 8.1).

THE PICTORIAL FIT-FRAIL SCALE (PFFS)

The PFFS was first introduced in 2019 as a visually based assessment designed to capture the multidimensional nature of frailty across 14 domains, including mobility, function, balance, cognition, mood, and social connection (Theou et al., 2019). Its visual approach was intended to overcome literacy, language, and cultural barriers, while being suitable for administration by patients, proxies, or healthcare professionals with minimal training (McGarrigle et al., 2019). Since then, the tool has been translated and validated internationally, including in Malaysia and Greece, demonstrating feasibility, validity, and good inter-rater reliability (Ahip et al., 2023; Voukelatou et al., 2023). In addition, it is designed to be highly practical, taking less than five minutes to complete when administered by a patient or caregiver. Unlike text-based instruments, it is not dependent on language skills or health literacy, making it accessible across diverse populations. Importantly, it does not require a physical examination by healthcare professionals, thereby reducing the potential for assessor-related bias (Theou et al., 2019; McGarrigle et al., 2019). Recent research has strengthened its evidence base. A 2025 single-centre Intensive care unit (ICU) study of 168 patients aged $\geq$70 years reported that 33.3% were non-frail, 48.2% had mild–moderate frailty, and 18.5% were severely frail (Statlender et al., 2025). The frailty status, as assessed by the PFFS, predicted 90-day mortality, with hazard ratios of 2.05 (95% CI 1.01–4.18) for mild–moderate frailty and 4.35 (95% CI 1.93–9.80) for severe frailty, compared to non-frail patients (Statlender et al., 2025). However, the study also found no association between PFFS status and ICU mortality or traditional prognostic indices such as Acute Physiology and Chronic Health Evaluation II (APACHE-II) or Sequential Organ Failure Assessment (SOFA) scores, suggesting that while the PFFS is valuable for longer-term prognostication, it may have limitations in short-term critical care outcomes. Despite this challenge, the PFFS remains a promising, feasible, and culturally adaptable frailty measure, offering unique advantages over text-based tools, particularly in diverse and resource-limited clinical environments (Figure 8.2).

THE FRAIL SCALE

The FRAIL scale was introduced in 2012 as a rapid screening instrument designed to integrate aspects of both the cumulative deficit and frailty phenotype models (Morley et al., 2012). It is composed of five self-report questions that address fatigue, resistance (ability to climb stairs), ambulation, multimorbidity, and unintentional weight loss, producing a score from 0 to 5 that categorises individuals as robust, pre-frail, or frail. Its major strengths lie in its simplicity, taking less than one minute to administer, requiring no equipment, and being feasible across diverse healthcare environments including primary care, acute hospital wards, rehabilitation settings, and nursing homes (Morley, 2012; Figure 8.3).

The 5-item FRAIL Scale is simple to administer (including remotely) and suitable for short pre-assessment screening; in surgical cohorts, a meta-analysis reported markedly higher 30-day mortality for those classified as frail (OR 6.62), supporting its prognostic utility (Gong et al., 2023). A systematic review and meta-analysis by Kojima (2018) examined studies, mainly in community settings, where frailty was defined using the FRAIL scale. The review found that both frail and pre-frail status were significantly associated with higher mortality compared with robust individuals. The authors highlighted the simplicity and feasibility of the FRAIL scale, which comprises only five yes/ no questions. It is quick to administer, can be self-reported or interviewer-administered, and requires no specialist equipment. In addition, the scale is useful for stratifying risk, as it distinguishes between robust, pre-frail, and frail individuals in relation to outcomes such as mortality. Recent international evidence reinforced both the practical value and the limits of the FRAIL Scale: a large community-based cohort study in China ($n = 5,402$) showed that the FRAIL Scale predicted incident disability,

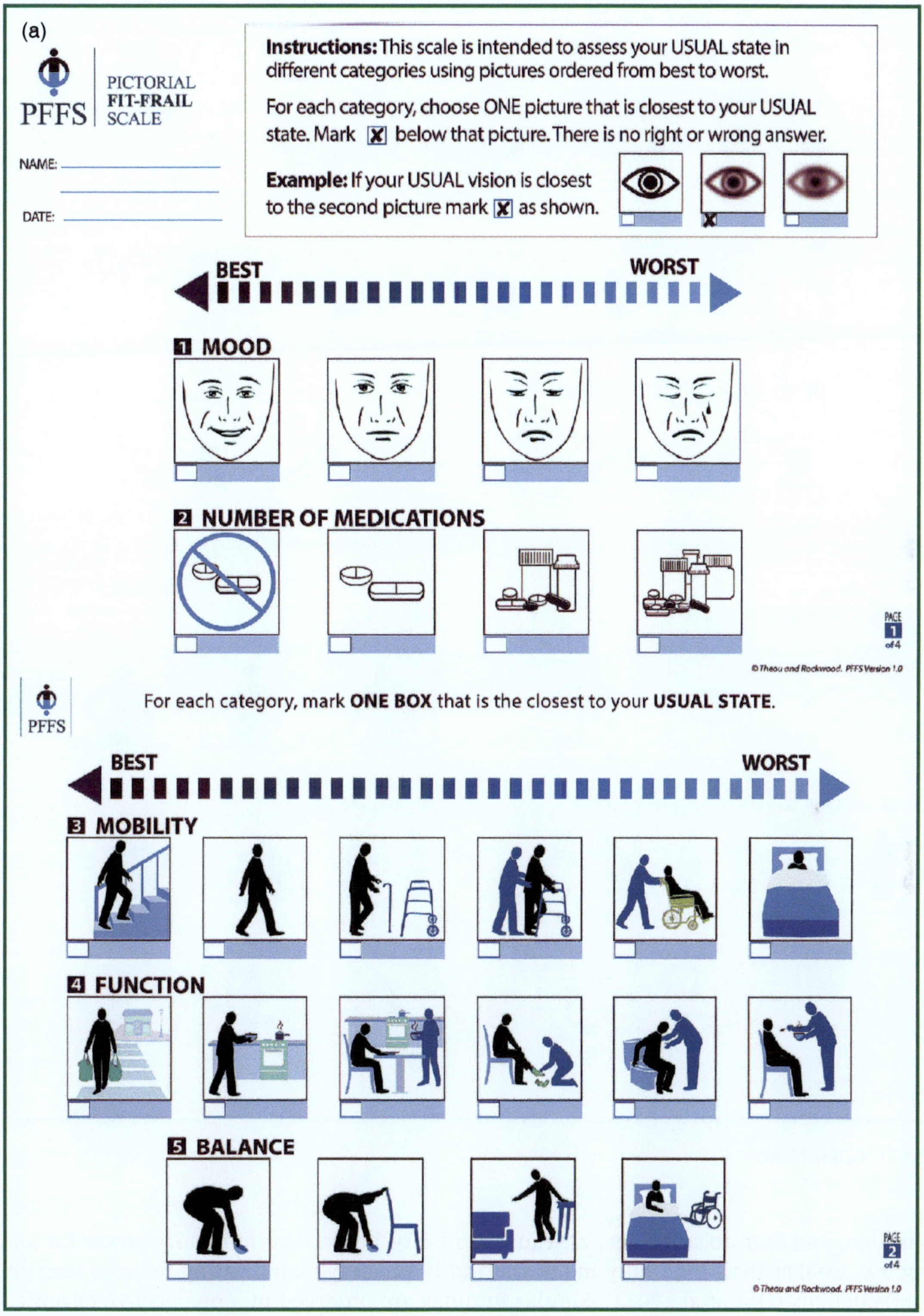

FIGURE 8.2 (a,b) The Pictorial Fit-Frail Scale. *Source*: Permission for reuse was taken.

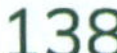

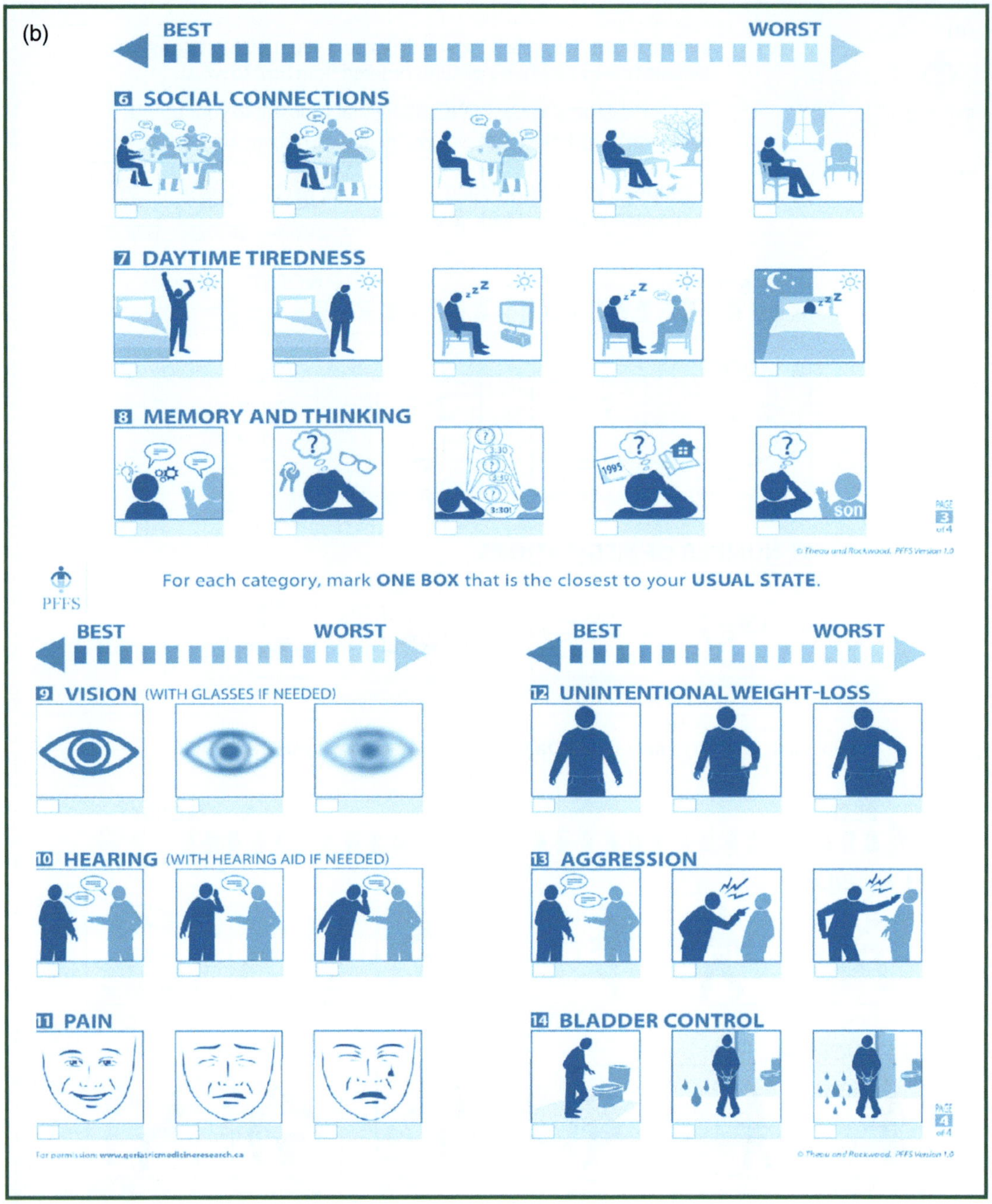

FIGURE 8.2   (Continued)

hospitalisation, and four- to seven-year all-cause mortality, but its discriminatory power for long-term mortality was weaker than the frailty index and frailty phenotype, indicating reduced sensitivity for more subtle deficits (Qin et al., 2023). Similar findings are observed in a prospective chronic kidney disease (CKD) outpatient cohort ($n = 153$), and the FRAIL Scale identified fewer frail cases than the physical frailty phenotype; in adults under 60 years, it showed a sensitivity of 41.3% and a specificity

FRAIL-NH

	0	1	2
Fatigue	No	Yes	PHQ-9 ≥10
Resistance	Independent transfer	Set up	Physical help
Ambulation	Independent	Walker	Not able/WC
Incontinence	None	Bladder	Bowel
Loss of weight	None	Yes	xxxx
Nutritional approach	Regular diet	Mechanically altered	Feeding tube
Help with dressing	Independent	Set up	Physical help
Total			0–13

Nonfrail (0–5), Prefrail (6–7), Frail (≥8)

Kaehr E, Visvanathan R, Malmstrom TK, Morley JE. Frailty in Nursing Homes: The FRAIL-NH Scale.
J Am Med Dir Assoc 2015;16(2):87.

FIGURE 8.3   The FRAIL Scale. *Source*: Kaehr et al. (2015)/with permission of Elsevier.

of 93.2%, and FRAIL-defined frailty independently predicted mortality (adjusted OR 6.8) (Rodrigues et al., 2024).

Nevertheless, recent psychometric syntheses have indicated that, while criterion validity and test–retest reliability are acceptable and feasibility is good (missing-data = 16.3%), evidence for construct validity, agreement with other instruments, and responsiveness to change remains limited or inconsistent across settings (Ng et al., 2024). Furthermore, the reliance on self-report introduces subjectivity and cut-off instability: in community data, the conventional threshold (≥3) shows low sensitivity (37%) against the Fried phenotype, whereas any positive item (≥1) improves sensitivity to ≈83% but yields many false positives, implying a two-step approach may be prudent (Rodríguez-Laso et al., 2022). However, the included studies varied in their methods, using different cut-points and definitions of pre-frail and frail, which makes pooling data and comparing results challenging (Kojima, 2018). Therefore, the FRAIL Scale is an efficient, scalable screen with a demonstrated prognostic signal, but it should be complemented by confirmatory assessment (e.g. performance-based measures or CGA) when diagnostic precision or monitoring of change is required (Gong et al., 2023).

EDMONTON FRAIL SCALE (EFS)

Developed in the early 2000s as a brief, multidimensional screen derived from CGA, the EFS was validated against geriatricians' clinical impressions and shown to be reliable in routine inpatient and outpatient practice (Rolfson et al., 2006). It samples nine domains (e.g. cognition, mood, continence, medication use, functional performance) and yields a 0–17 total score with standard severity bands (fit 0–3; vulnerable 4–5; mild 6–7; moderate 8–9; severe 10–17) (Edmonton Frail Scale, 2025).

One of the earliest adaptations was the Reported Edmonton Frail Scale (REFS), developed for acute inpatient use in 2009; it substituted the Timed Up and Go with self-reported functional items and adopted revised category thresholds suited to hospital settings (Hilmer et al., 2009). A subsequent modified REFS replaced the clock-drawing task with brief cognitive questions to improve practicality in acute care (Rose et al., 2018). A derivative Kyoto Frailty Scale distilled EFS content into a validated nine-item rapid screen (Kameda et al., 2021). An acute-care version (EFS-AC) is available under licence; it replaces performance items (e.g. Timed Up and Go test [TUG] and clock drawing) with self-report to emphasise baseline status, although formal validation against reference standards remains pending (Edmonton Frail Scale, 2025).

The EFS shows sound measurement performance when used as a screening instrument in stable settings, but its validity is less consistent in acutely unwell cohorts or when content is altered. A recent COSMIN-guided systematic review and meta-analysis (20 studies; n = 3,852) reported sufficient construct validity for the original EFS in most non-acute populations and adequate test–retest and inter-rater reliability. By contrast, modified versions—typically those omitting performance items—were significantly less likely to meet validity criteria, and results were more variable in acute care, underscoring the importance of using the unmodified tool or undertaking fresh validation when adaptations are necessary (Lee et al., 2025). In addition, in elective major abdominal surgery, a prospective observational study found that pre-operative EFS scores predicted post-operative morbidity, with 'fair' judgement for early and 30-day complications; feasibility and acceptability in clinic were good and inter-rater agreement was favourable, supporting EFS as a pragmatic pre-assessment screen rather than a stand-alone risk model (He et al., 2020). These findings are supported by other studies, a retrospective cohort analysis showed that higher EFS scores were associated with post-operative delirium in older surgical patients: while some literature suggests that phenotype-based frailty definitions can yield stronger delirium associations, EFS remains practical when a short, clinic-friendly tool is required.

For time-critical pathways, a self-report, acute-care variant (EFS-AC) has now been prospectively validated against the original instrument in 688 surgical patients ≥65 years, demonstrating excellent agreement for frailty status (AUC 0.971, 95% CI 0.958–0.983) and similar prediction of loss of independence; because it is self-administered, it permits screening in virtual clinics and on digital platforms, though services should audit local calibration. Earlier work also confirmed that the self-reported domains of EFS align well with clinician-administered scoring, strengthening the case for flexible delivery formats (Owodunni et al., 2024). Similarly, cardiovascular evidence indicates prognostic relevance but also highlights limits. In transcatheter aortic valve implantation, higher EFS scores are related to longer length of stay and higher mortality, supporting routine frailty screening before intervention (Holierook et al., 2024). Similarly, Ganesh et al. (2024) reported in a prospective single-centre elective Coronary artery bypass graft (CABG) cohort that both the EFS and EuroSCORE II showed only modest discrimination for short-term mortality (AUC 0.793 vs 0.752) and weak prediction of secondary complications, indicating the need for combined assessment and local recalibration. The study highlighted that adding the EFS to EuroSCORE II improved 30-day mortality prediction, supporting the EFS as an adjunct rather than a replacement for surgical risk scores.

Oncogeriatric data are concordant with this screening-first positioning. In a prospective radiotherapy cohort, EFS predicted overall survival and correlated strongly with the burden of geriatric impairments, helping to target CGA where it is most likely to influence care (Røyset et al., 2023). A broader oncogeriatrics analysis likewise found that higher EFS scores were independently associated with one-year mortality and with impairment load on comprehensive assessment, while also noting the need for further validation in patients who screen 'normal' on G8. Therefore, these findings suggest that EFS is an efficient front-door screen that should trigger fuller assessment when decisions with high consequences are contemplated.

THE TILBURG FRAILTY INDICATOR (TFI)

The Tilburg Frailty Indicator (TFI) was created in the Netherlands by Gobbens and colleagues in 2010 to provide a concise, self-report method of assessing frailty across physical, psychological, and social domains (Gobbens et al., 2010a). It is grounded in an integral conceptual model that links life-course determinants and disease to frailty and adverse outcomes (Gobbens et al., 2010b). The TFI comprises two sections: Part A records key determinants such as age, multimorbidity, and lifestyle, while Part B, containing 15 items, generates the frailty score used in research and practice. Evidence from multiple international validations shows strong internal consistency and good predictive validity for disability and quality-of-life outcomes (Gobbens and Uchmanowicz, 2021). Its strengths include a multidimensional approach, ease of administration without clinical examination, and suitability for diverse community and clinical settings. However, its reliance on self-report may introduce response bias, and it offers limited insight into dynamic or acute changes, meaning that CGA remains essential when complex care decisions are required.

Recent evidence confirmed both the value and the constraints of the TFI. Systematic review data show consistent internal consistency for the total score, typically with Cronbach's alpha above 0.70, and strong criterion validity for predicting disability and mortality (Gobbens et al., 2021). The tool has proved adaptable across cultures, with acceptable reliability demonstrated in new versions such as the Amharic translation (Kasa et al., 2023), and has predicted adverse outcomes in diverse clinical groups including oncology and cardiology patients. Similarly, Zhang et al. (2020) studied TFI in 2,250 community-dwelling older adults across Spain, Greece, Croatia, the Netherlands, and the United Kingdom. The full TFI showed satisfactory internal consistency (Cronbach's $\alpha \geq 0.70$) and good convergent, divergent, and concurrent validity, with most area-under-the-curve values above 0.70. However, the psychological and social subscales demonstrated weaker internal consistency. The authors concluded that the TFI is a reliable and valid tool for assessing frailty in diverse European community settings.

Its strengths lie in its multidimensional assessment covering physical, psychological, and social domains and its simple, self-administered format, which facilitates large-scale screening in community and outpatient settings. Nevertheless, some limitations recur across studies: weaker internal consistency in the psychological and social subscales, variable predictive value for healthcare utilisation, and limited evidence on responsiveness to clinical change (Balasch-Bernat et al., 2023). Exclusive reliance on self-report may introduce recall or desirability bias and can miss acute or fluctuating frailty. These considerations suggest that while the TFI is an efficient, validated screening instrument, it should complement rather than replace CGA when nuanced clinical decision-making is required (Figure 8.4).

Case Study 8.1   CFS in Acute Medicine

An 82-year-old man presents to the emergency department with pneumonia and delirium. The AP rapidly assesses baseline function and comorbidities, assigns a CFS score of 6 (moderately frail), and uses this to guide escalation decisions and early multidisciplinary input. By embedding the CFS into the acute admissions pathway and auditing outcomes, the AP demonstrates advanced clinical reasoning, interprofessional leadership, and service evaluation while teaching colleagues how to apply and interpret the scale.

Tilburg Frailty Indicator (TFI)*
Gobbens RJJ, van Assen MALM, Luijkx KG, Wijnen-Sponselee MTh, Schols JMGA. The Tilburg
Frailty Indicator: psychometric properties. J Am Med Dir Assoc 2010; 11(5):344-355.

Part A Determinants of frailty

1. Which sex are you?   0 male   0 female

2. What is your age?   .... years

3. What is your marital status?   0 married/living with partner
                                                               0 unmarried
                                                               0 separated/divorced
                                                               0 widow/widower

4. In which country were you born?   0 The Netherlands
                                                               0 Former Dutch East Indies
                                                               0 Suriname
                                                               0 Netherlands Antilles
                                                               0 Turkey
                                                               0 Morocco
                                                               0 Other, namely................

5. What is the highest level of education you have completed? 0 none or primary education
                                                               0 secondary education
                                                               0 higher professional or
                                                                  university education

6. Which category indicates your net monthly household income? 0 €600 or less
                                                               0 €601 - €900
                                                               0 €901 - €1200
                                                               0 €1201 - €1500
                                                               0 €1501 - €1800
                                                               0 €1801 - €2100
                                                               0 €2101 or more

7. Overall, how healthy would you say your lifestyle is?   0 healthy
                                                               0 not healthy, not unhealthy
                                                               0 unhealthy

8. Do you have two or more diseases and/or chronic disorders? 0 yes   0 no

9. Have you experienced one or more of the following events
    during the past year?
    -   the death of a loved one   0 yes   0 no
    -   a serious illness yourself   0 yes   0 no
    -   a serious illness in a loved one   0 yes   0 no
    -   a divorce or ending of an important intimate relationship   0 yes   0 no
    -   a traffic accident   0 yes   0 no
    -   a crime   0 yes   0 no

10. Are you satisfied with your home living environment?   0 yes   0 no

FIGURE 8.4   The Tilburg Frailty Indicator. *Source*: Gobbens et al. (2010a)/with permission of Elsevier.

Part B Components of frailty

B1   Physical components

11.	Do you feel physically healthy?	0 yes	0 no

12.   Have you lost a lot of weight recently without wishing   0 yes   0 no
      to do so?
      ('a lot' is: 6 kg or more during the last six months, or
      3 kg or more during the last month)

Do you experience problems in your daily life due to:

13.	..........difficulty in walking?	0 yes	0 no
14.	..........difficulty maintaining your balance?	0 yes	0 no
15.	..........poor hearing?	0 yes	0 no
16.	..........poor vision?	0 yes	0 no
17.	..........lack of strength in your hands?	0 yes	0 no
18.	..........physical tiredness?	0 yes	0 no

B2   Psychological components

19.	Do you have problems with your memory?	0 yes	0 sometimes	0 no
20.	Have you felt down during the last month?	0 yes	0 sometimes	0 no
21.	Have you felt nervous or anxious during the last month?	0 yes	0 sometimes	0 no
22.	Are you able to cope with problems well?	0 yes		0 no

B3   Social components

23.	Do you live alone?	0 yes		0 no
24.	Do you sometimes miss having people around you?	0 yes	0 sometimes	0 no
25.	Do you receive enough support from other people?	0 yes		0 no

* The TFI was translated into English using the method of back-translation.

Scoring Part B Components of frailty (range: 0 − 15)

Question 11:   yes = 0, no = 1

Question 12 − 18:   no = 0, yes = 1

Question 19:   no and sometimes = 0, yes = 1

Question 20 and 21:   no = 0, yes and sometimes = 1

Question 22:   yes = 0, no = 1

Question 23:   no = 0, yes = 1

Question 24:   no = 0, yes and sometimes = 1

Question 25:   yes = 0, no = 1

Cutpoint: 5

FIGURE 8.4   (Continued)

Case Study 8.2   PFFS in Culturally Diverse Primary Care

A 79-year-old woman with limited English attends a primary care clinic accompanied by her daughter. Using the Pictorial Fit-Frailty Scale, the AP overcomes language barriers and gains a multidimensional picture of frailty in less than five minutes. The results inform a tailored care plan including falls prevention and nutritional support. The AP mentors primary care staff in visual assessment methods and contributes data to a regional study on frailty and health inequalities, fulfilling education and research functions alongside clinical care.

Case Study 8.3   FRAIL Scale in Pre-Operative Assessment

A 70-year-old man scheduled for elective colorectal surgery completes the FRAIL Scale, scoring 3 (frail). The AP integrates this finding with surgical risk scores to inform shared decision-making about operative risk and post-operative support. Leading a quality improvement project to include FRAIL screening in all pre-assessment clinics, and training theatre staff to interpret results, demonstrates leadership and education capabilities, while a subsequent audit provides evidence for research and service development.

Case Study 8.4   EFS and TFI in Community Care

An AP conducting a home visit for an 85-year-old woman with multiple long-term conditions uses the Edmonton Frail Scale and Tilburg Frailty Indicator to capture physical, psychological, and social dimensions of frailty. The combined findings guide referrals to physiotherapy and social services and support a personalised anticipatory care plan. By supervising community nurses in applying these tools and leading an evaluation of their impact on unplanned admissions, the AP evidences clinical expertise, system leadership, team education, and practice-based research.

CONCLUSION

This chapter has outlined five validated frailty assessment tools including CFS, PFFS, FRAIL, EFS, and TFI, highlighting their theoretical basis, evidence, and practical application. Their use enables APs to deliver person-centred, safe, and effective care while evidencing competence across all four MPF pillars. Consistent, reflective application of these tools supports accurate risk stratification, proactive care planning, and improved outcomes for older adults living with frailty.

Take-Home Messages

1. Frailty is a multidimensional, progressive condition that requires structured, evidence-based assessment to guide timely and person-centred care.
2. CFS, PFFS, FRAIL, EFS, and TFI are well-validated instruments with differing strengths, limitations, and settings of best use; no single tool suits every clinical context.

3. Selection of an appropriate tool should be guided by patient population, purpose (screening, diagnosis, and prognostication), and available resources, with results interpreted alongside full clinical assessment.

4. Consistent use of these tools supports early identification of risk, more accurate care planning, and improved outcomes, including reduced unplanned hospital admissions and enhanced quality of life.

5. Integrating frailty assessment into routine practice helps standardise care, informs service planning, and provides data for ongoing quality improvement and research.

REFERENCES

Ahip, S.S., Ghazali, S.S., Theou, O. et al. (2023). The Pictorial Fit-Frail Scale—Malay version (PFFS-M): reliability and validity testing in Malaysian primary care. *Family Practice* 40 (2): 290–299.

Balasch-Bernat, M., Sentandreu-Mañó, T., Tomás, J.M. et al. (2023). Deepening the understanding of the structural validity of the Tilburg Frailty Indicator. *Aging Clinical and Experimental Research* 35 (6): 1263–1271.

Church, S., Rogers, E., Rockwood, K., and Theou, O. (2020). A scoping review of the clinical frailty scale. *BMC Geriatrics* 20 (1): 393.

Edmonton Frail Scale (2025). Edmonton Frail Scale (EFS). https://edmontonfrailscale.org (accessed 9 December 2025)

Ellis, H.L., Dunnell, L., Eyres, R. et al. (2025). What can we learn from 68 000 clinical frailty scale scores? Evaluating the utility of frailty assessment in emergency departments. *Age and Ageing* 54 (4): afaf093.

Ganesh, A., Ramnath, P., and Padmanabhan, C. (2024). Assessment of risk prediction Using Edmonton Frail Scale and European System for Cardiac Operative Risk Evaluation II among older patients undergoing coronary artery bypass graft surgery in a Tertiary Care Hospital in India. *Journal of the Indian Academy of Geriatrics* 20 (1): 30–33.

Gobbens, R.J. and Uchmanowicz, I. (2021). Assessing frailty with the Tilburg Frailty Indicator (TFI): a review of reliability and validity. *Clinical Interventions in Aging* 16: 863–875.

Gobbens, R.J., van Assen, M.A., Luijkx, K.G. et al. (2010a). The Tilburg frailty indicator: psychometric properties. *Journal of the American Medical Directors Association* 11 (5): 344–355.

Gobbens, R.J., Luijkx, K.G., Wijnen-Sponselee, M.T., and Schols, J.M. (2010b). Toward a conceptual definition of frail community dwelling older people. *Nursing Outlook* 58 (2): 76–86.

Gobbens, R.J., van Assen, M.A., Augustijn, H. et al. (2021). Prediction of mortality by the Tilburg Frailty Indicator (TFI). *Journal of the American Medical Directors Association* 22 (3): 607–e1.

Gong, S., Qian, D., Riazi, S. et al. (2023). Association between the FRAIL scale and postoperative complications in older surgical patients: a systematic review and meta-analysis. *Anesthesia & Analgesia* 136 (2): 251–261.

Granata, N., Vigoré, M., Steccanella, A. et al. (2022). The clinical frailty scale (CFS) employment in the frailty assessment of patients suffering from non-communicable diseases (NCDs): a systematic review. *Frontiers in Medicine* 9: 967952.

He, Y., Li, L.W., Hao, Y. et al. (2020). Assessment of predictive validity and feasibility of Edmonton Frail Scale in identifying postoperative complications among elderly patients: a prospective observational study. *Scientific Reports* 10 (1): 14682.

Hilmer, S.N., Perera, V., Mitchell, S. et al. (2009). The assessment of frailty in older people in acute care. *Australasian Journal on Ageing* 28 (4): 182–188.

Holierook, M., Henstra, M.J., Dolman, D.J. et al. (2024). Higher Edmonton Frail Scale prior to transcatheter Aortic Valve. Implantation is related to longer hospital stay and mortality. *International Journal of Cardiology* 399: 131637.

Hubbard, R.E., Maier, A.B., Hilmer, S.N. et al. (2020). Frailty in the face of COVID-19. *Age and Ageing* 49 (4): 499–500.

Kaehr, E., Visvanathan, R., Malmstrom, T.K., and Morley, J.E. (2015). Frailty in nursing homes: the FRAIL-NH scale. *Journal of the American Medical Directors Association* 16 (2): 87–89.

Kameda, M., Shibata, R., and Kondoh, H. (2021). Efficient and rapid assessment of multiple aspects of frailty using the Kyoto Frailty Scale, developed from the Edmonton Frail Scale. *Journal of Physical Therapy Science* 33 (3): 267–273.

Kasa, A.S., Drury, P., Chang, H.C.R. et al. (2023). Cross-cultural adaptation, validity, and reliability testing of the Tilburg Frailty Indicator (TFI) Amharic version for screening frailty in community-dwelling Ethiopian older people. *Clinical Interventions in Aging* 18: 1115–1127.

Kojima, G. (2018). Frailty defined by FRAIL scale as a predictor of mortality: a systematic review and meta-analysis. *Journal of the American Medical Directors Association* 19 (6): 480–483.

Ku, N.W., Hsu, Y.C., Mudhur, J. et al. (2025). The prognostic accuracy of frailty and vulnerability screening for older adults in the emergency department: a systematic review and meta-analysis. *Annals of Emergency Medicine* 86: 496–510.

Lee, J.H., Park, Y.S., Kim, M.J. et al. (2022). Clinical frailty scale as a predictor of short-term mortality: a systematic review and meta-analysis of studies on diagnostic test accuracy. *Academic Emergency Medicine* 29 (12): 1347–1356.

Lee, Z.R., Cheng, L.J., Yeo, Y.Y. et al. (2025). Measurement properties of the Edmonton frail scale in older adults: a systematic review and meta-analysis. *International Journal of Nursing Studies* 170: 105161.

McGarrigle, L., Squires, E., Wallace, L.M. et al. (2019). Investigating the feasibility and reliability of the Pictorial Fit-Frail Scale. *Age and Ageing* 48 (6): 832–837.

Morley, J.E., Malmstrom, T.K. and Miller, D.K. (2012). A simple frailty questionnaire (FRAIL) predicts outcomes in middle aged African Americans. *The Journal of Nutrition, Health & Aging* 16 (7): 601–608.

Ng, Y.X., Cheng, L.J., Quek, Y.Y. et al. (2024). The measurement properties and feasibility of FRAIL scale in older adults: a systematic review and meta-analysis. *Ageing Research Reviews* 95: 102243.

NHS England (2022). *Older people advanced practice area specific capability and curriculum framework*. NHS England. Available at: `https://advanced-practice.hee.nhs.uk/wp-content/uploads/sites/28/2025/01/Older-people-advanced-practice-area-specific-capability-and-curriculum-framework-NHSE.pdf` (accessed 30 January 2026).

NHS England (2023a). *Palliative and end of life care advanced practice area specific capability and curriculum framework*. NHS England. Available at: `https://advanced-practice.hee.nhs.uk/wp-content/uploads/sites/28/2025/01/Palliative-and-end-of-life-care-advanced-practice-area-specific-capability-and-curriculum-framework-NHSE.pdf` (accessed 30 January 2026).

NHS England (2023b). *Acute medicine advanced practice area specific capability and curriculum framework*. NHS England. Available at: `https://advanced-practice.hee.nhs.uk/wp-content/uploads/sites/28/2025/03/Acute-medicine-advanced-practice-area-specific-capability-and-curriculum-framework-NHSE.pdf` (accessed 30 January 2026).

NHS England (2025). *Multi-professional framework for advanced practice in England – Edition 2025*. NHS England. Available at: `https://advanced-practice.hee.nhs.uk/wp-content/uploads/sites/`

28/2025/05/Multi-professional-framework-for-advanced-practice-in-England---Edition-2025.pdf (accessed 29 January 2026).

Owodunni, O.P., Biala, E. Jr., Sirisegaram, L. et al. (2024). Validation of the self-reported Edmonton frail scale-acute care in patients ≥ 65 years undergoing surgery. *Perioperative Care and Operating Room Management* 35: 100383.

Qin, F., Guo, Y., Ruan, Y. et al. (2023). Frailty and risk of adverse outcomes among community-dwelling older adults in China: a comparison of four different frailty scales. *Frontiers in Public Health* 11: 1154809.

Rockwood, K. and Theou, O. (2020). Using the clinical frailty scale in allocating scarce health care resources. *Canadian Geriatrics Journal* 23 (3): 254–259.

Rockwood, K., Song, X., MacKnight, C. et al. (2005). A global clinical measure of fitness and frailty in elderly people. *Canadian Medical Association Journal* 173 (5): 489–495.

Rodrigues, H.C.N., Sousa, A.G.D.O., Preto, V.R.M. et al. (2024). FRAIL scale as a screening tool and a predictor of mortality in non-dialysis dependent patients. *Journal of Nephrology* 37 (4): 1085–1092.

Rodríguez-Laso, Á., Martín-Lesende, I., Sinclair, A. et al. (2022). Diagnostic accuracy of the FRAIL scale plus functional measures for frailty screening: a cross-sectional study. *BJGP Open* 6 (3).

Rolfson, D.B., Majumdar, S.R., Tsuyuki, R.T. et al. (2006). Validity and reliability of the Edmonton Frail Scale. *Age and Ageing* 35 (5): 526–529.

Rose, M., Yang, A., Welz, M. et al. (2018). Novel modification of the reported Edmonton Frail Scale. *Australasian Journal on Ageing* 37 (4): 305–308.

Røyset, I.M., Eriksen, G.F., Benth, J.Š. et al. (2023). Edmonton Frail Scale predicts mortality in older patients with cancer undergoing radiotherapy—a prospective observational study. *PLoS One* 18 (3): e0283507.

Statlender, L., Theou, O., Merchshiev, R. et al. (2025). The pictorial fit-frail scale: a novel tool for frailty assessment in critically ill older adults. *BMC Geriatrics* 25 (1): 105.

Theou, O., Andrew, M., Ahip, S.S. et al. (2019). The pictorial fit-frail scale: developing a visual scale to assess frailty. *Canadian Geriatrics Journal* 22 (2): 64–74.

Theou, O., Pérez-Zepeda, M.U., van der Valk, A.M. et al. (2021). A classification tree to assist with routine scoring of the clinical frailty scale. *Age and Ageing* 50 (5): 1406–1411.

Voukelatou, P., Kyvetos, A., Kollia, D. et al. (2023). Translation of the pictorial fit-frail scale into the Greek language and examination of its validity and reliability. *Cureus* 15 (7): e41553.

Wallis, S.J., Wall, J., Biram, R.W.S., and Romero-Ortuno, R. (2015). Association of the clinical frailty scale with hospital outcomes. *QJM: An International Journal of Medicine* 108 (12): 943–949.

Zhang, X., Tan, S.S., Bilajac, L. et al. (2020). Reliability and validity of the Tilburg frailty indicator in 5 European countries. *Journal of the American Medical Directors Association* 21 (6): 772–779.e6.

Zwawi, A., Wessman, T., Wändell, P. et al. (2025). A simplified clinical frailty scale predicts mortality in emergency department patients with acute dyspnea. *GeroScience*, published 11 September 2025 https://doi.org/10.1007/s11357-025-01864-7.

CHAPTER 9

Polypharmacy and Deprescribing

Aim

The aim of this chapter is to provide advanced practitioners (APs) with the knowledge and evidence-based strategies to identify, manage, and safely reduce problematic polypharmacy in frail older adults through structured, patient-centred deprescribing. It highlights relevant national policies, professional standards, and clinical tools to support safe and effective medicines optimisation.

LEARNING OUTCOMES

By the end of this chapter, readers will be able to:

1. Critically explain the concepts of polypharmacy, appropriate and problematic polypharmacy, overprescribing, and deprescribing in the context of frailty.
2. Apply national frameworks, professional standards, and validated deprescribing tools (e.g. STOPP/START, STOPPFrail, and Scottish 7-Step) to guide safe, patient-centred medication review.
3. Evaluate clinical scenarios to identify medications that may be reduced or stopped, balancing risks and benefits in line with individual goals of care.
4. Demonstrate how deprescribing can be embedded into multidisciplinary practice to reduce harm, improve quality of life, and align with the four pillars of advanced clinical practice.

SELF-ASSESSMENT QUESTIONS

1. When reviewing a frail older adult on multiple medications, how would you determine whether polypharmacy is appropriate, problematic, or a result of overprescribing?
2. How would you plan and monitor a structured deprescribing process for a patient taking several antihypertensive agents who is now experiencing recurrent falls?

> Thoughtful deprescribing turns the burden of many
> medicines into the balance of safer ageing.

INTRODUCTION

Deprescribing and the Role of Advanced Practitioners

Polypharmacy is a major challenge in the care of frail older adults, where multimorbidity often leads to complex prescribing and an increased risk of adverse drug events, hospitalisation, and functional decline (Alsararatee, 2025). Deprescribing, defined as the planned and supervised withdrawal of medicines that are no longer appropriate or may cause harm, is now recognised as a key element of medicines optimisation and person-centred care for older adults (Deprescribing.org, 2025a). Emerging evidence indicates that deprescribing interventions can improve patient outcomes, reduce drug burden, and prevent avoidable harm without compromising safety (Hurley et al., 2024; Linsky et al., 2024). This highlights the importance of integrating deprescribing into routine clinical practice, particularly for advanced practitioners (APs), who are often at the first line of managing polypharmacy in frail older adults.

In the United Kingdom, deprescribing is embedded within professional and legal frameworks that govern safe prescribing. The General Medical Council's Good Practice in Prescribing and Managing Medicines and Devices (GMC, 2021) requires prescribers to review treatment regularly and to discontinue medicines when risks outweigh benefits. The Health and Care Professions Council's Standards for Prescribing (HCPC, 2019) and the Royal Pharmaceutical Society's Prescribing Competency Framework (RPS, 2021) both emphasise that prescribing is a continuous cycle of initiation, monitoring, and, where appropriate, discontinuation. Similarly, the Care Quality Commission (CQC, 2019) identifies structured medication review, including deprescribing, as a marker of safe and high-quality care, while national policy from the Department of Health and Social Care (2021) positions deprescribing within its strategy to reduce overprescribing and medicines-related harm, aligning with the World Health Organization's Global Patient Safety Challenge (WHO, 2017).

APs are well positioned to lead this agenda. Their scope of practice, defined by the multi-professional framework (MPF) for advanced practice (NHS England, 2025), integrates expert clinical assessment, diagnostic reasoning, and prescribing authority with the leadership and education skills required to embed deprescribing into practice. This combination enables APs not only to make complex deprescribing decisions but also to lead multidisciplinary reviews and ensure decisions are aligned with patient goals and legal standards. This paper therefore provides practical guidance for APs in deprescribing commonly encountered medicines in frail older patients, drawing on national frameworks, validated tools, and evidence-based strategies to support safe, legalised, and person-centred care.

Multi-Professional Framework for Advanced Practitioners (NHS England, 2025)

This chapter maps to the following areas within the MPF:

1. Clinical practice: 1.1–1.11
2. Leadership and management: 2.1, 2.2, 2.3, 2.4, 2.5, 2.6, 2.7, 2.8
3. Education: 3.1, 3.3, 3.5, 3.8
4. Research: 4.1, 4.2, 4.3, 4.5, 4.6

Accreditation Consideration

This chapter maps to the statement with the following national accretional document:

Curriculum framework for advanced practice in the care of older people (NHS England, 2022):

1. Core CiPs: 1–6
2. Generic Clinical CiPs: 1, 2, 3, 4, 5, 6
3. Specialty Clinical CiPs (Older People): 3.1, 3.2, 3.3, 3.4, 3.5

Curriculum framework for advanced practitioners in the case of palliative and end-of-life care (NHS England, 2023a):

1. Clinical pillar: 1.1, 1.2, 1.3, 1.4
2. Leadership and management: 2.1
3. Education: 3.1
4. Research: 4.1

Curriculum for advanced practitioners in acute medicine (NHS England, 2023b):

1. Core CiPs: 1, 2, 3, 4, 5, 6
2. Generic Clinical CiPs: 1, 2, 3, 5, 6
3. Specialty Clinical CiPs (Acute Medicine): 1–5 and acute presentations

Polypharmacy

Polypharmacy refers to the use of multiple medications by a single individual, especially common in older adults with multimorbidity. This raises risks for adverse drug reactions, drug interactions, and increases complexity in monitoring and adherence (Varghese et al., 2023). According to the Specialist Pharmacy Service (SPS) the definition has evolved: rather than a fixed number of drugs alone, polypharmacy is now distinguished as appropriate versus problematic, reflecting whether the medication regimen is optimised for a patient's individual needs (SPS, 2025).

Appropriate Polypharmacy

Appropriate polypharmacy involves prescribing multiple medicines only when clinically indicated, tailored to the patient's condition, goals, and best available evidence (Cole and Wright, 2017). It aims to preserve quality of life, prolong lifespan where relevant, and reduce risk of harm. The SPS emphasises that this requires structured medication reviews, shared decision-making, and strategies like medicines optimisation, where the right medicine is given at the right time and dose for those individual circumstances (SPS, 2025).

Problematic Polypharmacy

Problematic polypharmacy arises when medicines are no longer appropriate, when harms outweigh benefits, or when the patient's capacity to manage the medication burden becomes compromised (Swinglehurst et al., 2023). Overprescribing overlaps with this: it describes prescribing medicines that are unnecessary, pose potential harm, or are not aligned with patient preferences (SPS, 2025). Both lead to increased risk of medication-related harms, hospital admissions, non-adherence, and impaired function (SPS, 2025). Cut-offs frequently used in practice are five or more drugs for polypharmacy and 10 or more for 'hyperpolypharmacy' or excessive burden (SPS, 2025).

Deprescribing

Deprescribing is the process of intentionally reducing or stopping medications that are no longer beneficial, are potentially harmful, or do not align with a patient's goals of care (Scott et al., 2015). The SPS describes deprescribing as patient-centred, involving shared decision-making with the patient (and carer if relevant), systematic review of the medicines, and appropriate follow-up to monitor effects and ensure safety (SPS, 2025).

DEPRESCRIBING TOOLS AVAILABLE TO SUPPORT DECISION-MAKING

Several structured tools have been developed to support clinicians in deprescribing and to ensure decisions are evidence-based and patient-centred. Deprescribing.org provides drug-specific algorithms and patient decision aids for commonly used medicines such as proton pump inhibitors (PPIs), antihyperglycemics, benzodiazepines, antipsychotics, and cholinesterase inhibitors, helping to guide both the deprescribing process and shared decision-making (Deprescribing.org, 2025b). Evidence from the *D-PRESCRIBE* trial demonstrated the effectiveness of this approach, with pharmacist-led use of these tools resulting in 43% of patients discontinuing inappropriate medicines compared with 12% under usual care at six months (Martin et al., 2018).

The STOPP/START criteria offer a widely validated method, providing explicit lists of potentially inappropriate prescriptions (STOPP) and prescribing omissions (START) for older adults; the updated version 3 now contains 190 criteria. STOPP has strong predictive validity: in a prospective cohort of 600 hospitalised older patients, STOPP-defined potentially inappropriate medicines were significantly associated with serious, avoidable adverse drug events contributing to hospital admission (adjusted OR 1.85, 95% CI 1.51–2.26, $p < 0.001$), whereas the Beers criteria did not show a significant association (Hamilton et al., 2011). For patients with advanced frailty and limited life expectancy, STOPPFrail provides explicit deprescribing criteria; in a prospective nursing-home study, pharmacist-guided STOPPFrail reviews reduced mean medicines from 16.0 to 14.6 immediately and 15.4 at six months without safety signals (Hurley et al., 2024).

The Scottish 7-Step approach offers a structured framework for medication review that incorporates treatment aims, clinical indication, dose, safety, interactions, and patient preferences (Scottish Government, 2018). Implementation in the real-world NHS Scotland context, aided by national decision support tools aligned with the 7-step polypharmacy review, is projected to yield substantial direct and indirect cost savings estimated at £2.1 million per annum from reductions in inappropriate prescribing (Wales and Mair, 2024). These tools provide robust, evidence-based methods to guide deprescribing in clinical practice, while supporting collaborative discussions that align with patient values and goals of care. Table 9.1 illustrates the common decision tool that can support prescribers.

TABLE 9.1 Deprescribing and medicines optimisation tools.

Tool/resource	How it can be used
Anticholinergic Burden (ACB) Calculator	Calculates cumulative anticholinergic effect of medicines and suggests lower-burden alternatives.
Medichec	Identifies drugs with anticholinergic, QTc, hyponatraemia, bleeding, dizziness, drowsiness, and constipation risks; highlights the cumulative impact of polypharmacy.
Medicines and Falls Guide (National Falls Prevention Coordination Group)	Supports medication reviews for people at risk of falls by identifying fall-risk-increasing drugs (FRIDs).
Medstopper	Ranks medicines by likelihood of benefit versus harm; provides tapering and discontinuation advice.
STOPPFrail (v2)	Identifies potentially inappropriate medicines in frail older adults with limited life expectancy; supports structured deprescribing in any setting.
STOPP/START (v3)	Provides explicit criteria to identify inappropriate medicines (STOPP) and omissions (START) in patients aged ≥65 years.
ThinkCascades	Outlines nine important prescribing cascades to help clinicians recognise when a medicine is prescribed to treat another's side effects.
Deprescribing.org Algorithms	Provides international evidence-based deprescribing guidance for PPIs, antihyperglycaemics, antipsychotics, benzodiazepines, and cholinesterase inhibitors/memantine.
Health Improvement Scotland—Right Decision Service	Digital decision-support system offering national polypharmacy guidance and tools for safe, evidence-based prescribing.
Health Improvement Scotland Polypharmacy Guides	Provide condition-specific strategies (e.g. antidepressants, respiratory, type 2 diabetes) to improve quality prescribing.
Manage My Meds (Scotland)	Patient-focused tool to help patients and carers understand medicines and prepare for medication reviews.
NHS Wales: Polypharmacy in Older People Guide	Practical deprescribing guides for stopping groups of medicines (e.g. acid suppressants, antihypertensives, opioids, benzodiazepines, bisphosphonates).
PrescQIPP IMPACT Tool	Helps clinicians identify priorities for deprescribing, highlighting issues to consider and recommendations for continuing or stopping medicines.
Ask 3 Questions (AQuA)	Supports shared decision-making by encouraging patients to ask about choices, pros/cons, and available support.
BRAN (Choosing Wisely UK)	Promotes shared decision-making by focusing on Benefits, Risks, Alternatives, and doing Nothing.
NICE Three-Talk Model	Guides shared decision-making through introducing choice, describing options, and exploring preferences.
Health Innovation Network Resources	Provides multilingual patient information materials to prepare for structured medication reviews.
SPS: Understanding Polypharmacy	Explains causes, consequences, and professional tools for managing polypharmacy and overprescribing.
SPS: Person-Centred Polypharmacy and Medication Review	Practical framework for identifying patients needing reviews and managing inappropriate polypharmacy with a patient-centred focus.
SPS: Resources to Support Medication Review	Provides tools and approaches for deprescribing and supports shared decision-making with patients.

Adapted from the Specialist Pharmacy Service (2025).

PRACTICAL GUIDANCE IN DEPRESCRIBING SOME MEDICATIONS IN CLINICAL PRACTICE

Reviewing the Ongoing Indication for Each Medicine

A fundamental element of safe prescribing, as required by the NMC Standards for Prescribing Practice (2023) and the RPS's Competency Framework (2021), is to ensure that every prescribed medicine continues to have a valid and evidence-based indication. Clinical circumstances evolve, and a medicine that was once justified may no longer be appropriate. For example, an individual who commenced atorvastatin for primary prevention two decades earlier may gain limited benefit in advanced age or in a palliative care context. The Medicines and Healthcare products Regulatory Agency (MHRA) regularly issues alerts about interactions such as the increased risk of myopathy when statins are co-prescribed with macrolide antibiotics (MHRA, 2014). This may require temporary suspension or permanent withdrawal. Although national policy sets the principle clearly, it does not mandate specific review intervals or provide detailed methodologies, which contributes to variation in practice between care settings. Therefore, it might be reasonable to hold statins such as atorvastatin for seven days while the frail patients complete their course of antibiotics.

Reducing Anticholinergic Burden

Medicines with anticholinergic activity, particularly when prescribed in combination, are strongly associated with adverse outcomes in frail older adults, including cognitive decline, constipation, urinary retention, delirium, and falls (Hilmer and Gnjidic, 2022). Prescribers can approach this risk systematically by using validated tools such as the Anticholinergic Cognitive Burden (ACB) Calculator or the Anticholinergic Drug Scale to quantify an individual's cumulative exposure (King and Rabino, 2024). For example, a frail patient receiving amitriptyline for neuropathic pain alongside oxybutynin for urinary incontinence would score highly on the ACB scale, highlighting a clinically significant risk. In such cases, safer alternatives might include substituting amitriptyline with gabapentin or pregabalin or considering non-pharmacological bladder training instead of oxybutynin. Deprescribing guided by these tools supports prescribers in making rational, patient-centred adjustments that reduce harm while maintaining therapeutic benefit, ensuring safer care for frail adults.

Individualising Antihypertensive Therapy

Deprescribing antihypertensive medication in frail older adults requires careful consideration of functional and cognitive status. Evidence from the Milan Geriatrics 75+ Cohort Study, which followed 1,587 outpatients aged 75 years and older over 10 years, demonstrated a U-shaped association between blood pressure and mortality: systolic blood pressure (SBP) of 165 mmHg and diastolic blood pressure of 85 mmHg were associated with the lowest mortality risk, while SBP below 120 mmHg increased mortality risk by 64% (HR 1.64, 95% CI 1.21–2.23) and SBP 120–139 mmHg increased risk by 32% (HR 1.32, 95% CI 1.10–1.60) compared to those with SBP 160–179 mmHg. Importantly, higher SBP was associated with lower mortality in those with impaired cognition and activities of daily living, but not in fitter individuals, underscoring the need for personalised prescribing (Ogliari et al., 2015). Current NICE guidance NICE HTN (2025a) recommends clinic blood pressure targets below 150/90 mmHg for adults aged 80 years and over, but also advises clinicians to apply judgement in frail or multimorbid patients, where treatment burden may outweigh benefit. For example, in a frail 85-year-old with recurrent falls, reducing or withdrawing an antihypertensive such as a calcium channel blocker may prevent hypotension-related syncope and preserve function. This illustrates that deprescribing in advanced age can be both safe and clinically advantageous when blood pressure management is aligned with frailty, cognition, and life expectancy.

Preventing Hyponatraemia Through Safe Prescribing and Deprescribing

Selective serotonin reuptake inhibitors (SSRIs), serotonin–noradrenaline reuptake inhibitors (SNRIs), and thiazide diuretics are well-established causes of hyponatraemia in older adults, with risk heightened by polypharmacy, frailty, and multimorbidity. NICE Guidance (2025b) advises baseline and follow-up sodium monitoring when initiating these agents; however, in clinical practice, hyponatraemia often develops after prolonged use. In such cases, deprescribing one or more causative drugs may represent the most effective harm-reduction strategy. For example, in an 82-year-old patient with recurrent mild hyponatraemia and falls while prescribed both citalopram and Bendroflumethiazide, deprescribing the thiazide and switching to an alternative antihypertensive could restore sodium balance and reduce fall risk.

Optimising Anticoagulant Use

The NICE NG196 (2021) recommends direct oral anticoagulants in preference to warfarin for many patients due to the reduced need for monitoring and fewer dietary interactions, although warfarin remains appropriate for some. Clinically significant drug interactions, such as between warfarin and macrolide antibiotics, may require a temporary hold or a long-term switch. Such decisions reflect the RPS competency to act promptly when the risks of treatment outweigh the benefits. However, this assumes ready access to INR testing and specialist advice, which is not universally available in all community settings.

When optimising anticoagulant use, clinicians must also weigh the competing risks of stroke versus bleeding, particularly in frail older adults with recurrent falls. For example, an 82-year-old patient with atrial fibrillation on Edoxaban who presents with repeated falls raises the dilemma of whether the risk of major bleeding, including intracranial haemorrhage, outweighs the benefits of continued stroke prophylaxis. Current NICE NG196 (2021) and European Society of Cardiology (ESC) guidance emphasise the use of validated tools such as CHA_2DS_2-VASc for stroke risk and HAS-BLED or ORBIT for bleeding risk to support shared decision-making and ensure patient involvement (Hindricks et al., 2021). Where uncertainty remains, clinicians are advised to seek specialist input according to the indication for anticoagulation, for example, referral to cardiology or stroke services in patients treated for atrial fibrillation.

SIMPLIFYING DIABETES THERAPY IN FRAIL OR END-OF-LIFE CONTEXTS

Strict glycaemic targets (e.g. $HbA_1c < 7\%$) may pose significant risks in older adults with frailty or limited life expectancy (Perry, 2024). A 2024 Canadian guideline endorses deprescribing hypoglycaemia-inducing medications, particularly insulin and sulphonylureas, in such populations, highlighting the need for individualised treatment goals based on frailty and comorbidity status (Farrell et al., 2017). Observational data support this approach: Mangé et al. (2021) found that 40.9% of frail older adults were potentially overtreated, with overly tight HbA_1c control; the study suggests an optimal target of 7–8% for frail patients compared to 6–7% for non-frail patients. Additionally, studies such as Sinclair et al. (2022) argue that an HbA_1c around 7.5% may best reduce hypoglycaemic risk and frailty-related complications. While many guidelines distinguish targets for healthier versus frail older adults, typically ± 8–9% for the latter, they lack detailed protocols for deprescribing complex regimens (Bolt ct al., 2024). In practice, clinicians may consider gradually tapering insulin or sulphonylureas in an 85-year-old experiencing recurrent hypoglycaemia with an HbA1c of 6.5%; this can reduce adverse events while maintaining acceptable glycaemic control. However, until more detailed frameworks exist, these decisions rely on informed clinical judgement, taking into account frailty severity, patient preference, and safety.

RATIONALISING IRON SUPPLEMENTATION

Lower-dose and non-daily oral iron regimens can be effective and are better tolerated in older adults (Uçan et al., 2023). Randomised and physiological studies show that alternate-day dosing improves absorption by avoiding hepcidin-mediated blockade, while split or consecutive-day high doses reduce fractional absorption and worsen tolerance (e.g. 60 mg on alternate days versus daily) (Stoffel et al., 2017). In octogenarians with iron-deficiency anaemia, low-dose elemental iron corrected anaemia effectively, supporting dose minimisation in later life (Rimon et al., 2005). Ferrous sulphate is consistently linked with increased gastrointestinal adverse effects, which can trigger prescribing cascades such as routine laxatives; reducing dose or stopping when no longer needed mitigates this risk (Tolkien et al., 2015). UK guidance advises one ferrous salt tablet once daily, with dose reduction to alternate days if not tolerated, checking haemoglobin at two to four weeks, and continuing therapy for about three months after correction to replete stores, after which ongoing need should be reviewed and long-term supplementation avoided unless a persistent indication exists (NICE, 2024). The British Society of Gastroenterology similarly supports once-daily or alternate-day dosing and continuation only long enough to restore stores, reinforcing deprescribing once objectives are achieved (Snook et al., 2021).

IDENTIFYING AND REVERSING PRESCRIBING CASCADES

A prescribing cascade occurs when a medicine is prescribed to manage the side effects of another. For instance, an older adult is prescribed naproxen for osteoarthritis. They subsequently develop gastritis and dyspepsia, which are recognised adverse effects of NSAIDs. Instead of addressing the NSAID as the cause, a clinician prescribes a PPI such as omeprazole to treat the gastric symptoms. The long-term PPI use then leads to iron and vitamin B12 deficiency and increases the risk of osteoporosis and fractures. The reversal of the cascade would involve stopping the NSAID (or using a safer alternative, such as topical analgesia), reassessing pain management strategies, and discontinuing unnecessary long-term PPI use once symptoms resolve.

Deprescribing the original causative medicine, when clinically appropriate, meets the national and international requirement of prescribing safely and effectively to avoid unnecessary harm. However, identification of cascades is often dependent on having access to comprehensive and longitudinal prescribing records, which may be unavailable across fragmented care systems.

USING A SINGLE DRUG TO ADDRESS MULTIPLE CONDITIONS SAFELY

When safe and evidence-based, using one medicine to manage multiple conditions can reduce the number of prescriptions, improve adherence, and lower the risk of adverse effects. For instance, beta-blockers can be used to manage hypertension, atrial fibrillation, and angina simultaneously. Despite this, national policy offers little guidance on determining when multi-condition prescribing is beneficial rather than potentially harmful, which leaves this decision to the prescriber's discretion.

MANAGING INSOMNIA WITHOUT LONG-TERM HYPNOTICS

NICE (2023) recommends cognitive behavioural therapy for insomnia (CBT-I) as the first-line treatment for long-term insomnia, with pharmacological options such as daridorexant considered only when CBT-I is ineffective, unavailable, or unsuitable. Where hypnotics such as zopiclone or benzodiazepines are already prescribed, gradual deprescribing minimises withdrawal and rebound insomnia (British National Formulary, 2025a). This approach aligns with the RPS competencies, supporting prescribing and care that are safe, effective, and evidence-based. In practice, however, access to cognitive behavioural therapy for insomnia is inconsistent, which may hinder the implementation of non-drug alternatives.

EMBEDDING DEPRESCRIBING INTO MULTIDISCIPLINARY POLYPHARMACY CLINICS

Polypharmacy clinics bring together nurse prescribers, pharmacists, and other healthcare professionals to undertake structured medication reviews. This model directly supports NHS England's structured medication review specification and the RPS's emphasis on collaborative prescribing. By institutionalising deprescribing within such clinics, the process becomes a standard element of medicines management rather than a reactive measure. However, provision across the United Kingdom remains inconsistent, and follow-up responsibilities after deprescribing decisions are not always clearly defined.

MANAGING CONSTIPATION IN FRAIL AND END-OF-LIFE PATIENTS

Constipation is highly prevalent in frail older adults and those receiving end-of-life care, where immobility, dehydration, neurological disease, and multiple medications all contribute (Gill et al., 2024). Opioids are a particularly common cause, acting on peripheral opioid receptors in the gastrointestinal tract to reduce motility. Consequently, constipation prophylaxis should be considered routine for any patient commenced on opioids. Management must be individualised according to the underlying cause, symptom severity, and patient comorbidities. Stimulant laxatives such as senna are often first-line and are particularly effective for opioid-induced constipation (OIC). However, these require to be used wisely as they are contraindicated in patients with abdominal pain as it can worsen their pain or bowel obstruction (BNF, 2025b).

Osmotic agents such as lactulose or macrogols (Laxido, Movicol) can be added, but they require good hydration to be effective. This may be unsuitable in patients with advanced frailty or fluid retention, for example, an older person with heart failure or renal impairment, where large fluid volumes needed for macrogols would worsen their condition. Or if the patient is dehydrated and septic, this option might not be successful. For faecal impaction, macrogols sachets dissolved in water may be prescribed, though again this requires caution in patients where fluid balance is restricted.

In such cases, suppositories, enemas, or digital rectal evacuation may be preferable, especially for distal constipation. For patients not responding to first-line agents, other options include lubiprostone, a chloride channel activator, or prucalopride, a selective serotonin (5-HT4) receptor agonist, both of which may be considered for refractory OIC. Non-drug approaches, such as ensuring optimal hydration, fibre intake where tolerated, and encouraging mobility, should be incorporated alongside pharmacological treatment (Chang et al., 2023). However, at the end of life, symptom relief takes priority, and the choice of agent should be tailored to what is most effective, feasible, and comfortable for the patient.

Learning Event

You are working in a multidisciplinary frailty clinic and asked to review an 83-year-old patient with multimorbidity, recurrent falls, and significant polypharmacy (15 regular medicines). You identify several drugs with no current indication and potential for harm, including duplicate antihypertensives and long-term PPI use. The patient is anxious about stopping medicines prescribed over many years. How would you apply a structured deprescribing process to ensure safety and shared decision-making? What validated tools (e.g. STOPP/START, STOPPFrail, Scottish 7-Step) would you use, and how would you monitor and document outcomes? How would you involve the wider team and demonstrate that your actions remain within professional standards and the four pillars of advanced practice?

Case Study 9.1   Polypharmacy and Deprescribing

1. **Falls, dizziness, and a long list of medicines**

   An 86-year-old woman with multimorbidity (HFpEF, T2DM, CKD3a, osteoarthritis) attends with recurrent falls and postural dizziness. She takes 12 regular medicines: ACE inhibitor, calcium-channel blocker, thiazide, loop diuretic PRN, metformin, gliclazide, simvastatin, omeprazole, amitriptyline 10 mg nocte, oxybutynin, codeine PRN, and senna. BP 108/58 mmHg sitting, orthostatic drop 24 mmHg; ACB score high; HbA1c 6.5%.

   - How will you structure a medication review (e.g. Scottish 7-Steps), identify prescribing cascades (NSAID-PPI-constipation-senna; amitriptyline-oxybutynin), and prioritise targets for deprescribing?
   - Which tools will you use (e.g. STOPP/START v3, STOPPFrail, ACB Calculator), and what immediate safety monitoring is required (hypotension, glycaemia, withdrawal)?
   - How will you conduct shared decision-making to agree goals (falls prevention over tight HbA1c), and document/review the taper plan (e.g. deprescribe amitriptyline → reassess nocturia → consider stopping oxybutynin; relax glycaemic target and reduce gliclazide)?
   - What criteria will indicate success or the need to reinstate therapy (falls rate, orthostatic BP, symptom scores, patient-reported outcomes)?

2. **Hyponatraemia on SSRI and thiazide (acute medical unit)**

   An 82-year-old man is admitted with confusion; Na^+ 126 mmol/L. Current medicines: citalopram 20 mg, bendroflumethiazide 2.5 mg, ramipril, alendronate, calcium/vitamin-D, paracetamol. He has had two similar admissions in six months.

   - How will you attribute causality and decide on deprescribing versus dose reduction (NICE CKS hyponatraemia; SPS guidance)?
   - Which medicine(s) will you stop first and why? What non-drug or alternative options will you offer (e.g. switch SSRI and review BP regimen)?
   - What monitoring and follow-up will you set (timing of repeat Na^+, mood surveillance, community phlebotomy, and safety-netting)?
   - How will you communicate the plan to primary care and the patient/carer to prevent re-challenge?

3. End-of-life care and treatment burden (care home MDT)

A 90-year-old with advanced frailty, dementia, and dysphagia is on 11 medicines, including a statin for primary prevention, a bisphosphonate, a tight BP regimen, and memantine. Aims of care focus on comfort and avoiding hospital conveyance.

- Using STOPPFrail, which medicines are candidates for discontinuation now, which to taper, and which to continue for symptom relief only?
- How will you balance risks (e.g. rebound phenomena) with likely time-to-benefit and align decisions with goals of care and best-interest processes?
- What is your stepwise deprescribing sequence and review interval, and how will you mitigate withdrawal or symptom recurrence?
- Which governance elements will you ensure (capacity assessment, documentation, MAR chart updates, anticipatory prescribing, and family communication)?

4. Anticoagulation in recurrent faller with AF (primary care review)

An 83-year-old with AF (CHA_2DS_2-VASc = 4) on a DOAC has three falls in two months. He also takes an SSRI and regular ibuprofen.

- How will you appraise stroke versus bleeding risk (HAS-BLED/ORBIT), address modifiable risks (stop NSAID and review SSRI), and decide whether to continue, switch, or dose-adjust the DOAC?
- What patient-centred discussion and documentation are needed to evidence shared decisions and safety-netting?

5. Proton pump inhibitor long-term use without indication (outpatient clinic)

A 78-year-old continues omeprazole 20 mg daily, which was started 'years ago' after NSAID-induced dyspepsia; NSAID stopped long ago. Iron deficiency persists despite oral iron.

- How will you confirm indication, plan a step-down/stop with rescue therapy, and monitor for recurrence while addressing potential PPI-related harms (iron/B12, fractures)?
- How will you avoid re-escalation without a clear indication (self-care plan, review date, letter to GP)?

CONCLUSION

Deprescribing is central to safe and effective care in frail older adults. The process should follow clear steps: review each medicine and its indication, assess risks and benefits, identify and prioritise drugs for withdrawal, taper where appropriate, and monitor closely with patient involvement. APs are well placed to lead this structured approach, ensuring that deprescribing reduces harm and aligns treatment with patient goals. Future work should focus on developing clearer deprescribing frameworks, improving access to decision-support tools, and embedding deprescribing into routine multidisciplinary practice across all care settings.

Take-Home Messages

1. Deprescribing should be approached as a systematic, patient-centred, and closely monitored process that involves structured medication review, assessment of indication and risk,

prioritisation of drugs for withdrawal, tapering where necessary, and ongoing follow-up with patient involvement.

2. In frail older adults, treatment goals should prioritise safety and quality of life over strict disease-specific targets, as rigid thresholds such as blood pressure or HbA1c can increase harm and compromise function.

3. Safe practice is best supported by the use of validated tools such as STOPP/START, STOPPFrail, and the Scottish 7-Step approach, alongside national frameworks from NICE, RPS, and NHS England that promote consistent, evidence-based deprescribing decisions.

4. APs working within multidisciplinary teams are well placed to lead deprescribing by applying prescribing authority, advanced clinical reasoning, and leadership skills to reduce treatment burden, prevent harm, and ensure care remains aligned with patient goals.

REFLECTIVE QUESTIONS

1. In what ways does your current approach to medication review enable or limit the identification of medications that could be safely deprescribed?

2. How do you recognise when treatment goals, such as tight blood pressure or glycaemic control, may be causing more harm than benefit in a frail older adult?

3. To what extent do you feel confident using tools such as STOPP/START or STOPPFrail, and what barriers might prevent you from applying them in daily practice?

4. How might your role within a multidisciplinary team influence the culture of deprescribing, and what more could you do to ensure prescribing decisions reflect patient goals and values?

REFERENCES

Alsararatee, H.H. (2025). Polypharmacy and deprescribing in clinical practice. *International Journal for Advancing Practice* 1–5. https://doi.org/10.12968/ijap.2024.0007.

BNF (2025a). *Hypnotics and Anxiolytics [Treatment Summary]*. NICE https://bnf.nice.org.uk/treatment-summaries/hypnotics-and-anxiolytics (accessed 26 August 2025).

BNF (2025b). *Senna*. BNF [Online]. https://bnf.nice.org.uk/drugs/senna (accessed 26 August 2025).

Bolt, J., Carvalho, V., Lin, K. et al. (2024). Systematic review of guideline recommendations for older and frail adults with type 2 diabetes mellitus. *Age and Ageing* 53 (11): afae259.

Care Quality Commission (2019). *Medicines in Health and Adult Social Care: Learning from Risks and Sharing Good Practice for Better Outcomes*. Newcastle: Care Quality Commission www.cqc.org.uk/sites/default/files/20190605_medicines_in_health_and_adult_social_care_report.pdf (accessed 16 August 2025).

Chang, L., Chey, W.D., Imdad, A. et al. (2023). American gastroenterological association–American college of gastroenterology clinical practice guideline: pharmacological management of chronic idiopathic constipation. *Gastroenterology* 164 (7): 1086–1106.

Cole, A. and Wright, H. (2017). The importance of 'appropriate' polypharmacy and the value of medicines. *European Journal of Hospital Pharmacy* 24 (1): 70–72.

Department of Health and Social Care (2021). *Good for You, Good for Us, Good for Everybody: A Plan to Reduce Overprescribing to Make Patient Care Better and Safer, Support the NHS, and Reduce Carbon Emissions.* London: DHSC https://www.gov.uk/government/publications/national-overprescribing-review-report (accessed 16 August 2025).

Deprescribing.org (2025a). What is deprescribing? https://deprescribing.org/what-is-deprescribing (accessed 26 August 2025).

Deprescribing.org (2025b). Deprescribing guidelines and algorithms. https://deprescribing.org/resources/deprescribing-guidelines-algorithms (accessed 26 August 2025).

Farrell, B., Black, C., Thompson, W. et al. (2017). Deprescribing antihyperglycemic agents in older persons: evidence-based clinical practice guideline. *Canadian Family Physician* 63 (11): 832–843.

General Medical Council (2021). *Good Practice in Prescribing and Managing Medicines and Devices.* London: GMC https://www.gmc-uk.org/ethical-guidance/ethical-guidance-for-doctors/prescribing-and-managing-medicines-and-devices (accessed 16 August 2025).

Gill, V., Badrzadeh, H., Williams, S. et al. (2024). A rapid review on the management of constipation for hospice and palliative care patients. *Journal of Hospice & Palliative Nursing* 26 (3): 122–131.

Hamilton, H., Gallagher, P., Ryan, C. et al. (2011). Potentially inappropriate medications defined by STOPP criteria and the risk of adverse drug events in older hospitalized patients. *Archives of Internal Medicine* 171 (11): 1013–1019. https://doi.org/10.1001/archinternmed.2011.215.

Health and Care Professions Council (2019). *Standards for Prescribing.* London: HCPC https://www.hcpc-uk.org/globalassets/standards/standards-for-prescribing/standards-for-prescribing2.pdf (accessed 16 August 2025).

Hilmer, S.N. and Gnjidic, D. (2022). The anticholinergic burden: from research to practice. *Australian Prescriber* 45 (4): 118–120.

Hindricks, G., Potpara, T., Dagres, N. et al. (2021). 2020 ESC guidelines for the diagnosis and management of atrial fibrillation developed in collaboration with the European Association for Cardio-Thoracic Surgery (EACTS). *European Heart Journal* 42 (5): 373–498.

Hurley, E., Dalton, K., Byrne, S. et al. (2024). Pharmacist-led deprescribing using STOPPFrail for frail older adults in nursing homes. *Journal of the American Medical Directors Association* 25 (9): 105122. https://doi.org/10.1016/j.jamda.2024.10.122.

King, R. and Rabino, S. (2024). Anticholinergic cognitive burden (ACB) calculator. https://www.acbcalc.com (accessed 16 August 2025).

Linsky, A.M., Motala, A., Lawson, E., and Shekelle, P. (2024). Deprescribing to reduce medication harms in older adults'. In: *Making Healthcare Safer IV: A Continuous Updating of Patient Safety Harms and Practices* [Internet] (ed. M. Maggard-Gibbons, E.B. Bass, P. Shekelle, and M.A. Rosen). Rockville, MD: Agency for Healthcare Research and Quality (US). Available at: https://www.ncbi.nlm.nih.gov/books/NBK600387/ (accessed 28 January 2026).

Mangé, A.S., Pagès, A., Sourdet, S. et al. (2021). Diabetes and frail older patients: glycemic control and prescription profile in real life. *Pharmacy* 9 (3): 115.

Martin, P., Tamblyn, R., Benedetti, A., and Tannenbaum, C. (2018). Effect of a pharmacist-led educational intervention on inappropriate medication prescriptions in older adults: the D-PRESCRIBE randomized clinical trial. *JAMA* 320 (18): 1889–1898. https://doi.org/10.1001/jama.2018.16131.

Medicines and Healthcare products Regulatory Agency (MHRA) (2014). Statins: interactions, and updated advice for atorvastatin. *Drug Safety Update* 8 (5): https://www.gov.uk/drug-safety-update/statins-interactions-and-updated-advice-for-atorvastatin (accessed 16 August 2025).

National Institute for Health and Care Excellence (2021). Atrial fibrillation: diagnosis and management (NICE guideline NG196). Published 27 April 2021, last updated 30 June 2021. www.nice.org.uk/guidance/ng196/chapter/Recommendations#anticoagulation (accessed 26 August 2025).

National Institute for Health and Care Excellence (2023). Daridorexant for treating long-term insomnia (technology appraisal guidance TA922). Published 18 October 2023. www.nice.org.uk/guidance/ta922 (accessed 26 August 2025).

National Institute for Health and Care Excellence (2024). CKS: anaemia – iron deficiency (management). Clinical Knowledge Summary. Last revised August 2024. London: NICE. https://cks.nice.org.uk/topics/anaemia-iron-deficiency/management/management (accessed 17 August 2025).

National Institute for Health and Care Excellence (2025a). *CKS: Hypertension – Management.* London: NICE https://cks.nice.org.uk/topics/hypertension/management/management (accessed 16 August 2025).

National Institute for Health and Care Excellence (2025b). Hyponatraemia: background information – causes. Clinical Knowledge Summaries. Last revised July 2025. https://cks.nice.org.uk/topics/hyponatraemia/background-information/causes (accessed 26 August 2025).

NHS England (2022). *Older people advanced practice area specific capability and curriculum framework.* NHS England. Available at: https://advanced-practice.hee.nhs.uk/wp-content/uploads/sites/28/2025/01/Older-people-advanced-practice-area-specific-capability-and-curriculum-framework-NHSE.pdf (accessed 30 January 2026).

NHS England (2023a). *Palliative and end of life care advanced practice area specific capability and curriculum framework.* NHS England. Available at: https://advanced-practice.hee.nhs.uk/wp-content/uploads/sites/28/2025/01/Palliative-and-end-of-life-care-advanced-practice-area-specific-capability-and-curriculum-framework-NHSE.pdf (accessed 30 January 2026).

NHS England (2023b). *Acute medicine advanced practice area specific capability and curriculum framework.* NHS England. Available at: https://advanced-practice.hee.nhs.uk/wp-content/uploads/sites/28/2025/03/Acute-medicine-advanced-practice-area-specific-capability-and-curriculum-framework-NHSE.pdf (accessed 30 January 2026).

NHS England (2025). *Multi-Professional Framework for Advanced Clinical Practice in England.* London: HEE https://advanced-practice.hee.nhs.uk (accessed 16 August 2025).

Nursing and Midwifery Council (2023). *Standards for prescribers.* Nursing and Midwifery Council. Available at: https://www.nmc.org.uk/standards/standards-for-post-registration/standards-for-prescribers/ (accessed 31 January 2026).

Ogliari, G., Westendorp, R.G.J., Muller, M. et al. (2015). Blood pressure and 10-year mortality risk in the Milan Geriatrics 75+ Cohort Study: role of functional and cognitive status. *Age and Ageing* 44 (6): 932–937. https://doi.org/10.1093/ageing/afv141.

Perry, T. (2024). Minimizing harms of tight glycemic control in older people with type 2 diabetes. *Therapeutics Letter* Vancouver: Therapeutics Initiative.

Rimon, E., Kagansky, N., Kagansky, M. et al. (2005). Are we giving too much iron? Low-dose iron therapy is effective in octogenarians. *The American Journal of Medicine* 118 (10): 1142–1147. https://doi.org/10.1016/j.amjmed.2005.01.065.

Royal Pharmaceutical Society (2021). *Competency Framework for all Prescribers*. London: Royal Pharmaceutical Society. Available at: `https://www.rpharms.com/resources/frameworks/prescribing-competency-framework/competency-framework` (accessed 31 January 2026).

Scott, I.A., Hilmer, S.N., Reeve, E. et al. (2015). Reducing inappropriate polypharmacy: the process of deprescribing. *JAMA Internal Medicine* 175 (5): 827–834. `https://doi.org/10.1001/jamainternmed.2015.0324`.

Scottish Government Polypharmacy Model of Care Group (2018). *Polypharmacy Guidance, Realistic Prescribing*, 3e. Scottish Government `http://therapeutics.scot.nhs.uk/wp-content/uploads/2018/04/Polypharmacy-Guidance-2018.pdf`.

Sinclair, A.J., Pennells, D., and Abdelhafiz, A.H. (2022). Hypoglycaemic therapy in frail older people with type 2 diabetes mellitus—a choice determined by metabolic phenotype. *Aging Clinical and Experimental Research* 34 (9): 1949–1967.

Snook, J., Bhala, N., Beales, I.L. et al. (2021). British Society of gastroenterology guidelines for the management of iron deficiency anaemia in adults. *Gut* 70 (11): 2030–2051.

Specialist Pharmacy Service (2025). Tools to support medication review. `https://www.sps.nhs.uk/articles/tools-to-support-medication-review` (accessed 26 August 2025).

Specialist Pharmacy Service (SPS) (2025). Understanding polypharmacy, overprescribing and deprescribing. `https://www.sps.nhs.uk/articles/understanding-polypharmacy-overprescribing-and-deprescribing` (accessed 12 September 2025).

Stoffel, N.U., Cercamondi, C.I., Brittenham, G. et al. (2017). Iron absorption from oral iron supplements given on consecutive versus alternate days and as single morning doses versus twice-daily split dosing in iron-depleted women: two open-label, randomised controlled trials. *The Lancet Haematology* 4 (11): e524–e533.

Swinglehurst, D., Hogger, L., and Fudge, N. (2023). Negotiating the polypharmacy paradox: a video-reflexive ethnography study of polypharmacy and its practices in primary care. *BMJ Quality and Safety* 32 (3): 150–159. `https://doi.org/10.1136/bmjqs-2022-014963`.

Tolkien, Z., Stecher, L., Mander, A.P. et al. (2015). Ferrous sulfate supplementation causes significant gastrointestinal side-effects in adults: a systematic review and meta-analysis. *PLoS One* 10 (2): e0117383.

Uçan, A., Kaya, Z.I., Yilmaz, E.Ö. et al. (2023). Comparing therapeutic effects of alternate day versus daily oral iron in women with iron deficiency anemia: a retrospective cohort study. *Medicine* 102 (30): e34421.

Varghese, D., Ishida, C., and Haseer Koya, H. (2023). Polypharmacy. In: *StatPearls*. Treasure Island, FL: StatPearls Publishing.

Wales, A. and Mair, A. (2024). Making the right decisions about medicines: national decision support for polypharmacy [poster]. Programme Lead, Knowledge and Decision Support, Digital Health & Care Innovation Centre & Head of Effective Prescribing & Therapeutics Division, Scottish Government. Right Decision Service. `https://rightdecisions.scot.nhs.uk/media/1778/rds-poster-5th-draft.pdf` (accessed 16 August 2025).

World Health Organization (2017). *Medication Without Harm: WHO Global Patient Safety Challenge*. Geneva: WHO `https://www.who.int/initiatives/medication-without-harm` (accessed 16 August 2025).

CHAPTER 10

Sarcopenia and Frailty

> **Aim**
>
> This chapter aims to provide an evidence-based overview of sarcopenia and its close relationship with frailty. It critically examines epidemiology, pathophysiology, diagnostic strategies, and current therapeutic interventions, highlighting the pivotal role of advanced practitioners (APs) in screening, prevention, and management. The chapter also explores emerging treatments and future research directions, supporting the integration of sarcopenia care into routine clinical practice.

LEARNING OUTCOMES

After reading this chapter, readers will be able to:

1. Explain the biological mechanisms and clinical significance of sarcopenia and its interaction with frailty.
2. Describe current epidemiological data on sarcopenia globally and within the United Kingdom.
3. Identify validated diagnostic criteria and tools, including those recommended by the European Working Group on Sarcopenia in Older People (EWGSOP2).
4. Appraise evidence-based interventions, including resistance training, nutritional strategies, and combined approaches, and recognise key implementation barriers.
5. Evaluate the impact of COVID-19 on sarcopenia and frailty and integrate these insights into practice.
6. Demonstrate how APs can lead screening, personalised management, multidisciplinary coordination, and service development to improve outcomes for older adults with sarcopenia.

SELF-ASSESSMENT QUESTIONS

1. When assessing an older adult with suspected sarcopenia, how would you integrate physical performance measures (e.g. gait speed and grip strength) with nutritional assessment to inform diagnosis and care planning?
2. As an AP leading a community frailty clinic, what steps would you take to embed sarcopenia screening and combined exercise–nutrition interventions into routine service pathways?

> Early recognition and action against sarcopenia preserve strength, independence, and dignity in ageing.

INTRODUCTION

The term sarcopenia was first introduced by Rosenberg in the late 1980s, deriving it from the Greek *sarx* (flesh) and *penia* (loss), to denote the age-related reduction in lean body mass and associated decline in physical function (Rosenberg, 1997). Early debate centred on whether sarcopenia should be viewed as part of normal ageing or as a medical condition and on identifying the point at which muscle loss becomes clinically significant. Over the last two decades, research has intensified and, in 2016, sarcopenia was officially recognised as a disease in the 10th edition of the International Classification of Diseases, yet it remains rarely diagnosed or recorded in clinical practice (Avgerinou, 2020). For APs, recognising sarcopenia within comprehensive frailty assessment is integral to anticipatory care planning and evidence-based intervention.

Multi-Professional Framework (MPF) for Advanced Practitioners

(Adapted from NHS England, 2025)

This chapter maps to the following areas within the MPF:

1. Clinical practice: 1.1, 1.4, 1.5, 1.7, 1.8, 1.9
2. Leadership and management: 2.1, 2.2, 2.5, 2.7
3. Education: 3.1, 3.3, 3.4, 3.5
4. Research: 4.1, 4.2, 4.3, 4.5

Accreditation Consideration

This chapter maps to the statement with the following national accretional document:
Curriculum framework for advanced practice in the care of older people (NHS England, 2022):

1. Core Capabilities CiPs: 1, 2, 3, 4, 5
2. Generic Clinical CiPs: 1, 2, 3, 4, 5
3. Specialty Clinical CiPs (Older People): 3.1, 3.2, 3.4, 3.5

Curriculum framework for APs in the case of palliative and end-of-life care (NHS England, 2023a):

1. Clinical pillar: 1.1, 1.2, 1.4
2. Leadership and management: 2.1
3. Education: 3.1, 3.4
4. Research: 4.1, 4.2

Curriculum for APs in acute medicine (NHS England, 2023b):

1. Core CiPs: 1, 2, 3, 4
2. Generic Clinical CiPs: 1, 2, 3, 4, 5
3. Specialty Clinical CiPs (Acute Medicine): 1–5 and acute presentations

The European Working Group on Sarcopenia in Older People (EWGSOP) first set out a consensus definition in 2010, describing sarcopenia as a condition marked by progressive, generalised loss of skeletal muscle mass and strength that raises the risk of disability, poor quality of life, and mortality (Cruz-Jentoft et al., 2010). In its 2018 update, EWGSOP2 placed primary emphasis on muscle strength as the key diagnostic criterion. Under the revised guidance, sarcopenia is considered probable when low muscle strength is found, confirmed when low muscle quantity or quality is also present, and severe when all three features, reduced strength, low muscle quantity or quality, and impaired physical performance, are demonstrated (Cruz-Jentoft et al., 2019).

Sarcopenia involves impaired neuromuscular signalling, disruptions in protein metabolism, compensatory changes in motor units, hormonal decline, and contributions from ongoing inflammation and oxidative stress (Dhillon and Hasni, 2017). With the continued ageing of the global population, sarcopenia is expected to become an increasingly significant contributor to morbidity, thereby placing growing demands on health services. Sarcopenia and frailty frequently occur together in older people, and the two syndromes share multiple biological mechanisms, suggesting overlapping and mutually reinforcing pathological processes (Narici and Maffulli, 2010). This chapter aims to summarise current knowledge about sarcopenia, examine recent therapeutic advances, and discuss how APs can lead in translating evidence into practice.

Types of Sarcopenias

Primary Sarcopenia

Primary sarcopenia refers to progressive and generalised loss of skeletal muscle mass and function that occurs with ageing in the absence of other identifiable causes. It is largely driven by age-related changes such as anabolic resistance, hormonal decline, and chronic low-grade inflammation, leading to reduced muscle strength and physical performance (Avgerinou, 2020).

Secondary Sarcopenia

Secondary sarcopenia develops when factors other than, or in addition to, ageing are evident. It may result from chronic systemic diseases, malignancy, organ failure, physical inactivity, or inadequate protein and energy intake, all of which accelerate muscle catabolism (Avgerinou, 2020).

Acute Sarcopenia

Acute sarcopenia describes a rapid decline in muscle mass and strength over less than six months, typically triggered by acute illness, surgery, or injury. It is often reversible with timely nutritional support, early mobilisation, and treatment of the underlying condition.

Chronic Sarcopenia

Chronic sarcopenia is diagnosed when muscle loss persists for six months or longer and is usually associated with long-term conditions such as chronic heart failure, chronic obstructive pulmonary disease, or neurodegenerative disease. It is progressive, increases frailty and mortality risk, and requires sustained multimodal interventions.

Sarcopenic Obesity

Sarcopenic obesity is defined by reduced lean body mass in the presence of excess adiposity. This dual burden exacerbates metabolic dysfunction, promotes fat infiltration of muscle, impairs mobility, and increases the risk of disability and death (Wei et al., 2023).

Malnutrition-associated Sarcopenia

Malnutrition-associated sarcopenia occurs when low dietary intake, impaired nutrient absorption, or increased nutrient demands lead to severe muscle wasting (Sieber, 2019). It is frequently seen in individuals with chronic inflammatory disease, cancer cachexia, or advanced organ failure, and requires prompt nutritional and medical management.

EPIDEMIOLOGY

The prevalence of sarcopenia varies greatly depending on the diagnostic criteria applied and the population studied. In community-dwelling older adults, assessments using the EWGSOP definitions have reported prevalence rates ranging from about 1% to nearly 30%, influenced by factors such as age, sex, comorbidities, and living environment (Cruz-Jentoft et al., 2014). The burden is even greater in acute-care settings. For example, a Norwegian multicentre observational study found that 37% of older adults admitted with hip fracture met the EWGSOP 2010 diagnostic criteria for sarcopenia, demonstrating a strong link between sarcopenia and fracture risk and reinforcing the need for systematic screening and targeted interventions in orthogeriatric services (Steihaug et al., 2017).

The consequences of sarcopenia are wide-ranging, including reduced mobility, increased risk of falls, delayed recovery from acute illness, prolonged hospitalisation, greater dependency, and higher mortality (Cruz-Jentoft and Sayer, 2019). Global data further illustrate the variability introduced by different diagnostic approaches. A large systematic review and meta-analysis of 151 studies ($n = 692{,}056$; mean age = 68.5 years) found worldwide prevalence estimates of 10–27%, with lower figures generally reported when the updated EWGSOP2 criteria were used (Petermann-Rocha et al., 2022). In the United Kingdom, the analysis of UK Biobank data showed that application of the original EWGSOP1 criteria gave a prevalence of 8.14%, whereas the use of the more stringent EWGSOP2 definition reduced this to just 0.36%, highlighting how diagnostic thresholds strongly influence prevalence estimates (Petermann-Rocha et al., 2020).

PATHOPHYSIOLOGY

Sarcopenia arises through interacting biological, metabolic, and environmental mechanisms. Loss of motor neurons reduces the number of functioning motor units; surviving neurons attempt reinnervation, yet the process is incomplete, leading to heterogeneous fibre sizes. There is preferential atrophy of fast-twitch (type II) muscle fibres, which are responsible for power and rapid movements, making older people more vulnerable to tasks demanding speed or suddenness (Evans and Lexell, 1995). In addition, muscle composition changes: accumulation of fat within and between muscle fibres, infiltration of non-contractile connective tissue, mitochondrial dysfunction, and oxidative stress degrade muscle quality and reduce strength relative to mass (Goodpaster et al., 2006).

Metabolically, hormonal changes including declines in testosterone, growth hormone, and insulin-like growth factor-1, reduce the anabolic drive. Systemic low-grade inflammation, elevated circulating cytokines such as interleukin-6 and tumour necrosis factor-α, contribute to catabolism. Nutritional deficiencies (especially protein and essential amino acids), physical inactivity, and sedentary behaviour further exacerbate the decline. Acute illnesses (e.g. infection, surgery) often trigger catabolic stress; in their aftermath, recovery is impaired when muscle reserves are already diminished (Figure 10.1).

IMPACT OF COVID-19 ON SARCOPENIA AND FRAILTY

The COVID-19 pandemic has drawn attention to musculoskeletal consequences that extend beyond respiratory disease. Evidence from a systematic review indicates that pre-existing sarcopenia increases the likelihood of severe infection, including higher rates of hospitalisation and intensive care admission (Halaweh and Ghannam, 2022). Sarcopenia and frailty may both worsen through mechanisms linked to

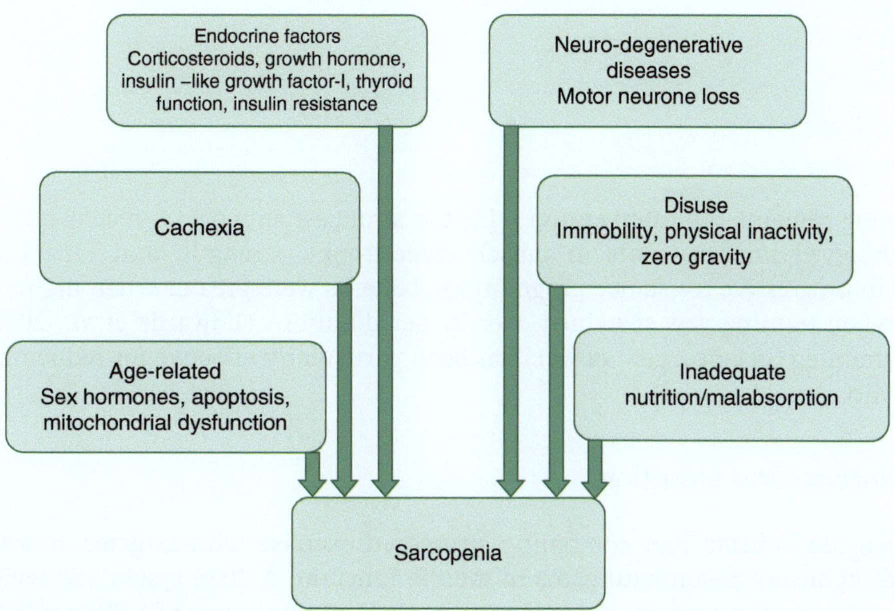

FIGURE 10.1   Aetiological factors and mechanisms of sarcopenia (*Source*: Martin and Ranhoff (2020) / with permission of Springer Nature).

post-COVID symptoms, extended hospital stays, and periods of enforced isolation, all of which can drive fatigue, reduced activity, and muscle loss (Martone et al., 2022; Welch et al., 2020). In addition, new data associating SARS-CoV-2 infection with cognitive impairment suggest a further route by which the virus may amplify the interplay between sarcopenia and frailty (Crivelli et al., 2022).

DIAGNOSTIC APPROACHES

Diagnosis of sarcopenia has become more standardised in recent years. The revised pathway from EWGSOP2 (2019) recommends a step-wise algorithm: first case finding (for example screening tools like SARC-F questionnaire or gait speed), then confirmation via assessment of muscle strength (grip strength or chair-rise), measurement of muscle quantity or mass (via Dual-energy X-ray absorpti-ometry (DXA), Magnetic Resonance Imaging (MRI), Computed Tomography (CT), or bioelectrical impedance), followed by measurement of physical performance (Short Physical Performance Battery [SPPB], timed up and go, gait speed) to stage severity (Cruz-Jentoft et al., 2019). This approach allows early detection and stratification of risk, which is essential for guiding intervention (Cruz-Jentoft et al., 2019).

Recent observational studies highlight the importance of protein intake in diagnosis and risk stratification. In a Korean randomised trial of frail and pre-frail older adults aged 70–85, protein intakes of 1.5 g/kg/day over 12 weeks led to improvements in muscle mass indicators compared to lower intake groups (0.8 and 1.2 g/kg/day) in men (Kim and Park, 2020). A cross-sectional Korean study also found that protein intake below about 1.0 g/kg/day was associated with significantly higher odds of low muscle mass compared to those consuming higher amounts (Huh and Son, 2022). These findings support adjusting diagnostic and preventive strategies to include nutritional assessment and dietary history routinely in older populations (Figure 10.2).

INTERVENTIONS

Exercise

Resistance training remains the intervention with the strongest support. A recent review of exercise interventions observed improvements in muscle hypertrophy, strength, and function when older adults engaged in progressive resistance programmes; benefits were greater when higher intensity was achieved, and when training was sustained over longer durations (Edwards et al., 2023). Resistance plus functional training (balance, gait, power) has been particularly effective for reducing falls risk and improving mobility.

Combined Exercise and Nutrition

Recent meta-analyses indicate that combining structured exercise with targeted nutritional supple-mentation yields clinically meaningful gains in muscle function. A 2025 systematic review and meta-analysis of 15 randomised controlled trials reported pooled improvements of 1.77 kg (95% CI 0.51–3.03) in handgrip strength, 0.22 kg/m^2 in skeletal muscle mass index (SMI), 0.09 m/s in usual gait speed, and a 1.38 second reduction in five-times Sit-to-Stand (STS) performance compared with control interventions

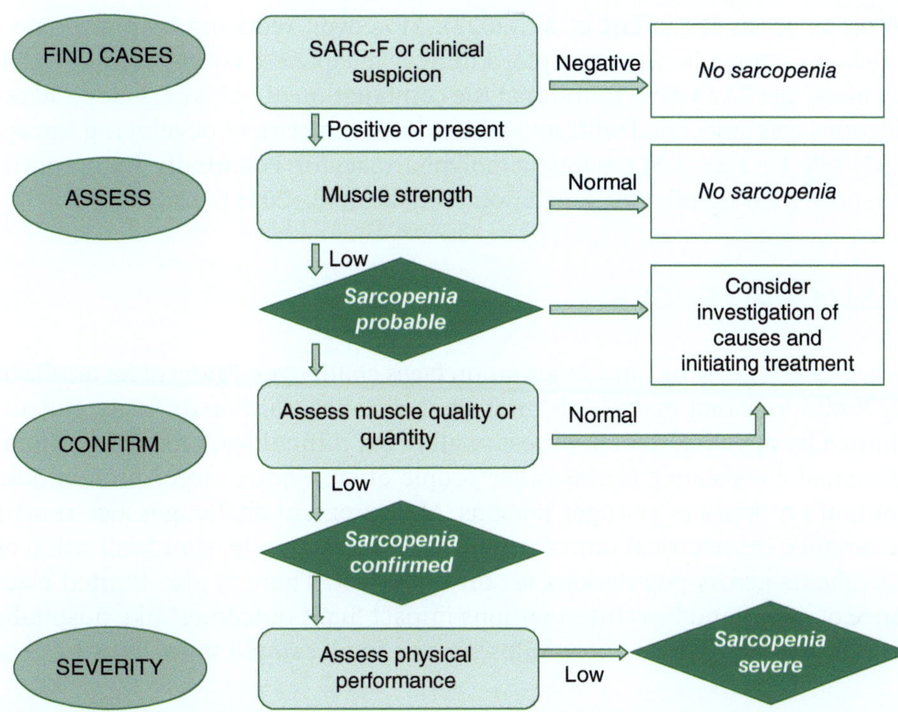

FIGURE 10.2 The EWGSOP algorithm for the diagnosis and grading of sarcopenia (*Source*: Martin and Ranhoff (2020) / with permission of Springer Nature).

(Yang et al., 2025). Furthermore, a recent Randomised Controlled Trials (RCT) in community settings found that combining protein supplementation with resistance training led to improvements in physical performance, grip strength, and muscle mass over 12 weeks (Ji et al., 2024).

Protein and Nutrition

Studies suggest that older adults require greater protein intake than standard adult recommendations. Kim and Park (2020) highlight that older adults consuming 0.8, 1.2, or 1.5 g/kg/day of protein over 12 weeks showed that an increase in absolute protein intake of more than 0.54 g/kg/day above habitual intake was positively associated with improvements in appendicular skeletal muscle mass indices in older men, whereas no significant effects were observed for gait speed, and no association with muscle mass was found in older women. In addition, supplementation with essential amino acids, whey protein, collagen peptides, or other high-biological value proteins in conjunction with exercise shows greater improvements than either intervention alone. For instance, in this trial, community-dwelling older adults underwent 16 weeks of resistance exercise plus leucine-enriched whey protein supplementation (about 1.5 g/kg/day), and improvements were reported in strength/functional outcomes (Kirk et al., 2021). Interventions lasting 10–24 weeks appear to produce measurable improvements in muscle mass and strength. However, heterogeneity in protocols (intensity, frequency, and nutritional composition), participant characteristics (baseline function, living setting, and comorbidities), and assessment tools leads to variability in outcomes (Yang et al., 2025; Whaikid and Piaseu, 2024). Correcting vitamin D deficiency in older adults may improve muscle strength and lower fracture risk, supporting its role in preventing both sarcopenia and osteoporosis (Beaudart et al., 2022). Moreover, reducing inappropriate polypharmacy may lower the risk of sarcopenia. For example, a nine-year Japanese cohort study of 1,549 community-dwelling adults (mean age 72.5 years) found that the combination of polypharmacy and potentially inappropriate medications was associated with more than double the risk of developing sarcopenia (adjusted hazard ratio 2.35; 95% CI 1.58–3.51), whereas polypharmacy or Potentially Inappropriate Medication (PIM) use alone showed no significant association (Tanaka et al., 2023).

BARRIERS AND CHALLENGES

While the evidence base is growing, implementation faces challenges. Many older adults have comorbidities or mobility limitations that make high-intensity resistance training difficult. Nutritional interventions may be limited by appetite, dental issues, swallowing difficulties, or socio-economic constraints. The concept of anabolic resistance means older people often require larger protein doses to elicit the same muscle protein synthesis as younger persons. Measurement challenges also remain, as access to DXA or MRI is variable; bioelectrical impedance may be less accurate; standardisation of strength and performance thresholds across populations is still imperfect. There is also limited evidence on long-term maintenance of gains, and how interventions impact 'hard outcomes' like hospitalisation, quality of life, or mortality. Some RCTs have short follow-ups or small sample sizes, limiting generalisability.

ROLE OF THE APs

APs are well placed to drive change in sarcopenia care. They can lead screening programmes in primary care, hospital outpatient clinics, or community settings, integrating strength and performance assessments into routine frailty or medicine reviews. For patients diagnosed with sarcopenia or 'possible sarcopenia', APs can design resistance-based exercise interventions, refer to physiotherapy, and liaise with dietetics to ensure adequate nutrition. APs should advocate for individualised care plans: assessing comorbidities, functional status, risk of falls, and patient goals. For nutritional interventions, they can oversee diet history, monitor protein intake, and address barriers (e.g. dental and appetite). Monitoring should include periodic measurements of strength (grip and leg), performance (gait speed and chair rise), and documentation of outcomes. Education of patients and caregivers about the importance of exercise and protein is critical. APs can deprescribe problematic polypharmacy where relevant to reduce the risk of sarcopenia.

Within service development, APs may establish multidisciplinary sarcopenia pathways: defining roles for screening, intervention, follow-up, and referral; embedding outcome audits; promoting access to suitable exercise programmes (community gyms and home-based resistance tools). They may also contribute to research, participating in or leading trials, or evaluating novel combination interventions or nutritional supplements.

RECENT ADVANCES AND EMERGING THERAPIES

Beyond resistance training and protein, new agents are under investigation. Supplementation with β-hydroxy-β-methylbutyrate (HMB) has shown promise in preserving lean body mass and strength in sarcopenic older adults, particularly in conjunction with exercise (Feng et al., 2024). Myokine modulation and anabolic hormone treatments are also areas of active research, though safety and long-term effects are still being established.

Digital health and telemedicine approaches are emerging. A telerehabilitation study using app-based or remote supervised exercise programmes has demonstrated feasibility and modest improvements in physical performance in older adults with sarcopenia. Such platforms may help overcome barriers of access, mobility, or geography. For instance, a recent RCT showed that a four-week remote resistance training delivered via a mobile app improved strength, balance, and instrumental activities of daily living in older adults with sarcopenia; its effects were comparable to those from in-person supervised rehabilitation (Zhang et al., 2025).

Focusing interventions for subpopulations (e.g. very old, institutionalised, cognitively impaired) is another area undergoing study. Evidence suggests that combined exercise–nutrition interventions are effective even in older adults with frailty or pre-sarcopenia in outpatient or community settings (Yang et al., 2025; Ji et al., 2024).

Best Practice Recommendations

Based on current evidence, best practice for managing sarcopenia might include:

- Routine screening for at-risk older adults (age, malnutrition, recent hospital admission, and low physical activity).
- Using simple tools like grip strength and gait speed in clinic, with confirmation of low muscle mass where feasible.
- Prescribing resistance training programmes tailored to ability (progressive load and frequency 2–3×/week) and supported balance/functional training.
- Ensuring nutritional adequacy: protein intake of ~1.2–1.5 g/kg/day for those with sarcopenia; attention to protein quality (Essential Amino Acids [EAAs] and leucine-rich sources); correction of vitamin D deficiency.
- Combining exercise and nutrition interventions where possible yields superior results.
- Conduct comprehensive geriatric assessment to ensure multidisciplinary input.

FUTURE RESEARCH DIRECTIONS

Key areas for future work include:

- Establishing standardised diagnostic thresholds adapted to diverse populations (different ethnicities and body compositions).
- Large-scale RCTs with long follow-ups to assess maintenance of gains, impact on frailty trajectory, hospitalisation, and quality of life.
- Comparative trials of nutritional supplement types (e.g. whey, casein, collagen, and HMB) and dosing strategies.
- Evaluations of digital/remote delivery models (telehealth, apps, and wearable technologies) to extend reach.
- Health services research to understand how best to integrate sarcopenia care pathways into routine practice, including resource, training, and funding implications.

CONCLUSION

Sarcopenia is a common, disabling condition for older adults, but one for which effective interventions exist. Current evidence supports combined resistance training and nutritional strategies (particularly higher protein intake) as central to prevention and treatment. APs are well placed to lead screening, individualised intervention, multidisciplinary coordination, and ongoing monitoring. As the population ages, integrating sarcopenia care into routine clinical pathways is both a clinical and ethical imperative.

Take-Home Messages

1. Sarcopenia is common, tightly linked to frailty, and drives falls, disability, admissions, and mortality.
2. Diagnose with EWGSOP2: low muscle strength (grip or 5 × STS >15 seconds or unable), confirm low muscle mass, grade severity with SPPB ≤8, gait speed, or Timed Up and Go test (TUG) ≥20 seconds.
3. Most effective treatment is progressive resistance training 2–3×/week plus protein about 1.2–1.5 g/kg/day; correct vitamin D and add balance/gait work.
4. Combine exercise and nutrition for bigger gains, tackle malnutrition, inactivity, and harmful polypharmacy.
5. APs lead screening and pathways using grip, 5 × STS, gait speed, SPPB, and TUG; personalise plans, review regularly, and coordinate Multidisciplinary Team (MDT) care.

REFERENCES

Avgerinou, C. (2020). Sarcopenia: why it matters in general practice. *The British Journal of General Practice* 70 (693): 200.

Beaudart, C., Buckinx, F., Rabenda, V. et al. (2022). The role of vitamin D in the prevention and management of sarcopenia: a systematic review and meta-analysis. *Journal of Cachexia, Sarcopenia and Muscle* 13 (1): 164–179.

Crivelli, L., Palmer, K., Calandri, I. et al. (2022). Changes in cognitive functioning after COVID-19: a systematic review and meta-analysis. *Alzheimer's & Dementia* 18 (5): 1047–1066.

Cruz-Jentoft, A.J. and Sayer, A.A. (2019). Sarcopenia. *The Lancet* 393 (10191): 2636–2646.

Cruz-Jentoft, A.J., Baeyens, J.P., Bauer, J.M. et al. (2010). Sarcopenia: European consensus on definition and diagnosis: report of the European Working Group on Sarcopenia in Older People. *Age and Ageing* 39 (4): 412–423.

Cruz-Jentoft, A.J., Landi, F., Schneider, S.M. et al. (2014). Prevalence of and interventions for sarcopenia in ageing adults: a systematic review. Report of the International Sarcopenia Initiative (EWGSOP and IWGS). *Age and Ageing* 43 (6): 748–759.

Cruz-Jentoft, A.J., Bahat, G., Bauer, J. et al. (2019). Sarcopenia: revised European consensus on definition and diagnosis. *Age and Ageing* 48 (1): 16–31.

Dhillon, R.J.S. and Hasni, S. (2017). Pathogenesis and management of sarcopenia. *Clinics in Geriatric Medicine* 33 (1): 17–26.

Edwards, H.R., Jones, H., Moseley, J. et al. (2023). Exercise interventions for the management of sarcopenia: possibilities and challenges. *Physical & Occupational Therapy in Geriatrics* 41 (4): 654–677.

Evans, W.J. and Lexell, J. (1995). Human aging, muscle mass, and fiber type composition. *The Journals of Gerontology Series A: Biological Sciences and Medical Sciences* 50 (Special_Issue): 11–16.

Feng, Y., Chen, P., Li, T. et al. (2024). Effects of exercise with or without β-hydroxy-β-methylbutyrate supplementation on muscle mass, muscle strength, and physical performance in patients with sarcopenia: a systematic review and meta-analysis. *Frontiers in Nutrition* 11: 1460133.

Goodpaster, B.H., Park, S.W., Harris, T.B. et al. (2006). The loss of skeletal muscle strength, mass, and quality in older adults: the health, aging and body composition study. *The Journals of Gerontology Series A: Biological Sciences and Medical Sciences* 61 (10): 1059–1064.

Halaweh, H. and Ghannam, I. (2022). The devastating trio of sarcopenia, frailty, and COVID-19 – a systematic review and meta-analysis. *Clinical Nutrition* 51: 143–151.

Huh, Y. and Son, K.Y. (2022). Association between total protein intake and low muscle mass in Korean adults. *BMC Geriatrics* 22 (1): 319.

Ji, W., Lee, D., Kim, M. et al. (2024). Efficacy of a combined exercise and nutrition intervention study for outpatients with possible sarcopenia in community-based primary care clinics (ENdSarC): study protocol for a multicenter single-blinded randomized controlled trial. *BMC Geriatrics* 24 (1): 861.

Kim, D. and Park, Y. (2020). Amount of protein required to improve muscle mass in older adults. *Nutrients* 12 (6): 1700.

Kirk, B., Mooney, K., Vogrin, S. et al. (2021). Leucine-enriched whey protein supplementation, resistance-based exercise, and cardiometabolic health in older adults: a randomized controlled trial. *Journal of Cachexia, Sarcopenia and Muscle* 12 (6): 2022–2033.

Martin, F.C. and Ranhoff, A.H. (2020). Frailty and sarcopenia. In: *Orthogeriatrics: The Management of Older Patients with Fragility Fractures* (ed. P. Falaschi and D. Marsh), 53–65. Cham: Springer.

Martone, A.M., Tosato, M., Ciciarello, F. et al. (2022). Sarcopenia as potential biological substrate of long COVID-19 syndrome: prevalence, clinical features, and risk factors. *Journal of Cachexia, Sarcopenia and Muscle* 13 (4): 1974–1982.

Narici, M.V. and Maffulli, N. (2010). Sarcopenia: characteristics, mechanisms and functional significance. *British Medical Bulletin* 95 (1): 139–159.

NHS England (2022). *Older people advanced practice area specific capability and curriculum framework.* NHS England. Available at: `https://advanced-practice.hee.nhs.uk/wp-content/uploads/sites/28/2025/01/Older-people-advanced-practice-area-specific-capability-and-curriculum-framework-NHSE.pdf` (accessed 30 January 2026).

NHS England (2023a). *Palliative and end of life care advanced practice area specific capability and curriculum framework.* NHS England. Available at: `https://advanced-practice.hee.nhs.uk/wp-content/uploads/sites/28/2025/01/Palliative-and-end-of-life-care-advanced-practice-area-specific-capability-and-curriculum-framework-NHSE.pdf` (accessed 30 January 2026).

NHS England (2023b). *Acute medicine advanced practice area specific capability and curriculum framework.* NHS England. Available at: `https://advanced-practice.hee.nhs.uk/wp-content/uploads/sites/28/2025/03/Acute-medicine-advanced-practice-area-specific-capability-and-curriculum-framework-NHSE.pdf` (accessed 30 January 2026).

NHS England (2025). *Multi-professional framework for advanced practice in England – Edition 2025.* NHS England. Available at: `https://advanced-practice.hee.nhs.uk/wp-content/uploads/sites/`

28/2025/05/Multi-professional-framework-for-advanced-practice-in-England---Edition-2025.pdf (accessed 29 January 2026).

Petermann-Rocha, F., Chen, M., Gray, S.R. et al. (2020). New versus old guidelines for sarcopenia classification: what is the impact on prevalence and health outcomes? *Age and Ageing* 49 (2): 300–304.

Petermann-Rocha, F., Balntzi, V., Gray, S.R. et al. (2022). Global prevalence of sarcopenia and severe sarcopenia: a systematic review and meta-analysis. *Journal of Cachexia, Sarcopenia and Muscle* 13 (1): 86–99.

Rosenberg, I.H. (1997). Sarcopenia: origins and clinical relevance. *The Journal of Nutrition* 127 (5): 990S–991S.

Sieber, C.C. (2019). Malnutrition and sarcopenia. *Aging Clinical and Experimental Research* 31 (6): 793–798.

Steihaug, O.M., Gjesdal, C.G., Bogen, B. et al. (2017). Sarcopenia in patients with hip fracture: a multicenter cross-sectional study. *PLoS One* 12 (9): e0184780.

Tanaka, T., Akishita, M., Kojima, T. et al. (2023). Polypharmacy with potentially inappropriate medications as a risk factor of new onset sarcopenia among community-dwelling Japanese older adults: a 9-year Kashiwa cohort study. *BMC Geriatrics* 23 (1): 390.

Wei, S., Nguyen, T.T., Zhang, Y. et al. (2023). Sarcopenic obesity: epidemiology, pathophysiology, cardiovascular disease, mortality, and management. *Frontiers in Endocrinology* 14: 1185221.

Welch, C., Greig, C., Masud, T. et al. (2020). COVID-19 and acute sarcopenia. *Aging and Disease* 11 (6): 1345.

Whaikid, P. and Piaseu, N. (2024). The effectiveness of protein supplementation combined with resistance exercise programs among community-dwelling older adults with sarcopenia: a systematic review and meta-analysis. *Epidemiology and Health* 46: e2024030.

Yang, Y., Pan, N., Luo, J. et al. (2025). Exercise and nutrition for sarcopenia: a systematic review and meta-analysis with subgroup analysis by population characteristics. *Nutrients* 17 (14): 2342.

Zhang, L., Ge, Y., Zhao, W. et al. (2025). A 4-week mobile app–based telerehabilitation program vs conventional in-person rehabilitation in older adults with sarcopenia: randomized controlled trial. *Journal of Medical Internet Research* 27: e67846.

CHAPTER 11

Ageing and Physiological Changes

Aim

This chapter provides advanced practitioners (APs) with an overview understanding of the physiological changes associated with ageing and frailty across major organ systems. It highlights how these changes interact with multimorbidity, polypharmacy, and social determinants to influence clinical assessment, decision-making, and management in older adults.

LEARNING OUTCOMES

By the end of this chapter, APs will be able to:

1. Critically explain age-related physiological changes in the nervous, respiratory, cardiovascular, gastrointestinal, genitourinary, endocrine, integumentary, and haematology–immune systems, and their relevance to frailty.
2. Apply this knowledge to improve assessment, differential diagnosis, and treatment planning, recognising when symptoms are more likely to reflect disease than normal ageing.
3. Integrate awareness of system-specific ageing with frailty screening, polypharmacy review, and anticipatory care to prevent decompensation during acute illness or stress.
4. Formulate evidence-informed, person-centred management strategies that enhance resilience and quality of life for older adults.

SELF-ASSESSMENT QUESTIONS

1. How confident are you in distinguishing between normal age-related physiological change and early signs of disease when assessing an older adult?
2. In what ways do you currently integrate knowledge of system-specific ageing and frailty into your clinical decision-making and anticipatory care planning?

> To master the care of older adults, every healthcare professional must see ageing not as decline but as transformation, where recognising physiological change becomes the key to preserving dignity, function, and life itself.

INTRODUCTION

Ageing represents a gradual, intrinsic, and time-related reduction in physiological performance and systemic resilience, distinct from specific disease processes (Guo et al., 2022). It is characterised by reduced homeostatic reserve, slower cellular repair, and increased susceptibility to internal and external stressors (Ukraintseva et al., 2021). Chronological age alone is an imprecise guide, as biological ageing varies widely between individuals, with marked differences in physiological capacity and functional reserve (Chen et al., 2023). Consequently, clinical decisions should consider multimorbidity, polypharmacy, social context, and functional status rather than age in isolation.

Frailty is now recognised as a discrete clinical entity arising from cumulative physiological decline (British Geriatrics Society, 2014). It is commonly accompanied by sarcopenia, involuntary weight loss, fatigue, cognitive changes, and reduced physical activity. Conceptual frameworks such as the frailty phenotype (Fried et al., 2001) and the cumulative deficit model (Rockwood and Mitnitski, 2006) capture both the biological deterioration and the functional dependence that develop over time. Understanding the system-level physiological alterations underpinning frailty is therefore central to anticipating complications and guiding preventive and therapeutic strategies (Figure 11.1). Despite increasing clinical awareness, detailed knowledge of organ-specific physiological changes that heighten vulnerability in frailty remains incomplete.

Multi-Professional Framework (MPF) for Advanced Practitioners

(NHS England, 2025)
This chapter maps to the following areas within the MPF:

1. Clinical practice: 1.1, 1.3, 1.4, 1.5, 1.7, 1.8, 1.9
2. Leadership and management: 2.1, 2.2, 2.3, 2.5, 2.7
3. Education: 3.1, 3.3, 3.4, 3.5
4. Research: 4.1, 4.2, 4.3, 4.5

Accreditation Consideration

This chapter maps to the statement with the following national accretional document:
Curriculum framework for advanced practice in the care of older people (NHS England, 2022):

1. Core CiPs: 1, 2, 3, 4, 5
2. Generic Clinical CiPs: 1, 2, 3, 4, 5
3. Specialty Clinical CiPs (Older People): 3.1, 3.2, 3.4, 3.5

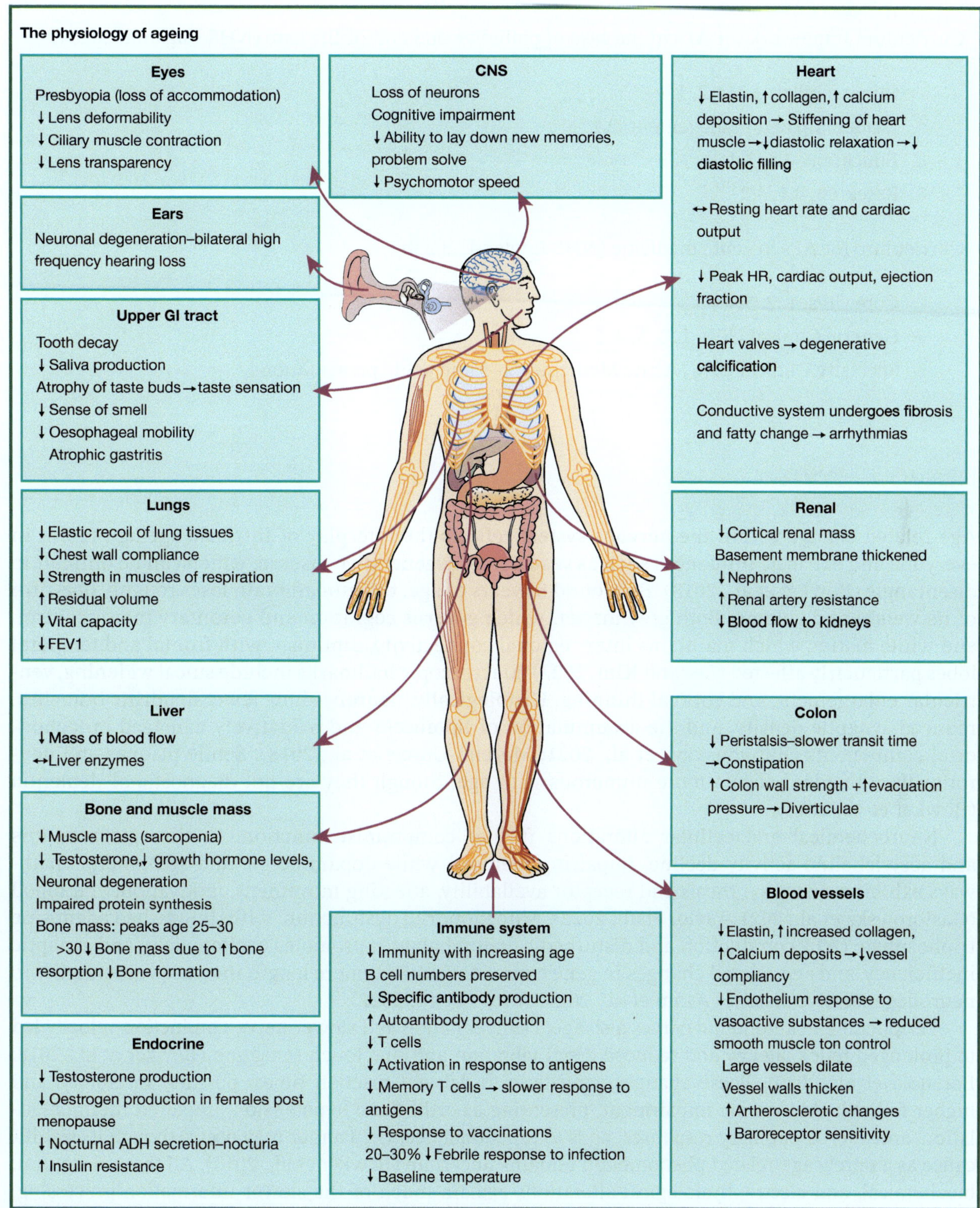

FIGURE 11.1 Overview of physiological. *Source*: Adapted from Blundell and Gordon (2015) Wiley.

Curriculum framework for APs in the case of palliative and end-of-life care (NHS England, 2023a):

1. Clinical pillar: 1.1, 1.2, 1.4
2. Leadership and management: 2.1
3. Education: 3.1, 3.4
4. Research: 4.1, 4.2

Curriculum for APs in acute medicine (NHS England, 2023b):

1. Core CiPs: 1, 2, 3, 4
2. Generic Clinical CiPs: 1, 2, 3, 4, 5
3. Specialty Clinical CiPs (Acute Medicine): 1–5 and acute presentations

NERVOUS SYSTEM

Age-related change within the nervous system reflects the interplay of intrinsic ageing present in everyone and extrinsic influences such as vascular or degenerative disease, which can be difficult to disentangle (Bowker et al., 2018). By around 85 years of age, the human brain loses roughly one-fifth of its weight and volume. Both grey matter, which governs cognition and voluntary motor control, and white matter, which maintains inter-regional connectivity, diminish, with frontal and temporal lobes particularly affected (Lee and Kim, 2022). Macroscopic hallmarks include sulcal widening, ventricular enlargement, and cortical thinning. Histologically, neurons show fewer dendritic branches, reduced synaptic density, and the accumulation of lipofuscin and oxidatively damaged mitochondrial components (Blinkouskaya et al., 2021; Moreno-García et al., 2018). Senile plaques and neurofibrillary tangles become more numerous with age, though they are not diagnostic of dementia (Bowker et al., 2018).

Neurochemical and cellular alterations further compromise function. Cholinergic receptors and acetylcholine activity decline, impairing memory, while dopaminergic and serotonergic pathways exhibit reduced synthesis and receptor availability, affecting movement, motivation, and mood (Gasiorowska et al., 2021; Taylor et al., 2022). Mitochondrial dysfunction, with diminished adenosine triphosphate (ATP) production and disturbed calcium balance, promotes excitotoxicity and synaptic inefficiency, and age-related changes in gene expression and telomere length increase vulnerability to neurodegenerative disease (Azam et al., 2021; Jurcău et al., 2022).

Peripheral and autonomic nerves also age. Demyelination and slower nerve-conduction velocity led to prolonged reflex latency and reduced distal vibration and fine touch sensation (Bowker et al., 2018; Borzuola et al., 2020). These changes contribute to delayed reaction times, postural instability, and higher fall risk. Autonomic impairment, presenting as orthostatic hypotension, impaired thermoregulation, and altered pupillary responses, adds to functional decline. Tremor may occur, though its significance as a purely age-related phenomenon remains uncertain (Bowker et al., 2018). All these structural, biochemical, and electrophysiological alterations explain much of the slower information processing, executive dysfunction, and increased sensitivity to neuromodulating drugs observed in later life, while also setting the stage for neurodegenerative disorders such as Alzheimer's disease (Figure 11.1).

RESPIRATORY SYSTEM

Physiological ageing of the respiratory system produces progressive structural and functional changes that reduce pulmonary reserve and heighten vulnerability to decompensation during illness (Takla et al., 2024). Loss of elastic recoil, caused by degeneration of elastin fibres and enlargement of alveolar spaces, leads to small-airway closure at low lung volumes, increased residual volume (Figure 11.1), and a steady decline in forced expiratory volume in one second (FEV_1) of roughly 25–30 mL per year from the mid-thirties, with steeper falls after 70 years (Physiopedia, 2025). Arterial oxygen tension decreases almost linearly, from about 12.7 kPa at age 30 to around 10 kPa by age 60, reflecting widening of the alveolar–arterial oxygen gradient and impaired ventilation–perfusion matching (Physiopedia, 2025).

Stiffening of the chest wall is another hallmark, arising from calcification of costal cartilages, degenerative changes in intercostal, intervertebral and costovertebral joints, and kyphoscoliosis related to osteoporosis (Chaddha et al., 2023; Bowker et al., 2018). Concomitant sarcopenia weakens the diaphragm and accessory respiratory muscles, lowering maximal minute ventilation and increasing the work of breathing. Although lung compliance may rise because of reduced elastic recoil, the net effect of parenchymal stiffening and thoracic rigidity is impaired overall mechanics. Chemoreceptor sensitivity to hypoxia and hypercapnia is blunted, resulting in a weaker ventilatory response to falling oxygen or rising carbon dioxide levels (Bowker et al., 2018).

Airway defence mechanisms also deteriorate. Degeneration of bronchial epithelium and submucosal glands diminishes mucociliary clearance, while a less sensitive cough reflex and weaker expiratory muscles impede clearance of secretions (Schneider et al., 2021; Bowker et al., 2018). These factors increase the risk of retained secretions, underventilation of dependent lung zones, and lower respiratory tract infections, particularly aspiration pneumonia. During acute insults such as pneumonia, limited pulmonary reserve can precipitate rapid respiratory failure and more severe presentations even when pre-existing disease is stable (Bowker et al., 2018).

In healthy non-smokers, these intrinsic changes rarely cause symptoms at rest, and exercise tolerance usually remains adequate because oxygen consumption and cardiac output decline in parallel with lung function. However, in smokers or those with chronic respiratory conditions such as emphysema, the same age-related changes amplify symptoms and accelerate functional decline (Bowker et al., 2018). Breathlessness in later life is frequently multifactorial, reflecting combined effects of lung ageing, reduced fitness, musculoskeletal problems, obesity, or coexisting cardiac disease. Chronic dyspnoea may reflect reduced physical fitness, obesity, musculoskeletal problems such as osteoarthritis or spinal deformity, prior lung damage (for example, apical fibrosis after tuberculosis), and the modest effects of intrinsic ageing. Acute breathlessness often arises from a combination of conditions such as pneumonia, rapid atrial fibrillation, and heart failure, where combined therapy (e.g. digoxin, diuretics, and antibiotics) may be indicated.

All these structural and physiological alterations, including loss of elastic recoil, chest wall stiffening, reduced chemoreceptor responsiveness, and impaired airway defence, explain the increased susceptibility of older adults to respiratory infection, aspiration, and ventilatory failure, and highlight the importance of preventive strategies and vigilant clinical assessment.

CARDIOVASCULAR SYSTEM

Cardiovascular ageing reflects interacting processes of intrinsic cellular change, lifelong exposure to risk factors, and acquired disease. Large arteries become thicker, elongated, and less elastic (Figure 11.1), raising systolic pressure and peripheral vascular resistance and predisposing to isolated systolic hypertension and aortic 'unfolding' visible on chest X-ray (Bowker et al., 2018; Singam et al., 2020). Intimal thickening favours atheroma formation. The left ventricle compensates through concentric hypertrophy, which increases filling pressures and reduces diastolic compliance, limiting the ability to augment cardiac output during stress (Ding et al., 2024). With advancing age, the left atrium dilates, further increasing the risk of atrial fibrillation.

Electrical conduction also changes. Fibrosis and fatty infiltration of the sinoatrial (SA) node and conduction pathways slow impulse generation and transmission, making first-degree heart block, bundle branch block, and left axis deviation more common (Bowker et al., 2018). Maximum heart rate declines by roughly 10% at rest and 25% under stress, while β-adrenergic receptor down-regulation and altered calcium handling blunt contractile reserve and catecholamine responsiveness (Moghtadaei et al., 2016; Bowker et al., 2018). These changes reduce cardiac reserve, so tachycardia is a less reliable sign of acute illness. The progressive loss of pacemaker cells weakens SA node control, allowing ectopic atrial foci to trigger atrial fibrillation, which markedly increases the risk of embolic stroke (British Geriatrics Society, 2025).

Heart failure with preserved ejection fraction (HFpEF) is predominantly a disorder of older adults and now represents more than half of all heart failure diagnoses. Early stages feature subclinical cardiac remodelling such as left atrial enlargement, increased left ventricular mass, impaired diastolic function, and raised E/e' ratios, which can evolve into overt atrial fibrillation, coronary artery disease, and decompensated heart failure if unrecognised (Upadhya and Kitzman, 2020; Ijaz et al., 2025; Gharagozloo et al., 2024).

Ageing also impairs circulatory reflexes. Baroreceptor sensitivity declines, and venous capacitance vessels lose compliance, reducing orthostatic compensation and predisposing to postural hypotension, which affects about one in five community-dwelling older people (Bencivenga et al., 2022; Bhanu et al., 2024). Autonomic dysfunction limits compensatory tachycardia, so symptoms may include dizziness, syncope, or falls, particularly in the context of antihypertensives, diuretics, or psychoactive medicines (Rivasi et al., 2020).

While intrinsic ageing alone rarely causes symptoms in fit older adults, its impact is amplified by cumulative exposure to cardiovascular risk factors and by disease acquisition. Smoking, hypertension, diabetes, and dyslipidaemia accelerate vascular stiffening and atheroma. Nevertheless, cardiovascular ageing is modifiable: sustained exercise, weight management, and good control of risk factors can preserve cardiac reserve and blunt age-related change, so that a healthy, active older adult may exhibit less functional impairment than a sedentary younger person (Bowker et al., 2018). Therefore, arterial stiffening, myocardial and conduction system remodelling, reduced baroreceptor sensitivity, and diminished β-adrenergic responsiveness together reduce cardiovascular reserve. These alterations increase the likelihood of hypertension, atrial fibrillation, heart failure, and orthostatic hypotension, and they magnify the haemodynamic impact of acute illness. Early detection and management of risk factors, structured exercise, and careful medication review remain key strategies for maintaining cardiovascular health in later life.

Frailty and Age-Related Cardiovascular Changes

Ageing produces progressive alterations in cardiac structure and function that predispose older adults to frailty and cardiovascular disease. As explained earlier, these changes include left ventricular hypertrophy, left atrial enlargement, and arterial stiffening, which collectively represent subclinical

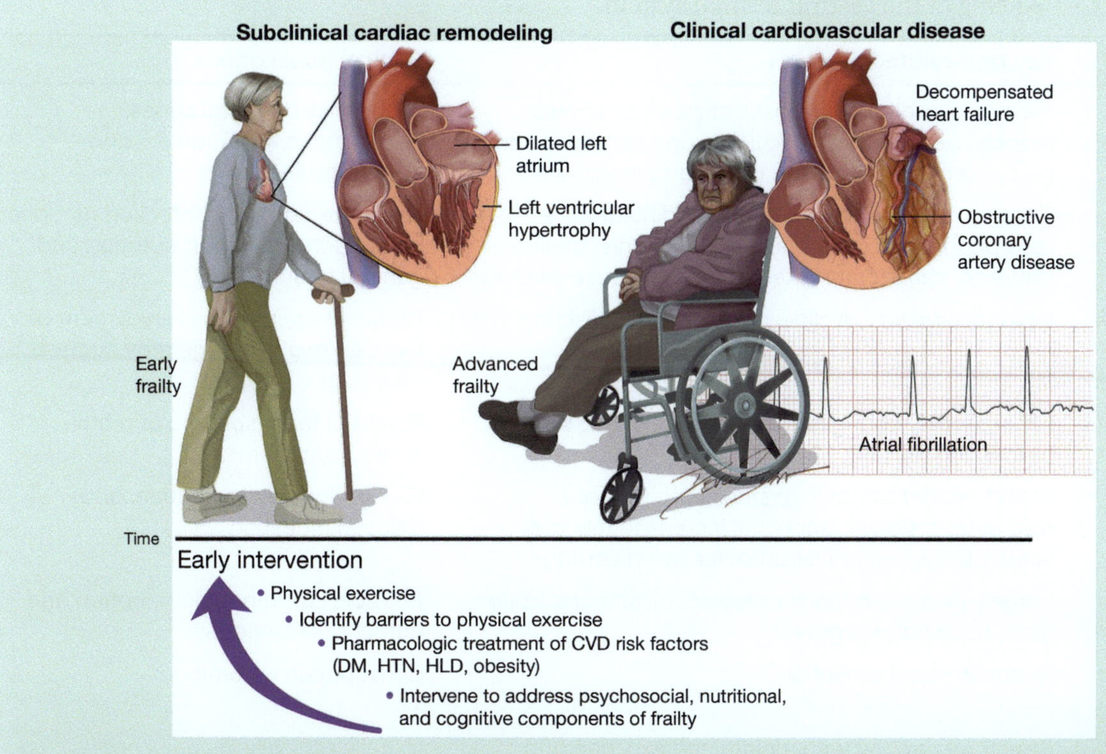

FIGURE 11.2   Progress of frailty and cardiovascular disease. *Source*: Ijaz et al. (2025)/American College of Cardiology Foundation/CC BY 4.0.

cardiac remodelling. In this phase, physiological reserve is reduced, yet overt symptoms may be absent. Figure 11.2 demonstrates this transition, showing an older adult with early frailty exhibiting compensatory cardiac changes such as left ventricular hypertrophy and atrial dilatation. As these changes advance, they culminate in clinical cardiovascular disease, characterised by decompensated heart failure, obstructive coronary artery disease, and atrial fibrillation (features illustrated in the second stage of the figure).

Figure 11.2 emphasises opportunities for early intervention to prevent progression. These include promoting physical activity, addressing barriers to exercise, optimising management of cardiovascular risk factors such as diabetes, hypertension, dyslipidaemia, and obesity, and providing psychosocial, nutritional, and cognitive support. These measures can slow the physiological decline associated with ageing and reduce the burden of frailty-related cardiovascular morbidity.

GASTROINTESTINAL SYSTEM

Ageing affects the gastrointestinal (GI) tract from the oral cavity to the liver, bringing structural and functional changes that can compromise nutrition, immunity, and drug handling (Hinssen et al., 2024; Figure 11.1 and Table 11.1).

TABLE 11.1   Ageing of the gastrointestinal system.

Region	Key age-related changes	Clinical implications
Teeth	Yellowing and loss of translucency, enamel wear, reduced dentine/pulp vascularity and sensitivity, and gum recession with risk of caries and tooth loss	Higher risk of dental caries, periodontitis, malnutrition, and systemic infection
Mouth	Thinner, more fragile mucosa; mandibular bone resorption; reduced orofacial muscle tone causing dribbling; xerostomia, often drug- or disease-related	Greater trauma and infection risk; poor oral health can impair nutrition and general health
Taste/smell	Gradual olfactory decline, reducing taste discrimination	Reduced appetite and enjoyment of food; an acute change may suggest neurological disease
Oesophagus	Minor motility changes; increased incidence of hiatus hernia and reflux	Potential for dysphagia or reflux-related symptoms
Stomach	More frequent atrophic gastritis with reduced acid output; slower emptying; increased mucosal vulnerability; higher *Helicobacter pylori* carriage	Risk of gastritis, ulceration, and delayed digestion
Small intestine	Largely preserved function; lower calcium absorption; more bacterial overgrowth	Possible calcium malabsorption and nutrient deficiencies
Large intestine	Reduced rectal sensation	Constipation is common
Pancreas	Structural atrophy with maintained exocrine and endocrine function	Usually clinically insignificant functional impact
Liver	Around 25% reduction in weight and volume; lipofuscin deposition; liver function usually normal	Mild biochemical changes, usually within normal limits; interpret tests cautiously
Gallbladder	Higher prevalence of gallstones, particularly in women over 80	Risk of gallstone complications despite frequent absence of symptoms

Ageing brings structural and functional alterations throughout the gastrointestinal system, influencing oral health, motility, absorption, and metabolic processes.

Oral Cavity and Dentition

Teeth become more yellow and less translucent as enamel thins and cannot regenerate. Dentine and pulp lose vascularity and sensitivity, and gums recede with periodontal disease, producing the classic 'long in the tooth' appearance (Bowker et al., 2018). Caries, periodontitis, and tooth loss are frequent but not inevitable, while bone resorption in the mandible, accelerated by tooth loss and osteoporosis, alters facial structure. Salivary glands generally retain the ability to secrete, yet xerostomia is common due to chronic disease or medications. Thinning of oral mucosa, reduced taste and smell, and declining orofacial muscle tone can impair chewing and swallowing, affecting dietary intake and medication administration (De Sire et al., 2022).

Oesophagus and Stomach

Ageing leads to subtle changes in oesophageal innervation and peristalsis, and the lower oesophageal sphincter becomes less competent, increasing the risk of gastro-oesophageal reflux, aspiration, and hiatal hernia (Andrade and Herbella, 2024; Bowker et al., 2018). Gastric emptying slows, and atrophic gastritis becomes more prevalent, reducing production of hydrochloric acid and intrinsic factor. This impairs absorption of vitamin B12, iron, and calcium, while increased *Helicobacter pylori* carriage adds to mucosal vulnerability.

Small and Large Intestine

Small-bowel function is largely preserved, but calcium absorption diminishes, and bacterial overgrowth becomes more common, leading to diarrhoea, malnutrition, and weight loss (Vara-Luiz et al., 2025; Bowker et al., 2018). In the colon, weaker peristalsis, reduced rectal sensation, inactivity, and the effects of drugs—particularly opioids and anticholinergics—contribute to constipation (Gallo et al., 2024).

Pancreas, Liver, and Gallbladder

The pancreas undergoes modest atrophy without major functional loss. By contrast, the liver shows a progressive fall in mass and blood flow of around 25–30% compared with younger adults, with accumulation of lipofuscin pigment (Drenth-Van Maanen et al., 2020; Bowker et al., 2018). Phase I metabolic pathways (oxidation and reduction) are most affected, while phase II conjugation remains relatively intact. This increases the bioavailability of drugs with high first-pass metabolism, such as opioids and metoclopramide, and heightens sensitivity to medicines with a narrow therapeutic index, including benzodiazepines and warfarin (Ngcobo, 2025). Standard liver function tests, such as alanine aminotransferase and alkaline phosphatase, may remain within normal limits, masking reduced metabolic reserve. The gallbladder shows a higher incidence of gallstones affecting up to 40% of women over 80 years, although most remain asymptomatic (Bowker et al., 2018).

In health, these intrinsic changes rarely cause overt symptoms, but they lower the threshold for decompensation during illness or polypharmacy. Collectively, they explain the increased risks of malnutrition, aspiration, infection, constipation, and adverse drug reactions in older adults, and underline the importance of preventive dental care, tailored nutrition, and careful prescribing.

GENITOURINARY SYSTEM

Age-related changes in the genitourinary tract arise from gradual structural and physiological decline, compounded by frailty, multimorbidity, and medication effects. Diminished functional reserve limits the ability to cope with illness, dehydration, or polypharmacy (Figure 11.1).

Kidneys and Renal Function

Glomerular filtration rate (GFR) falls by about 1 mL/min each year after the age of 40 because of nephron loss, glomerulosclerosis, and reduced renal perfusion (American Society of Nephrology, 2011). Sarcopenia can keep serum creatinine deceptively normal; therefore, creatinine clearance or cystatin C is more reliable for estimating renal function (Wang et al., 2023). The ageing kidney also shows weaker concentrating ability, reduced vasopressin responsiveness, and greater susceptibility to nephrotoxins and haemodynamic changes (Docherty et al., 2021). These factors increase the risk of hyponatraemia, hypernatraemia, and acute kidney injury. Slower clearance of renally excreted drugs such as digoxin, lithium, aminoglycosides, and certain opioids further heightens toxicity risk, so prescribing should follow a 'start low and go slow' approach with regular monitoring (British Geriatrics Society, 2020).

Lower Urinary Tract

Bladder capacity and compliance decrease with age, while detrusor overactivity and reduced urinary flow rate lead to urgency, frequency, nocturia, and incontinence. These symptoms can limit mobility, discourage adequate hydration, and predispose to falls and acute kidney injury. Urinary tract infections (UTIs) are common, often presenting with non-specific features such as confusion or sudden functional decline (Godbole et al., 2020). Good hydration, appropriate catheter management, and tailored continence care help reduce risk.

Sex-specific Changes

In women, the post-menopausal fall in oestrogen leads to thinning of the vaginal epithelium, reduced lubrication, increased acidity, and greater vulnerability to vaginal and urinary infection (Bowker et al., 2018). The uterus and ovaries atrophy, and the vagina becomes smaller and less elastic. Hormone replacement therapy can relieve menopausal symptoms but carries important risks that limit long-term use.

In men, testicular mass and sperm production gradually decline, and semen quality diminishes. The prostate enlarges and fibroses, producing benign prostatic hyperplasia (BPH), which is common in later life and can cause bladder outflow obstruction, incomplete emptying, and recurrent UTIs (Fiard et al., 2021; Liu et al., 2023; Sandhu et al., 2024; Wei et al., 2025). Although erection becomes less sustained and the refractory period lengthens, severe erectile dysfunction is usually due to disease or medication rather than ageing alone. Testosterone levels remain stable or fall slightly; a more pronounced deficiency can present with fatigue, muscle loss, osteoporosis, reduced sexual function, and cognitive changes. Carefully monitored testosterone replacement may offer symptomatic benefit in confirmed hypogonadism but requires vigilance for adverse effects such as rising haematocrit and prostatic enlargement (Bowker et al., 2018).

Sexual Health in Both Sexes

Cross-sectional studies suggest a marked decline in sexual activity with age, but longitudinal data show smaller changes, implying that social and cultural factors strongly influence late-life sexuality. Physical illness (e.g. arthritis, cardiovascular disease), depression, and bereavement also play major roles, and many of these factors are modifiable (Bowker et al., 2018). Taken together, these renal, urinary, and reproductive changes explain the increased incidence of UTIs, voiding dysfunction, sexual health concerns, and drug-related complications in later life. Comprehensive assessment, including renal monitoring, continence support, and sensitive discussion of sexual health, is essential for maintaining quality of life in older adults.

ENDOCRINE SYSTEM

Endocrine ageing is characterised by gradual alterations in hormone secretion, metabolism, and target-tissue responsiveness, which interact with frailty, chronic disease, and lifestyle factors to influence clinical outcomes (Figure 11.1).

Hypothalamic Pituitary Axis

With age, growth hormone secretion and insulin-like growth factor-1 (IGF-1) production decline, contributing to sarcopenia, reduced bone mass, and frailty (Gupta and Kumar, 2022). Circadian rhythms become less robust, leading to altered sleep patterns and impaired stress responses. Chronic, low-grade activation of the hypothalamic–pituitary–adrenal axis can result in sustained cortisol elevations, affecting cognition, mood, and immune function (Stamou et al., 2023).

Thyroid Function

In healthy older adults, overall thyroid function is usually preserved. Median thyroid-stimulating hormone (TSH) levels drift slowly upwards but remain within the reference range (Bowker et al., 2018). Subclinical hypothyroidism is common and often asymptomatic (Guan et al., 2022). Lower T3 and TSH values may occur in very advanced age or during acute illness, typically reflecting non-thyroidal illness (sick euthyroid syndrome) rather than true hypothyroidism. In such cases, thyroid function tests (TFTs) should be repeated after recovery before considering treatment. Distinguishing this transient pattern from primary or secondary hypothyroidism is essential to avoid unnecessary hormone replacement.

Glucose Metabolism

Ageing is associated with delayed and reduced insulin secretion in response to glucose, slower suppression of hepatic glucose output, and diminished peripheral (muscle and fat) insulin sensitivity (Bowker et al., 2018). Together with lower physical activity and lean body mass, these changes lead to more frequent impaired glucose tolerance (IGT). Although IGT increases macrovascular risk, only a minority of older people progress to overt diabetes.

Gonadal Hormones

In women, menopause typically occurs around age 50 years, leading to a sharp fall in oestrogen, with consequent atrophy of the vaginal epithelium, decreased lubrication, and greater susceptibility to vaginal and urinary infection. Oestrogen deficiency also heightens the risk of osteoporosis and cardiovascular disease (Kojima et al., 2022; Bowker et al., 2018). In men, testosterone declines more gradually, and most remain fertile. Testicular mass, sperm production, and semen quality decrease; erections may be less firm and the refractory period longer. Severe erectile dysfunction usually indicates comorbidity or drug effects rather than normal ageing. A minority of men experience clinically significant hypogonadism with fatigue, muscle wasting, osteoporosis, and reduced sexual function. Testosterone replacement may alleviate symptoms but carries risks such as raised haematocrit and prostatic enlargement, and requires close monitoring (Gregori et al., 2021; Bowker et al., 2018).

Energy Balance and Appetite Regulation

Altered secretion of leptin, ghrelin, and cholecystokinin affects satiety and appetite, predisposing to anorexia of ageing and involuntary weight loss (Moss et al., 2012).

Overall, endocrine ageing involves subtle but clinically significant changes across multiple axes. Most are asymptomatic in health but can amplify frailty, impair recovery from illness, and increase vulnerability to metabolic and cardiovascular disease. Regular review of thyroid status, glucose tolerance, bone health, and reproductive hormone effects supports early recognition and appropriate intervention.

INTEGUMENTARY SYSTEM

Ageing skin shows progressive thinning of the epidermis, reduced dermal collagen, and loss of subcutaneous fat, making it fragile and less elastic (Nigam and Knight, 2017). Sebaceous and sweat gland activity decline, leading to dryness (xerosis) and impaired thermoregulation (Eidt, 2023). Cumulative ultraviolet exposure and reduced deoxyribonucleic acid (DNA) repair increase the lifetime risk of skin malignancy (Haisma, 2022). Wound healing slows, and the incidence of pressure ulcers and skin tears rises (Sandoz, 2024).

Frailty amplifies these changes. Immobility, incontinence, and polypharmacy further compromise the skin barrier. Flattening of the dermal–epidermal junction reduces mechanical resilience and promotes shear-related injuries such as skin tears (Roig-Rosello and Rousselle, 2020). Loss of collagen and elastin weakens structural support (Gohil et al., 2022). Immunosenescence and chronic low-grade inflammation delay tissue repair, and abnormal neutrophil responses can worsen injury (Drew et al., 2017). Pretibial lacerations, common in frail older women, particularly those on anticoagulants, are increasingly recognised as serious wounds with significant morbidity and mortality (Paavana et al., 2023).

Risk assessment and early prevention are essential. Tools such as PURPOSE-T for pressure ulcer risk and the Integrated Same-day Treatment and Assessment Pathway (ISTAP) classification for skin tears help identify individuals at high risk and guide targeted interventions (LeBlanc et al., 2018; National Wound Care Strategy Programme, 2024). As frailty advances, regular skin assessment should form part of comprehensive frailty evaluation and care planning to reduce preventable skin injury and support optimal healing.

HAEMATOLOGY AND IMMUNE SYSTEM

Ageing and frailty are accompanied by profound but heterogeneous changes in blood formation, immune regulation, and coagulation, which together heighten susceptibility to anaemia, infection, thrombosis, and malignancy.

Haematopoiesis and Anaemia

Bone marrow stem cells become functionally exhausted and increasingly biased towards myeloid cell production, with reduced lymphoid output (Sun et al., 2025). Population studies show a gradual fall in haemoglobin from about 60 years of age, and 10–20% of older adults have levels below 12 g/dL in women or 13 g/dL in men (Bowker et al., 2018). Nevertheless, age itself rarely causes significant anaemia; most cases are due to chronic disease, renal impairment, nutrient deficiency, or occult blood loss. Anaemia of chronic inflammation is common and usually normocytic, driven by impaired erythropoietin response, iron sequestration, and diminished marrow reserve (Lee et al., 2021). Clinically, anaemia is linked to fatigue, reduced physical performance, cognitive decline, and increased mortality. Investigation should be based on clinical context rather than a single haemoglobin threshold.

Coagulation and Inflammatory Milieu

Ageing is associated with 'inflammageing' a persistent, low-grade inflammatory state characterised by raised interleukin-6, C-reactive protein, and tumour necrosis factor-alpha (Ferrucci and Fabbri, 2018). This promotes myelopoiesis and contributes to anaemia as well as vascular disease. Platelet hyper-reactivity and endothelial changes create a prothrombotic state, raising the risk of venous thromboembolism, particularly in immobilised or acutely unwell, frail patients (Akrivou et al., 2022). Erythrocyte sedimentation rate (ESR) rises with age and can be mildly elevated in the absence of disease, but a marked increase (>90 mm/h) usually reflects serious pathology such as paraproteinaemia, chronic infection, or giant cell arteritis (Bowker et al., 2018).

Immune Ageing (Immunosenescence)

The immune system does not simply 'wear out'; it becomes dysregulated. Memory T lymphocytes and autoantibodies increase, while production of new T cells, key interleukins, and high-affinity antibodies to novel antigens declines (Bowker et al., 2018). Macrophage antigen clearance and complement activation are less efficient, and vaccine responses are weaker. These changes increase vulnerability to infection, malignancy, and impaired wound healing. Reactivation of latent infections such as varicella zoster (shingles) and tuberculosis is more likely, and pneumonia, influenza, and bacterial endocarditis carry higher mortality. Figure 11.1 provides an overview of the other key physiological changes that occur across the major organ systems with ageing.

Clinical Consequences

Infection in older adults often presents atypically with non-specific deterioration, falls, delirium, or incontinence. Fever may be absent or delayed, and classical laboratory markers such as leucocytosis, raised C-reactive protein, or complement activation may appear late. Diagnostic tests can be misleading; for example, urine dipsticks frequently show colonisation without true infection. Because sepsis may be advanced before it is clinically obvious, treatment is often empirical and delayed recognition increases complications.

Overall, age-related haematological and immune changes exacerbated by frailty, comorbidity, and malnutrition demand careful clinical evaluation. Regular blood monitoring, cautious interpretation of inflammatory markers, and vigilant infection surveillance are essential to maintain health and reduce preventable morbidity and mortality in later life.

Case Study 11.1   A Complex Presentation with Advanced Ageing

Mr H, an 86-year-old man with known frailty (Clinical Frailty Scale 6), heart failure with preserved ejection fraction, stage 3 chronic kidney disease, and mild cognitive impairment, was assessed by an AP on an acute medical unit. His carer reported two days of increasing confusion, poor oral intake, and a fall that morning.

Assessment by the AP

- History and examination: Mr H complained of dizziness and abdominal discomfort. He was mildly hypotensive (BP 94/60 mmHg) with an irregular heart rate of 110 bpm, dry mucous membranes, and reduced skin turgor. Cardiovascular examination revealed an irregularly irregular pulse and mild ankle oedema. Chest auscultation showed bibasal crackles.
- Investigations: Electrocardiogram (ECG) confirmed atrial fibrillation with a rapid ventricular response. Blood tests demonstrated:
  - eGFR 32 mL/min/1.73 m^2 (baseline 48)
  - Haemoglobin 9.8 g/dL (previously 11.5)
  - C-reactive protein 84 mg/L
  - Serum sodium 128 mmol/L
  - B-type natriuretic peptide (BNP) markedly elevated
  - Urinalysis: positive for nitrites and leucocytes
  - Chest X-ray: pulmonary congestion with no focal pneumonia

Clinical reasoning and management
The AP identified multiple interacting problems:

- Cardiovascular: atrial fibrillation with fast ventricular response and decompensated heart failure due to reduced diastolic compliance and blunted β-adrenergic responsiveness.
- Renal and fluid balance: acute kidney injury on chronic kidney disease, complicated by hyponatraemia and risk of fluid overload.
- Infection and haematology: probable UTI presenting as delirium, with anaemia of chronic inflammation.
- Frailty and nutrition: poor oral intake and immobility increasing risk of further functional decline.

A comprehensive plan was initiated: cautious intravenous hydration with strict input/output monitoring, empirical intravenous antibiotics, rhythm and rate control in consultation with cardiology, temporary suspension of nephrotoxic medicines, and iron studies to guide anaemia management. Early involvement of physiotherapy, dietetics, and social services supported rehabilitation and discharge planning.

This case illustrates the complexity of acute presentations in advanced age, where age-related changes in the cardiovascular, renal, immune, and haematological systems converge with frailty to produce rapid decompensation. The AP's role in synthesising multisystem information, prioritising interventions, and coordinating multidisciplinary input is critical for stabilisation, prevention of further decline, and shared decision-making about ongoing care.

CONCLUSION

Ageing is a universal, intrinsic process but its clinical impact is highly variable and often masked by disease and social factors. Across every organ system, gradual structural and functional decline reduces physiological reserve, rendering older adults more vulnerable to illness, iatrogenic harm, and delayed recovery. APs who understand these mechanisms can better distinguish normal ageing from pathology, anticipate complications, and lead proactive, preventive care that supports healthy ageing and mitigates frailty.

Take-Home Messages

1. Normal ageing involves predictable, system-wide physiological changes, but significant symptoms usually signal disease or modifiable risk factors.

2. Frailty represents the cumulative effect of these changes, lowering resilience and increasing susceptibility to acute illness and functional decline.

3. Skilled assessment, early detection of reversible factors, and careful medication management are essential AP competencies to reduce avoidable harm.

4. Holistic, person-centred strategies incorporating physical activity, nutrition, psychosocial support, and anticipatory care are key to preserving independence and quality of life in later years.

REFERENCES

Akrivou, D., Perlepe, G., Kirgou, P. et al. (2022). Pathophysiological aspects of aging in venous thromboembolism: an update. *Medicina* 58 (8): 1078.

American Society of Nephrology (ASN) (2011). Aging and the kidney: physiology and pathophysiology. *Kidney News* 3 (2): 1–6. https://www.asn-online.org/publications/kidneynews/archives/2011/KN_2011_02_feb.pdf (accessed 26 July 2025).

Andrade, M.L. and Herbella, F.A. (2024). The sequel of age and frailty on the pathophysiology and treatment of surgical esophageal diseases. *Annals of Esophagus* 7: 5.

Azam, S., Haque, M.E., Balakrishnan, R. et al. (2021). The ageing brain: molecular and cellular basis of neurodegeneration. *Frontiers in Cell and Developmental Biology* 9: 683459.

Bencivenga, L., Barreto, P.D.S., Rolland, Y. et al. (2022). Blood pressure variability: a potential marker of aging. *Ageing Research Reviews* 80: 101677.

Bhanu, C., Petersen, I., Orlu, M. et al. (2024). Drug-induced orthostatic hypotension: cluster analysis of co-prescription patterns in older people in UK primary care. *Pharmacoepidemiology and Drug Safety* 33 (1): e5730.

Blinkouskaya, Y., Caçoilo, A., Gollamudi, T. et al. (2021). Brain aging mechanisms with mechanical manifestations. *Mechanisms of Ageing and Development* 200: 111575.

Blundell, A. and Gordon, A. (2015). *Geriatric Medicine at a Glance*, 1e. Chichester: Wiley Blackwell.

Borzuola, R., Giombini, A., Torre, G. et al. (2020). Central and peripheral neuromuscular adaptations to ageing. *Journal of Clinical Medicine* 9 (3): 741.

Bowker, L.K., Price, J.D., Shah, K.S., and Smith, S.C. (2018). *Oxford Handbook of Geriatric Medicine*, 3e. Oxford: Oxford University Press.

British Geriatrics Society (2014). *Introduction to Frailty.* https://www.bgs.org.uk/introduction-to-frailty (accessed 29 July 2025).

British Geriatrics Society (2020). *End of Life Care in Frailty: Pain.* https://www.bgs.org.uk/end-of-life-care-in-frailty-pain (accessed 31 July 2025).

British Geriatrics Society (2025). *Atrial Fibrillation, TIA and Stroke.* https://www.bgs.org.uk/atrial-fibrillation-tia-and-stroke (accessed 26 July 2025).

Chaddha, R., Agrawal, G., Koirala, S., and Ruparel, S. (2023). Osteoporosis and vertebral column. *Indian Journal of Orthopaedics* 57 (Suppl. 1): 163–175.

Chen, R., Wang, Y., Zhang, S. et al. (2023). Biomarkers of ageing: current state-of-art, challenges, and opportunities. *MedComm - Future Medicine* 2 (2): e50.

De Sire, A., Ferrillo, M., Lippi, L. et al. (2022). Sarcopenic dysphagia, malnutrition, and oral frailty in elderly: a comprehensive review. *Nutrients* 14 (5): 982.

Ding, C.C.A., Dokos, S., Bakir, A.A. et al. (2024). Simulating impaired left ventricular–arterial coupling in aging and disease: a systematic review. *Biomedical Engineering Online* 23 (1): 24.

Docherty, N.G., Delles, C., D'Haese, P. et al. (2021). Haemodynamic frailty—a risk factor for acute kidney injury in the elderly. *Ageing Research Reviews* 70: 101408.

Drenth-Van Maanen, A.C., Wilting, I., and Jansen, P.A. (2020). Prescribing medicines to older people—how to consider the impact of ageing on human organ and body functions. *British Journal of Clinical Pharmacology* 86 (10): 1921–1930.

Drew, W., Wilson, D., and Sapey, E. (2017). Frailty and the immune system. *Journal of Aging Research and Healthcare* 2 (1): 1–14.

Eidt, L.M. (2023). Cutaneous aging and dermatosis in geriatric patients. In: *Dermatology in Public Health Environments: A Comprehensive Textbook* (ed. R.R. Bonamigo), 967–1001. Cham: Springer International Publishing.

Ferrucci, L. and Fabbri, E. (2018). Inflammageing: chronic inflammation in ageing, cardiovascular disease, and frailty. *Nature Reviews Cardiology* 15 (9): 505–522.

Fiard, G., Stavrinides, V., Chambers, E.S. et al. (2021). Cellular senescence as a possible link between prostate diseases of the ageing male. *Nature Reviews Urology* 18 (10): 597–610.

Fried, L.P., Tangen, C.M., Walston, J. et al. (2001). Frailty in older adults: evidence for a phenotype. *The Journals of Gerontology Series A: Biological Sciences and Medical Sciences* 56 (3): M146–M157.

Gallo, A., Pellegrino, S., Pero, E. et al. (2024). Main disorders of gastrointestinal tract in older people: an overview. *Gastrointestinal Disorders* 6 (1): 313–336.

Gasiorowska, A., Wydrych, M., Drapich, P. et al. (2021). The biology and pathobiology of glutamatergic, cholinergic, and dopaminergic signaling in the aging brain. *Frontiers in Aging Neuroscience* 13: 654931.

Gharagozloo, K., Mehdizadeh, M., Heckman, G. et al. (2024). Heart failure with preserved ejection fraction in the elderly population: basic mechanisms and clinical considerations. *Canadian Journal of Cardiology* 40 (8): 1424–1444.

Godbole, G.P., Cerruto, N., and Chavada, R. (2020). Principles of assessment and management of urinary tract infections in older adults. *Journal of Pharmacy Practice and Research* 50 (3): 276–283.

Gohil, K., Varma, P., Byford, G. et al. (2022). Pretibial lacerations. *British Journal of Hospital Medicine* 83 (12): 1–7.

Gregori, G., Celli, A., Barnouin, Y. et al. (2021). Cognitive response to testosterone replacement added to intensive lifestyle intervention in older men with obesity and hypogonadism: prespecified secondary analyses of a randomized clinical trial. *The American Journal of Clinical Nutrition* 114 (5): 1590–1599.

Guan, B., Luo, J., Huang, X. et al. (2022). Association between thyroid hormone levels and frailty in the community-dwelling oldest-old: a cross-sectional study. *Chinese Medical Journal* 135 (16): 1962–1968.

Guo, J., Huang, X., Dou, L. et al. (2022). Aging and aging-related diseases: from molecular mechanisms to interventions and treatments. *Signal Transduction and Targeted Therapy* 7 (1): 391.

Gupta, P. and Kumar, S. (2022). Sarcopenia and endocrine ageing: are they related? *Cureus* 14 (9): e28787.

Haisma, M.S. (2022) *Keratinocyte carcinoma – risk factors for development and progression: focus on tumor-related factors, medication and frailty.* Doctor of Philosophy thesis, University of Groningen. Available at: https://research.rug.nl/en/publications/keratinocyte-carcinoma-risk-factors-for-development-and-progressi/ (accessed 1 January 2026).

Hinssen, F., Mensink, M., Huppertz, T., and van der Wielen, N. (2024). Impact of aging on the digestive system related to protein digestion in vivo. *Critical Reviews in Food Science and Nutrition* 1–17.

Ijaz, N., Nanna, M.G., and Damluji, A.A. (2025). *Prevent frailty, prevent cardiovascular disease: early identification of patients at risk. JACC: Advances* 4 (6 Pt 2): 101701. https://doi.org/10.1016/j.jacadv.2025.101701.

Jurcău, M.C., Andronie-Cioara, F.L., Jurcău, A. et al. (2022). The link between oxidative stress, mitochondrial dysfunction and neuroinflammation in the pathophysiology of Alzheimer's disease: therapeutic implications and future perspectives. *Antioxidants* 11 (11): 2167.

Kojima, G., Taniguchi, Y., Ogawa, K. et al. (2022). Age at menopause is negatively associated with frailty: a systematic review and meta-analysis. *Maturitas* 165: 94–99.

LeBlanc, K., Campbell, K.E., Wood, E., and Beeckman, D. (2018). Best practice recommendations for the prevention and management of skin tears in aged skin: an overview. *Wounds International* https://woundsinternational.com/journal-articles/best-practice-recommendations-for-the-prevention-and-management-of-skin-tears-in-aged-skin-an-overview/ (accessed 19 July 2025).

Lee, J. and Kim, H.J. (2022). Normal aging induces changes in the brain and neurodegeneration progress: review of the structural, biochemical, metabolic, cellular, and molecular changes. *Frontiers in Aging Neuroscience* 14: 931536.

Lee, C.T., Chen, M.Z., Yip, C.Y.C. et al. (2021). Prevalence of anemia and its association with frailty, physical function and cognition in community-dwelling older adults: findings from the HOPE study. *The Journal of Nutrition, Health and Aging* 25 (5): 679–687.

Liu, D., Li, C., Li, Y. et al. (2023). Benign prostatic hyperplasia burden comparison between China and United States based on the Global Burden of Disease Study 2019. *World Journal of Urology* 41 (12): 3629–3634.

Moghtadaei, M., Jansen, H.J., Mackasey, M. et al. (2016). The impacts of age and frailty on heart rate and sinoatrial node function. *The Journal of Physiology* 594 (23): 7105–7126.

Moreno-García, A., Kun, A., Calero, O. et al. (2018). An overview of the role of lipofuscin in age-related neurodegeneration. *Frontiers in Neuroscience* 12: 464.

Moss, C., Dhillo, W.S., Frost, G., and Hickson, M. (2012). Gastrointestinal hormones: the regulation of appetite and the anorexia of ageing. *Journal of Human Nutrition and Dietetics* 25 (1): 3–15.

National Wound Care Strategy Programme (2024). *Pressure Ulcer Recommendations and Clinical Pathway.* https://www.nationalwoundcarestrategy.net/wp-content/uploads/2024/07/NWCSPPU-Clinical-Recommendations-andpathway-Updated-21st-May-2024.pdf (accessed 20 July 2025).

Ngcobo, N.N. (2025). Influence of ageing on the pharmacodynamics and pharmacokinetics of chronically administered medicines in geriatric patients: a review. *Clinical Pharmacokinetics* 64 (3): 335–367.

NHS England (2022). *Older people advanced practice area specific capability and curriculum framework.* NHS England. Available at: https://advanced-practice.hee.nhs.uk/wp-content/uploads/sites/28/2025/01/Older-people-advanced-practice-area-specific-capability-and-curriculum-framework-NHSE.pdf (accessed 30 January 2026).

NHS England (2023a). *Palliative and end of life care advanced practice area specific capability and curriculum framework*. NHS England. Available at: `https://advanced-practice.hee.nhs.uk/wp-content/uploads/sites/28/2025/01/Palliative-and-end-of-life-care-advanced-practice-area-specific-capability-and-curriculum-framework-NHSE.pdf` (accessed 30 January 2026).

NHS England (2023b). *Acute medicine advanced practice area specific capability and curriculum framework*. NHS England. Available at: `https://advanced-practice.hee.nhs.uk/wp-content/uploads/sites/28/2025/03/Acute-medicine-advanced-practice-area-specific-capability-and-curriculum-framework-NHSE.pdf` (accessed 30 January 2026).

NHS England (2025). *Multi-professional framework for advanced practice in England – Edition 2025*. NHS England. Available at: `https://advanced-practice.hee.nhs.uk/wp-content/uploads/sites/28/2025/05/Multi-professional-framework-for-advanced-practice-in-England---Edition-2025.pdf` (accessed 29 January 2026).

Nigam, Y. and Knight, J. (2017). Anatomy and physiology of ageing 11: the skin. *Nursing Times* 113 (12): 51–55.

Paavana, T., Banks, T., Ford, D., and Singh, R. (2023). Pretibial haematoma in the elderly: a review of management and mortality. *Journal of Surgery* 3 (2): 1112.

Physiopedia (2025). Ageing and the Cardiorespiratory System. `https://www.physio-pedia.com/Ageing_and_the_Cardiorespiratory_System` (accessed 26 July 2025).

Rivasi, G., Rafanelli, M., Mossello, E. et al. (2020). Drug-related orthostatic hypotension: beyond anti-hypertensive medications. *Drugs & Aging* 37 (10): 725–738.

Rockwood, K. and Mitnitski, A. (2006). Limits to deficit accumulation in elderly people. *Mechanisms of Ageing and Development* 127 (5): 494–496.

Roig-Rosello, E. and Rousselle, P. (2020). The human epidermal basement membrane: a shaped and cell instructive platform that aging slowly alters. *Biomolecules* 10 (12): 1607.

Sandhu, J.S., Bixler, B.R., Dahm, P. et al. (2024). Management of lower urinary tract symptoms attributed to benign prostatic hyperplasia (BPH): AUA guideline amendment 2023. *The Journal of Urology* 211 (1): 11–19.

Sandoz, H. (2024). Frailty and the ageing skin: understanding skin tears. *Journal of Community Nursing* 38 (5): 20–26.

Schneider, J.L., Rowe, J.H., Garcia-de-Alba, C. et al. (2021). The aging lung: physiology, disease, and immunity. *Cell* 184 (8): 1990–2019.

Singam, N.S.V., Fine, C., and Fleg, J.L. (2020). Cardiac changes associated with vascular aging. *Clinical Cardiology* 43 (2): 92–98.

Stamou, M.I., Colling, C., and Dichtel, L.E. (2023). Adrenal aging and its effects on the stress response and immunosenescence. *Maturitas* 168: 13–19.

Sun, N., Lin, C.H., Li, M.Y. et al. (2025). Clusterin drives myeloid bias in aged hematopoietic stem cells by regulating mitochondrial function. *Nature Aging* 1–18.

Takla, M., Mele, M., and Takla, T. (2024). Anatomical and physiological changes in aging. In: *Geriatric Anesthesia: A Practical Guide* (ed. B. Gourkanti, D. Chaudhry, I. Gratz, et al.), 10–22. Sharjah: Bentham Science Publishers.

Taylor, W.D., Zald, D.H., Felger, J.C. et al. (2022). Influences of dopaminergic system dysfunction on late-life depression. *Molecular Psychiatry* 27 (1): 180–191.

Ukraintseva, S., Arbeev, K., Duan, M. et al. (2021). Decline in biological resilience as key manifestation of aging: potential mechanisms and role in health and longevity. *Mechanisms of Ageing and Development* 194: 111418.

Upadhya, B. and Kitzman, D.W. (2020). Heart failure with preserved ejection fraction: new approaches to diagnosis and management. *Clinical Cardiology* 43 (2): 145–155.

Vara-Luiz, F., Mendes, I., Palma, C. et al. (2025). Age-related decline of gastric secretion: facts and controversies. *Biomedicines* 13 (7): 1546.

Wang, C., Guo, X., Xu, X. et al. (2023). Association between sarcopenia and frailty in elderly patients with chronic kidney disease. *Journal of Cachexia, Sarcopenia and Muscle* 14 (4): 1855–1864.

Wei, J.T., Dauw, C.A., and Brodsky, C.N. (2025). Lower urinary tract symptoms in men: a review. *Journal of the American Medical Association*.

GERIATRIC MEDICINE

WHY GERIATRIC MEDICINE IS DIFFERENT?

Geriatric medicine focuses on the care of older adults who are typically characterised by frailty, multi-morbidity, and functional decline rather than chronological age alone. This field is unique because ageing itself interacts with chronic disease, acute illness, and social vulnerability, creating a pattern of interdependence rarely seen in younger adults (Figure 1). These overlapping influences result in the loss of physiological reserve, impaired homeostasis, and an increased risk of atypical or non-specific clinical presentations such as falls, confusion, or general functional decline.

The Figure 1 illustrates how physiological ageing reduces adaptability, while social and environmental factors such as isolation, poverty, or inadequate housing further compromise resilience. Superimposed chronic diseases, polypharmacy, and cognitive impairment intensify this fragility. The culmination of these processes is expressed through the so-called Geriatric Giants: immobility, instability, incontinence, intellectual impairment, iatrogenesis, and inanition. Consequently, geriatric medicine should adopt a holistic, person-centred approach through comprehensive geriatric assessment (CGA) rather than focusing on single pathologies. Its goal is not merely to treat disease but to restore and preserve function, dignity, and quality of life within the context of multimorbidity and frailty.

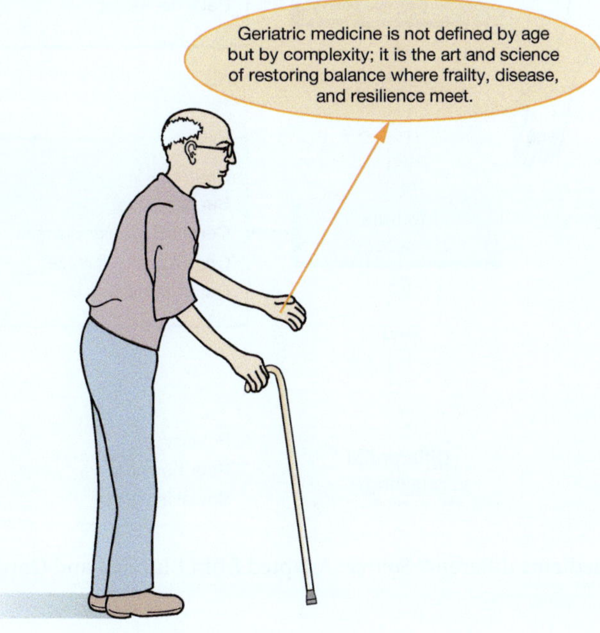

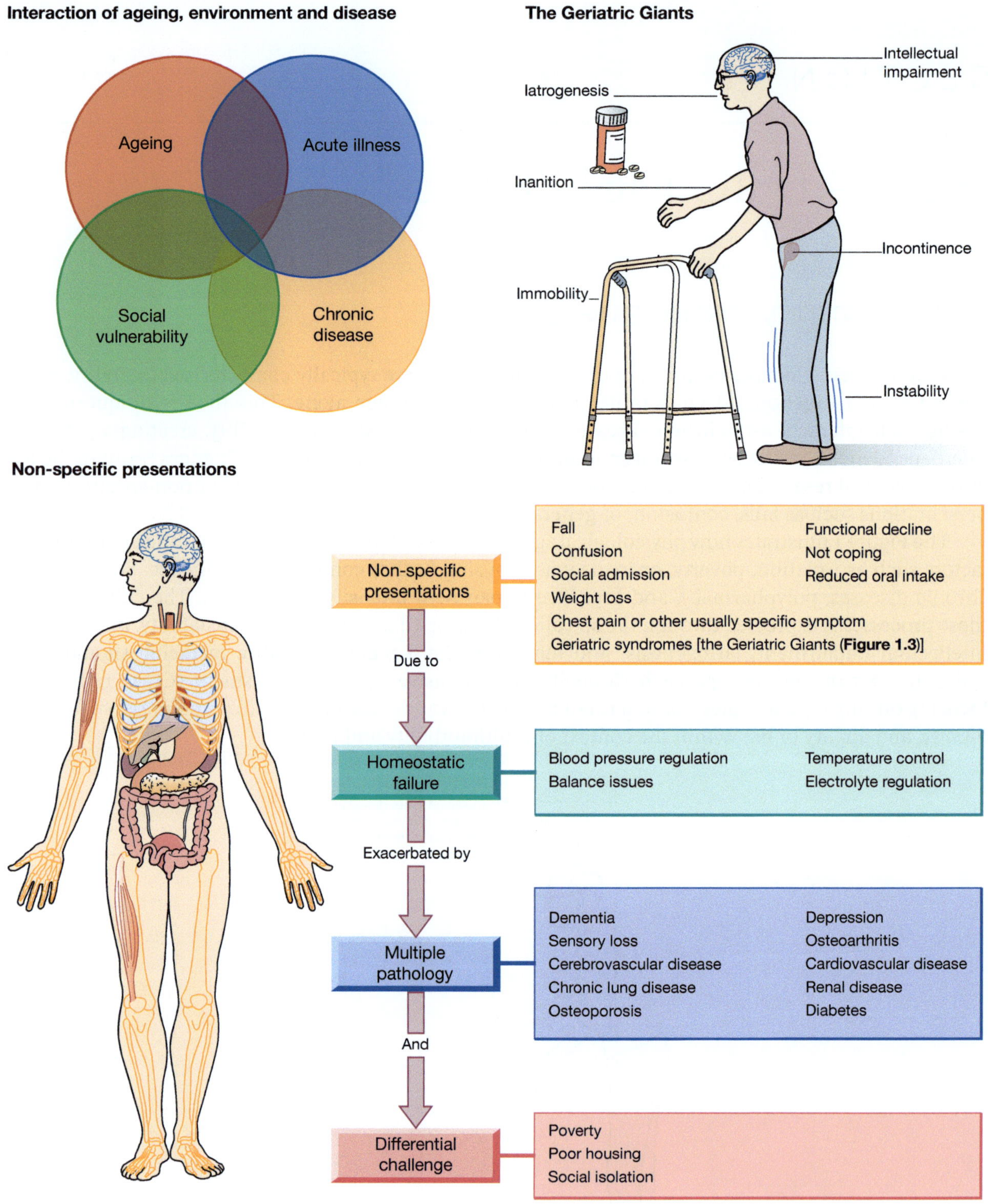

Interaction of ageing, environment and disease

The Geriatric Giants

Non-specific presentations

FIGURE 1   Why is geriatric medicine different? *Source*: Adapted from Blundell and Gordon (2015) (Wiley).

MPF CAPABILITIES AND GERIATRIC MEDICINE

MPF pillar	Capability number(s)	How demonstrated across section 3 (Geriatric Medicine)
Clinical practice	1.1–1.11	APs deliver accountable and autonomous care within professional and legal boundaries (1.1), apply clinical reasoning in complex, uncertain multimorbidity (1.2), and demonstrate reflective awareness of limits of competence (1.3). They undertake comprehensive, holistic assessment and diagnostic synthesis across systems (CGA, CFS, and FI/eFI) (1.4, 1.6), employ advanced communication to support shared decision-making (1.5), and initiate, evaluate, and modify interventions—covering medication review, falls prevention, nutrition, and end-of-life planning (1.7). They manage clinical risk and safety in unpredictable frailty deterioration (1.8), collaborate across organisational and professional boundaries (1.9), act as clinical role models for frailty-informed care (1.10), and evidence subject-specific competence through specialist knowledge of geriatric medicine and frailty mechanisms (1.11).
Leadership and management	2.1–2.11	Section 3 exemplifies inclusive and relational leadership (2.1), alignment with organisational values and person-centred service delivery (2.2), and evaluation of service outcomes (2.3). APs engage in peer review to improve practice (2.4), lead frailty-specific pathway redesigns (HF, COPD, AKI, and falls) (2.5), and co-produce service improvements with patients and carers (2.6). They provide consultancy across professional and organisational boundaries (2.7), demonstrate resilience and adaptability within complex geriatric systems (2.8), continually develop practice in response to changing population health and demographic trends (2.9), constructively challenge unsafe or inequitable practice (2.10), and negotiate an ethical and legally sound individual scope of practice that prioritises safety and governance (2.11).
Education	3.1–3.8	APs critically assess and address their own learning needs (3.1), pursue self-directed learning in emerging frailty science (3.2), and promote patient and carer health literacy to support shared management (3.3). They advocate for organisational learning cultures (3.4), facilitate interprofessional learning and reflective peer review (3.5), identify and address developmental needs within teams (3.6), build workforce capacity through work-based and interprofessional learning (3.7), and act as role models, supervisors, and mentors within frailty education programmes (3.8).
Research	4.1–4.8	Section 3 embeds research literacy across systems. APs critically engage with frailty and geriatric research (4.1), evaluate and audit clinical practice such as readmissions, medication burden, and pressure-injury rates (4.2), and synthesise findings from large cohort studies and guidelines to inform practice (4.3). They identify evidence gaps in frailty biomarker validation or psychosocial domains (4.4); propose and contribute to research to strengthen frailty management (4.5); establish robust governance and documentation processes for QI (4.6); disseminate findings through presentations, teaching, and publications (4.7); and build academic–clinical networks linking practice with research institutions (4.8).

ADVANCED CLINICAL PRACTICE FRAMEWORK FOR ELDERLY PEOPLE

Framework domain	Relevant CiPs	How section 3 demonstrates alignment
Core CiPs	1–6	Section 3 embeds professional autonomy and ethical reasoning in complex frailty care. It demonstrates inclusive communication, quality improvement, supervision, and research engagement across all organ-system chapters.
Generic Clinical CiPs	1–6	Chapters on neurology, cardiology, respiratory, and renal care evidence advanced assessment, multidisciplinary management, and safe discharge planning. Frailty is used as the unifying framework for long-term condition management and risk stratification.
Specialty Clinical CiPs (Older People/Frailty)	1–4	Section 3 reflects the comprehensive management of frail older adults, including anticipatory and advance care planning, frailty assessment (CGA, eFI, and FI), communication with patients and families, and interdisciplinary leadership.
Overall Mapping Summary	—	Section 3 equips APs to function as clinical leaders within frailty care, blending system-specific geriatric knowledge with advanced decision-making, inclusive leadership, reflective education, and a research-informed approach to service improvement.

ADVANCED CLINICAL PRACTICE FRAMEWORK FOR PALLIATIVE AND END-OF-LIFE MEDICINE

Category	Relevant CiPs	How section 3 demonstrates alignment
Core CiPs	1–6	Section 3 evidence autonomy, ethical reasoning, and advanced communication in managing progressive, life-limiting conditions, such as advanced heart failure, COPD, and dementia. It shows reflective practice, quality improvement in symptom control, and research engagement to enhance end-of-life outcomes.
Generic Clinical CiPs	1–4	The section demonstrates holistic palliative assessment, collaborative care planning, and management of complex symptoms. It addresses continuity of care, carer engagement, and coordination of multidisciplinary support for dying patients.
Specialty Clinical CiPs (Palliative and End-of-Life)	Clinical Pillars 1–4	Section 3 reflects therapeutic communication, differential diagnosis in complex palliative presentations, collaborative care planning, and leadership in symptom management and bereavement care. It reinforces multidisciplinary and intersectoral collaboration.
Summary	—	The section demonstrates alignment with the Palliative and End-of-Life Framework through integration of anticipatory care, ethical practice, symptom management, and inclusive leadership across all system-based geriatric chapters.

ADVANCED CLINICAL PRACTICE FRAMEWORK FOR ACUTE MEDICINE

Category	Relevant CiPs	How section 3 demonstrates alignment
Core CiPs	1–6	Section 3 demonstrates advanced-level functioning in acute care by applying ethical and legal frameworks to frailty-related emergencies. APs are shown to lead service improvement, mentor colleagues, and undertake research on acute presentations in older adults.
Generic Clinical CiPs	1–6	The chapters on acute deterioration, infection, falls, and delirium illustrate critical assessment under uncertainty, rapid intervention, escalation decisions, and safe discharge coordination in dynamic and high-risk settings.
Specialty Clinical CiPs (Acute Medicine Services) and acute presentations	1–5	Section 3 demonstrates active engagement in acute service development and evaluation, leadership of same-day emergency care (SDEC) models, prioritisation of patients based on illness severity, integration with critical care and other specialties, and coordination of complex discharges.
Summary	—	The section aligns closely with the Acute Medicine Framework, evidencing advanced practitioners' capacity to lead, assess, and manage frail or acutely ill older adults within dynamic clinical systems.

REFERENCE

Blundell, A. and Gordon, A. (2015). *Geriatric Medicine at a glance*. John Wiley & Sons.

CHAPTER 12

Neurology System

Aim

To critically explores the common neurological changes and major neurological disorders in older adults including Parkinson's disease, epilepsy, and motor neurone disease highlighting their interplay with frailty and outlining evidence-based approaches to assessment, diagnosis, and management within advanced practice.

LEARNING OUTCOMES

After studying this chapter, readers will be able to:

1. Critically appraise the pathophysiology, epidemiology, and clinical presentation of Parkinson's disease, epilepsy, and motor neurone disease in older adults.
2. Apply evidence-based strategies for assessment, diagnosis, and management of these conditions, integrating frailty considerations and multidisciplinary care.
3. Evaluate the role of the advanced practitioners (APs) in early recognition of neurological decline, holistic care planning, and patient and carer education.
4. Reflect on ethical, safety, and quality-improvement aspects of neurological care in frailty and end of life practice.

SELF-ASSESSMENT QUESTIONS

1. In an older adult, how would you distinguish an epileptic seizure from convulsive syncope at the bedside, and which first-line tests would you order immediately?

2. What key motor and non-motor features point to Parkinson's disease, and why are time-critical dopaminergic medicines (and alternatives if nil by mouth) essential for safety?

PARKINSON'S DISEASE

Parkinson's disease (PD) is a chronic, progressive neurodegenerative disorder characterised by the selective loss of dopamine-producing neurons in the substantia nigra, resulting in a cardinal syndrome of bradykinesia, rigidity, resting tremor, and postural instability. Diagnosis remains clinical, relying on a detailed history and neurological examination because no definitive biomarker can reliably differentiate PD from vascular parkinsonism, drug-induced parkinsonism, or atypical parkinsonian disorders such as progressive supranuclear palsy and multiple system atrophy (NICE, 2017; Kalia and Lang, 2015). In the United Kingdom, the prevalence is approximately 150–160 per 100,000, with an annual incidence of 15–20 per 100,000, increasing steeply with advancing age (Parkinson's UK, 2025).

Approximately 166,000 people in the United Kingdom are currently diagnosed with PD, and numbers are projected to rise as the population ages and diagnostic recognition improves (Parkinson's UK, 2025). Globally, an estimated 11.77 million people were living with PD in 2021, equating to a standardised prevalence of around 139 per 100,000 (Luo et al., 2025). Modelling studies predict that by 2050 the worldwide number will reach about 25.2 million, corresponding to an all-age prevalence of approximately 267 per 100,000 and an age-standardised prevalence of about 216 per 100,000 (Su et al., 2025). Frailty is common in PD and strongly influences outcomes. A meta-analysis found a pooled frailty prevalence of around 38%, with individual studies reporting ranges between 24% and 55% (McMillan et al., 2021). UK data show that among hospitalised patients aged 75 years or older, about 84% were classified as frail, and severe or very severe frailty was associated with markedly higher inpatient mortality (Neurology Academy, 2023). In a hospital cohort, severe frailty conferred markedly increased odds of death during admission compared with less frail counterparts (Hewitt *et al.*, 2020; Hewitt *et al.*, 2019; Rockwood *et al.*, 2005).

PD is now recognised as a multisystem disease with prominent non-motor manifestations— including depression, cognitive decline, autonomic dysfunction, sleep disturbance, and pain that frequently precede or overshadow motor symptoms. These features interact with the physiology of ageing and contribute directly to the frailty phenotype. For example, impaired mobility, orthostatic hypotension, sarcopenia, and swallowing difficulties accelerate functional decline, heighten the risk of falls and malnutrition, and increase vulnerability to minor stressors. As a result, PD can both precipitate and intensify frailty, leading to greater morbidity, earlier dependency, and higher rates of hospitalisation and mortality (Kouli et al., 2020; Hernández-Triana et al., 2025).

Early recognition of frailty in PD is therefore essential. Comprehensive geriatric assessment, proactive bone health and falls prevention, and advance care planning should be embedded within routine management to preserve autonomy and optimise quality of life for patients and their carers.

CLINICAL PRESENTATION

Diagnosis is clinical and follows the UK Parkinson's Disease Society Brain Bank criteria, which require bradykinesia, slowness in initiating and executing movement, plus at least one of rigidity, rest tremor, or postural instability. The classic rest tremor is often described as 'pill-rolling' and typically begins asymmetrically. Additional motor manifestations include hypomimia, micrographia, shuffling gait with reduced arm swing, and episodes of freezing. Reflexes remain normal, and pyramidal signs are absent (NICE, 2017).

Non-motor symptoms are frequent and may precede motor signs. They encompass depression, anxiety, psychosis, cognitive impairment, sleep disturbance, autonomic dysfunction (orthostatic hypotension, constipation, urinary problems, drooling), and sensory complaints such as anosmia (NICE, 2017). Their recognition is critical for holistic management.

INVESTIGATIONS

The diagnosis is clinical but should be confirmed or reviewed by a specialist in movement disorders. Neuroimaging, such as MRI or CT, helps exclude vascular or structural mimics. Dopamine transporter imaging (e.g. 123I-FP-CIT SPECT or DaTSCAN™) may support diagnosis when uncertainty remains, but it is not routinely required (NICE, 2017).

MANAGEMENT

Management is best delivered by a multidisciplinary team, ideally within a specialist Parkinson's clinic. Individualised pharmacological treatment aims to optimise motor function while limiting long-term complications.

- Levodopa combined with a peripheral decarboxylase inhibitor remains the most effective agent for motor symptoms.
- Dopamine agonists (e.g. ropinirole and pramipexole) and monoamine oxidase-B inhibitors (e.g. selegiline and rasagiline) may be preferred initially in younger patients or used in combination as the disease advances.
- Adjunctive therapies include catechol-*O*-methyltransferase inhibitors (e.g. entacapone), amantadine for dyskinesia, and intermittent subcutaneous apomorphine for refractory motor fluctuations.

When oral intake is compromised, dispersible levodopa preparations via nasogastric tube, transdermal rotigotine, or subcutaneous apomorphine can maintain dopaminergic stimulation. Deep brain stimulation or ablative procedures may be appropriate for selected patients with disabling motor complications unresponsive to medication (Mouchaileh and Cameron, 2025).

SUPPORTIVE AND MULTIDISCIPLINARY CARE

Specialist Parkinson's nurses, physiotherapists, occupational therapists, speech and language therapists, and dietitians all contribute to sustaining function and quality of life. Attention to bone health, falls prevention, mood disorders, and cognitive change are integral. Advanced care planning, including palliative approaches, becomes important as motor and non-motor symptoms progress.

Case Study 12.1 Parkinson's Disease

Mr A, a 74-year-old retired engineer with a six-year history of idiopathic Parkinson's disease, was referred to Same Day Emergency Care after several early-morning falls and increasing difficulty initiating movement.

He reported light-headedness on standing, disturbed sleep, and a two-week history of low mood and loss of appetite. His prescribed treatment included co-careldopa 125 mg four times daily and ropinirole 6 mg at night.

The AP undertook a full history covering motor fluctuations, orthostatic symptoms, nutrition, bowel and bladder function, cognition and mood, and specifically excluded acute infection, stroke, and syncope.

Examination confirmed bradykinesia and cogwheel rigidity, with postural blood pressure showing a 25-mmHg systolic fall on standing; cardiovascular, respiratory and musculoskeletal systems were also examined to identify comorbid contributors to falls. Bedside tests (lying and standing blood pressure, electrocardiogram (ECG), urinalysis) and laboratory investigations, including full blood count, urea and electrolytes, thyroid profile, and vitamin B12/folate, were arranged, while a recent MRI ruled out structural lesions. Synthesising these findings, the AP identified neurogenic orthostatic hypotension as the principal cause of the falls, with nocturnal 'off' periods as a contributory factor.

Management combined complex clinical reasoning with all four pillars of advanced practice. The AP modified Mr A's treatment by adding a night-time modified-release levodopa preparation and initiated midodrine for orthostatic hypotension after specialist discussion, while prescribing vitamin D and bisphosphonate prophylaxis for fracture prevention. Multidisciplinary input was coordinated with neurology, pharmacy, physiotherapy, occupational therapy, and dietetics, and a detailed care plan was created to prevent future falls and ensure time-critical administration of Parkinson's medication during hospital admissions.

Patient and carer education addressed postural blood-pressure management, compression stockings, and safe positional changes, and ward nurses received teaching on recognising 'off' periods and administering medicines on time.

Evidence-based guidance, including NICE NG71, informed each decision, and the AP documented outcomes for inclusion in the hospital's frailty quality-improvement audit. Over the subsequent four weeks, Mr A experienced no further falls and improved mobility, illustrating how advanced assessment, diagnostic reasoning, leadership, education, and research can be integrated to deliver high-quality, person-centred care for a person living with Parkinson's disease complicated by frailty.

EPILEPSY

Epilepsy is a disorder of recurrent, unprovoked seizures arising from abnormal electrical activity within the brain. While primary (idiopathic) epilepsy often begins in adolescence, new-onset seizures are more common in later life, with an incidence exceeding 100 per 100,000 in those over 70 years (Liu et al., 2016). This rise reflects the greater frequency of secondary epilepsy caused by conditions such as cerebral ischaemia, subdural haematoma, and intracranial tumours (Bowker et al., 2012). In older adults, seizures may also be provoked by acute metabolic disturbances such as hyponatraemia or hypoglycaemia, infection, including meningitis or encephalitis, withdrawal from alcohol or benzodiazepines, certain medicines (e.g. fluoroquinolones, tricyclic antidepressants), and nutritional deficiency such as thiamine deficiency leading to Wernicke's encephalopathy. Ageing itself lowers the seizure threshold, further increasing susceptibility (Figure 12.1).

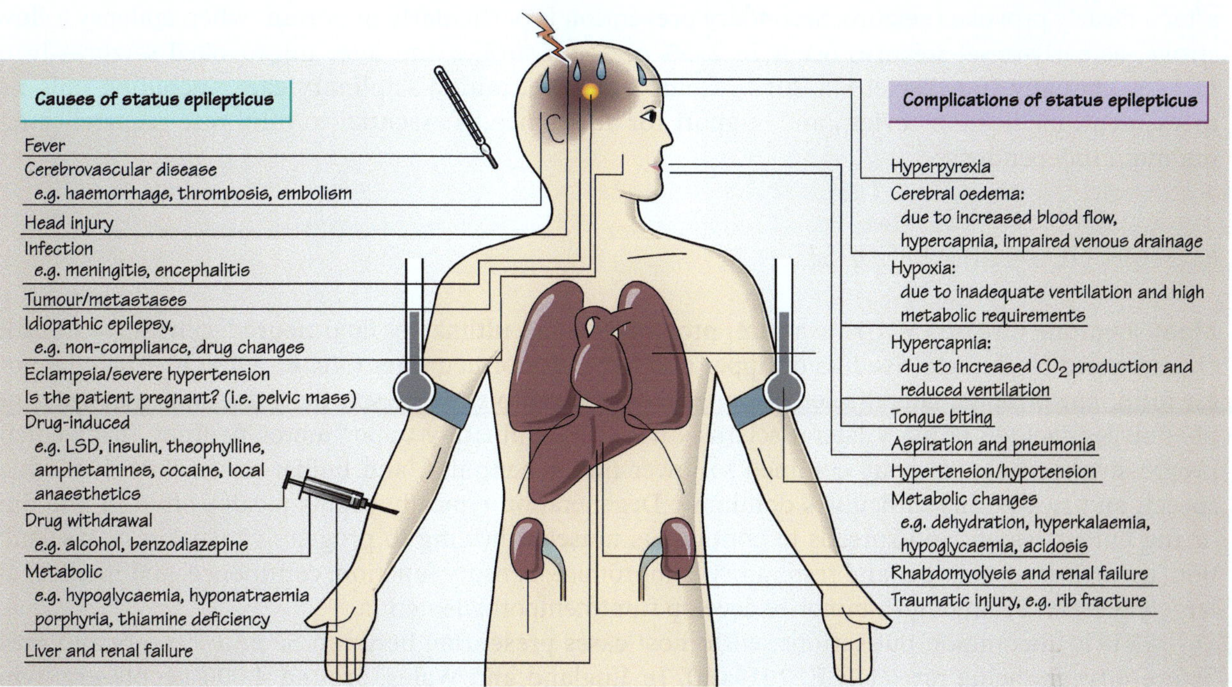

FIGURE 12.1   Causes of status epilepsy. *Source*: Leach (2014)/John Wiley & Sons.

DIAGNOSIS

Diagnosis relies on a thorough clinical history and a detailed account from a witness. Features such as tongue-biting, urinary incontinence, and post-ictal confusion, while helpful, may be less discriminatory in older adults, where cardiovascular causes of transient loss of consciousness are common (NICE, 2025). Cerebral hypoperfusion, for example, due to bradyarrhythmia, can precipitate convulsive syncope and may coexist with epilepsy, so assessment must include cardiovascular evaluation. Routine blood tests, chest radiography, and electrocardiography are essential to identify precipitating or alternative causes. Neuroimaging, typically a computed tomography (CT) brain scan, is important to exclude acute structural lesions, while electroencephalography (EEG) can support the diagnosis if positive, though a normal EEG does not rule out epilepsy (NICE, 2025).

Management starts with addressing reversible factors, such as correcting electrolyte imbalance, treating infection, or withdrawing offending drugs. Acute seizures are treated with benzodiazepines (e.g. intravenous or rectal lorazepam or diazepam); persistent seizures may require intravenous phenytoin with cardiac monitoring, and in rare cases, airway protection and intubation (NICE, 2025). Long-term antiepileptic medication is usually considered after a second unprovoked seizure, or sooner when a structural brain lesion is identified or when early return to driving is necessary. Commonly used agents include carbamazepine, sodium valproate, lamotrigine, and levetiracetam, each chosen according to seizure type, comorbidity, and potential drug interactions. Regular monitoring is needed to balance efficacy against adverse effects such as sedation, cognitive change, and haematological or hepatic toxicity.

Older adults with epilepsy require advice on driving, with notification of the Driver and Vehicle Licensing Agency (DVLA) mandatory. After a first unprovoked seizure, a seizure-free period of at least one year is generally required before driving can resume, although shorter intervals may be considered after a clearly provoked seizure. Secondary prevention is particularly important when epilepsy follows stroke, as early-onset seizures occur in 2–5% of acute strokes and later unprovoked seizures in up to 1.5% annually (Bowker et al., 2012). Comprehensive, multidisciplinary care, including falls risk assessment, medication review, and support for adherence, is essential to minimise recurrence and maintain independence.

MOTOR NEURONE DISEASE

Motor neurone disease (MND) is a rare, progressive, and ultimately fatal neurodegenerative disorder characterised by the selective loss of upper and lower motor neurones (NICE, 2019a,b). The commonest form, amyotrophic lateral sclerosis, produces a mixed picture of spasticity and wasting, but other phenotypes include primary lateral sclerosis with predominantly upper motor neurone involvement, progressive muscular atrophy confined to lower motor neurones, and bulbar-onset disease in which speech and swallowing difficulties dominate. Degeneration typically begins focally, often in one limb or the bulbar region, and spreads to contiguous muscles, leading to progressive weakness, fasciculation, dysarthria, dysphagia, and respiratory compromise. Sensory function, continence, and intellect are largely preserved, although a minority develop frontotemporal dementia.

MND is uncommon but serious, with most cases presenting between 55 and 79 years and onset before 40 years being rare (NICE, 2019a,b). In England and Wales, around 4,000 people are living with the condition at any time. About 5–10% of cases show a familial pattern linked to identifiable gene variants, while the remainder are sporadic (NICE, 2019a,b). Survival is limited: most people die within 2–3 years of symptom onset, about 25% live to 5 years, and only 5–10% survive for 10 years (NICE, 2019a,b).

DIAGNOSIS

Diagnosis can be delayed or missed because early manifestations may mimic cervical myelopathy, cerebrovascular disease, myasthenia gravis, or peripheral neuropathies. Clinical recognition rests on the coexistence of upper motor neurone signs such as brisk reflexes, spasticity, and extensor plantar responses with lower motor neurone features of wasting and fasciculation. Electromyography provides supportive evidence of widespread denervation, while neuroimaging is undertaken to exclude structural lesions.

MANAGEMENT

Management is largely supportive but requires skilled multidisciplinary care. Riluzole, a sodium channel blocker, modestly prolongs survival in amyotrophic lateral sclerosis and is recommended under specialist supervision with monitoring for hepatotoxicity and neutropenia (NICE, 2019a,b). Respiratory support with non-invasive ventilation, timely speech and language therapy, nutritional interventions including gastrostomy, and optimal symptom control with agents such as baclofen for spasticity or low-dose opioids for dyspnoea are central to care. Early advance care planning, psychological support, and engagement with specialist MND nurses and patient-support organisations are essential to maintain quality of life (Figure 12.2 and Table 12.1).

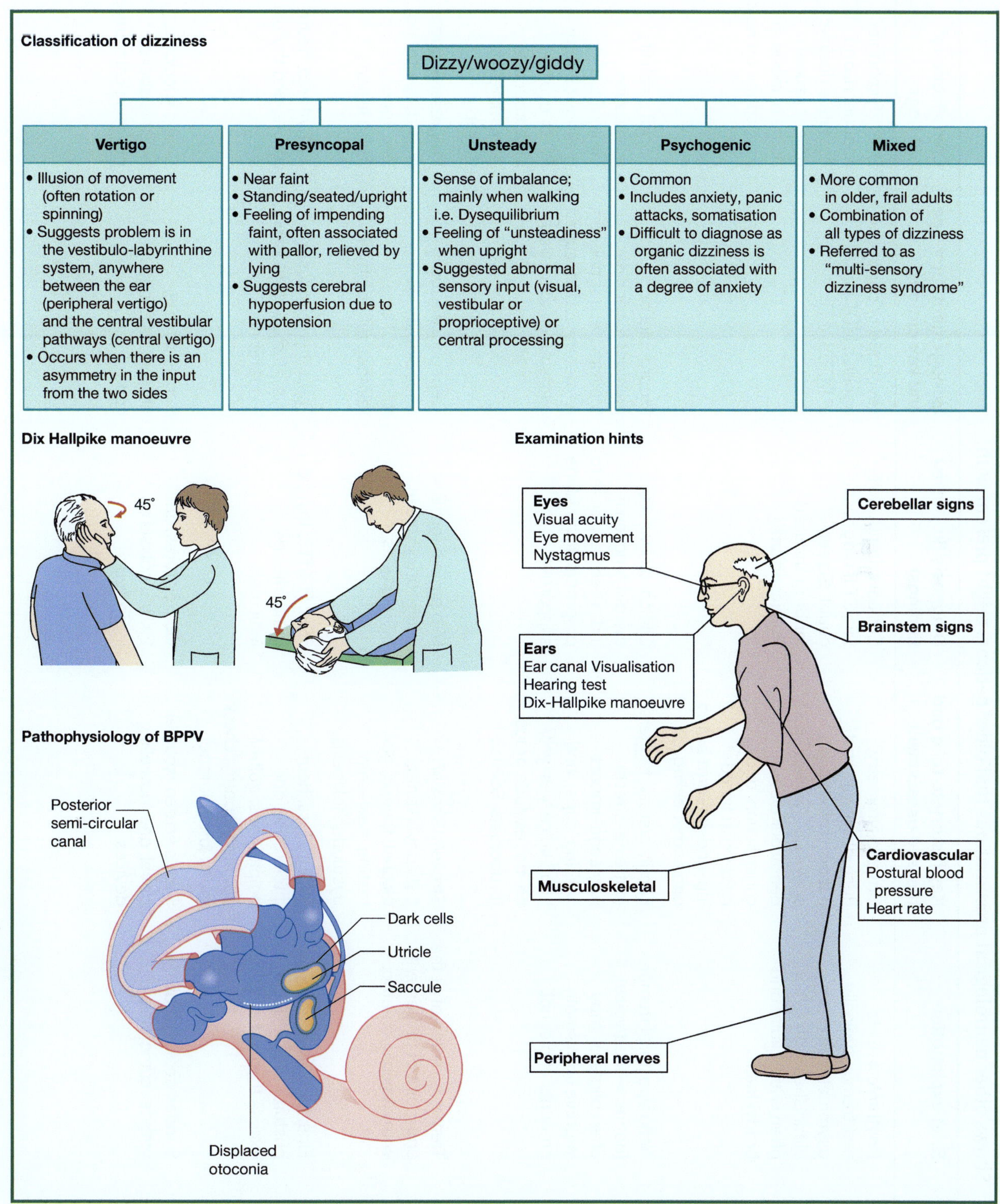

FIGURE 12.2   Classification of dizziness. *Source*: Blundell and Gordon (2015)/John Wiley & Sons.

TABLE 12.1 Shows other neurological presentations that older patients might present with.

Condition	Brief explanation	Key history to take and focused assessment	Diagnosis (key tests/findings)	Management (first-line and key options)	Complications/red flags
Rest tremor (Parkinsonian tremor)	Rhythmic 4–6 Hz rest tremor, typically asymmetrical; diminishes with action; often with rigidity and bradykinesia.	Onset/asymmetry, fluctuation with rest/action, stiffness, slowness, REM sleep behaviour disorder, constipation, and hyposmia; timed 'up-and-go', arm swing, and cogwheeling.	Clinical criteria; DaT-SPECT if diagnostic doubt. Screen for drug-induced Parkinsonism.	Levodopa or dopamine agonist; MDT input (PT/OT/SALT).	Falls, dysphagia/aspiration, and cognitive decline; urgent review if acute akinesia or medication omission.
Postural tremor—Essential tremor (ET)	Action/postural tremor (hands > head/voice), often bilateral; may improve with small amounts of alcohol.	Family history, triggers (caffeine, stress), functional impact (writing, cups), and head/voice 'yes–yes/no–no'; exclude drugs (β-agonists, SSRIs).	Clinical diagnosis; thyroid function if indicated; response to propranolol/primidone supportive.	Propranolol or primidone; consider topiramate, gabapentin; refractory: DBS/focused ultrasound (specialist).	Social disability, medication intolerance; distinguish from PD to avoid inappropriate dopaminergic therapy.
Action/intention tremor—Cerebellar	Tremor is maximal at the end-point of movement; with ataxia/dysmetria.	Stroke/MS/toxin/anticonvulsants; alcohol; thyroid; gait testing, heel–shin, dysdiadochokinesis.	MRI brain if focal/acute; drug screen; thyroid tests.	Treat cause (stop offending drugs, thiamine if alcohol-related), rehab/physio.	Progressive gait ataxia, dysarthria; look for posterior fossa lesions.
Thyrotoxic tremor	Fine, high-frequency postural tremor due to excess thyroid hormone.	Weight loss, heat intolerance, and palpitations; goitre/ophthalmopathy; check meds (amiodarone).	TSH, fT4/fT3; thyroid antibodies as indicated.	Treat thyrotoxicosis; symptomatic β-blocker if appropriate.	Arrhythmia, heart failure, and thyroid storm.
Rigors (infection-related shaking)	Sudden coarse shaking with fever/malaise.	Sepsis screen (source), travel, and indwelling devices.	Obs, cultures, and CXR/urinalysis as indicated.	Sepsis bundle, antibiotics per source control.	Septic shock; do not mislabel as neurological tremor.

Asterixis/ metabolic tremor	Negative myoclonus with metabolic failure (hepatic/uraemic/ respiratory).	Encephalopathy features, toxin/meds, and liver/ renal history.	U&E, LFTs, ABG, and ammonia.	Treat underlying failure; supportive care.	Cerebral oedema, arrhythmia, and respiratory failure.
Drug/alcohol withdrawal tremor	Coarse postural tremor after cessation or dose change.	Alcohol/benzodiazepine use; timing of last dose; autonomic symptoms, seizures.	CIWA-Ar scoring; tox screen.	Benzodiazepine protocol; thiamine; supportive care.	Delirium tremens; Wernicke's encephalopathy (give parenteral thiamine).
Drug-induced tremor	Tremor from lithium, valproate, SSRIs, TCAs, β-agonists, etc.	Full medication list (including OTC/herbals, caffeine), onset versus dose changes.	Drug level where relevant (lithium, valproate); TFTs if implicated.	Reduce/stop culprit; switch agent; symptomatic β-blocker if suitable.	Toxicity (e.g. lithium).
Orthostatic tremor	Rapid (13–18 Hz) leg tremor only on standing, relieved by walking/ sitting.	Unsteadiness on standing, better when moving; palpate thigh/ calf tremor.	Surface EMG if needed.	Clonazepam/ gabapentin (specialist); pacing, stools/rails for standing tasks.	Falls, anxiety, and avoidance of standing.
Post-herpetic neuralgia (PHN)	Persistent neuropathic pain after shingles in dermatomal distribution.	Zoster history, allodynia, and sleep/mood impact.	Clinical; exclude secondary infection.	First-line: gabapentin/ pregabalin or TCAs; topical lidocaine/ capsaicin; consider antivirals within 72 h of rash for prevention.	Chronic pain, depression, and deconditioning.
Trigeminal neuralgia (TN)	Paroxysmal, unilateral facial pain (V2/V3 > V1), triggerable.	Dental triggers, chewing/ talking, weight loss, and red flags (sensory loss, bilateral).	MRI to exclude secondary causes; multidisciplinary dental input.	Carbamazepine/ oxcarbazepine first-line; consider microvascular decompression/ablative procedures if refractory (specialist).	Malnutrition, depression/suicide risk; secondary TN (tumour/MS)—urgent work-up.
Peripheral neuropathies (general)	Symmetrical distal sensory ± motor loss ('glove-and-stocking') or focal mononeuropathies.	Diabetes, alcohol, renal/ thyroid disease, B12, toxins/drugs, cancer symptoms, and family history; falls risk.	B12, glucose/HbA1c, TFTs, SPEP/UPEP, and ESR/CRP; NCS/EMG if unclear.	Treat cause; neuropathic pain regimen; foot care, physio, and safety adaptations.	Ulcers, falls, and Charcot joints; acute weakness → consider GBS.

(Continued)

TABLE 12.1 (Continued)

Condition	Brief explanation	Key history to take and focused assessment	Diagnosis (key tests/ findings)	Management (first-line and key options)	Complications/ red flags
Guillain–Barré syndrome (GBS)	Acute immune-mediated polyradiculoneuropathy with ascending weakness ± autonomic dysfunction.	Recent infection/vaccine; progression hours–days; respiratory or bulbar symptoms; autonomic features.	Clinical + NCS; CSF albumino-cytological dissociation (often after 1 week). Monitor FVC serially.	IVIg or plasma exchange; VTE prophylaxis; airway/ITU if needed; early rehab.	Respiratory failure, dysautonomia (arrhythmias, BP lability); need for urgent escalation.
Subdural haematoma (SDH)	Venous bleed between dura and arachnoid, often after minor head injury; commoner in older adults/ anticoagulated.	Head trauma/falls (may be remote), new confusion/drowsiness, focal deficits, and gait change; anticoagulants.	Urgent CT head; consider MRI if equivocal; repeat imaging if deterioration.	Neurosurgical discussion; reversal of anticoagulation where appropriate; burr-hole drainage for symptomatic/large SDH; close observation if small/stable.	Raised ICP, cerebral herniation and seizures, with high mortality if recognition and imaging are delayed; therefore, a low threshold for scanning is required.
Neuroleptic malignant syndrome (NMS)	Life-threatening reaction to dopamine blockade (antipsychotics); hyperthermia, 'lead-pipe' rigidity, altered mental state, autonomic instability, ↑CK.	Recent start/dose increase/long-acting depot; dehydration, agitation; rule out infection/serotonin syndrome.	Clinical diagnosis; CK, U&E, and LFTs; exclude other causes; ECG; consider ICU.	Immediate stop antipsychotic; aggressive supportive care (IV fluids, cooling); consider dantrolene, bromocriptine/ amantadine in severe cases; ICU if needed.	Rhabdomyolysis, renal failure, DIC, and arrhythmias; mortality if delayed treatment.
Serotonin syndrome (SS)	Excess serotonergic activity: triad of mental status change, autonomic instability, neuromuscular hyperactivity; classically after serotonergic drug change/interaction.	Medication review (SSRIs, MAOIs, tramadol, linezolid, triptans, MDMA), timing (<24 h), and clonus/hyperreflexia.	Clinical diagnosis (Hunter criteria); exclude NMS/ infection; obs, ECG, and CK.	Stop serotonergic agents; supportive care (IV fluids, cooling, benzodiazepines); consider cyproheptadine in moderate–severe cases; ICU if severe.	Hyperthermia, rhabdomyolysis, seizures, and arrhythmias; rapid escalation needed.
Insomnia in older adults	Reduced sleep efficiency with age; often multifactorial and exacerbated by comorbidity/medicines.	Sleep diary, caffeine/ alcohol, pain, LUTS/ nocturia, reflux, depression/anxiety, and OSA risk; ward environment factors.	Primarily clinical; screen for secondary causes; consider CBT-I tools.	First-line CBT-I (including digital CBT-I such as Sleepio where suitable); short courses of hypnotics only, if necessary, at the lowest effective dose.	Falls, cognitive impairment from sedatives; dependence with prolonged benzodiazepine/ Z-drug use.

Sleep disorders in older people	Sleep becomes lighter and more fragmented with age, and disorders such as insomnia, restless legs syndrome, circadian rhythm disturbance, obstructive/central sleep apnoea, and REM sleep behaviour disorder are common. Benzodiazepine use can worsen dependence, cognitive impairment, and falls risk.	Sleep diary; onset/duration of symptoms; review of comorbidities (pain, heart or lung disease, neurological disease); medication and alcohol/caffeine history; partner observations for apnoea, limb jerks, or dream-enacting movements.	First-line non-pharmacological measures (sleep hygiene, cognitive behavioural therapy for insomnia, gradual light therapy for circadian disorders). Avoid long-term benzodiazepines. Use dopamine agonists for restless legs if needed; CPAP or other positive pressure therapy for sleep apnoea; clonazepam may help REM sleep behaviour disorder.	Falls, confusion, depression, and road-traffic accidents from sedative use; respiratory or cardiovascular complications from untreated sleep apnoea; progression to Parkinson's or Lewy body disease in some REM sleep behaviour disorder cases	Sleep problems are common in older adults, with causes including insomnia, restless legs, circadian rhythm disturbance, sleep apnoea, and REM sleep behaviour disorder. Management emphasises treating underlying factors, using behavioural strategies, and avoiding long-term benzodiazepines due to risks of dependence, falls and cognitive decline (Harbison 2002).

Abbreviations: ABG, arterial blood gas; BP, blood pressure; CBT-I, cognitive behavioural therapy for insomnia; CK, creatine kinase; CPAP, continuous positive airway pressure; CRP, C-reactive protein; CSF, cerebrospinal fluid; CXR, chest X-ray; DaT-SPECT, dopamine transporter single-photon emission computed tomography; DBS, deep brain stimulation; DIC, disseminated intravascular coagulation; EMG, electromyography; ESR, erythrocyte sedimentation rate; FVC, forced vital capacity; ICU, Intensive care unit; ICP, Intracranial pressure; ITU, intensive therapy unit; IVIg, intravenous immunoglobulin; LFTs, liver function tests; LUTS, Lower urinary tract symptoms; MAOIs, Monoamine oxidase inhibitors; MDT, multidisciplinary team; MDMA, 3,4-methylenedioxymethamphetamine; MRI, magnetic resonance imaging; NCS, nerve conduction studies; NMS, neuroleptic malignant syndrome; OT, occupational therapy; OSA, obstructive sleep apnoea; OTC, over-the-counter; PD, Parkinson's disease; PT, physiotherapy; REM, rapid eye movement; SALT, speech and language therapy; SPEP/UPEP, serum/urine protein electrophoresis; SS, serotonin syndrome; SSRIs, selective serotonin reuptake inhibitors; TCA, tricyclic antidepressant; TFTs, thyroid function tests; TSH, thyroid-stimulating hormone; U&E, urea and electrolytes; VTE, venous thromboembolism.

STROKE

A stroke is the abrupt onset of a focal neurological syndrome lasting ≥24 hours or causing death, due to a vascular cause (ischaemia or spontaneous intracranial haemorrhage, including subarachnoid haemorrhage but excluding subdural/extradural). A transient ischaemic attack (TIA) produces identical focal symptoms but resolves within 24 hours; early management should not differ at first contact because urgent treatment reduces harm. The 'time-is-brain' principle remains quantified: untreated large-vessel ischaemia is associated with an estimated loss of ~1.9 million neurons per minute on average (Risitano and Toni, 2020).

Classification

The Oxfordshire Community Stroke Project (OCSP), often referred to as the Bamford classification, is a clinically based system that helps to infer the vascular territory affected and to estimate early prognosis (Andrade et al., 2021). It distinguishes between four main syndromes: Total Anterior Circulation Stroke (TACS), which typically combines motor or sensory loss with homonymous hemianopia and higher cortical dysfunction; Partial Anterior Circulation Stroke (PACS), which presents with two of these three features or with isolated cortical disturbance; Lacunar Stroke (LACS), usually caused by small-vessel occlusion and characterised by pure motor or sensory deficits without cortical signs; and Posterior Circulation Stroke (POCS), which reflects vertebrobasilar disease and often manifests with brainstem or cerebellar features such as diplopia, vertigo or ataxia. Alongside this, the Trial of ORG 10172 in Acute Stroke Treatment (TOAST) classification provides an aetiological framework for ischaemic stroke, categorising cases into large-artery atherosclerosis, cardioembolism, small-vessel occlusion, other determined causes, and undetermined causes. Both OCSP and TOAST remain recommended in UK guidance as practical tools for structuring initial clinical assessment, supporting diagnostic reasoning, and planning investigations.

History Taking in Suspected Stroke/TIA

Structure the history to confirm focal neurology, define onset, and surface red flags, risk, premorbid function, and treatment windows (NICE, 2019a,b):

1. Presenting features and tempo:
   - Exact time last seen well; mode of onset (sudden versus stepwise progression).
   - Nature of deficit: weakness, speech/language disturbance, visual loss (including monocular amaurosis), ataxia, hemisensory change, diplopia, and vertigo.
   - Headache at onset (especially severe/thunderclap) or early reduced consciousness suggests haemorrhage or subarachnoid haemorrhage (SAH).
   - Seizure at onset raises alternative diagnoses and affects thrombolysis decisions.
2. Stroke mimics and precipitants:
   - Hypoglycaemia (check capillary glucose immediately).
   - Recent head injury (consider SDH).
   - Migraine with aura, seizure with post-ictal paresis, functional neurological disorder, sepsis, and electrolyte disturbance.

3. Vascular risk and embolic sources:
   - Atrial fibrillation, recent myocardial infarction, valvular disease, endocarditis symptoms, carotid territory TIA, known carotid stenosis, and prior stroke/TIA.
   - Hypertension, diabetes, dyslipidaemia, smoking, harmful alcohol use, and obstructive sleep apnoea.
   - Oestrogen exposure (combined oral contraceptive; post-menopausal hormone replacement therapy [HRT]).
4. Antithrombotics and contraindications:
   - Current antiplatelet/anticoagulant therapy (including direct oral anticoagulants [DOACs]), last dose/time, and any bleeding history.
   - Recent surgery, active bleeding, or uncontrolled hypertension. https://www.nice.org.uk/guidance/ng128/chapter/recommendations?utm_source=chatgpt.com
5. Functional baseline and supports:
   - Premorbid independence, cognition, communication, continence, mobility aids, living situation, and carers are vital for decisions on thrombolysis/thrombectomy, imaging, swallow safety, and discharge planning.
6. TIA specific:
   - Treat as a medical emergency; do not use ABCD2 to defer urgent assessment, as lower scores can still conceal high early risk. Arrange a same-day specialist assessment if symptoms are ongoing/fluctuating or within 24 hours if high risk is suspected (NICE, 2019a,b).

Examination in Suspected Stroke/TIA

Perform and document a standardised neurological and general examination, then quantify severity (NICE, 2019a):

A. Immediate safety checks:
   - Airway, breathing, and circulation; oxygen saturation (supplement only if hypoxic).
   - Capillary glucose (exclude hypoglycaemia).
   - Temperature; treat pyrexia and search for infection if present.
B. Standardised severity score:
   - Use the NIH Stroke Scale (NIHSS) at first assessment to quantify deficits and support reperfusion decisions; repeat to track change.
C. Level of consciousness and higher cortical function:
   - Glasgow Coma Scale (GCS) (or Alert, Voice, Pain, Unresponsive [AVPU]) and orientation.
   - Language: distinguish dysphasia (receptive/expressive) from dysarthria. Test one-step then multistep commands (avoid demonstration), naming (common then less common items), repetition, reading, and writing if feasible.
   - Neglect/inattention: confirm intact primary sensation/fields to each side separately, then apply simultaneous bilateral stimuli to detect extinction; observe for gaze preference and personal neglect.
D. Cranial nerves and visual system:
   - Visual acuity if possible; confrontational fields for hemianopia; pupils; eye movements for gaze palsy/internuclear signs; facial symmetry and power; bulbar function, including cough and voice quality, as a pre-screen to formal swallow testing.

E. Motor system:
- Tone (often reduced acutely); power with Medical Research Council grades; pronator drift for subtle pyramidal weakness; observe characteristic patterns (arm flexors > extensors; leg extensors > flexors in corticospinal lesions). Assess coordination, mindful that weakness limits testing.

F. Sensory system:
- Light touch, pin-prick if available, and proprioception; screen for hemisensory loss and sensory extinction with bilateral simultaneous stimulation.

G. Cerebellar/brainstem signs (posterior circulation):
- Nystagmus, dysmetria, dysdiadochokinesis, and truncal ataxia; severe gait imbalance out of keeping with limb weakness suggests posterior circulation involvement.

H. Gait and function:
- If safe, observe sit-to-stand and first steps; otherwise, assess sitting balance and transfers. Document the need for immediate fall precautions.

I. General examination for cause/complications:
- Pulse and rhythm (irregularly irregular suggests atrial fibrillation [AF]); blood pressure in both arms; cardiac examination (murmur, heart failure).
- Respiratory examination (aspiration risk, pneumonia).
- Hydration status; abdominal palpation for urinary retention.

J. Swallow screening (pre-SALT):
- Patients with suspected stroke should have prompt swallow screening before oral intake; high-risk findings (drowsiness, wet voice, weak cough, coughing after sips) mandate nil by mouth, intravenous or NG hydration, and urgent SALT review. Early enteral feeding via NG is associated with better outcomes when oral intake is unsafe.

Bedside Investigation Priorities (To Support History/Examination)

- Immediate: capillary glucose; 12-lead ECG (AF/ischaemia); observations including temperature and oxygen saturation.
- First bloods: FBC, U&E, glucose/HbA1c, lipids, and CRP; consider ESR/blood cultures if vasculitis or endocarditis suspected.
- Brain imaging urgently: non-contrast CT to exclude haemorrhage and major mimics; do not delay referral for reperfusion therapy when eligible. Vascular imaging and carotid imaging follow local pathways.

Examination Findings That Change Pathways Rapidly

- Decreased consciousness, malignant hypertension, thunderclap headache, meningism, or rapidly worsening neurology (urgent imaging and specialist input).
- Severe hemiparesis with gaze deviation and cortical signs (consider large-vessel occlusion → thrombectomy pathway if within window).
- Posterior circulation 'red flag' cluster (acute severe imbalance, dysarthria, diplopia, haemodynamic instability).

Prevention of Early Complications That Can Be Initiated at the Bedside

- Early mobilisation when safe; intermittent pneumatic compression for immobile patients to reduce deep vein thrombosis (DVT) risk; avoid graduated compression stockings.

Take-Home Messages

1. Normal ageing of the nervous system involves neuronal loss, demyelination, and altered neurotransmission, which reduce neurological resilience and increase drug sensitivity.
2. PD is a multisystem disorder whose non-motor features often drive frailty and functional decline; timely recognition and specialist-led, multidisciplinary management are crucial.
3. Epilepsy in later life commonly reflects secondary causes and requires careful differentiation from cardiovascular events, with treatment focused on reversible precipitants and appropriate antiepileptic therapy.
4. MND demands early multidisciplinary intervention, symptom control, and advance care planning to preserve quality of life despite limited survival.
5. Early, structured assessment of suspected stroke using validated frameworks such as OCSP for clinical classification and TOAST for aetiology, alongside urgent imaging and risk factor evaluation, enables APs to guide timely intervention and improve patient outcomes.

CONCLUSION

Neurological ageing is marked by structural and biochemical changes that lower the reserve of the nervous system and predispose older adults to disorders such as PD, epilepsy, and MND. These conditions often interact with frailty, increasing vulnerability to falls, cognitive decline, and hospitalisation. Comprehensive, multidisciplinary assessment and evidence-based management grounded in the four pillars of advanced practice are essential to sustain function, prevent complications, and support patients and carers in complex decision-making and advance care planning.

REFERENCES

Andrade, J.B.C.D., Mohr, J.P., Timbó, F.B. et al. (2021). Oxfordshire community stroke project classification: a proposed automated algorithm. *European Stroke Journal* 6 (2): 160–167.

Blundell, A. and Gordon, A. (2015). *Geriatric Medicine at a Glance*, 1e. Chichester: Wiley Blackwell.

Bowker, L., Price, J., and Smith, S. (2012). *Oxford Handbook of Geriatric Medicine*. Oxford: Oxford University Press.

Harbison, J. (2002). Sleep disorders in older people. *Age and Ageing* 31 (Suppl_2): 6–9. `https://doi.org/10.1093/ageing/31.suppl_2.6` (accessed 21 September 2025).

Hernández-Triana, D., Páez-García, S., Mena, A. et al. (2025). Parkinson's disease and frailty: a two-way link across aging. *Journal of Clinical Medicine* 15 (1): 63.

Hewitt, J., Carter, B., McCarthy, K. et al. (2019). Frailty predicts mortality in all emergency surgical admissions regardless of age. An observational study. *Age and Ageing* 48 (3): 388–394.

Hewitt, J., Carter, B., Vilches-Moraga, A. et al. (2020). *The effect of frailty on survival in patients with COVID-19 (COPE): a multicentre, European, observational cohort study. The Lancet Public Health* 5 (8): e444–e451.

Kalia, L.V. and Lang, A.E. (2015). Parkinson's disease. *Lancet* 386 (9996): 896–912.

Kouli, A., Torsney, K.M., and Kuan, W.-L. (2020). *Parkinson's Disease: Etiology, Neuropathology, and Pathogenesis.* In: *Parkinson's Disease: Non-Motor and Non-Dopaminergic Features: Advances in Experimental Medicine and Biology* (ed. E. Marras and S. Chaudhuri), 1–22. Cham: Springer.

Leach, R. (2014). *Critical Care Medicine at a Glance*, 3e. Chichester: Wiley-Blackwell.

Liu, S., Yu, W., and Lü, Y. (2016). The causes of new-onset epilepsy and seizures in the elderly. *Neuropsychiatric Disease and Treatment* 12: 1425–1434.

Luo, Y., Qiao, L., Li, M. et al. (2025). Global, regional, national epidemiology and trends of Parkinson's disease from 1990 to 2021: findings from the Global Burden of Disease Study 2021. *Frontiers in Aging Neuroscience* 16: 1498756.

McMillan, J.M., Michalchuk, Q., and Goodarzi, Z. (2021). Frailty in Parkinson's disease: a systematic review and meta-analysis. *Clinical Parkinsonism & Related Disorders* 4: 100095.

Mouchaileh, N. and Cameron, J. (2025). Device-assisted therapies for Parkinson disease. *Australian Prescriber* 48 (1): 10.

National Institute for Health and Care Excellence (NICE) (2017). Parkinson's disease in adults: diagnosis and management. NG71 – context. `https://www.nice.org.uk/guidance/ng71/chapter/Context` (accessed 21 September 2025).

National Institute for Health and Care Excellence (NICE) (2019a). Stroke and transient ischaemic attack in over 16s: diagnosis and initial management (NG128). `https://www.nice.org.uk/guidance/NG128` (accessed 1 October 2025).

National Institute for Health and Care Excellence (NICE) (2019b). Motor neurone disease: assessment and management. NG42 – context. `https://www.nice.org.uk/guidance/ng42/chapter/Context` (accessed 21 September 2025).

National Institute for Health and Care Excellence (NICE) (2025). Epilepsies: diagnosis and management (NG217). `https://www.nice.org.uk/guidance/ng217` (accessed 21 September 2025).

Neurology Academy (2023). *A Geriatrician's Approach to Frailty in Parkinson's [Webinar].* Neurology Academy, 7 July. `https://neurologyacademy.org/events/webinar/a-geriatricians-approach-to-frailty-in-parkinsons` (accessed 21 September 2025).

Parkinson's UK (2025). *Reporting on Parkinson's: Information for Journalists.* Parkinson's UK `https://www.parkinsons.org.uk/about-us/reporting-parkinsons-information-journalists` (accessed 21 September 2025).

Risitano, A. and Toni, D. (2020). Time is brain: timing of revascularization of brain arteries in stroke. *European Heart Journal Supplements* 22 (Supplement_L): L155–L159.

Rockwood, K., Song, X., MacKnight, C. et al. (2005). *A global clinical measure of fitness and frailty in elderly people. Canadian Medical Association Journal* 173 (5): 489–495.

Su, D., Cui, Y., He, C. et al. (2025). Projections for prevalence of Parkinson's disease and its driving factors in 195 countries and territories to 2050: modelling study of Global Burden of Disease Study 2021. *BMJ* 388, bmj-2024-080952. `https://www.bmj.com/content/388/bmj-2024-080952`: (accessed 21 September 2025).

CHAPTER 13

Psychiatry

> **Aim**
>
> The aim of this chapter is to provide a psychiatry framework for recognising, assessing, and managing late-life cognitive impairment, delirium, dementia, depression, and anxiety in older adults, minimising misattribution to 'normal ageing' and reducing harm.

LEARNING OUTCOMES

By the end of this chapter, readers will be able to:

1. Distinguish normal ageing from mild cognitive impairment, dementia, delirium, and depressive/anxiety disorders using phenomenology, time course, and collateral information.
2. Conduct a structured psychiatric assessment, including mental state examination, capacity and risk appraisal, and appropriate screening for cognition and mood.
3. Formulate biopsychosocial management plans that address sensory loss, medicines, pain, environment, and carer factors, with clear thresholds for referral to old age psychiatry.
4. Initiate proportionate non-pharmacological and pharmacological treatments in frailty, employing 'start low, review often' and time-limited trials for psychotropics.
5. Lead sensitive communication about diagnosis, driving, advance planning, and safeguarding, documenting decisions clearly.

SELF-ASSESSMENT QUESTIONS

1. An older adult presents with a two-day history of fluctuation in attention and new visual misperceptions: which bedside screen will you use first, what immediate causes will you prioritise, and how will you manage risk in the first hour?

2. A patient with probable Lewy body dementia has distressing hallucinations: outline three non-drug strategies; name medicines you will avoid and why; and set a review plan for any short, cautious pharmacological trial.

INTRODUCTION

Psychological health in older adults is often under-assessed, overlooked, or misattributed to the ageing process itself (Devita et al., 2022). Forgetfulness, apathy, or withdrawal is too frequently labelled as 'normal ageing' rather than being recognised as symptoms of underlying cognitive impairment, depression, or delirium (Care UK, 2025). This misattribution leads to under-diagnosis, delays in treatment, and avoidable deterioration in health outcomes. Advanced practitioners (APs) are ideally placed to detect these concerns, given their sustained contact with older patients in both acute and community settings.

COGNITIVE IMPAIRMENT

Prevalence and Impact

Cognitive impairment is not an inevitable feature of ageing, yet its prevalence increases significantly with age (Han et al., 2022). It is highly prevalent among older adults and is closely associated with frailty. Globally, a recent systematic review and meta-analysis estimated that 23.7% of the geriatric population experience mild cognitive impairment (MCI) (Salari et al., 2025). Another review reported a median prevalence of 19.0%, although estimates ranged from 5.1% to 41.0% across different community-based studies, reflecting variation in diagnostic criteria and methodology (Pais et al., 2020). In Europe, the prevalence of cognitive frailty defined as the coexistence of physical frailty and cognitive impairment was estimated at 16% when broad criteria were applied and 6% when stricter diagnostic definitions were used, based on pooled international data (Zhang et al., 2022).

There are currently estimated to be 982,000 people with dementia in the United Kingdom, but more than a third of people with the condition do not have a diagnosis. The number is expected to rise to 1.4 million by 2040 (Alzheimer's Society, 2024). In addition, the cost of dementia in the United Kingdom was predicted to be £42 billion in 2024, increasing to £90 billion by 2040 (Alzheimer's Society, 2024). Many more live with mild cognitive impairment, which may not meet criteria for dementia but still has considerable impact on daily function, decision-making, and engagement with care. Cognitive decline has profound consequences for autonomy. It can increase the risk of medication errors, poor nutrition, falls, hospitalisation, and premature institutionalisation. When integrated into comprehensive geriatric assessment (CGA), assessment of cognitive function helps to inform realistic care planning, advance care discussions, and appropriate risk management (British Geriatric Society {BGS}, 2025a).

Clinical Presentation

Patients with mild cognitive impairment (MCI) frequently present with vague and subjective complaints of declining cognitive performance, which can be difficult to separate from the gradual changes observed in healthy ageing (Galati et al., 2025). Memory loss is often the most common symptom, but patients may also experience problems with concentration, decision-making, or language, alongside difficulties in planning or organising everyday tasks.

Distinguishing these cognitive symptoms from issues attributable to coexisting conditions is challenging. Sensory deprivation, such as hearing loss or reduced visual acuity, is common in older adults and can mimic or exacerbate cognitive difficulties (Ge et al., 2023). Likewise, motor deficits, for example, tremor or impaired mobility, may further complicate the clinical picture, creating uncertainty about whether changes are primarily neurological, sensory, or functional in origin. Behavioural changes may accompany early cognitive decline, including irritability, suspicion, withdrawal from social activities, or apathy (Alzheimer's Society, 2025). APs should remain cautious for subtle cues such as repeated questioning within short timeframes, frequent misplacement of personal belongings, or errors in handling finances.

In memory clinics, such signs are usually corroborated by collateral history from relatives or carers; however, in acute or community settings, professionals must be particularly proactive in identifying these indicators (British Geriatrics Society [BGS], 2025a). The assessment should extend beyond symptom recognition to consider safety. While safety-related questioning is essential in dementia care, it may also be appropriate for patients with MCI. Clinicians should explore risks around driving, cooking, smoking, or the use of heating appliances, as these activities may pose hazards even in the earlier stages of cognitive decline. These areas will be explored in depth in part three of this series. Such proactive assessment enables timely interventions that support independence while safeguarding well-being.

Although no specific physical signs are diagnostic of cognitive impairment, a through physical examination remains an essential component of assessment. The purpose is not to identify cognitive impairment (CI) directly but to exclude or detect underlying conditions that may mimic or contribute to cognitive decline. Endocrine disorders such as thyroid disease, nutritional deficiencies including low vitamin B12, and infections such as syphilis can all present with cognitive symptoms and must be considered. Equally important is the evaluation of sensory and motor function. Hearing and visual impairments are highly prevalent in older adults and may exacerbate or be mistaken for cognitive difficulties, while motor deficits, such as tremor or gait instability, can further complicate presentation. Identifying and addressing these factors ensures that symptoms are not wrongly attributed solely to cognitive decline. Therefore, a structured mental status examination should be undertaken to document the degree and pattern of cognitive dysfunction. This provides a baseline for future comparison and guides decisions on further investigations and management within the framework of CGA.

Assessment Tools

Structured screening is essential. Commonly used tools are attached in Table 13.1. Each tool has strengths and limitations; choice depends on time, clinical setting, and patient capacity. Importantly, these tools are screening instruments and not diagnostic in isolation. Formal diagnosis requires a combination of neuropsychological testing, blood investigations (full blood count (FBC), urea and electrolytes (U+Es), serum calcium, liver function tests (LFTs), thyroid function tests (TFTs), serum vitamin B12, and serum folate) and, in many cases, neuroimaging. APs should be familiar with the limits of screening and ensure that abnormal results trigger further investigation and referral. Figure 13.1 demonstrates an algorithm to conduct a Capacity Assessment (CA) assessment.

Early recognition supports risk reduction through vascular risk management, physical and cognitive activity, social engagement, and correction of sensory deficits (NICE, 2025). Ongoing review, typically every 6–12 months, aids timely detection of progression and facilitates care planning, including discussions about driving and legal considerations. Within CGA, cognition remains central to delivering safe, person-centred care.

TABLE 13.1 Common cognitive screening tools.

Tool	Purpose	Time to administer
Three-Item Recall Test	Quick screening for short-term memory	10 minutes
Clock Drawing Test	Screening for cognitive dysfunction secondary to dementia, delirium, or neurological/psychiatric illness	Variable
Mini-Cog (Mini Cognitive Assessment)	Brief screening for early cognitive impairment	5–10 minutes
BIMS (Brief Interview for Mental Status)	Short screening tool for general mental status	5–10 minutes
GPCOG (General Practitioner Assessment of Cognition)	Screening for dementia in primary care/general practice	10 minutes
MoCA (Montreal Cognitive Assessment)	Rapid screening for mild cognitive impairment	10 minutes
XpressO by MoCA (XpressO by Montreal Cognitive Assessment)	Self-administered digital pre-screening to distinguish subjective vs objective cognitive impairment	7 minutes

DELIRIUM

Definition and Significance

Delirium is an acute, fluctuating disturbance of attention and cognition, usually precipitated by underlying causes such as infection, dehydration, pain, medication, or environmental change (National Institute for Health and Care Excellence [NICE], 2023). It is particularly common in older adults with frailty and is associated with serious consequences, including increased mortality, functional decline, prolonged hospital stays, and greater risk of institutionalisation (Cechinel et al., 2022). Despite this, delirium is frequently under-recognised, particularly in its hypoactive form where patients present as withdrawn or drowsy rather than overtly agitated. For instance, in a cohort study, Al Farsi et al. (2023) reported that hypoactive delirium was the most common subtype, with 35.4% of cases going unrecognised. Failure to detect and treat delirium promptly can result in lasting cognitive impairment and poor long-term outcomes, which is why it is regarded as a medical emergency requiring urgent assessment and intervention.

Globally, among medically hospitalised older patients, the pooled prevalence of delirium is estimated at 23.6% (95% CI 19–29%), with an incidence of 13.5% during hospital admission (Wu et al., 2025). Comparable figures have been reported in European inpatient settings, where around 23% of older patients are affected, though estimates vary according to diagnostic criteria (Bellelli et al., 2021). In the United Kingdom, a large point-prevalence study across 45 hospitals found that 14.7% of inpatients aged 65 years and older presented with delirium at admission. Those living with frailty were at significantly greater risk and experienced poorer outcomes, including longer hospitalisation and increased mortality (Geriatric Medicine Research Collaborative, 2019).

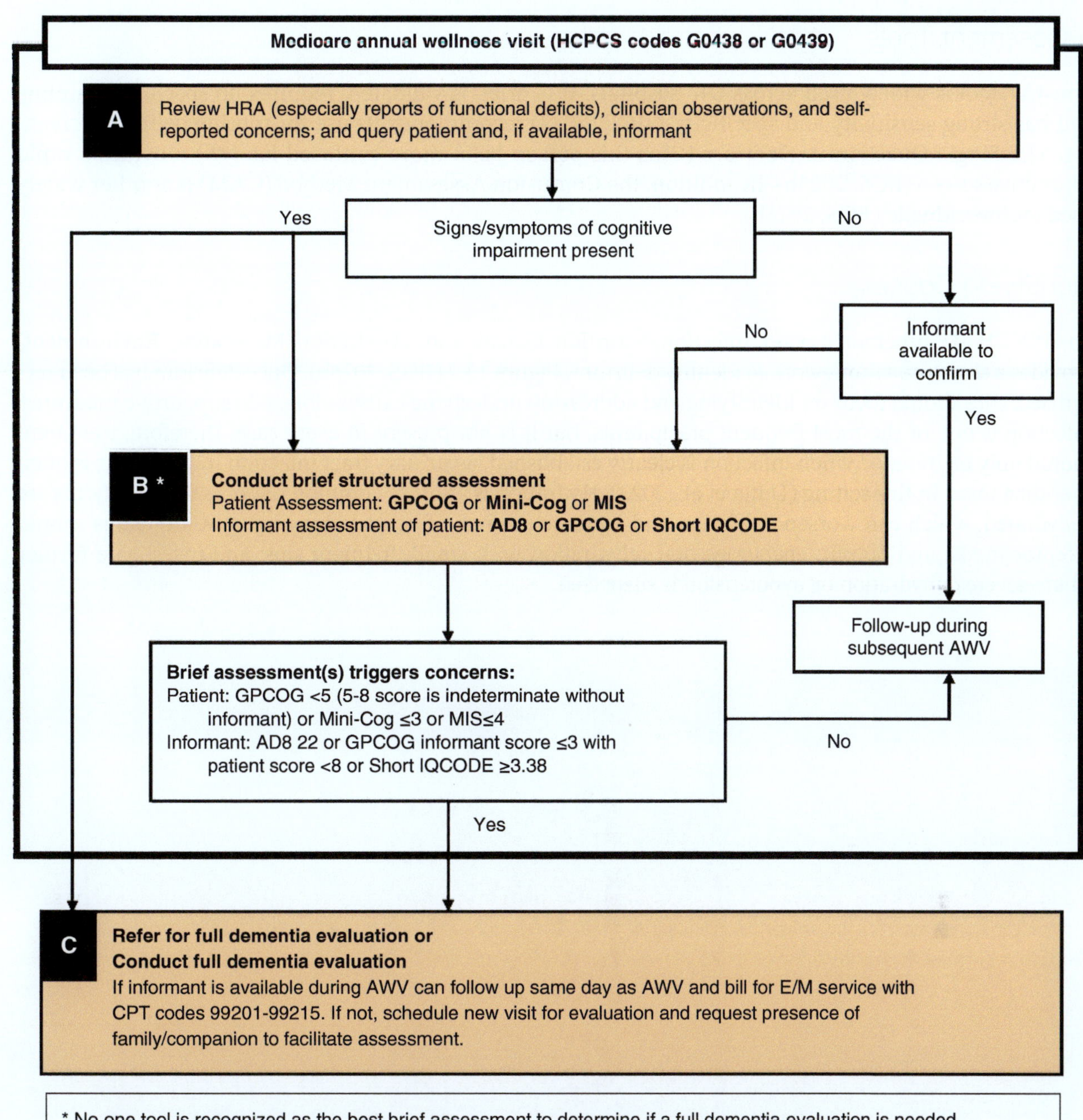

FIGURE 13.1 Algorithm for assessment of cognition. *Source*: Cordell et al. (2013)/with permission of Elsevier.

Assessment Tools

The 4AT tool is widely used across UK hospitals. It is brief, is validated, requires no specialist training, and has strong sensitivity and specificity. NICE (2023) recommends its use for routine delirium screening. The Single Question in Delirium ('Has this person been more confused lately?') provides a rapid adjunctive screen (BGS, 2025b). In addition, the Confusion Assessment Method (CAM) is another widely used tool worldwide (BGS, 2025b).

Identifying Causes

The PINCH ME mnemonic (Pain, Infection, Nutrition, Constipation, Hydration, Medication, Environment) provides a structured framework to identify delirium, Figure 13.2 (BGS, 2025b). Once delirium has been recognised, care should focus on identifying and addressing underlying causes alongside supportive measures. Infection is one of the most frequent precipitants, but it is not present in every case; therefore, treatment should only be initiated when infection is clearly established, as urinary tract infection in particular is often over-diagnosed in this setting (Dutta et al., 2022). Hydration is another common issue, as many patients are dehydrated, which can worsen confusion and increase the risk of acute kidney injury. Care teams should monitor intake and output; encourage oral rehydration with small, frequent sips; and investigate further where severe dehydration or hypotension is suspected.

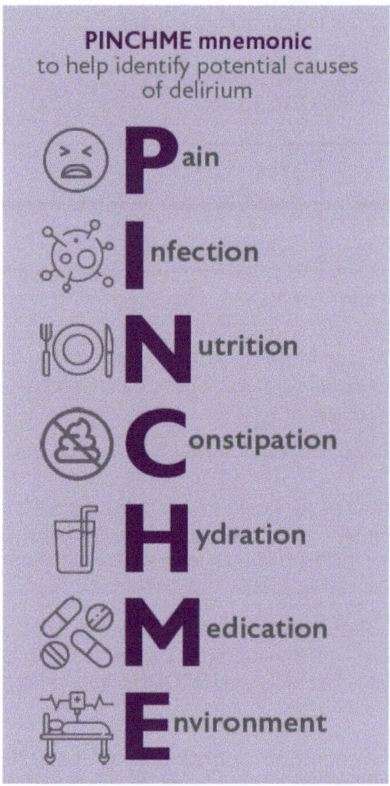

FIGURE 13.2   PINCH ME mnemonic. *Source*: British Geriatric Medicine (2025b)/British Geriatrics Society.

Nutritional support is also essential, as patients with delirium often eat poorly (BGS, 2020). High-calorie foods that are familiar and acceptable to the patient should be offered, weight should be monitored, and dietetic referral considered where needed. Reduced intake of food and fluids may also cause constipation, which can aggravate delirium and should be managed with appropriate laxatives tailored to the patient's preferences. Unrecognised pain is another contributor that requires routine assessment and treatment. Paracetamol should form the basis of analgesia, with weak opioids added only if necessary and used cautiously due to their sedative and cognitive side effects. Urinary retention may also complicate delirium, even when patients appear to be voiding regularly, and bladder assessment should be considered; catheterisation should be avoided unless unavoidable and discontinued at the earliest opportunity.

Mobility should be encouraged to maintain function and reduce complications, while a full medication review is crucial to identify possible drug-related causes. Medicines with anticholinergic effects, sedatives, opioids, and some antidepressants and antihistamines are well recognised for their role in precipitating delirium, and both newly prescribed and long-standing therapies should be critically assessed (Weidmann et al., 2025). Withdrawal from alcohol or other substances may also act as a trigger and should not be overlooked. Sleep disturbance is common, and promoting a regular sleep-wake cycle through non-pharmacological measures is preferable, as hypnotics may prolong or worsen delirium.

Patients and families should receive education about delirium and simple reorientation strategies should be used, such as providing regular reminders of time, date, and place. Supportive environments that reduce noise, ensure adequate lighting, and make clocks and calendars visible can assist, as can encouraging the use of sensory aids such as hearing aids and spectacles. Continuity of care with familiar staff or relatives may also help lessen anxiety and confusion.

Sedation should be avoided wherever possible, but in cases of severe distress or risk to self or others, low-dose antipsychotics may be required. Haloperidol is recommended as first line (NICE, 2023), usually in small, divided doses not exceeding 5 mg in 24 hours, with prior electrocardiogram (ECG) monitoring due to the risk of QTc prolongation (Norfolk and Norwich University Hospitals, 2024). Haloperidol is contraindicated in conditions such as Parkinson's disease or significant cardiac disease (British National Formulary, 2025). If unsuitable, lorazepam may be used in low doses, not exceeding 3 mg in 24 hours. Any sedative therapy should be reviewed frequently, with plans to reduce and stop treatment ideally within 24–48 hours and certainly within one week.

APs play a central role in early recognition. Observing for new-onset confusion, inattention, or perceptual disturbance is vital. Collateral information from relatives or carers can confirm whether a change is acute. Once delirium is suspected, rapid communication with the wider multidisciplinary team is required to ensure timely diagnosis and management.

DEMENTIA

A careful history remains the cornerstone of dementia assessment. Information should be sought from the person and those who know them well to establish the timing, pace of decline, and nature of symptoms (NICE, 2025). Medication review must cover prescribed, over-the-counter, and recreational substances, including alcohol. Enquiries about a family history of early-onset dementia and any previous psychiatric illness, such as depression, are essential.

Dementia is typically a progressive disorder leading to increasing dependency and, ultimately, death, often through complications such as malnutrition, dehydration, or infection. The pattern of deterioration can give diagnostic clues: Alzheimer's disease usually presents insidiously; vascular dementia may show stepwise decline after cerebrovascular events; abrupt onset may follow a single major stroke; and rapid progression over weeks or months should prompt consideration of drug toxicity, metabolic derangement, neoplasia, or subdural haematoma.

Cognitive changes often involve marked impairment of short-term memory, difficulty performing complex tasks such as managing finances, language disturbance with word-finding problems, behavioural changes (apathy, irritability, aggression, and wandering), disorientation, and later failure to recognise people or familiar environments. Agnosia (loss of object recognition), apraxia (inability to carry out coordinated actions), and poor judgement or reasoning can also occur. Self-care skills gradually decline, leading to loss of continence and basic personal care.

PHYSICAL AND MENTAL EXAMINATION

Physical examination helps identify contributory or reversible conditions. Findings may include evidence of vascular disease, neuropathy, parkinsonian features, thyroid disease, malignancy, or chronic liver disease related to alcohol. In advanced stages, primitive reflexes (such as grasp or sucking) and global hyperreflexia with extensor plantar responses may appear. Mental state examination is crucial to rule out delirium—characterised by acute onset, fluctuating attention, and altered consciousness—and depression, for which tools such as the Geriatric Depression Scale can be used.

COGNITIVE TESTING

Standardised tools such as the Mini-Mental State Examination (MMSE), Montreal Cognitive Assessment (MoCA), Mini-Cog, or clock drawing test provide a baseline and allow monitoring of change. Repeat testing can help confirm progressive decline. In complex or uncertain cases, detailed neuropsychological assessment may clarify the diagnosis, distinguish dementia from depression, identify specific subtypes, and track treatment response.

COMMUNICATING THE DIAGNOSIS

Whenever possible, the diagnosis should be shared with the patient in a sensitive manner. Early disclosure supports autonomy, enables medical and financial planning (including advance directives and power of attorney), and facilitates treatment decisions and participation in research. Any risk of distress can be mitigated through multidisciplinary support that focuses on therapeutic options and available services.

INVESTIGATIONS

While fully reversible causes of dementia are uncommon, screening for them is vital. Recommended baseline blood tests include full blood count, erythrocyte sedimentation rate, vitamin B12 and folate, urea and electrolytes, calcium, liver and thyroid function, C-reactive protein, and random glucose. Syphilis or HIV serology is reserved for cases with specific risk factors or atypical presentations. An ECG and chest X-ray can detect cardiac disease or occult malignancy (NICE, 2025).

All patients should be considered for brain imaging at some point. Early imaging is essential for those with onset before 60 years, sudden or rapidly progressive symptoms, a history of cancer or head injury, or focal neurological signs. Computed tomography (CT) is commonly used and can assess medial temporal lobe volume, while magnetic resonance imaging (MRI) provides greater structural detail. Functional imaging, such as single-photon emission computed tomography (SPECT) or positron emission tomography (PET), is largely restricted to specialist centres to refine differential diagnosis between Alzheimer's and vascular dementia. Electroencephalography (EEG) may help diagnose frontotemporal dementia, Creutzfeldt-Jakob disease, or seizure disorders. Lumbar puncture is reserved for suspected central nervous system infection (NICE, 2025).

DEPRESSION

Epidemiology and Risk Factors

Depression is highly prevalent among older adults and is strongly associated with frailty (BGS, 2025b). Studies show that with increasing frailty severity, the likelihood of depression also rises (Feng et al., 2014; Marconcin et al., 2022). There is a reciprocal relationship: depression accelerates functional decline and cognitive deterioration, while frailty increases vulnerability to depression. Globally, a systematic review and meta-analysis reported a pooled prevalence of depression of 38.6% among frail older adults (95% CI 30.1–47.1) (Soysal et al., 2017). In the United Kingdom, analysis of 69,178 residents aged $\geq$65 years in the UK Biobank demonstrated that 46% of frail participants met a broad definition of depression at baseline (Kim et al., 2025). European data from the 17-country Survey of Health, Ageing and Retirement in Europe (SHARE) cohort similarly indicate that between 69.6% and 72.5% of frail older adults scored above the EURO-D threshold for clinically relevant depressive symptoms between 2015 and 2020 (Marconcin et al., 2022). These findings highlight the consistency of the association across different populations and health systems. For healthcare professionals, this underlines the importance of routinely identifying and screening for depressive symptoms in frail older adults, using validated tools within CGA. Early detection not only supports timely intervention but may also mitigate further functional decline and preserve quality of life.

Clinical Presentation

Depression in older people may present differently compared to younger adults. Instead of expressing sadness, patients may report somatic complaints such as fatigue, gastrointestinal discomfort, poor sleep, or weight loss (Nelson et al., 2018). Symptoms may also include irritability, apathy, slowed responses, or loss of interest in previously valued activities. APs must remain alert to these atypical presentations, which can easily be mistaken for 'normal ageing' or physical illness.

Late-life depression carries grave risks. In 2022, of the 49,449 suicides reported in the United States, 10,433 (21%) occurred in people aged 65 years and older (Cleveland Clinic, 2023). Older adults tend to plan suicide more carefully; are more likely to use highly lethal methods; and, due to frailty and comorbidities, are less likely to survive attempts (National Council on Aging, 2025). Among those who attempt suicide, approximately one in four older adults will die compared with one in 200 young people (National Council on Aging, 2025). Risk factors include male sex, bereavement, social isolation, chronic illness, and history of prior attempts. Early detection is therefore paramount.

Assessment should also incorporate collateral history, given that many older adults under-report or minimise psychological symptoms due to stigma. APs must use open and non-judgemental language, for example, asking 'Have you been finding less joy in things recently?' rather than 'Are you depressed?' (BGS, 2025b). One widely tool that used in clinical settings is the two-question screener, valued for its brevity and sensitivity. It asks (1) 'During the last month, have you often been bothered by feeling down, depressed, or hopeless?' and (2) 'During the last month, have you been bothered by having little interest or pleasure in doing things?' A positive response to either question indicates the need for further, more detailed assessment (BGS, 2025b). Table 13.2 shown the most common screening tools that can be used to identify depression.

Management of depression requires a focused approach. Mild symptoms may respond to psychological therapies, behavioural activation, reminiscence therapy, or social interventions. Moderate-to-severe depression may require pharmacological treatment, but antidepressants should be prescribed with caution due to risks of polypharmacy, falls, and side effects. In all cases, support for carers and family is crucial, as is referral to mental health services when risk is significant. Table 13.3 explains the most common depression screening tools.

TABLE 13.2 Key clinical features that aid in differentiating delirium from dementia in older adults.

Feature	Delirium	Dementia
Onset	Develops suddenly or over days	Evolves slowly over months or years
Potential for reversal	Frequently resolves when the precipitating cause is treated	Rarely reversible
Fluctuation in symptoms	Pronounced variation through the day or even within hours	Symptoms usually stable within a day; evening deterioration ('sundowning') or day-to-day fluctuation may occur, especially in Lewy body dementia
Attention	Marked and variable inattention	Often intact until advanced stages
Level of consciousness	Often reduced or fluctuating	Typically normal
Hallucinations and misinterpretation	Visual hallucinations and misperceptions common	Hallucinations tend to appear late; early visual hallucinations with fluctuating cognition point to Lewy body dementia
Behavioural disturbance	Fear, restlessness, or aggression frequent	Less common in early disease
Thought processes	Disorganised thinking and unreal ideas frequent	Slowed or impoverished thinking occurs later
Motor signs	Tremor, asterixis, or myoclonus may be present	Usually absent until advanced disease
Speech	May show slurring or word-finding difficulty	Speech generally preserved until late
Writing ability (dysgraphia)	May deteriorate early	Decline generally late
Memory	Short-term memory severely impaired; long-term memory also affected	Long-term memory often preserved until later stages

Source: Adapted from NICE (2025) and Bowker et al. (2018).

TABLE 13.3   Depression screening tools.

Tool	Purpose/use	Time to administer
GDS-4 (Geriatric Depression Scale-4 items)	Quick screening for depressive symptoms in older adults	3 minutes
GDS-15 (Geriatric Depression Scale-15 items)	Evaluates severity of depression and monitors treatment response	10 minutes
GDS-30 (Geriatric Depression Scale-30 items)	Original full version; comprehensive evaluation of depression	20 minutes
HAM-D/HDRS (Hamilton Depression Rating Scale)	Assesses signs and severity of depression; used to track treatment outcomes	10–20 minutes
HAM-A/HARS (Hamilton Anxiety Rating Scale)	Rates severity of anxiety; useful for GAD and for evaluating treatment	15–20 minutes
PHQ-9 (Patient Health Questionnaire-9 items)	Screens for depression, supports tentative diagnosis, and measures severity	15–20 minutes
GAD-7 (Generalised Anxiety Disorder Questionnaire-7 items)	Brief screening for GAD and monitoring of treatment outcomes	5 minutes
DSM-IV Criteria for Depression	Diagnostic framework for depression, considering symptom count and functional impairment	(Clinical interview)

ANXIETY AND EMOTIONAL WELL-BEING

Anxiety is another important but often under-recognised psychological condition in older adults (Johnco et al., 2024). It may manifest as excessive worry, restlessness, agitation, or avoidance behaviour. In frail individuals, anxiety often coexists with depression or cognitive impairment and contributes to functional decline (Pinton et al., 2023). Older adults may present with health-related anxiety, fear of falling, or panic symptoms. These can restrict mobility, increase dependency, and lead to social withdrawal. Tools, such as the Geriatric Anxiety Inventory (GAI), provide structured assessment (Champagne et al., 2021).

Management of anxiety in older adults prioritises non-pharmacological strategies such as reassurance, psychoeducation, and cognitive-behavioural therapy (CBT) specifically adapted for later life. Pharmacotherapy, particularly using benzodiazepines, is approached with caution due to increased risks of sedation, falls, functional decline, and cognitive impairment in this population (Neil-Sztramko et al., 2025; Shapoval et al., 2025). The psychological domain of CGA also addresses emotional well-being, which is shaped by loss, loneliness, bereavement, and lived experience of ageing with chronic illness. Grief, fatigue, pain, and sensory impairment may all mimic psychological conditions or contribute to emotional distress. Table 13.4 shows the other psychiatric presentations.

PERSON-CENTRED APPROACHES

Holistic interventions include meaningful activity, reminiscence therapy, music, social engagement, and supportive routines. Carer education is also vital, particularly in dementia, where behavioural and psychological symptoms can otherwise cause strain and misunderstanding. APs should adopt a biopsychosocial approach, integrating physical health, environmental context, and social networks into care

TABLE 13.4 Other psychologist presentations.

Presentation	Typical onset/course	Hallmark clinical features	Distinguish from	Initial tests (screen)	First-line management (setting-agnostic)
Alzheimer's disease	Insidious; slow progression over years	Early episodic memory loss → multidomain impairment; normal neurology	Vascular dementia, DLB, depression	Cognitive screen (MMSE/MoCA), routine bloods; MRI (medial temporal atrophy)	Cholinesterase inhibitor (donepezil, rivastigmine, galantamine) if indicated; support carers; risk reduction for comorbidity.
Vascular dementia	Stepwise or abrupt decline; may follow stroke/TIA	Executive dysfunction, gait disturbance, mood lability; focal neurology	Alzheimer's disease, mixed AD/vascular	Vascular risk review; MRI/CT (strategic infarcts, white matter disease)	Aggressive vascular risk modification; consider AChE inhibitor in mixed pictures as per local policy.
Dementia with Lewy bodies (DLB)	Insidious; often faster than AD	Fluctuating cognition/alertness, well-formed visual hallucinations, parkinsonism; rapid eye movement (REM) sleep behaviour disorder	Parkinson's disease dementia (timing of motor vs cognitive >1 year), delirium	Cognitive screen; meds review (neuroleptic sensitivity); MRI to exclude alternatives	Avoid typical antipsychotics; consider rivastigmine for cognition/behaviour; cautious quetiapine only if necessary.
Parkinson's disease dementia (PDD)	Dementia developing >1 year after motor Parkinson's disease (PD)	Executive/visuospatial deficits; hallucinations can occur; motor PD prominent	DLB (dementia first or within 1 year), medication-induced psychosis	Review dopaminergic load; cognitive screen	Optimise PD meds (reduce triggers of psychosis), consider rivastigmine; use antipsychotics with great caution.
Frontotemporal dementia (FTD)	Younger onset (often <70); gradual	Early personality/behaviour change (bvFTD) or primary language syndromes; insight poor; memory relatively spared early	Depression, bipolar disorder, AD	Cognitive screen may be 'normal'; MRI (frontal/temporal atrophy)	Behavioural/environmental strategies; carer support; refer to specialist services.

Normal-pressure hydrocephalus (NPH)	Subacute–chronic	Triad: gait disturbance (early, broad-based), urinary urgency/incontinence, cognitive slowing/apathy	Parkinsonism, vascular gait disorder, AD	MRI/CT (ventriculomegaly out of proportion to atrophy); consider cerebrospinal fluid (CSF) drainage response	Neurosurgical assessment for shunt if appropriate; gait benefits > cognitive gains on average.
Depression (late-life)/pseudodementia'	Weeks–months; may be abrupt	Low mood/anhedonia, poor concentration; frequent 'don't know' in testing; memory improves with cueing	Early dementia	GDS or PHQ-9; rule out hypothyroidism, B12/folate deficiency	Psychological therapy ± SSRI; reassess cognition after mood improves.
Late-life psychosis	Variable	Delusions/hallucinations; often sensory impairment or organic drivers	DLB, delirium, depression with psychosis	Screen for infection, metabolic disturbance, meds; hearing/vision check	Treat cause; cautious antipsychotic use; address sensory deficits; follow-up.
Alcohol-related cognitive disorder/withdrawal states	Variable; withdrawal hours–days after cessation	Confusion, tremor, autonomic signs; Wernicke triad (confusion, ataxia, ophthalmoplegia)	Delirium from other causes, depression	Glucose, electrolytes, LFTs; thiamine status (clinical); collateral history	Thiamine replacement, managed withdrawal (benzodiazepine protocol), rehabilitation support.

Source: Adapted from NICE (2025) and Bowker et al. (2018).

planning. Assessment should also be culturally sensitive. Some older adults may describe psychological distress through physical metaphors such as 'my heart feels heavy' or may minimise mental health concerns due to cultural stigma. Respect for these perspectives, alongside rigorous assessment, enhances therapeutic engagement and trust.

Case Study 13.1   Acute Confusion in a Person with Suspected Dementia

Mrs H, a 79-year-old retired teacher, was brought to the same-day emergency care unit by her daughter after a sudden episode of confusion and fall at home. The daughter reported that over the previous two months Mrs H had experienced fluctuating alertness, vivid visual hallucinations, and disturbed sleep, including acting out dreams. Her medical history included hypertension, atrial fibrillation treated with apixaban, and suspected early Alzheimer's disease.

On assessment, Mrs H was alert but easily distracted, disorientated to time and place, and described seeing 'children playing in the room'. Physical examination revealed mild bradykinesia and rigidity but no focal neurological deficit or fever. Bedside tests showed mild hyponatraemia; all other routine blood investigations and an urgent head CT were unremarkable. The AP considered differentials including delirium, dementia with Lewy bodies, Parkinson's disease with dementia, and late-onset psychosis. The pattern of fluctuating cognition, well-formed hallucinations, REM sleep behaviour disorder, and subtle parkinsonism strongly supported a diagnosis of dementia with Lewy bodies with a mild superimposed delirium.

The AP provided immediate management by ensuring hydration, correcting electrolyte imbalance, optimising sensory input with hearing aids and spectacles, and creating a calm environment. Antipsychotic medication was avoided because of the high risk of worsening motor symptoms; instead, low-dose rivastigmine was initiated after discussion with the memory clinic. Driving cessation was addressed sensitively. Mrs H lacked capacity to make an informed decision on driving, so in line with the Mental Capacity Act 2005, a best interests decision was made to notify the driver and vehicle licensing agency.

Psychosocial support included referral to community dementia services, carer support groups, and social services for home safety assessment. Advance care planning was started, covering future treatment preferences and lasting power of attorney. The AP documented all discussions and capacity assessments, ensuring that decisions complied with legal requirements and professional standards on consent and confidentiality.

Mrs H was discharged home the same day with a clear plan for community follow-up, including repeat cognitive assessment and monitoring of electrolytes. This case illustrates how an advanced clinical practitioner integrates complex clinical reasoning, psychosocial assessment, and a sound understanding of ethical and legal frameworks to deliver safe, person-centred dementia care.

CONCLUSION

Psychiatric care of older adults demands precise syndromic diagnosis; early recognition of organic precipitants; and proportionate, person-centred interventions. Consistent use of brief screening, collateral history, targeted investigations, careful prescribing, and clear documentation reduces harm, supports autonomy, and sustains quality of life for patients and carers.

Take-Home Messages

1. Treat new cognitive or behavioural change as a clinical syndrome to explain, not an artefact of age.
2. Think delirium first in acute change; identify and treat causes promptly.
3. In cognition, use brief tools to screen; abnormal results require further enquiry and escalation.
4. In Lewy body disease, avoid typical antipsychotics; prefer non-drug measures and cautious alternatives if needed.
5. For depression and anxiety in frailty, prioritise psychological therapies; if prescribing, start low and review early for falls, hyponatraemia, and QTc effects.
6. Reassess at defined intervals or sooner after any safety incident; involve carers and record capacity and best interests decisions clearly.

REFERENCES

Al Farsi, R.S., Al Alawi, A.M., Al Huraizi, A.R. et al. (2023). Delirium in medically hospitalized patients: prevalence, recognition and risk factors: a prospective cohort study. *Journal of Clinical Medicine* 12 (12): 3897. https://doi.org/10.3390/jcm12123897.

Alzheimer's Society (2024). *How Many People Have Dementia in the UK?* Alzheimer's Society [Online]. https://www.alzheimers.org.uk/blog/how-many-people-have-dementia-uk (accessed 30 August 2025).

Alzheimer's Society (2025). Symptoms of dementia. https://www.alzheimers.org.uk/about-dementia/symptoms-and-diagnosis/symptoms (accessed 30 August 2025).

Bellelli, G., Brathwaite, J.S., and Mazzola, P. (2021). Delirium: a marker of vulnerability in older people. *Frontiers in Aging Neuroscience* 13: 626127. https://doi.org/10.3389/fnagi.2021.626127.

Bowker, L.K., Price, J.D., Shah, K.S., and Smith, S.C. (2018). *Oxford Handbook of Geriatric Medicine*, 3e. Oxford University Press.

British Geriatrics Society (2020). *End of Life Care in Frailty: Delirium.* London: BGS https://www.bgs.org.uk/resources/end-of-life-care-in-frailty-delirium (accessed 30 August 2025).

British Geriatrics Society (2025a). Comprehensive Geriatric Assessment (CGA) Hub. https://www.bgs.org.uk/CGA (accessed 30 August 2025).

British Geriatrics Society (2025b). *Comprehensive Geriatric Assessment (CGA): Psychological Domain.* British Geriatrics Society [Online]. Published 18 June 2025. https://www.bgs.org.uk/cga-psychological-domain (accessed 30 August 2025).

British National Formulary (BNF) (2025). *Haloperidol: Contra-Indications.* BNF–NICE https://bnf.nice.org.uk/drugs/haloperidol/#contra-indications.assets.publishing.service.gov.uk+13bnf.nice.org.uk+13en.wikipedia.org+13 (accessed 30 August 2025).

Care UK (2025). Signs of ageing or dementia? https://www.careuk.com/help-advice/signs-of-ageing-or-dementia (accessed 30 August 2025).

Cechinel, C., Lenardt, M.H., Rodrigues, J.A.M. et al. (2022). Frailty and delirium in hospitalized older adults: a systematic review with meta-analysis. *Revista Latino-Americana de Enfermagem* 30: e3687. https://doi.org/10.1590/1518-8345.5767.3687.

Champagne, A., Landreville, P., and Gosselin, P. (2021). A systematic review of the psychometric properties of the geriatric anxiety inventory. *Canadian Journal on Aging/La Revue Canadienne du Vieillissement* 40 (3): 376–395. https://doi.org/10.1017/S0714980820000212.

Cleveland Clinic (2023). What to know about older adults and suicide risk. April 4, 2023. Found on the Internet at `https://health.clevelandclinic.org/suicide-in-older-adults` (accessed 30 August 2025).

Cordell, C.B., Borson, S., Boustani, M. et al. (2013). Alzheimer's Association recommendations for operationalizing the detection of cognitive impairment during the Medicare Annual Wellness Visit in a primary care setting. *Alzheimer's & Dementia* 9 (2): 141–150. `https://doi.org/10.1016/j.jalz.2012.09.011` (accessed 30 August 2025).

Devita, M., De Salvo, R., Ravelli, A. et al. (2022). Recognizing depression in the elderly: practical guidance and challenges for clinical management. *Neuropsychiatric Disease and Treatment* 18: 2867–2880. `https://doi.org/10.2147/NDT.S372850`.

Dutta, C., Pasha, K., Paul, S. et al. (2022). Urinary tract infection induced delirium in elderly patients: a systematic review. *Cureus* 14 (12): e32321.

Feng, L., Nyunt, M.S.Z., Feng, L. et al. (2014). Frailty predicts new and persistent depressive symptoms among community-dwelling older adults: findings from Singapore longitudinal aging study. *Journal of the American Medical Directors Association* 15 (1): 76–e7.

Galati, S., Rossi, M., Del Signore, F. et al. (2025). Conventional and neuropsychological criteria for mild cognitive impairment show similar prognostic value for dementia across 12 years in a non-clinical setting. *Scientific Reports* 15: 19827. `https://doi.org/10.1038/s41598-025-19827-2`.

Ge, S., Pan, W., Wu, B. et al. (2023). Sensory impairment and cognitive decline among older adults: an analysis of mediation and moderation effects of loneliness. *Frontiers in Neuroscience* 16: 1092297. `https://doi.org/10.3389/fnins.2023.1092297`.

Geriatric Medicine Research Collaborative (2019). Delirium is prevalent in older hospital inpatients and associated with adverse outcomes: results of a prospective multi-centre study on World Delirium Awareness Day. *BMC Medicine* 17: 229. `https://doi.org/10.1186/s12916-019-1458-7`.

Han, F., Luo, C., Lv, D. et al. (2022). Risk factors affecting cognitive impairment of the elderly aged 65 and over: a cross-sectional study. *Frontiers in Aging Neuroscience* 14: 903794. `https://doi.org/10.3389/fnagi.2022.903794`.

Johnco, C.J., Matovic, D., and Wuthrich, V.M. (2024). Anxiety disorders in later life. *Psychiatric Clinics* 47 (4): 741–752. `https://doi.org/10.1016/j.psc.2023.08.004`.

Kim, J., Kenyon, J., Lu, J. et al. (2025). Among 69, 178 UK residents ages 65+ years, frailty associates significantly with lifestyle behaviours and depression: a cross-sectional study. *Health Science Reports* 8 (3): e70593.

Marconcin, P., Ihle, A., Gouveia, É.R. et al. (2022). Prevalence of frailty and its association with depressive symptoms among European older adults from 17 countries: a 5-year longitudinal study. *International Journal of Environmental Research and Public Health* 19 (21): 14055.

National Council on Aging (2025). *Suicide and Older Adults: What You Should Know*. National Council on Aging [Online]. `https://www.ncoa.org/article/suicide-and-older-adults-what-you-should-know` (accessed 30 August 2025).

National Institute for Health and Care Excellence (NICE) (2023). Delirium: prevention, diagnosis and management in hospital and long-term care [CG103]. `https://www.nice.org.uk/guidance/cg103/chapter/Recommendations#think-delirium` (accessed 30 August 2025).

National Institute for Health and Care Excellence (NICE) (2025). Clinical knowledge summaries: dementia. `https://cks.nice.org.uk/topics/dementia/` (accessed 24 September 2025).

Neil-Sztramko, S.E., Levy, A., Flint, A.J. et al. (2025). Pharmacological treatment of anxiety in older adults: a systematic review and meta-analysis. *The Lancet Psychiatry* 12 (6): 421–432. `https://doi.org/10.1016/S2215-0366(25)00123-4`.

Nelson, B.D., Kessel, E.M., Klein, D.N., and Shankman, S.A. (2018). Depression symptom dimensions and asymmetrical frontal cortical activity while anticipating reward. *Psychophysiology* 55 (1): e12892.

Norfolk and Norwich University Hospitals (2024). Acute management of delirium in older patients [Online]. `https://www.nnuh.nhs.uk/publication/download/acute-delirium-in-older-patients-management-of-ca4047v9/` (accessed 30 August 2025).

Pais, R., Ruano, L., Carvalho, O.P., and Barros, H. (2020). Global cognitive impairment prevalence and incidence in community dwelling older adults—a systematic review. *Geriatrics* 5 (4): 84. `https://doi.org/10.3390/geriatrics5040084`.

Pinton, A., Wroblewski, K., Schumm, L.P. et al. (2023). Relating depression, anxiety, stress and loneliness to 5-year decline in physical function and frailty. *Archives of Gerontology and Geriatrics* 115: 105199. `https://doi.org/10.1016/j.archger.2023.10.199`.

Salari, N., Lotfi, F., Abdolmaleki, A. et al. (2025). The global prevalence of mild cognitive impairment in geriatric population with emphasis on influential factors: a systematic review and meta-analysis. *BMC Geriatrics* 25 (1): 313. `https://doi.org/10.1186/s12877-025-05806-1`.

Shapoval, V., de Saint Hubert, M., Evrard, P. et al. (2025). Barriers to deprescribing benzodiazepines in older adults in a survey of European physicians. *JAMA Network Open* 8 (3): e2459883. `https://doi.org/10.1001/jamanetworkopen.2024.59883`.

Soysal, P., Veronese, N., Thompson, T. et al. (2017). Relationship between depression and frailty in older adults: a systematic review and meta-analysis. *Ageing Research Reviews* 36: 78–87.

Weidmann, A.E., Proppé, G.B., Matthíasdóttir, R. et al. (2025). Medication-induced causes of delirium in patients with and without dementia: a systematic review of published neurology guidelines. *International Journal of Clinical Pharmacy* 1–18.

Wu, C.R., Chang, K.M., Traynor, V., and Chiu, H.Y. (2025). Global incidence and prevalence of delirium and its risk factors in medically hospitalized older patients: a systematic review and meta-analysis. *International Journal of Nursing Studies* 162: 104959. `https://doi.org/10.1016/j.ijnurstu.2025.104959`.

Zhang, T., Ren, Y., Shen, P. et al. (2022). Prevalence and associated risk factors of cognitive frailty: a systematic review and meta-analysis. *Frontiers in Aging Neuroscience* 13: 755926. `https://doi.org/10.3389/fnagi.2021.755926`.

CHAPTER 14

Cardiology

Aim

The aim of this chapter is to provide advanced practitioners (APs) with an in-depth understanding of how frailty influences the presentation, diagnosis, management, and outcomes of key cardiovascular conditions including acute coronary syndrome, arrhythmias, heart failure, and hypertension in order to support safe, individualised, and patient-centred care.

LEARNING OUTCOMES

After studying this chapter, readers will be able to:

1. Explain how frailty modifies the pathophysiology, presentation, and prognosis of acute coronary syndrome (ACS), arrhythmias (including atrial fibrillation), heart failure, and hypertension.
2. Critically appraise diagnostic and management strategies for these conditions, integrating comprehensive geriatric assessment and shared decision-making.
3. Formulate individualised management plans that balance cardiovascular risk reduction with quality of life, functional status, and patient's goals of care.
4. Anticipate common complications such as bleeding, delirium, falls, and arrhythmic events and implement preventative and responsive measures in acute and community settings.

SELF-ASSESSMENT QUESTIONS

1. How does frailty influence the clinical presentation and risk stratification of acute coronary syndrome compared with non-frail older adults?
2. In a frail patient with atrial fibrillation and recurrent gastrointestinal bleeding, how would you weigh the competing risks of thromboembolism and haemorrhage when deciding on anticoagulation?

ACUTE CORONARY SYNDROME IN FRAIL OLDER ADULTS

What Is ACS in the Context of Frailty

Definition of acute coronary syndrome (ACS): Unstable angina, evolving myocardial infarction (MI), with underlying pathologies such as plaque rupture, thrombosis, and inflammation; may present as ST-segment elevation MI (STEMI) or non-ST-segment elevation ACS (NSTE-ACS) (National Institute for Health and Care Excellence [NICE], 2025a).

Frailty: Frailty is a syndrome of impaired physiological reserve and increased vulnerability to stressors, characterised by multisystem decline including reduced physical strength, mobility, weight loss, and exhaustion (Kim and Rockwood, 2024). In older patients with ACS, frailty alters clinical presentation and heightens the risk of complications, poor recovery, cardiovascular events, major bleeding, rehospitalisation, and both short- and long-term mortality (Jiménez-Salva et al., 2025). Even mild frailty significantly increases these risks (Bebb et al., 2018). There is a limited number of randomised controlled trials exploring frailty and ACS; therefore, future studies should investigate this area (Chad et al., 2024).

Risk Factors

Risk factors for ACS in frail older people largely overlap with those in younger populations but have additional modifiers (Table 14.1).

Signs and Symptoms

Frail older adults often manifest ACS differently; recognition can be more difficult. Key points:

- Typical symptoms may be blunted or absent: Less chest pain, more 'silent' infarctions; elderly may present with dyspnoea, fatigue, sweating, syncope, and confusion.
- Atypical or non-cardiac symptoms: Epigastric discomfort, nausea or vomiting, acute confusion/delirium, weakness, and/or collapse.

TABLE 14.1   Risk factors for ACs.

Category	Standard risks	Frailty-related modifiers
Non-modifiable	Age, male sex, family history of ischaemic heart disease	Biological rather than chronological age more predictive; higher baseline vulnerability with advancing frailty.
Modifiable cardiovascular	Hypertension, diabetes mellitus, dyslipidaemia, smoking, obesity, sedentary lifestyle	Reduced physiological reserve means a smaller margin between compensation and decompensation; comorbidity burden intensifies risk; polypharmacy may lead to drug interactions or under-treatment.
Frailty-specific factors	Sarcopenia, malnutrition, cognitive impairment, impaired mobility, decreased physical activity	These contribute both to increased risk of ACS (via inflammation, reduced cardiac/pulmonary reserve, etc.) and worse outcomes (greater mortality, bleeding, and rehospitalisation) in the ACS setting.

- Signs: Tachycardia or bradycardia, hypotension, signs of heart failure (pulmonary oedema, raised jugular venous pressure [JVP], and basal crepitations), diaphoresis, and pallor. Because of frailty, these signs may be subtle or delayed. Some frail patients may have low fever and peripheral oedema.

ASSESSMENT IN FRAIL PATIENTS

To properly evaluate a frail older person with suspected ACS, assessment needs to be broader than in robust patients. Components include:

1. Clinical history and electrocardiogram (ECG)/biomarkers
   - As usual, history of chest pain and risk factor inquiry. But also enquire about functional baseline, cognition, prior mobility, and nutritional state.
   - ECG may show ST elevation, new bundle branch block, or non-specific changes. Biomarkers (troponin and CK-MB) as per local guidelines.
2. Frailty assessment tools
   - Use validated tools: Fried Phenotype (≥3 of 5 criteria: weight loss, exhaustion, low physical activity, slow gait, and weak grip).
   - Clinical Frailty Scale, Edmonton Frail Scale, and Hospital Frailty Risk Score. These help predict prognosis and risk of complications.
3. Comorbidity, cognitive, and functional status
   - Assess for renal impairment, pulmonary disease, and stroke.
   - Cognitive impairment/delirium baseline; capacity.
   - Baseline functional ability: activities of daily living (ADLs), mobility, and frailty reserve.
4. Risk stratification
   - Standard ACS risk scores (e.g. GRACE and TIMI) but recognise limitations: high age, frailty, comorbidity often not fully accounted, may overestimate or misclassify risk in frailty.
   - Assess bleeding risk (including frailty, renal function, or previous bleeding).

DIAGNOSIS

- Diagnostic criteria: As per ACS definitions: presence of chest pain or equivalent, ECG changes, and cardiac enzyme rise such as troponin. In frail patients, enzyme rise may be delayed or blunted; ECG may show more non-specific changes.
- Use of imaging/further tests: Echocardiography to assess wall motion and left ventricle (LV) function; cardiac imaging if needed (but balanced against patient's ability to tolerate) (Figure 14.1).

MANAGEMENT OF ACS IN FRAIL OLDER ADULTS

Management aims to limit myocardial damage, relieve symptoms, and reduce recurrence, while tailoring interventions to frailty, comorbidity, and patient's goals of care.

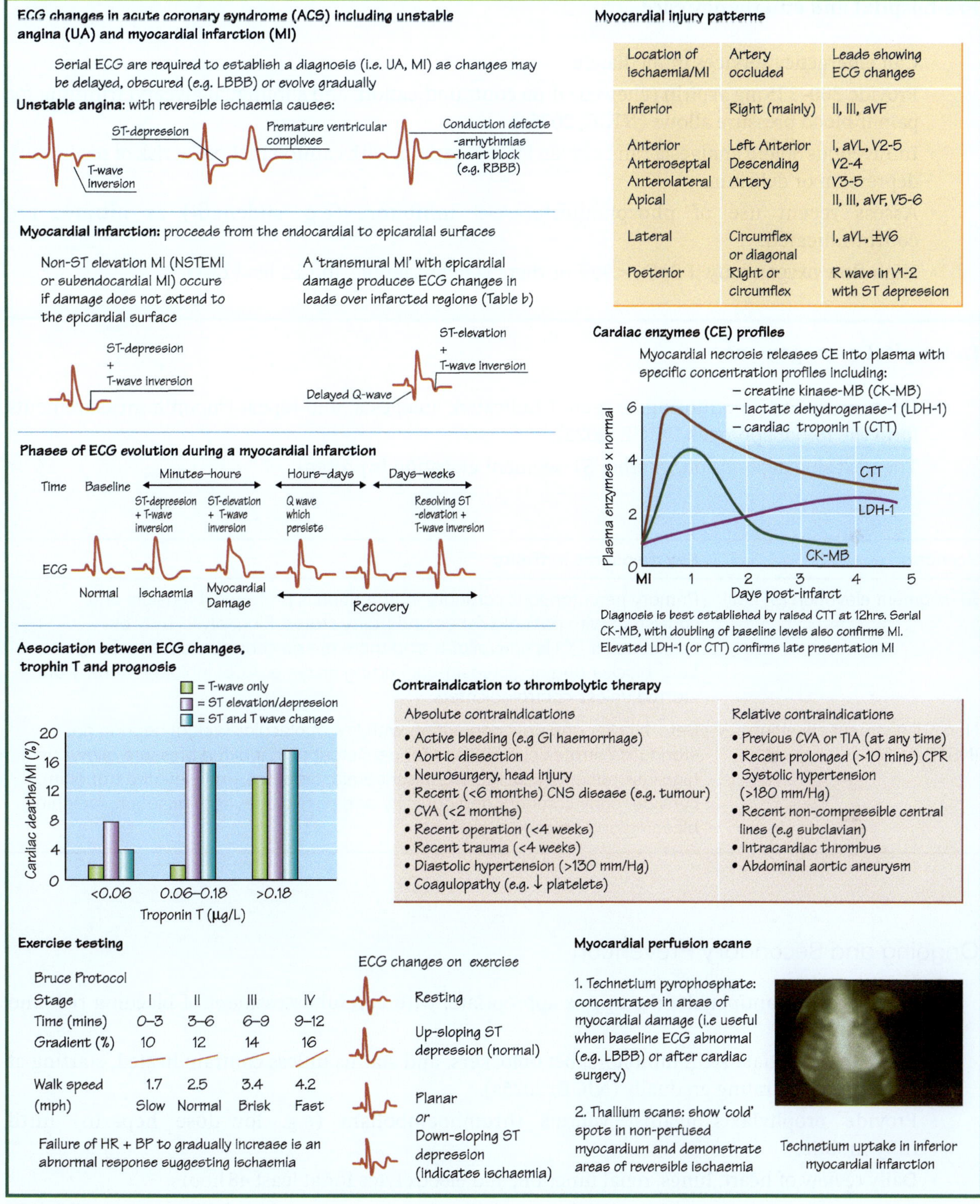

Location of ischaemia/MI	Artery occluded	Leads showing ECG changes
Inferior	Right (mainly)	II, III, aVF
Anterior	Left Anterior	I, aVL, V2-5
Anteroseptal	Descending	V2-4
Anterolateral	Artery	V3-5
Apical		II, III, aVF, V5-6
Lateral	Circumflex or diagonal	I, aVL, ±V6
Posterior	Right or circumflex	R wave in V1-2 with ST depression

Absolute contraindications	Relative contraindications
• Active bleeding (e.g GI haemorrhage)	• Previous CVA or TIA (at any time)
• Aortic dissection	• Recent prolonged (>10 mins) CPR
• Neurosurgery, head injury	• Systolic hypertension (>180 mm/Hg)
• Recent (<6 months) CNS disease (e.g. tumour)	• Recent non-compressible central lines (e.g subclavian)
• CVA (<2 months)	• Intracardiac thrombus
• Recent operation (<4 weeks)	• Abdominal aortic aneurysm
• Recent trauma (<4 weeks)	
• Diastolic hypertension (>130 mm/Hg)	
• Coagulopathy (e.g. ↓ platelets)	

FIGURE 14.1 Investigation and management of ACS. *Source:* Leach (2014)/John Wiley & Sons.

Pre-hospital and emergency care

- Call emergency services immediately.
- Provide 300–325 mg aspirin (chewed) if no contraindication, and sublingual glyceryl trinitrate for pain if blood pressure allows (NICE, 2025a).
- Intravenous opioid analgesia can be given for severe pain, with caution in those at risk of respiratory depression or delirium.
- Assess recent use of phosphodiesterase-5 inhibitors (e.g. sildenafil) as nitrates are contraindicated.
- High-flow oxygen only if SpO_2 <90% or there is hypoxaemia, and 12-lead ECG.

In-hospital management

- Continuous ECG monitoring, oxygen if indicated, analgesia, and repeat troponin measurements form the initial approach (NICE, 2025).
- The next step depends on whether ST-segment elevation is present.

Scenario	Key measures in frailty
ST-segment elevation (STEMI)	Primary percutaneous coronary intervention is preferred if feasible and consistent with patient wishes and frailty status. Fibrinolysis may be considered if PCI is unavailable and there are no contraindications. Early beta-blocker and angiotensin-converting enzyme (ACE) inhibitor therapy are started unless contraindicated.
Non-ST-segment elevation (NSTE-ACS)	Beta-blocker and anticoagulation with low-molecular-weight heparin are standard. Nitrates can be used for persistent pain if blood pressure allows. In high-risk patients (e.g. recurrent ischaemia, diabetes, and elevated troponin), consider early coronary angiography and possible revascularisation, weighing bleeding and procedural risk.

Ongoing and Secondary Prevention

- Continue dual-antiplatelet therapy as appropriate, with careful assessment of bleeding risk and renal function.
- Maintain or initiate ACE inhibitors, beta-blockers, and statins unless contraindicated, starting at low dose and titrating gradually (NICE, 2025a).
- Provide prophylaxis against venous thromboembolism (e.g. low-dose heparin) until fully mobile.
- Daily review of heart, lungs, renal function, and electrolytes for at least 48 hours.
- Offer smoking cessation, optimal diabetes and blood pressure control, and dietary advice (high in fibre, fruits and vegetables, low in saturated fat).

Frailty-specific Considerations

- Engage the patient and family in shared decision-making, incorporating comprehensive geriatric assessment to guide intensity of treatment.
- Prioritise early mobilisation, delirium prevention, nutrition, and rehabilitation to reduce functional decline.
- For very frail or terminal patients, a conservative or palliative approach may be more appropriate, focusing on comfort and symptom relief.

Discharge and Long-term Care

- Gradual resumption of activity is encouraged; most can return to light work within 4–12 weeks if recovery is uncomplicated.
- Sexual activity can usually resume after about one month if the patient is symptom free.
- Advise avoiding long-haul air travel for approximately two months.

Complication

Complications following MI can affect several organ systems and occur at different stages of recovery. Early complications include cardiac arrest, cardiogenic shock, and unstable angina. Disturbances of heart rhythm are frequent: bradyarrhythmia such as sinus bradycardia or atrioventricular (AV) block may necessitate pacing, while ventricular tachycardia, ventricular fibrillation, and atrial fibrillation can lead to sudden deterioration and require prompt antiarrhythmic therapy. Left or right ventricular failure may develop, causing pulmonary oedema or low-output shock (NICE, 2025b).

Pericarditis and cardiac tamponade can arise due to pericardial inflammation or effusion. Thromboembolic events, such as deep vein thrombosis, pulmonary embolism, and systemic embolism, are also recognised risks. Structural complications include acute mitral regurgitation from papillary muscle rupture, ventricular septal defect, and late left ventricular aneurysm. Dressler's syndrome, a post-MI inflammatory reaction, presents later with fever, pericardial pain, and effusion. Each of these complications carries significant morbidity or mortality and requires timely recognition and targeted management (NICE, 2025b).

Arrhythmias

Cardiac arrhythmias are disturbances of impulse formation or conduction leading to abnormal heart rhythms (Antzelevitch and Burashnikov, 2011). They range from benign isolated ectopics to severe forms that compromise cardiac output and can be fatal. Arrhythmias may present as bradyarrhythmias (heart rate <60 bpm), tachyarrhythmias (heart rate >100 bpm), or irregular rhythms such as atrial fibrillation.

Arrhythmias are common across all age groups and may occur in healthy individuals or in association with structural heart disease. Cardiac causes include MI, ischaemic heart disease, cardiomyopathies, valvular lesions, myocarditis, and pericarditis. Non-cardiac precipitants are equally important and encompass electrolyte imbalances (potassium, calcium, and magnesium), thyroid dysfunction, hypoxia, acidosis, fever, and a variety of drugs such as β-agonists and certain antidepressants (Flynn et al., 2013). Lifestyle factors such as caffeine, alcohol, and smoking can trigger episodes (Lim and Kalman, 2024).

CLINICAL PRESENTATION, ASSESSMENT, AND DIAGNOSIS

Symptoms depend on the type and rate of rhythm disturbance. Palpitations, chest discomfort, breathlessness, presyncope, syncope (Figure 14.2), and sudden fatigue are frequent. Some patients remain asymptomatic and are diagnosed incidentally. Severe arrhythmias can present with hypotension, pulmonary oedema, or cardiac arrest.

A careful history should include onset, duration, precipitating factors, associated chest pain or dyspnoea, and relevant drug or family history. Examination may reveal an irregular pulse, signs of heart failure, or thyrotoxicosis. Investigations begin with a 12-lead ECG to identify ischaemia, conduction defects, or characteristic

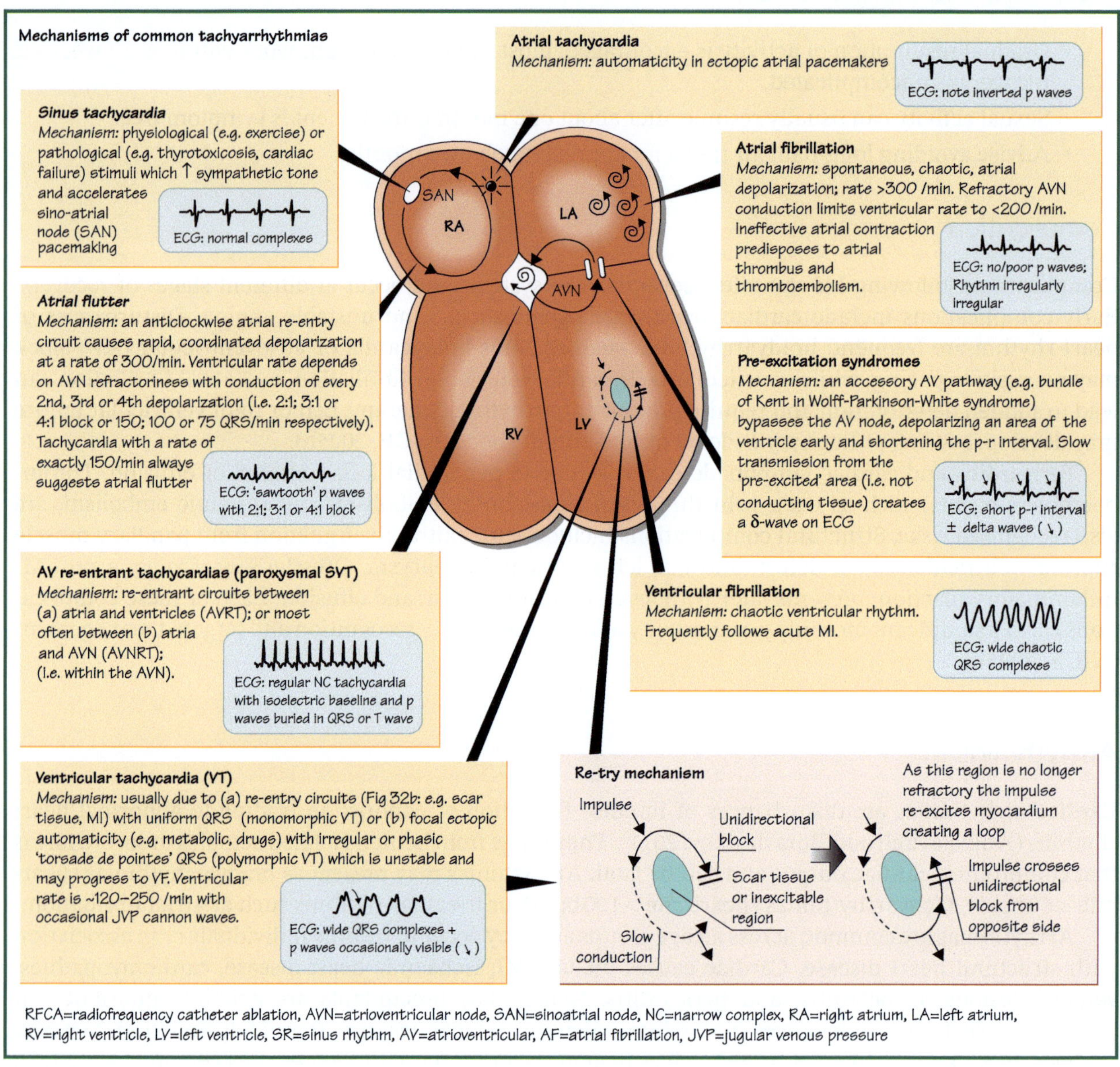

FIGURE 14.2 Tachyarrhythmia. *Source*: Leach (2014)/John Wiley & Sons.

features such as short PR interval or long QT. Because many arrhythmias are paroxysmal, ambulatory ECG (24-hour or longer) is often needed. Echocardiography assesses underlying structural disease, while blood tests for electrolytes, calcium, magnesium, and thyroid function help detect reversible causes.

MANAGEMENT

Treatment is focused to the specific arrhythmia and clinical context. Bradyarrhythmias are observed if asymptomatic and rate is >40 bpm. Symptomatic cases require intravenous atropine and, if unresponsive, temporary or permanent pacing. Supraventricular tachycardias are initially treated with vagal manoeuvres and adenosine with β-blockers or calcium channel blockers for maintenance. Atrial fibrillation and flutter require rate or rhythm control and thromboembolic prophylaxis with anticoagulation. Ventricular tachycardia and ventricular fibrillation are medical emergencies managed with intravenous amiodarone or lidocaine and often electrical cardioversion or defibrillation. Correcting underlying precipitants such as electrolyte disturbance, hypoxia, or drug toxicity is essential. For recurrent or high-risk arrhythmias, implantable cardioverter-defibrillators or permanent pacemakers improve survival.

COMPLICATIONS AND PROGNOSIS

Untreated arrhythmias can lead to thromboembolism, heart failure, syncope with trauma, or sudden cardiac death. Prognosis varies widely: isolated ectopics are usually benign, whereas sustained ventricular arrhythmias carry high mortality without prompt treatment. Early recognition of warning signs and prompt ECG evaluation are crucial. Structured safety-netting advice, for example, using a traffic light framework, helps patients understand when urgent reassessment is needed. For clinicians in acute and community settings, vigilant monitoring and timely referral reduce complications and improve outcomes (Figure 14.3).

ATRIAL FIBRILLATION AND FLUTTER IN FRAIL OLDER ADULTS

Definition and Clinical Relevance

Atrial fibrillation (AF) is the most common sustained arrhythmia in later life. It is characterised by rapid, disorganised atrial electrical activity, producing an irregularly irregular ventricular rate. Flutter is a related macro-re-entrant rhythm, usually with a more organised atrial rate. Both markedly increase the risk of thromboembolism and stroke, which is accentuated in frail older adults because of coexisting comorbidity and impaired physiological reserve. Public Health England (PHE) estimated, using age-sex-specific data from a northern Sweden population study, that 1,496,972 people in England were living with AF in 2019 at both GP practice and local population levels (PHE, 2020). In addition, the European Society of Cardiology (ESC) guidelines highlight that AF is the most prevalent sustained arrhythmia globally, affecting an estimated 2–4% of adults. Its incidence and prevalence rise with age and are consistently higher in men than in women, with overall numbers projected to increase as populations age and detection improves (Table 14.2) (Hindricks et al., 2021).

Syncope

History

- Age
- Precipitants, position (lying, standing), and activity at time of event
- Prodromal symptoms such as nausea, pallor, light-headedness
- Collateral history from eye witness about duration of event or associated movements (myoclonus, seizure activity)
- Past medical history
- Family history of sudden death or fainting
- Drug history (antihypertensives, antiarrhythmics, drugs affecting QT interval)

Cardiac syncope arises as a consequence of haemodynamic compromise in the setting of cardiac arrhythmias or structural heart disease. It is the second most common cause of syncope

Arrhythmias			Structural heart disease	
Bradycardia	**Tachycardia**	**Drug-induced**	**Cardiac**	**Other**
Sinus node disease Atrio-ventricular conduction defects	Supraventricular tachycardia Ventricular tachycardia	Antiarrhythmics Antianginals Antiemetics Antipsychotics Inotropes	Valve disease Acute myocardial infarction Hypertrophic cardiomyopathy Pericardial disease/ cardiac tamponade Congenital abnormalities	Pulmonary embolus Severe pulmonary hypertension Acute aortic dissection

- **Orthostatic hypotension** defined as a symptomatic systolic blood pressure (BP) drop of 20 mm Hg or diastolic BP drop of 10 mm Hg within 3 minutes of standing. It occurs as a consequence of impaired vasoconstriction due to chronic impairment of autonomic sympathetic activity

Drug induced	**Primary autonomic failure**	**Secondary autonomic failure**	**Volume depletion**
Antihypertensives (in particular short acting medications) Diuretics Vasodilators Phenothiazines Antidepressants	Pure autonomic failure Parkinson's disease with autonomic failure Multi-system atrophy Dementia with Lewy bodies	Diabetes mellitus Amyloidosis Spinal cord injuries Uraemia	Haemorrhage Diarrhoea Vomiting Dehydration

Reflex syncope : transient loss of consciousness due to inappropriate cardiovascular responses of vasodilatation or bradycardia, leading to systemic hypotension and cerebral hypoperfusion. It is the most common cause of syncope

Vasovagal	**Situational**	**Carotid sinus syndrome**	**Atyical/other**
Mediated by: Emotional stress (fear, pain) Orthostatic stress	After eating (post prandial) Cough/sneeze Post micturition Post-exercise Playing wind instrument Weightlifting	3 subtypes Cardioinhibitory Vasodepressor Mixed	No apparent trigger Atypical presentation

Examination

- Cardiac examination: pulse rate and rhythm, murmurs
- Neurological examination: usually normal
- Physical features of associated disease e.g. Parkinson's disease
- Lying and standing BP

Causes-COR

- Cardiac
- Orthostatic hypotension
- Reflex syncope

Investigations

- Basic bloods checking for anaemia, dehydration
- ECG: baseline rhythm, rate, QRS morphology, QT interval, axis
- 24 hour ECG monitoring: arrhythmia, cardiac slowing or pause, atrioventricular conduction defects

If diagnosis is uncertain following initial evaluation, further testing is guided by suspected underlying aetiology

- Echocardiography: structural heart disease
- Implantable loop recorder: subcutaneous monitoring device for arrhythmia
- Electrophysiological studies if arrhythmia suspected but standard testing has not demonstrated it
- Exercise stress test
- Cardiac catheterisation
- Head up tilt table test +/– carotid sinus

FIGURE 14.3 Syncope. *Source*: Blundell and Gordon (2015)/John Wiley & Sons.

TABLE 14.2 Difference between valvular and non-valvular AF.

Feature	Valvular AF	Non-valvular AF
Definition	AF in the presence of moderate-to-severe mitral stenosis or any mechanical valve	AF without moderate-to-severe mitral stenosis or a mechanical heart valve
Possible valve status	Mechanical valve (open/closed), valve stenosis	May include mild mitral stenosis, valve repair, mitral regurgitation, or aortic stenosis
Stroke-risk scoring	CHA_2DS_2-VASc not applicable	CHA_2DS_2-VASc applicable
Preferred anticoagulant	Warfarin (dabigatran linked to higher stroke risk than warfarin)	Direct oral anticoagulants or warfarin as clinically indicated

Algorithm: Classification of AF

1. Assess duration of AF episode

   If < 7 days → paroxysmal AF

   If ≥ 7 days → go to Step 2

2. If continuous AF > 7 days

   If duration ≤ 1 year → persistent AF

   If duration > 1 year → go to Step 3

3. If continuous AF > 1 year

   If rhythm control interventions are still being considered → long-standing persistent AF

   If no further rhythm control intervention is planned → permanent AF

Causes and Risk Factors of AF

See Table 14.3.

TABLE 14.3 Risk factors and cases of AF.

Category	Risk factors/causes
Cardiac or valvular	Hypertension (1.7-fold higher AF risk), ischaemic heart disease, heart failure with reduced ejection fraction, valvular heart disease, atrial/ventricular dilatation or hypertrophy, pre-excitation syndromes (e.g. Wolff-Parkinson-White), sick sinus syndrome, congenital heart disease, pericarditis, amyloidosis, myocarditis, recent cardiothoracic or other surgery
Non-cardiac	Acute infections (e.g. pneumonia), pulmonary embolism, chronic obstructive pulmonary disease (COPD), chronic kidney disease (CKD), electrolyte disturbance (e.g. hypokalaemia and hyponatraemia), cancer (e.g. lung cancer), thyrotoxicosis, diabetes mellitus (≥2-fold higher AF prevalence), obstructive sleep apnoea
Lifestyle and other	Increasing age, excessive alcohol intake, obesity (risk rises with BMI), long-term vigorous or endurance exercise, cigarette smoking, certain medications (e.g. thyroxine, lithium, and beta-2 agonist bronchodilators)

Source: Adapted from NICE (2025).

Clinical Presentation

The principal manifestation is a fast, irregular pulse exceeding 100 beats per minute, accompanied by tiredness, breathlessness, dizziness, and chest pain. The inefficient cardiac contractions impair circulatory performance, potentially causing hypotension and heart failure. However, AF in frailty may be silent or manifest atypically. While palpitations, dyspnoea, chest discomfort, or presyncope are typical, older frail individuals often present with non-specific symptoms such as fatigue, confusion, falls, or worsening heart failure. The hallmark finding is an irregularly irregular pulse, with an apical rate exceeding the radial rate.

Assessment and Investigations

Diagnosis is confirmed by a 12-lead ECG showing absent P-waves with irregular QRS complexes. Laboratory tests should include renal and thyroid function, electrolytes, and cardiac biomarkers. Echocardiography helps to identify left atrial enlargement, left ventricular dysfunction, and structural valve disease. Stroke risk and bleeding risk should be estimated using validated tools such as CHA_2DS_2-VASc and HAS-BLED, while frailty assessments (e.g. Clinical Frailty Scale) guide therapeutic intensity.

MANAGEMENT

Acute (Onset ≤48 hours)

- Treat precipitating factors such as infection or acute coronary syndrome.
- Control ventricular rate with a beta-blocker or non-dihydropyridine calcium channel blocker (e.g. diltiazem), given intravenously if necessary. Digoxin may be used if there is severe left ventricular impairment.
- In haemodynamically unstable patients, immediate electrical cardioversion is indicated. In selected stable cases, pharmacological cardioversion (e.g. intravenous amiodarone) can be considered.
- Anticoagulation is recommended unless AF is of very recent onset and no structural heart disease is evident.

Chronic or Persistent AF

- Rate control remains the preferred strategy in older frail patients, using beta-blockers or calcium channel blockers. Digoxin can be added if monotherapy is inadequate.
- Rhythm control (e.g. amiodarone) is reserved for symptomatic patients where rate control fails and comorbidity allows.
- Oral anticoagulation with a direct oral anticoagulant or warfarin (target INR 2.0–3.0) reduces stroke risk and is generally indicated unless contraindicated. The decision must weigh frailty, fall risk, renal function, and patient preferences.

Paroxysmal AF

- Antiarrhythmic drugs may help maintain sinus rhythm if symptoms are troublesome and contraindications are absent.
- Anticoagulation is guided by the same stroke-risk criteria as for chronic AF.

Special Considerations in Frailty

- Comprehensive geriatric assessment is crucial to balance stroke prevention with bleeding and fall risks.
- Medication optimisation is essential: start low, titrate slowly, and monitor renal and hepatic function.
- Shared decision-making should clarify goals of care, especially in advanced frailty where quality of life may outweigh rhythm control.

Case Study 14.1 Management of Permanent AF and Recurrent Lower Gastrointestinal Bleeding

An 80-year-old patient with permanent AF and a CHA_2DS_2-VASc score of 4 presented with repeated episodes of fresh per-rectal bleeding requiring multiple blood transfusions. Previous upper and lower gastrointestinal endoscopies had revealed angiodysplasia of the bowel, and angiographic imaging confirmed recurrent bleeding from angiodysplastic lesions. Despite endoscopic interventions, the patient continued to experience clinically significant haemorrhage.

The patient had been maintained on apixaban for stroke prevention. Given the ongoing gastrointestinal bleeding, a multidisciplinary team (MDT) discussion by the AP was arranged involving cardiology, gastroenterology, stroke medicine, and the AP. During this meeting, the AP contributed observations from the patient's clinical course, emphasising the frequency and severity of bleeding episodes, transfusion requirements, and the impact on functional status and quality of life.

The discussion was about the CHA_2DS_2-VASc score, indicating a substantial risk of thromboembolic stroke, alongside the Outcomes Registry for Better Informed Treatment (ORBIT) bleeding risk score, which was markedly higher and indicated very high haemorrhagic risk. After shared decision-making and detailed counselling about the competing risks of stroke and major bleeding, the patient opted to discontinue apixaban.

The AP clearly documented the decision and their own observations within the medical record. A formal clinical letter, summarising the MDT deliberations and the patient's preferences, was sent to the patient's general practitioner and uploaded to the electronic record to ensure all healthcare professionals could access the rationale for discontinuation of anticoagulation if future review was required. This case illustrates the complexity of balancing thromboembolic and bleeding risks in frail older adults with AF and highlights the central role of APs in multidisciplinary decision-making and comprehensive documentation.

HEART FAILURE IN FRAILTY

Heart failure is a syndrome characterised by typical signs and symptoms arising from structural or functional cardiac impairment that leads to diminished cardiac output. Around one million people in the United Kingdom are affected, and prevalence is rising globally. Management is complicated by an ageing population with multiple comorbidities, while the condition contributes to about 5% of emergency hospital admissions and 2% of overall NHS spending, representing a significant and increasing economic burden (British Geriatrics Society, 2020).

DEFINITION, CAUSES, AND CLINICAL FEATURES

Heart failure may involve left ventricular dysfunction, right ventricular dysfunction, or both and is classified according to ejection fraction into reduced (HFrEF) or preserved (HFpEF) categories. Myocardial ischaemia, hypertension, valvular heart disease, and cardiomyopathy are frequent underlying causes, while acute precipitants include arrhythmia, infection, anaemia, and uncontrolled blood pressure. Frail older adults often present with atypical or subtle symptoms. Breathlessness on exertion, orthopnoea, paroxysmal nocturnal dyspnoea, and fatigue are classical, but confusion, anorexia, falls, and weight loss may predominate. Physical findings can include tachycardia, displaced apex beat, pulmonary crackles, elevated jugular venous pressure, hepatomegaly, ascites, and peripheral oedema.

Diagnosis rests on careful history and examination supported by investigations. Natriuretic peptides (BNP or NT-proBNP) are valuable screening tools; a 12-lead ECG may reveal ischaemia, arrhythmia or conduction defects; chest radiography can demonstrate cardiomegaly or pulmonary congestion; and echocardiography confirms left ventricular dysfunction and identifies structural causes. New York Heart Association functional classes I–IV describe the impact of symptoms on daily activity.

MANAGEMENT

Treatment integrates standard heart failure therapies with the principles of comprehensive geriatric assessment. General measures include smoking cessation, vaccination, dietary sodium restriction, fluid balance monitoring, and graded exercise. Loop diuretics such as furosemide relieve congestion and are titrated carefully in renal impairment. ACE inhibitors or angiotensin receptor blockers reduce mortality and hospitalisation and are introduced at low dose with gradual up-titration. Evidence supports the use of beta-blockers (bisoprolol, carvedilol, or slow-release metoprolol) in stable HFrEF and mineralocorticoid receptor antagonists such as spironolactone in New York Heart Association class II–IV if renal function and potassium levels allow. SGLT2 inhibitors (e.g. dapagliflozin) now form part of core therapy irrespective of diabetes. Other options for selected patients include ivabradine, sacubitril/valsartan, or, when ACE inhibitors are not tolerated, hydralazine with isosorbide dinitrate. Device therapies such as implantable cardioverter defibrillator or cardiac resynchronisation can be beneficial when life expectancy and functional reserve are sufficient. Acute decompensation requires hospital care with intravenous diuretics, oxygen if hypoxic, and, in refractory cases, vasodilators or inotropes (Figure 14.4).

FRAILTY CONSIDERATIONS

Frailty powerfully predicts mortality, hospital readmission, and adverse reactions to therapy. Management therefore demands early multidisciplinary input, medication review, and careful monitoring of renal function, blood pressure, and electrolytes. Goals of care, including the balance between longevity and quality of life, should be established with patients and families. In advanced or end-stage disease, symptom-focused or palliative approaches may better reflect patient preferences than maximal disease-directed treatment.

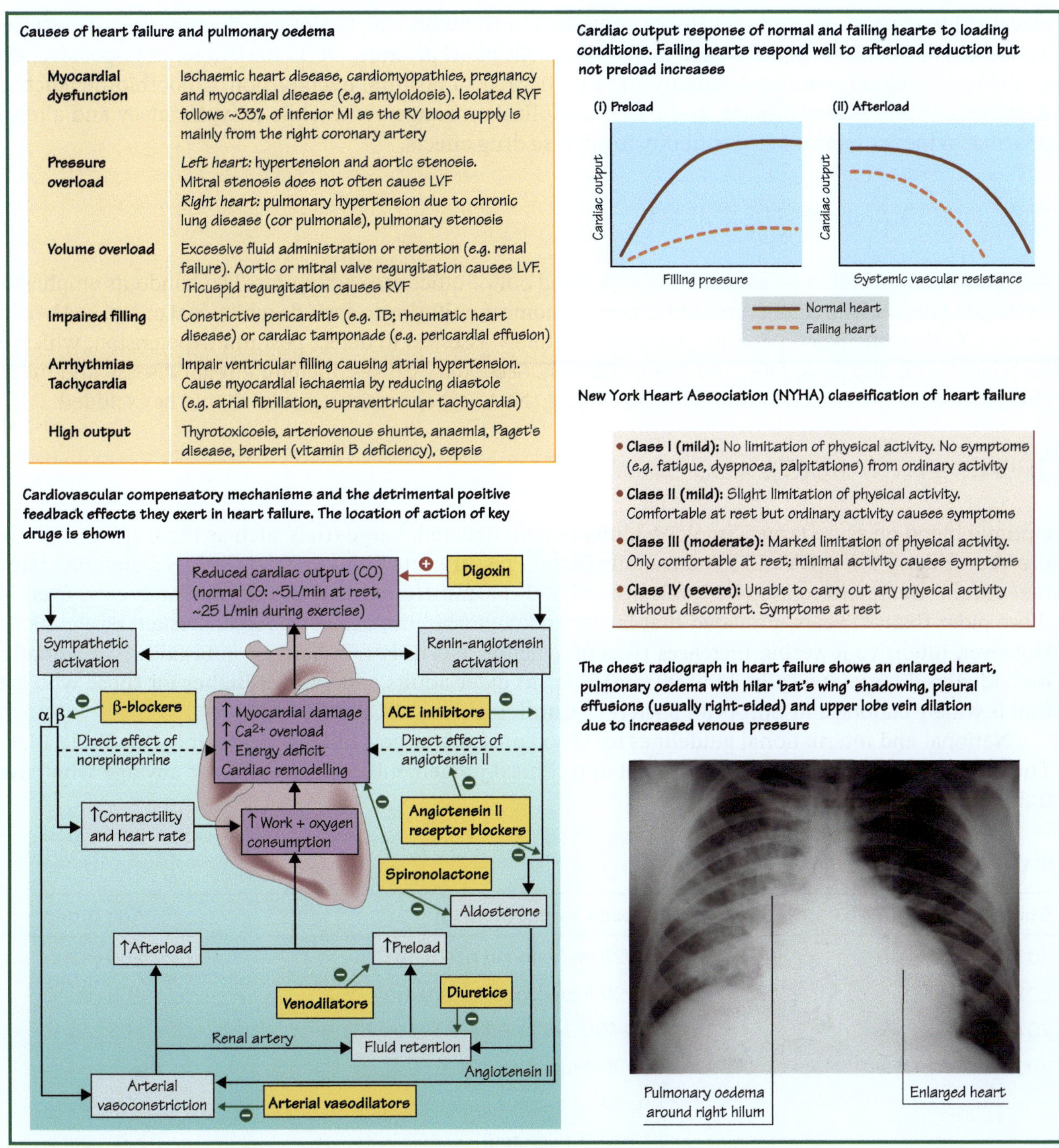

FIGURE 14.4 Heart failure and pulmonary oedema management. *Source*: Leach (2014)/John Wiley & Sons.

HYPERTENSION IN OLDER ADULTS

Hypertension is highly prevalent in later life and represents a major modifiable risk factor for stroke, MI, heart failure, cognitive decline, and renal disease. Ageing is associated with arterial stiffening and reduced baroreceptor sensitivity, resulting in a predominantly systolic pattern of hypertension with widened pulse pressure. In the United Kingdom, over two-thirds of adults older than 65 years live with elevated blood pressure, and prevalence continues to rise with age. Structural changes in large arteries lead to loss of vascular compliance and increased systolic blood pressure. Declining baroreflex responsiveness contributes to blood pressure variability and a higher risk of postural hypotension. Comorbidities such as diabetes, chronic kidney disease, and frailty complicate management, while polypharmacy and altered pharmacokinetics increase susceptibility to adverse drug effects.

DIAGNOSIS AND ASSESSMENT

Accurate diagnosis relies on standardised office and out-of-office measurements. The handouts emphasise repeated seated measurements and ambulatory or home monitoring to exclude white-coat or masked hypertension. Orthostatic blood pressure should be routinely assessed to detect postural hypotension, which is associated with dizziness, falls, and hospitalisation. Secondary causes, including renal disease and medicines such as non-steroidal anti-inflammatory drug (NSAIDs) or corticosteroids, should be excluded.

TREATMENT TARGETS AND EVIDENCE

Optimal blood pressure targets in older adults remain debated. Large trials such as the Hypertension in the Very Elderly Trial (HYVET) and Systolic Blood Pressure Intervention Trial (SPRINT) demonstrated that careful treatment to systolic levels around 130–140 mmHg reduces cardiovascular events, even in those older than 80 years, provided that frailty and comorbidities are considered (Beckett et al., 2008). However, intensive lowering increases risks of syncope, electrolyte imbalance, and falls. A pragmatic, individualised target typically <140/90 mmHg for fit older adults and slightly higher for those who are frail is widely endorsed in European Society of Cardiology and NICE guidance.

National and international guidelines for blood pressure targets differ considerably (see Table 14.4). The 2019 NICE guidance emphasises applying clinical judgement for individuals of any age who have frailty or multimorbidity.

TABLE 14.4   Hypertension guidelines.

Guideline (year)	Proposed target (mmHg)	Age group
2017 ACC/AHA	<130/80 (Whelton et al. 2018)	≥65 years
2017 ACP/AAFP	<150/90 (Qaseem et al. 2017)	≥60 years
2018 ESC/ESH	130–140/70–80 (Williams et al. 2018)	≥65 years
2019 Chinese	<140/90 (Hua et al. 2019)	≥65 years
	<150/90	≥80 years
	<140/90 (if tolerated)	≥80 years
UK (NICE) 2023	<150/90 Use clinical judgement for people of any age with frailty or multimorbidity (NICE 2025).	≥80 years
2020 Canadian	<120 (Rabi et al. 2020)	≥75 years
2021 WHO	<140/90 (without comorbidity) (Campbell et al. 2022)	—
British and Irish Hypertension Society (recent position statement, 2025)	<140/90 mmHg	<80 years old
	High target is acceptable and use 'clinical judgement' (Faconti et al. 2025).	>80 years old

MANAGEMENT PRINCIPLES

Management combines lifestyle modification and pharmacotherapy. Salt restriction, weight optimisation, regular physical activity, moderation of alcohol intake, and smoking cessation remain cornerstones. Pharmacological therapy usually starts with a thiazide-type diuretic, calcium channel blocker, ACE inhibitor, or angiotensin receptor blocker, guided by comorbidities and tolerability. It is important to consider practical steps such as 'start low, titrate slow', acknowledging increased drug sensitivity in older age. Combination therapy is frequently required to achieve targets.

CHALLENGES ENCOUNTERED IN TREATING HYPERTENSIVE ELDERLY

Treating hypertension in older adults presents complex clinical challenges. Age-related changes in pharmacokinetics and pharmacodynamics heighten sensitivity to many drugs, while cognitive impairment can hinder adherence and increase the risk of errors. Multiple long-term conditions and high prevalence of polypharmacy amplify the likelihood of adverse drug interactions. Orthostatic hypotension is common, raising the risk of dizziness and falls, and necessitates routine postural blood pressure monitoring. Reduced gait speed and lower quality of life may complicate lifestyle interventions. The financial burden of medication, side effects such as constipation or incontinence, and sensory deficits can further reduce treatment acceptability. Effective care also depends on social support and may generate significant caregiver costs. Frailty compounds these issues, requiring individualised blood pressure targets and shared decision-making to balance the benefits of cardiovascular protection with the risk of harm.

Special Considerations

Frailty and multimorbidity: Frail older adults are vulnerable to adverse effects of aggressive therapy. Blood pressure should be reviewed at every contact, with careful balance of cardiovascular benefit against risk of falls and functional decline.

Postural and postprandial hypotension: A fall of ≥ 20 mmHg systolic pressure within two hours after meals is common (Ringer et al., 2025). Advice on smaller, more frequent meals and review of antihypertensives can help.

Cognitive impairment: Midlife hypertension is a risk factor for dementia, and SPRINT-MIND suggests that treatment may delay cognitive decline (Williamson et al., 2019). Yet established dementia may limit adherence and heighten sensitivity to hypotension.

Adherence and health literacy: Poor understanding of hypertension and complex regimens often reduce adherence. Simple dosing schedules, patient education, and regular review improve control.

Integration with comprehensive care: Management of hypertension in later life should form part of a holistic assessment addressing comorbidities, frailty, polypharmacy, and patient goals. Shared decision-making ensures that treatment intensity aligns with life expectancy and functional priorities.

Learning Event 1: Individualising Blood Pressure Targets in Frailty

Mr B, an 84-year-old man with frailty and type 2 diabetes, was referred to urgent care service following three falls in six weeks. His seated blood pressure averaged 130/72 mmHg while taking amlodipine 10 mg, perindopril 4 mg, and indapamide 2.5 mg daily. Orthostatic measurement revealed a 25-mmHg systolic drop on standing.

The AP undertook a comprehensive review, including medication reconciliation, frailty scoring, and discussion with the patient and family regarding goals of care. Drawing on NICE (2019) recommendations and the principle, start low, titrate slow. The AP decided to decrease amlodipine. Thus, amlodipine was reduced to 5 mg daily, while continuing other agents.

At two-month follow-up, the AP documented a stable seated systolic pressure of 145 mmHg, minimal orthostatic change, and only one minor, non-injurious fall. The AP also provided education on postural safety and arranged community physiotherapy.

This case illustrates how AP integrate assessment, shared decision-making, and medicine optimisation to achieve safe, individualised blood pressure targets and reduce falls in frail older adults.

Learning Event 2: Falls Associated with Environmental Change and Antihypertensive Therapy

A 78-year-old adult with a history of hypertension and heart failure experienced a fall while passing urine. Earlier in the day, they had been walking a dog in cold, snowy conditions and developed acute urinary urgency.

Current medicines included furosemide 40 mg twice daily, ramipril 10 mg once daily, bisoprolol 10 mg once daily, and isosorbide mononitrate 120 mg once daily.

On assessment in the same-day emergency care unit, orthostatic blood pressure testing demonstrated a postural drop of 25 mmHg systolic. The AP considered the combined effects of environmental temperature change, diuretic-related volume depletion, and α-blocker-induced vasodilatation. After discussion with the patient and family, adjustments were made to diuretic timing and tamsulosin was reviewed. Advice was given on gradual position changes and ensuring warmth before toileting.

Learning Point

Rapid transition from cold outdoor temperatures to a warm indoor environment can exacerbate dysfunctional blood pressure autoregulation, particularly in those taking multiple antihypertensives or α-blockers. Comprehensive medication review and environmental safety advice are essential to reduce recurrent falls.

CONCLUSION

Frailty profoundly alters cardiovascular disease trajectories, affecting presentation, treatment tolerance, and prognosis. Incorporating frailty assessment and patient-centred goals into every stage of care enables safer, more effective, and individualised management for older adults with cardiac conditions.

Take-Home Messages

1. Frailty is an independent determinant of cardiovascular risk, shaping presentation, therapeutic tolerance, and outcomes in ACS, arrhythmias, heart failure, and hypertension.

2. Management requires comprehensive geriatric assessment, cautious prescribing, and early multidisciplinary involvement to balance longevity with quality of life.

3. Shared decision-making and careful documentation of patient preferences are essential, particularly when considering invasive procedures or anticoagulation.

4. Prevention of complications including delirium, bleeding, falls, and functional decline should underpin all diagnostic and therapeutic decisions.

REFERENCES

Antzelevitch, C. and Burashnikov, A. (2011). Overview of basic mechanisms of cardiac arrhythmia. *Cardiac Electrophysiology Clinics* 3 (1): 23.

Bebb, O., Smith, F.G., Clegg, A. et al. (2018). Frailty and acute coronary syndrome: a structured literature review. *European Heart Journal: Acute Cardiovascular Care* 7 (2): 166–175.

Beckett, N.S., Peters, R., Fletcher, A.E. et al. (2008). Treatment of hypertension in patients 80 years of age or older. *New England Journal of Medicine* 358 (18): 1887–1898.

Blundell, A. and Gordon, A. (2015). *Geriatric Medicine at a Glance*, 1e. Chichester: Wiley Blackwell.

British Geriatrics Society Cardiovascular SIG, Barton, C., and Roshan, S. (2020). *Cardiovascular Care in the Older Adult: Heart Failure*. British Geriatrics Society https://www.bgs.org.uk/cardiovascular-care-in-the-older-adult-heart-failure (accessed 20 September 2025).

Campbell, N.R., Burnens, M.P., Whelton, P.K. et al. (2022). 2021 World Health Organization guideline on pharmacological treatment of hypertension: policy implications for the region of the Americas. *The Lancet Regional Health –Americas* 9: 100219.

Chad, T., Koulouroudias, M., Layton, G.R. et al. (2024). Frailty in acute coronary syndromes. A systematic review and narrative synthesis of frailty assessment tools and interventions from randomised controlled trials. *International Journal of Cardiology* 399: 131764.

Faconti, L., Tantirige, N., Poulter, N.R. et al. (2025). Call to action: British and Irish hypertension society position statement on blood pressure treatment thresholds and targets. *Journal of Human Hypertension* 39 (8): 537–540.

Flynn, J.A., Choi, M.J., and Wooster, L.D. (2013). *Oxford American Handbook of Clinical Medicine*. Oxford: Oxford University Press.

Hindricks, G., Potpara, T., Dagres, N. et al. (2021). 2020 ESC Guidelines for the diagnosis and management of atrial fibrillation developed in collaboration with the European Association for Cardio-Thoracic Surgery (EACTS) The Task Force for the diagnosis and management of atrial fibrillation of the European Society of Cardiology (ESC) Developed with the special contribution of the European Heart Rhythm Association (EHRA) of the ESC. *European Heart Journal* 42 (5): 373–498.

Hua, Q., Fan, L., and Li, J. (2019). 2019 Chinese guideline for the management of hypertension in the elderly. *Journal of Geriatric Cardiology (JGC)* 16 (2): 67.

Jiménez-Salva, M., Carmona-Segovia, A., Molina-Ramos, A.I. et al. (2025). Older adults with acute coronary syndrome: the impact of frailty and nutritional status on in-hospital complications. *European Journal of Cardiovascular Nursing* 24 (4): 595–605.

Kim, D.H. and Rockwood, K. (2024). Frailty in older adults. *New England Journal of Medicine* 391 (6): 538–548.

Leach, R. (2014). *Critical Care Medicine at a Glance*, 3e. Chichester: Wiley-Blackwell.

Lim, M.W. and Kalman, J.M. (2024). The impact of lifestyle factors on atrial fibrillation. *Journal of Molecular and Cellular Cardiology* 193: 91–99.

National Institute for Health and Care Excellence (NICE) (2019). *Hypertension in Adults: Diagnosis and Management (Guideline NG136).* London: NICE https://www.nice.org.uk/guidance/ng136/chapter/recommendations (accessed 20 September 2025).

National Institute for Health and Care Excellence (NICE) (2025) *Hypertension — management.* Available at: https://cks.nice.org.uk/topics/hypertension/management/management/ (accessed 1 February 2026).

National Institute for Health and Care Excellence (NICE) (2025a). *Acute Coronary Syndromes: Treatment Summaries.* BNF https://bnf.nice.org.uk/treatment-summaries/acute-coronary-syndromes/ (accessed 18 September 2025).

National Institute for Health and Care Excellence (NICE) (2025b). MI – secondary prevention: complications. Clinical Knowledge Summaries. Last revised in May 2025. https://cks.nice.org.uk/topics/mi-secondary-prevention/background-information/complications/ (accessed 18 September 2025).

National Institute for Health and Care Excellence (NICE) Clinical Knowledge Summaries (CKS) (2025). Atrial fibrillation: causes and risk factors. https://cks.nice.org.uk/topics/atrial-fibrillation/background-information/causes-risk-factors/ (accessed 20 September 2025).

Public Health England (2020). *Atrial fibrillation prevalence estimates for local populations.* London: Public Health England. Available at: https://www.gov.uk/government/publications/atrial-fibrillation-prevalence-estimates-for-local-populations (accessed 1 February 2026).

Qaseem, A., Wilt, T.J., Rich, R. et al. (2017). Pharmacologic treatment of hypertension in adults aged 60 years or older to higher versus lower blood pressure targets: a clinical practice guideline from the American College of Physicians and the American Academy of Family Physicians. *Annals of Internal Medicine* 166 (6): 430–437.

Rabi, D.M., McBrien, K.A., Sapir-Pichhadze, R. et al. (2020). Hypertension Canada's 2020 comprehensive guidelines for the prevention, diagnosis, risk assessment, and treatment of hypertension in adults and children. *Canadian Journal of Cardiology* 36 (5): 596–624. https://hypertension.ca/wp-content/uploads/2020/10/2020-22-HT-Guidelines-E-WEB_v3b.pdf (accessed 20 September 2025).

Ringer, M., Hashmi, M.F., and Lappin, S.L. (2025). Orthostatic hypotension. In: *StatPearls* [Internet]. Treasure Island, FL: StatPearls Publishing https://www.ncbi.nlm.nih.gov/books/NBK448192/ (accessed 20 September 2025).

Whelton, P.K., Carey, R.M., Aronow, W.S. et al. (2018). 2017 ACC/AHA/AAPA/ABC/ACPM/AGS/APhA/ASH/ASPC/NMA/PCNA guideline for the prevention, detection, evaluation, and management of high blood pressure in adults: a report of the American College of Cardiology/American Heart Association Task Force on Clinical Practice Guidelines. *Journal of the American College of Cardiology* 71 (19): e127–e248.

Williams, B., Mancia, G., Spiering, W., and ESC Scientific Document Group (2018). ESC/ESH guidelines for the management of arterial hypertension. *European Heart Journal* 39 (33): 3021–3104.

Williamson, J.D., Pajewski, N.M., Auchus, A.P. et al. (2019). Effect of intensive vs standard blood pressure control on probable dementia: a randomized clinical trial. *JAMA* 321 (6): 553–561.

CHAPTER 15

Respiratory Medicine

> **Aim**
>
> The aim of this chapter is to provide advanced practitioners (APs) and other healthcare professionals with an evidence-based understanding of age-related respiratory physiology and the assessment and management of key respiratory conditions in frail older adults. It integrates current guidance to support comprehensive, person-centred care that balances disease-directed treatment with quality of life and patient preferences.

LEARNING OUTCOMES

After engaging with this chapter, readers will be able to:

1. Recognise the atypical presentations of respiratory infection, asthma, chronic obstructive pulmonary disease (COPD), lung cancer, pulmonary embolism, and COVID-19 in older people living with frailty.
2. Apply current national guidance to the diagnosis and management of these conditions, including the use of frailty assessment tools such as the Clinical Frailty Scale.
3. Integrate non-pharmacological, palliative, and multidisciplinary approaches to optimise symptom control, maintain function, and respect patient goals.
4. Critically appraise complex cases and make shared decisions about investigation, treatment escalation, and end-of-life care.

SELF-ASSESSMENT QUESTIONS

1. How does frailty modify the presentation, investigation, and management of community-acquired pneumonia in older adults?
2. What key clinical indicators should prompt suspicion of pulmonary embolism in a frail older patient presenting with unexplained breathlessness and a normal chest X-ray?

RESPIRATORY TRACT INFECTIONS IN OLDER ADULTS

Cough (with or without sputum), breathlessness, fever, and pleuritic chest discomfort are frequent reasons for presentation of respiratory tract infections in later life. Precise anatomical diagnosis is essential because infection in different parts of the respiratory tract carries distinct microbiological implications, prognoses, and therapeutic implications. The non-specific label 'chest infection' should therefore be avoided.

Infections of the Upper Airways

In later life, infections of the upper respiratory tract (nasopharynx, sinuses, and larynx) are typically viral, with rhinovirus, seasonal coronaviruses, and influenza viruses among the common causes. They may present with nasal obstruction, rhinorrhoea, pharyngeal discomfort, and fever and can extend to the lower tract to trigger cough, wheeze, or an exacerbation of chronic respiratory or cardiac conditions.

With advancing age, these infections tend to be less frequent but more clinically significant. The likelihood of complications increases, including:

- Spread to the lower respiratory tract, producing tracheobronchitis or pneumonia.
- Exacerbation of pre-existing conditions such as chronic heart failure or asthma.
- Extra-respiratory manifestations such as falls, acute confusion, or sudden immobility.
- Prolonged recovery with lingering fatigue, anorexia, or deconditioning lasting weeks.
- Higher rates of hospitalisation and mortality than in younger adults.

Preventive measures, including annual influenza and COVID-19 vaccination, thorough hand hygiene, and prompt treatment of comorbid illness, are particularly valuable in reducing severity and complications.

Acute Tracheobronchitis

Acute tracheobronchitis is defined by inflammation of the conducting airways with little or no involvement of lung parenchyma. It is common in people with chronic airway disease (for example, chronic obstructive pulmonary disease [COPD] or bronchiectasis). Compared with community-acquired pneumonia, it generally causes less systemic disturbance and carries a better prognosis. Typical features include a prominent cough, expiratory wheeze, and chest tightness, without pleuritic pain or focal crackles on auscultation.

Chest radiograph is not routinely required unless pneumonia is suspected. The condition is usually viral and therefore self-limiting. Management is mainly supportive, focusing on adequate hydration, relief of bronchospasm with inhaled bronchodilators if needed, and judicious use of antipyretics. Antibacterial therapy should be reserved for patients with evidence of bacterial infection or significant risk factors such as structural lung disease or marked immunosuppression; doxycycline or macrolide antibiotics may be appropriate when indicated.

Influenza and Influenza-like Illness in Older Adults

Influenza is the most clinically significant viral infection of the respiratory tract, often presenting as a severe systemic disease that can predispose to secondary bacterial pneumonia, commonly with *Staphylococcus aureus*, *Haemophilus influenzae*, or *Streptococcus pneumoniae*. Seasonal peaks usually occur in the winter months, and major global outbreaks may follow antigenic shift in the circulating virus.

The illness typically begins abruptly with fever, chills, headache, pronounced myalgia, and profound fatigue. Gastrointestinal features such as nausea, vomiting, and diarrhoea, together with photophobia and other ocular symptoms, are relatively frequent. Rhinorrhoea, by contrast, is less prominent than with common cold viruses. Compared with younger adults, older people may exhibit similar cardinal symptoms but are more vulnerable to complications such as secondary bacterial infection, myocarditis, or neurological manifestations including meningoencephalitis. Mild meningeal irritation is relatively common and, in the presence of confusion or other neurological signs, should prompt consideration of cerebrospinal fluid analysis.

Diagnosis rests on careful clinical assessment supported by current surveillance data. Because a number of respiratory viruses can cause an identical acute febrile syndrome, and serological confirmation is delayed, clinicians often use the pragmatic term influenza-like illness during the initial assessment. Virological confirmation, when available, is particularly valuable during outbreaks in community or residential care settings, as it guides infection control and targeted use of antivirals and vaccines.

Preventive strategies including annual influenza vaccination, early antiviral therapy where appropriate, and strict infection control measures remain key to reducing morbidity, hospitalisation, and mortality among older adults.

PNEUMONIA IN OLDER ADULTS

Pneumonia is an acute infection of the lung parenchyma producing new radiological shadowing and a variable clinical picture. It may follow a lobar, bronchial, or mixed distribution. Symptoms are often subtle or non-specific in later life, with presentations ranging from mild malaise and loss of appetite to severe systemic illness.

PRESENTATION, ASSESSMENT, AND MICROBIOLOGY

Older people often present with cough that may be dry, confusion or delirium, new functional decline, falls, or worsening frailty rather than with classic pleuritic pain or high fever. Hypoxaemia and tachypnoea are more reliable indicators of severity than pyrexia, which may be absent. Some patients arrive in shock or with features of acute respiratory distress syndrome, but this is uncommon.

Initial evaluation should include pulse oximetry and clinical scoring systems such as the CURB-65 to guide the need for hospital care (Lim et al., 2003). Arterial blood gas analysis is usually reserved for those with oxygen saturation below about 90%. Routine blood tests including renal function and C-reactive protein (CRP) help assess disease severity and guide fluid management. Markedly raised CRP may indicate pneumococcal infection or severe sepsis (Figure 15.1).

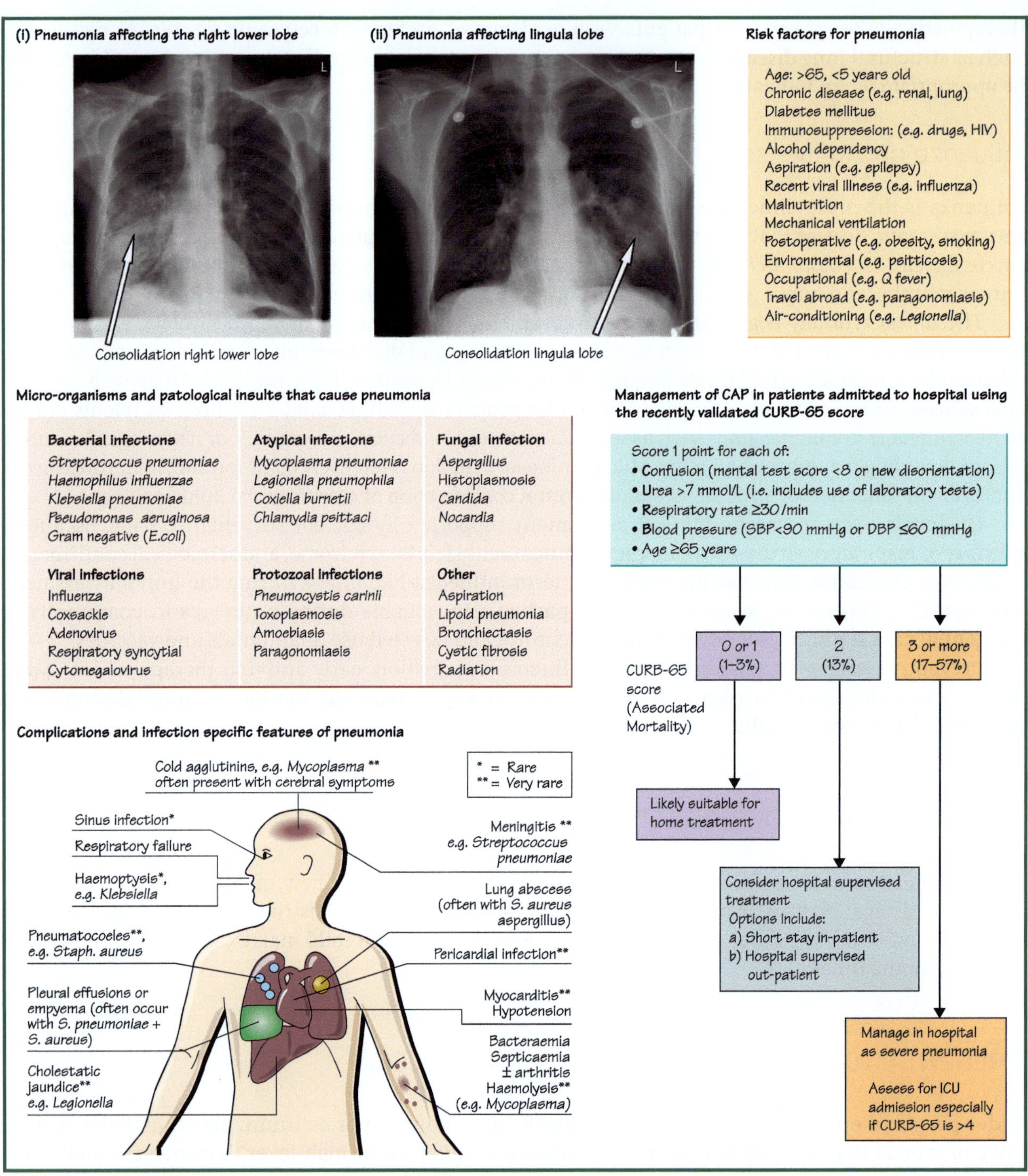

FIGURE 15.1 Community-acquired pneumonia. *Source*: Leach (2014)/John Wiley & Sons.

Chest radiograph is essential to confirm parenchymal involvement and to identify possible alternative or coexisting conditions such as pleural effusion, heart failure, or lung malignancy. Blood cultures are recommended, but sputum cultures are rarely contributory unless tuberculosis or unusual organisms are suspected.

A causative organism is not identified in many cases. *Streptococcus pneumoniae* remains the most frequent pathogen across community, care-home, and hospital settings. Viruses, particularly influenza and respiratory syncytial virus, are increasingly recognised as primary causes or facilitators of secondary bacterial disease. Other relevant pathogens include *Haemophilus influenzae*, *Staphylococcus aureus*, *Legionella pneumophila*, *Mycoplasma pneumoniae*, and Gram-negative bacilli such as *Klebsiella* and *Pseudomonas aeruginosa*, especially in frail, institutionalised, or previously treated patients. Aspiration pneumonia, involving anaerobic bacteria, is an important consideration in individuals with swallowing difficulties or prolonged immobility.

MANAGEMENT AND PROGNOSIS

Management extends beyond antimicrobial therapy. Key measures include careful assessment of hydration with oral, subcutaneous, or intravenous fluids; oxygen supplementation for symptomatic hypoxaemia; early mobilisation and upright positioning; physiotherapy and saline nebulisers to aid clearance of secretions; and judicious use of small-dose opioids for distressing dyspnoea or pain.

The choice of antimicrobial depends on clinical context and local resistance patterns. In uncomplicated community-acquired pneumonia, oral amoxicillin is usually appropriate; macrolides such as clarithromycin may be added when atypical infection is suspected or during mycoplasma outbreaks. For those at risk of aspiration or Gram-negative infection, co-amoxiclav or an equivalent broader spectrum agent may be indicated. Hospitalised or severely ill patients may require initial intravenous therapy (for example, a second-generation cephalosporin with a macrolide), de-escalated once culture results are available to minimise complications such as *Clostridioides* difficile infection. When methicillin-resistant *Staphylococcus aureus* is suspected, vancomycin or linezolid should be considered.

Renal impairment, advanced age, multiple comorbidities, and high CURB-65 scores all predict poorer outcomes. Discussion with the patient and family about ceilings of treatment, including ventilatory support and cardiopulmonary resuscitation, is best undertaken early. After clinical recovery, follow-up imaging may be appropriate to exclude underlying malignancy, particularly in those with a history of smoking or when radiographic resolution is incomplete (Figure 15.2).

Case Study 15.1   Non-Resolving Pneumonia in an Older Adult Managed in SDEC

An 82-year-old man with known chronic obstructive pulmonary disease (COPD) and type 2 diabetes attended the Same Day Emergency Care (SDEC) unit with a five-day history of cough, fever, and increasing breathlessness. He had been started on oral amoxicillin by his general practitioner, but remained pyrexial with worsening dyspnoea. On assessment by the AP, he was tachypnoeic at 28 breaths/min with oxygen saturation of 89% on room air and a CURB-65 score of 3, indicating high risk.

The AP undertook a full review to explain the lack of improvement. Potential alternative or coexisting diagnoses including pulmonary embolism, heart failure, and pleural effusion were considered.

Repeat chest radiography demonstrated an enlarging right lower-zone consolidation with a moderate pleural effusion. Blood cultures were repeated, and a Legionella urinary antigen test was requested. The patient's family confirmed full adherence to his antibiotic regimen and no swallowing problems.

In view of persistent hypoxaemia and suspected complicated pneumonia, the AP commenced intravenous co-amoxiclav and clarithromycin according to local protocol, arranged urgent thoracic ultrasound, and liaised with the respiratory team for possible drainage. Supportive care included controlled oxygen, careful fluid balance, and early mobilisation where possible.

The AP discussed escalation of care with the patient and family, outlining options for ward admission if respiratory function declined, and documented the agreed plan in the shared electronic record. Microbiology results later confirmed *Streptococcus pneumoniae* resistant to first-line oral therapy. The patient stabilised after intravenous treatment and drainage of the effusion, and was discharged after 48 hours on a step-down oral antibiotic course with community follow-up.

This case highlights the essential role of SDEC and advanced practice in rapidly re-evaluating pneumonia that fails to respond to oral antibiotics, ensuring early recognition of complications, prompt intravenous therapy, and coordinated multidisciplinary care for frail older adults.

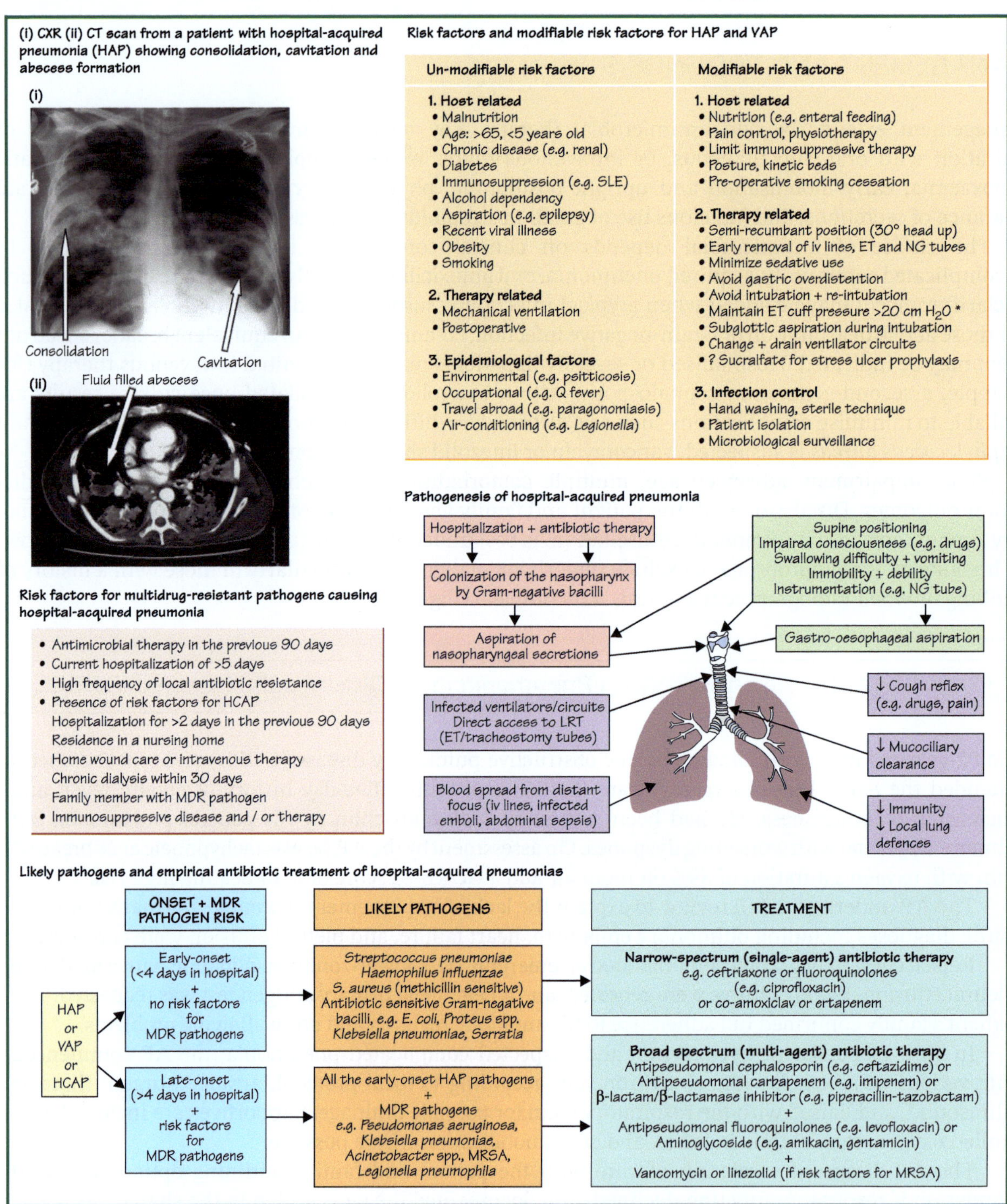

FIGURE 15.2 Hospital-acquired pneumonia. *Source*: Leach (2014)/John Wiley & Sons.

ASPIRATION PNEUMONIA AND CHEMICAL PNEUMONITIS IN OLDER ADULTS

Aspiration of oropharyngeal or gastric material into the lower airways is a frequent problem in later life. It ranges from silent micro-aspiration of saliva to major inhalation of gastric contents and may lead to chemical pneumonitis, infective pneumonia, or both.

Risk Factors

Situations that increase the likelihood of aspiration include:

- Neurological or structural swallowing impairment, for example, after stroke or in advanced Parkinson's disease.
- Severe gastro-oesophageal reflux or vomiting disorders.
- Depressed consciousness due to seizures, sedative medication, or acute illness.
- Previous episodes of aspiration or recurrent lower respiratory infection.
- Enteral feeding via nasogastric or gastrostomy tube.

Diagnosis

A clinical history of cough or respiratory distress in the context of one or more of these risk factors should raise suspicion. Chest radiography often shows consolidation in dependent lung regions, commonly the right lower lobe, although any area may be involved. The clinical picture may vary from subtle deterioration to severe sepsis.

Management

The inflammatory reaction to inhaled gastric material is often chemical rather than purely bacterial, so the need for antibiotics must be judged carefully. Where infection is likely—such as in frail or acutely unwell patients, those in high-dependency settings, or after large-volume aspiration—broad-spectrum intravenous antibiotics active against Gram-negative and anaerobic organisms may be required. Less severe cases often respond to oral agents such as amoxicillin or co-amoxiclav.

It is equally important to address predisposing factors. A formal swallowing assessment can guide safer nutrition strategies such as thickened fluids, modified-texture diets, and assisted upright feeding. When risk remains high, temporary cessation of oral intake or modification of enteral feeding may be appropriate until swallowing safety improves.

In palliative or advanced dementia care, comfort and dignity take precedence. Food and drink should not be withheld if they give pleasure, even when aspiration is likely, provided that risks and benefits are clearly discussed with family or carers. Measures such as careful supervision, small boluses, and upright positioning can reduce distress while supporting quality of life.

FRAILTY AND COVID-19 IN OLDER ADULTS

Frailty, reflecting diminished physiological reserve and vulnerability to stressors, is a key predictor of adverse outcomes in older adults with COVID-19. Both the British Geriatrics Society (BGS) and the National Institute for Health and Care Excellence (NICE) recommend formal frailty assessment—most often with the Clinical Frailty Scale (CFS)—to inform comprehensive, individualised care rather than to restrict treatment on the basis of age alone (BGS, 2021; NICE, 2025).

Presentation and Assessment

Older adults with COVID-19 frequently present atypically. Rather than the classical triad of fever, cough, and breathlessness, first manifestations may include delirium, falls, acute loss of mobility, or sudden functional decline (NICE, 2025). Pulse oximetry should be performed even when respiratory distress is not apparent, and clinicians should consider alternative or concomitant pathologies such as pulmonary embolism (PE), bacterial pneumonia, or heart failure. The CFS, a nine-point measure based on premorbid mobility, independence, and cognition, is the most widely used tool. BGS and NICE recommend assessing baseline status over the two weeks before illness to guide treatment planning (Rockwood et al., 2005; BGS, 2021).

Evidence on Outcomes

A large and consistent evidence base shows that frailty is strongly and independently associated with mortality in COVID-19. Systematic reviews and meta-analyses demonstrate a near-linear increase in death rates with a rising CFS score: People with mild or moderate frailty (CFS 4–5) have about twice the risk of death compared with those who are fit (CFS 1–3), while those with more advanced frailty (CFS 6–9) face a threefold or higher risk (Kastora et al., 2021; Pranata et al., 2021). Frailty is also linked to higher rates of delirium, longer hospital stays, and reduced likelihood of intensive care admission (Cosco et al., 2021). These associations persist after adjusting for age and comorbidity, indicating that frailty provides prognostic information beyond chronological age.

Management and Ongoing Care

NICE's living guideline on managing COVID-19 (NG191) and BGS statements advise that frailty assessment should feed into a holistic care plan (BGS, 2021; NICE, 2025). Supportive measures include carefully titrated oxygen, thromboembolism prophylaxis, nutritional and hydration support, and early mobilisation. Where indicated, antiviral treatment (for example, nirmatrelvir-ritonavir) and appropriate use of corticosteroids or other immunomodulators remain essential, irrespective of frailty status. Clear, timely discussions with patients and families about treatment preferences are encouraged, with plans reviewed as clinical circumstances evolve.

Recovery and Long-term Impact

Many older adults who survive acute COVID-19 experience prolonged effects such as fatigue, breathlessness, cognitive impairment, and reduced exercise capacity features often termed long COVID. These sequelae can exacerbate pre-existing frailty or lead to new functional dependence. NICE recommends structured follow-up, rehabilitation, and multidisciplinary support to limit long-term disability (NICE, 2025).

PULMONARY EMBOLISM IN OLDER ADULTS

PE is a frequent and potentially fatal cause of acute or subacute respiratory compromise in later life (Alsararatee, 2024). It is often called the great pretender because it can mimic or coexist with other disorders such as pneumonia, heart failure, and COPD. In consequence, it is underdiagnosed and sometimes omitted from death certification.

Presentation and Assessment

The classic triad of pleuritic pain, dyspnoea, and haemoptysis is uncommon in older people. Presentations may instead include (Alsararatee, 2025):

- Sudden or episodic breathlessness, unexplained tachypnoea, or hypoxia.
- Syncope, presyncope, collapse, or even cardiac arrest.
- Progressive, unexplained right heart strain or pulmonary hypertension.
- Non-specific or misleading features such as fever, new arrhythmia, resistant heart failure, delirium, or unexplained functional decline.

Because these features overlap with other acute conditions common in later life, diagnosis relies on combining careful clinical evaluation with appropriate imaging. A normal chest radiograph in a breathless patient, or only minor changes such as atelectasis or small effusions, should heighten suspicion. Computed tomographic pulmonary angiography (CTPA) is the gold-standard investigation where available; a ventilation-perfusion scan is an alternative when CTPA is contraindication (Alsararatee, 2025).

D-dimer testing has limited specificity in the elderly because infection, inflammation, and malignancy frequently elevate levels. Arterial blood gas analysis typically shows hypoxaemia and a widened alveolar-arterial oxygen gradient, but these changes are neither sensitive nor specific. Echocardiography may reveal acute right ventricular strain or pulmonary hypertension and can support early treatment when CTPA is not immediately feasible.

Key diagnostic pointers in older adults include:

- Breathlessness with clear lung fields on chest X-ray.
- Unexplained or worsening right heart failure.
- Lack of response to standard therapy for pneumonia, COPD exacerbation, or cardiac failure.

Management

Once PE is confirmed, the Pulmonary Embolism Severity Index (PESI) or its simplified form (sPESI) should be calculated to determine whether outpatient management is appropriate (Aujesky et al., 2005). It is also essential to establish whether the PE is provoked (for example, after surgery or prolonged immobility) or unprovoked, as unprovoked PE generally warrants haematology referral for further investigation and long-term follow-up. Patients with a high PESI/sPESI score should be admitted for inpatient care and managed according to local hospital protocols.

Anticoagulation remains the mainstay of therapy. Low-molecular-weight heparin (for example, enoxaparin or dalteparin) or a direct oral anticoagulant is usually started immediately once PE is suspected, provided that there is no major bleeding risk. Warfarin may be chosen for longer-term treatment when reversal or monitoring is desirable. Baseline renal function, haemoglobin, and coagulation studies should always be checked, as older patients are more prone to occult gastrointestinal bleeding and drug interactions.

Thrombolysis may be lifesaving in cases of massive PE with shock or severe right ventricular strain. Although bleeding risk rises with age, advanced age alone is not a contraindication; decisions should be based on overall clinical context and patient preferences (Alsararatee, 2025). Moreover, inferior vena cava filters may be indicated when anticoagulation is impossible, for example, because of active bleeding or when embolic events continue despite adequate anticoagulation. Newer filters can sometimes be retrieved once the acute risk has resolved.

Special Considerations in Later Life

- Higher diagnostic challenge: Overlapping symptoms, atypical presentations, and frequent comorbidities make early recognition difficult.
- Increased treatment risk: Frailty, polypharmacy, and renal impairment raise the likelihood of anticoagulant-related bleeding.
- Need for holistic care: Decisions on investigation and treatment should consider the patient's baseline frailty, functional goals, and quality of life and involve the person and their family wherever possible.

ASTHMA AND COPD IN FRAILTY: ASSESSMENT AND MANAGEMENT

Asthma and COPD are frequent respiratory conditions in older adults living with frailty, often presenting as overlapping syndromes of airflow limitation (Figure 15.3). Both disorders may be underdiagnosed because breathlessness, cough, or hypoxaemia can be misattributed to ageing, deconditioning, heart failure, or anaemia (NICE, 2019; NICE, 2024). In frail people, diminished physiological reserve and altered inflammatory responses can blunt symptom recognition and delay care. Comorbidities such as cardiovascular disease, osteoporosis, depression, and malnutrition can worsen respiratory impairment and complicate management (Tarazona-Santabalbina et al., 2023).

Asthma may persist from childhood or arise de novo in later life. Compared with younger individuals, older adults more often report persistent cough than episodic wheeze, and allergic triggers are less evident. Nocturnal symptoms may present as breathlessness or paroxysmal nocturnal dyspnoea, and medicines such as non-steroidal anti-inflammatory drugs or β-blockers can provoke bronchospasm (NICE, 2024). COPD is strongly linked to cumulative smoking exposure but may progress even in long-term ex-smokers. Symptoms are typically slowly progressive with limited day-to-day variability, and chronic bronchitis can lead to fatigue, poor sleep, and weight loss (NICE, 2019).

Accurate diagnosis relies on pulse oximetry, spirometry, and, where feasible, serial peak expiratory flow readings. However, frailty, cognitive impairment, and reduced hand strength can hinder technique, increasing the value of experienced respiratory physiology support. Chest imaging and blood tests remain essential to exclude alternative or coexisting conditions such as PE or malignancy (NICE, 2019).

Treatment principles mirror those for younger adults but must account for frailty-related vulnerabilities. Inhaled bronchodilators and corticosteroids remain first line; long-acting preparations and large-volume spacers may enhance adherence and drug delivery. Regular review of inhaler technique and early involvement of community pharmacists or respiratory nurses help maintain effectiveness. Oral theophyllines should be used cautiously because altered pharmacokinetics, drug interactions, and infection can precipitate toxicity. Vaccination against influenza and pneumococcus is recommended (NICE, 2019).

Non-pharmacological measures are central to improving outcomes. Pulmonary rehabilitation, combining tailored exercise, education, and behavioural support, is as effective as inhaler therapy and reduces exacerbations (NICE, 2019). Nutritional assessment, smoking cessation support, and social

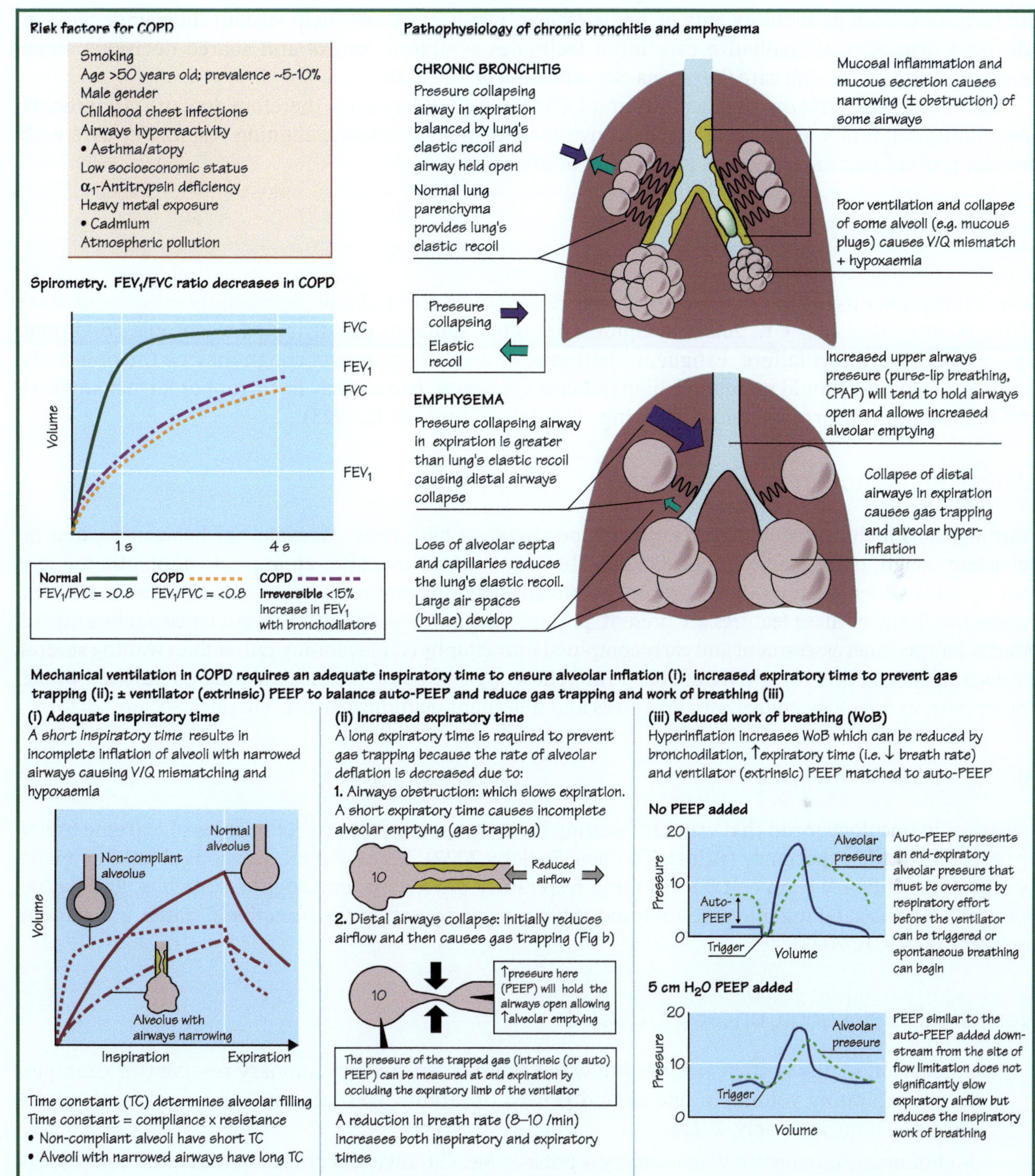

FIGURE 15.3   COPD. *Source:* Leach (2014)/John Wiley & Sons.

interventions, such as mobility aids or home oxygen when indicated, help sustain independence. For advanced disease, early palliative care input facilitates symptom control and shared decisions about ventilation and end-of-life care (Tarazona-Santabalbina et al., 2023).

Recognition and treatment of asthma and COPD in frail older adults therefore demand comprehensive, multidisciplinary assessment and sensitive management strategies, aligning respiratory care with broader goals of comfort, function, and quality of life.

LUNG CANCER IN LATER LIFE

Lung cancer remains the leading cause of cancer-related mortality and is predominantly a disease of older adults (Cancer Research UK, 2025). Symptoms are often subtle or misattributed to chronic conditions such as COPD or heart failure. Fatigue, weight loss, or a slowly changing cough may be the only early features. Clinicians should maintain a high index of suspicion, particularly in current or former smokers and in those with recurrent or slow-resolving chest infections (NICE, 2023).

Clinical Presentation and Assessment

Warning signs include haemoptysis (especially persistent or with clots), unexplained hoarseness, new or persistent cough, chest pain, or consolidation that does not resolve after appropriate antibiotic therapy (NICE, 2023). Older adults may present with functional decline or confusion rather than classical respiratory symptoms. If any of these features are present, prompt imaging is essential. NICE guidance advises urgent referral for specialist assessment and early computed tomography (CT) scanning rather than waiting several weeks to repeat a chest X-ray (NICE, 2023). Bronchoscopy and tissue diagnosis should be pursued where appropriate, as histology guides both prognosis and treatment planning (British Thoracic Society, 2022).

Management Principles

Advances in oncology mean that watchful waiting is rarely appropriate, except in cases of extreme frailty or very limited life expectancy (British Thoracic Society, 2022). Management decisions should be made by a multidisciplinary team (MDT) including respiratory physicians, oncologists, surgeons, and palliative care specialists, taking into account tumour type, stage, comorbidities, functional status, and patient preferences (NICE, 2023).

Non-Small-Cell Lung Cancer (NSCLC)

- Surgery offers the best chance of cure when there is adequate pulmonary reserve (for example, forced expiratory volume in one second [FEV_1] of around 1.5 L or more) and no distant spread (British Thoracic Society, 2022).
- Radiotherapy is indicated when surgery is not feasible. Curative schedules such as continuous hyper-fractionated accelerated radiotherapy (CHART) may be offered to fit patients; palliative radiotherapy helps relieve symptoms such as haemoptysis, chest pain, or bronchial obstruction (NICE, 2023).
- Systemic therapy including targeted agents (e.g. epidermal growth factor receptor [EGFR] inhibitors) or immunotherapy is increasingly used according to tumour genetics and patient tolerance (NICE, 2023).

Small-Cell Lung Cancer (SCLC)

SCLC accounts for about one-fifth of lung cancers and is relatively more common in later life (Cancer Research UK, 2025). Most cases present with extensive disease. Chemotherapy remains the main treatment and can achieve rapid tumour shrinkage, but the intensity and number of cycles are tailored to frailty and performance status (British Thoracic Society, 2022). Surgery is rarely an option because localised disease at diagnosis is uncommon.

Palliative and Supportive Care

Many older adults will require symptom control even when disease-directed treatment is undertaken. Options include palliative radiotherapy for airway obstruction, chest wall pain, or bony metastases; endobronchial interventions such as stenting or thermal therapy to relieve obstruction and cough; aspiration or indwelling catheter for recurrent pleural effusion; and opioids for distressing cough or pain (NICE, 2023).

Key Considerations in Older Adults

- Comorbidity and frailty influence investigation and treatment tolerance. Early comprehensive geriatric assessment helps match interventions to goals of care (BTS, 2022; NICE, 2023).
- Under-diagnosis and under-treatment remain common; decisions should be based on function and preferences rather than age alone (Cancer Research UK, 2025).
- Shared decision-making is essential to balance potential survival benefit with treatment-related burdens (NICE, 2023).

CONCLUSION

Respiratory disorders in later life rarely occur in isolation. Normal ageing leads to modest changes in lung mechanics, but frailty, multimorbidity, and environmental exposures create significant vulnerability to acute illness and functional decline. Conditions such as pneumonia, COPD, asthma, lung cancer, and PE often present atypically, and timely recognition relies on a high index of suspicion and structured frailty assessment. Management should combine accurate diagnosis; guideline-based pharmacological therapy; and non-drug strategies including pulmonary rehabilitation, vaccination, and early palliative involvement. Central to best practice is a holistic, multidisciplinary approach that addresses physical, psychological, and social needs while aligning care with individual priorities.

Take-Home Messages

1. Frailty independently predicts poor outcomes in all major respiratory illnesses, including COVID-19 and COPD.
2. Presentations are frequently non-specific; unexplained functional decline or delirium may signal serious pulmonary disease.
3. Early, comprehensive assessment using tools such as CURB-65 for pneumonia or the Clinical Frailty Scale guides appropriate treatment and escalation planning.

4. Evidence-based management combines accurate diagnosis; optimised inhaler or systemic therapy; vaccination; pulmonary rehabilitation; and careful attention to nutrition, mobility, and psychosocial support.

5. Palliative care should be integrated early to relieve symptoms and support shared decision-making about treatment intensity and end-of-life care.

REFERENCES

Alsararatee, H.H. (2024). Atypical presentation of pulmonary embolism masquerading as abdominal pain. *Open Journal of Clinical and Medical Images* 4 (1): 1167.

Alsararatee, H.H. (2025). Assessment, diagnosis and management of pulmonary embolism. *International Journal for Advancing Practice* 1–9.

Aujesky, D., Obrosky, D.S., Stone, R.A. et al. (2005). Derivation and validation of a prognostic model for pulmonary embolism. *American Journal of Respiratory and Critical Care Medicine* 172 (8): 1041–1046.

BGS (2021). *COVID-19: Frailty Scores and Outcomes in Older People*. British Geriatrics Society (updated 24 June 2021). https://www.bgs.org.uk/covidfrailty (accessed 20 September 2025).

British Thoracic Society (2022). Guideline for the investigation and management of pulmonary nodules and lung cancer in adults. *Thorax* 77 (Suppl. 1): 1–44. https://doi.org/10.1136/thorax-2021-218915.

Cancer Research UK (2025). Lung cancer statistics and outlook. https://www.cancerresearchuk.org/health-professional/cancer-statistics/statistics-by-cancer-type/lung-cancer (accessed 20 September 2025).

Cosco, T.D., Best, J., Davis, D. et al. (2021). What is the relationship between validated frailty scores and mortality for adults with COVID-19 in acute hospital care? A systematic review. *Age and Ageing* 50 (3): 608–616.

Kastora, S., Kounidas, G., Perrott, S. et al. (2021). Clinical frailty scale as a point of care prognostic indicator of mortality in COVID-19: a systematic review and meta-analysis. *EClinicalMedicine* 36: 100896.

Leach, R. (2014). *Critical Care Medicine at a Glance*, 3e. Chichester: Wiley-Blackwell.

Lim, W.S., Van der Eerden, M.M., Laing, R. et al. (2003). Defining community acquired pneumonia severity on presentation to hospital: an international derivation and validation study. *Thorax* 58 (5): 377–382.

National Institute for Health and Care Excellence (NICE) (2023). Lung cancer: diagnosis and management (NG122). https://www.nice.org.uk/guidance/ng122 (accessed 20 September 2025).

NICE (2019). *Chronic Obstructive Pulmonary Disease in Over 16s: Diagnosis and Management (NG115)*. London: National Institute for Health and Care Excellence https://www.nice.org.uk/guidance/ng115.

NICE (2024). *Asthma: Diagnosis, Monitoring and Chronic Asthma Management (NG245)*. London: National Institute for Health and Care Excellence https://www.nice.org.uk/guidance/ng245.

NICE (2025). *COVID-19 Rapid Guideline: Managing COVID-19 (NG191)*. National Institute for Health and Care Excellence https://www.nice.org.uk/guidance/ng191 (accessed 20 September 2025).

Pranata, R., Henrina, J., Lim, M.A. et al. (2021). Clinical frailty scale and mortality in COVID-19: a systematic review and dose–response meta-analysis. *Archives of Gerontology and Geriatrics* 93: 104324.

Rockwood, K., Song, X., MacKnight, C. et al. (2005). A global clinical measure of fitness and frailty in elderly people. *CMAJ* 173 (5): 489–495.

Tarazona-Santabalbina, F.J., Naval, E., la Cámara-de, D. et al. (2023). Is frailty diagnosis important in patients with COPD? A narrative review of the literature. *International Journal of Environmental Research and Public Health* 20 (3): 1678.

CHAPTER 16

Gastroenterology

Aim

The aim of this chapter is to provide a concise, evidence-based account of gastrointestinal disorders in older adults, linking age-related physiological changes, frailty, nutrition, and hydration and outlining safe, person-centred assessment and management.

LEARNING OUTCOMES

By the end of this chapter, readers will be able to:

1. Explain how ageing alters gastrointestinal structure and function and how this reshapes symptom profiles.
2. Differentiate common conditions in later life (e.g. dysphagia, GORD, peptic ulcer disease, constipation, and bowel obstruction) and recognise red-flag features.
3. Select appropriate first-line investigations (including endoscopy, manometry, imaging, and nutrition screening tools) and interpret results in context.
4. Formulate pragmatic management plans that balance benefit, burden, and patient goals, including safe use of PPIs, laxatives, and indications for enteral feeding.

SELF-ASSESSMENT QUESTIONS

1. How do age-related changes in gastrointestinal structure and function contribute to the atypical presentation of common disorders such as peptic ulcer disease and constipation in older adults?
2. What key ethical and clinical considerations should guide decisions on clinically assisted nutrition and hydration in frail older patients with advanced dysphagia?

NUTRITION, HYDRATION, AND WEIGHT LOSS IN OLDER ADULTS

Normal ageing is associated with lower energy needs because of reduced physical activity and a slower resting metabolic rate from loss of lean muscle. Appetite often diminishes and reserves of macro- and micronutrients fall, increasing vulnerability to malnutrition. Illness compounds these risks: Undernutrition affects around 15% of community-dwelling older adults, 5–12% of housebound people with multiple morbidities, 35–65% of acutely hospitalised patients, and up to 60% of those in institutions (Bowker et al., 2012). Malnutrition predicts adverse outcomes including greater dependency, morbidity, mortality, and health service use.

As explained within the comprehensive geriatric assessment (CGA) (Chapter 7) guidance on nutrition and hydration, malnutrition and frailty are closely interrelated, with malnourished individuals being approximately four times more likely to develop frailty (Laur et al., 2017). The CGA endorsed the importance of routine screening for undernutrition, overnutrition, and sarcopenia using validated tools, with muscle strength regarded as a practical marker of frailty (Khor et al., 2022). Key factors to assess include appetite, fluid intake, polypharmacy, psychological well-being, ability to shop and cook, socioeconomic circumstances, sensory loss, oral health, gastrointestinal symptoms, dysphagia, falls risk, and vitamin D status (British Geriatrics Society, 2025). Evidence suggests that food-based strategies to improve nutrition and muscle health are essential, while oral nutritional supplements have limited proven benefit in frail older adults (Thomson et al., 2022).

Assessment begins with careful documentation of weight trends and dietary intake. Body mass index can be estimated using alternative measurements such as ulnar length or mid-arm circumference when standing height is unobtainable. Rapid unintentional weight loss of more than 2.3 kg in a month or 4.5 kg in six months is of clinical concern. Nutritional risk-screening tools such as the Malnutrition Universal Screening Tool (MUST) are recommended in UK clinical practice.

Management requires early recognition and a multidisciplinary approach. Contributing factors may include medical conditions (e.g. chronic infection and malignancy), psychological issues (e.g. depression and dementia), social difficulties (e.g. isolation and poverty), and age-related changes in hunger or taste. Practical measures include protected mealtimes, assistance with feeding, food fortification, and high-energy oral supplements when acceptable. In selected cases, enteral feeding using nasogastric or percutaneous gastrostomy routes may be appropriate, with careful monitoring for complications such as aspiration and refeeding syndrome.

Decisions about clinically assisted nutrition and hydration should be guided by a thorough capacity assessment and, where capacity is lacking, by best interest principles in line with the Mental Capacity Act 2005. Advanced care plans and any advanced decisions to refuse treatment must be reviewed. Discussions should include the aims of treatment, realistic outcomes, and review points, ensuring that the patient, relatives, and the multidisciplinary team share a clear understanding. Where disagreement persists or withdrawal of long-term feeding is proposed, advice from ethics committees or the Court of Protection may be required (Bowker et al., 2012).

Case Study 16.1   AP Decision-Making in Clinically Assisted Nutrition and Hydration

Mrs H, an 86-year-old woman with advanced Parkinson's disease and dementia, was admitted from a nursing home following recurrent aspiration pneumonia and significant weight loss. She was drowsy but occasionally responsive. The AP undertook a comprehensive geriatric assessment: reviewing her medical history, medication, swallowing studies, nutritional intake, and prior advanced care plan. Collateral history from family and nursing home staff confirmed that Mrs H had consistently expressed a wish to avoid burdensome interventions and valued comfort over life prolongation.

The AP led a structured multidisciplinary meeting involving the family, speech and language therapist, acute medicine consultants, dietitian, palliative care team, and ward nurses. The clinical examination and investigations confirmed progressive dysphagia and ongoing aspiration risk. Using the Mental Capacity Act 2005 framework, the AP documented that Mrs H lacked decision-making capacity and that best interest decisions must reflect her known preferences and values.

Balancing clinical evidence and ethical principles of autonomy, beneficence, non-maleficence, and justice, the AP recommended a comfort-focused plan: careful hand feeding with accepted aspiration risk, thorough mouth care, and palliative support, while withholding nasogastric or gastrostomy feeding. The family agreed after clear explanation of risks, benefits, and the option for review. The decision and rationale were recorded, and regular reassessment was planned.

OESOPHAGEAL DISEASE

Disorders of the oesophagus are common in older adults and may arise from both structural and functional changes. Gastro-oesophageal reflux disease (GORD) is the most frequent presentation. It typically causes retrosternal burning discomfort, acid regurgitation, and sometimes atypical chest pain or bloating, but these symptoms often bear little relation to the severity of mucosal damage. The presence of red-flag features such as recent or rapid onset, progressive swallowing difficulty, unexplained vomiting, weight loss, or iron deficiency anaemia should prompt urgent endoscopic investigation to rule out malignancy. When such warning signs are absent, a therapeutic trial of proton pump inhibitors (PPIs) is appropriate and often highly effective. It is important to discontinue or reduce medicines that exacerbate reflux, including non-steroidal anti-inflammatory drugs, corticosteroids, and bisphosphonates.

Hiatus hernia becomes increasingly prevalent with age as connective tissues supporting the gastro-oesophageal junction weaken. While it may remain asymptomatic, it frequently coexists with GORD and can occasionally cause dysphagia or, if very large, respiratory compromise or gastric strangulation. Diagnosis can be confirmed by endoscopy, contrast imaging, or chest radiography. Management usually begins with lifestyle modification, weight reduction, smaller meals, avoidance of alcohol and caffeine, and elevation of the bed head alongside PPIs; surgical repair is reserved for severe or refractory disease.

Achalasia, an uncommon degenerative disorder of oesophageal innervation, leads to failure of lower oesophageal sphincter relaxation and absent peristalsis, producing slowly progressive dysphagia for solids and liquids. Although endoscopy is performed to exclude cancer, manometry provides the definitive diagnosis. Treatments aim to relax the sphincter and may include pharmacological agents such as calcium channel blockers or nitrates, botulinum toxin injection, endoscopic balloon dilation, or surgical myotomy.

A range of other motility disorders may also affect older adults. These include diffuse oesophageal spasm, nutcracker oesophagus, and hypertensive lower sphincter, which can cause chest pain and intermittent dysphagia. They may occur in isolation or secondary to systemic illnesses such as diabetes or systemic sclerosis. Manometry remains the diagnostic gold standard and drug therapy such as calcium channel blockers or low-dose tricyclic antidepressants may provide relief. Furthermore, oesophageal candidiasis should be considered in frail or immunocompromised patients, particularly when oral thrush is present. Symptoms include odynophagia and dysphagia. Diagnosis is usually made endoscopically and treatment with oral fluconazole is effective. All these conditions illustrate how age-related physiological change, comorbidity, and polypharmacy increase the complexity of diagnosis and management of oesophageal disease in older people, requiring a holistic, multidisciplinary approach.

DYSPHAGIA IN OLDER ADULTS

Swallowing problems are frequent in later life and often signal significant underlying disease. An accurate history is essential, focusing on which consistencies cause difficulty, where the sensation of blockage is felt (mouth, throat, behind the sternum, or upper abdomen), and whether swallowing weakens during a meal, a feature suggestive of neuromuscular disorders such as myasthenia gravis. A history of coughing, wheezing, or recurrent chest infection may indicate silent aspiration. Physical assessment should look for loss of weight, oral or pharyngeal infection, cervical or supraclavicular lymphadenopathy, and any clinical sign of gastric outlet obstruction. Watching the patient drink or eat can yield important diagnostic clues.

Structural disorders, which usually obstruct solids first, include cancers of the oesophagus or stomach, benign strictures from chronic inflammation or systemic sclerosis, pharyngeal pouches, severe oesophagitis or fungal infection, and external compression from mediastinal lesions or cervical osteophytes. Food impaction or bezoars are additional risks in frail or cognitively impaired people.

Functional disorders, often more troublesome with liquids, may arise from cerebrovascular accidents, Parkinson's disease, motor neuron disease, myasthenia gravis, or multiple sclerosis or from primary oesophageal motility disturbances such as achalasia or diffuse spasm.

Upper gastrointestinal endoscopy is the investigation of choice because it allows visual assessment, tissue sampling, and therapeutic dilation when needed. A contrast swallow may precede endoscopy if perforation risk is suspected, and videofluoroscopy can help evaluate the mechanics of swallowing, although radiographic aspiration does not always translate into clinical harm. Treatment depends on cause and overall health status. Short empirical courses of proton pump inhibitors may be tried when invasive testing is unsuitable. Antifungal agents are prescribed if candidiasis is evident. Endoscopic dilation or stent insertion can relieve strictures, while speech and language therapists advise on safe textures and feeding positions in functional disease. For oesophageal dysmotility, selected patients may benefit from smooth muscle relaxants such as calcium channel blockers or nitrates.

Malnutrition and aspiration are common complications. Early dietetic input, use of high-energy oral supplements, and when oral intake is inadequate, timely initiation of nasogastric or percutaneous endoscopic gastrostomy feeding can be life-saving. If aspiration pneumonitis occurs, management includes careful airway protection, supplemental oxygen, chest physiotherapy, and appropriate antibiotics.

PEPTIC ULCER DISEASE IN LATER LIFE

Peptic ulcer disease is now far less common than in previous decades largely because of improved pharmacological management, yet it remains an important diagnosis in older adults. Current studies found that non-steroidal anti-inflammatory drug (NSAID) use and infection with *Helicobacter pylori* remain the two major causes of peptic ulcer disease. Global infection rates have declined over the past three decades but remain substantial. A recent global meta-analysis estimated an overall prevalence of about 43.9% (Chen et al., 2024). UK data indicate a prevalence of roughly 35% in adults (UK Biobank, 2025), while population studies from East Asia still report higher levels of 50–60% in older people (Kang et al., 2025). These findings highlight that *H. pylori* infection remains a clinically important risk factor in older adults despite falling worldwide prevalence. Although infection is frequently asymptomatic, it is the most frequent infective cause of dyspepsia in older populations and is strongly associated with duodenal ulceration.

Clinical presentation varies. Some patients experience classic epigastric pain, heartburn, or retrosternal discomfort, while others present with anaemia, weight loss, or acute complications such as gastrointestinal bleeding (Figure 16.1) or perforation. Atypical or subtle symptoms, such as loss of appetite or vague abdominal discomfort, are not uncommon in frail older adults and may delay recognition.

Upper gastrointestinal endoscopy remains the investigation of choice because it is safe, well tolerated, and permits tissue sampling and therapeutic intervention. *H. pylori* can be confirmed via rapid urease testing, histology, breath testing, or serology. When ulcers are found, discontinuing NSAIDs and

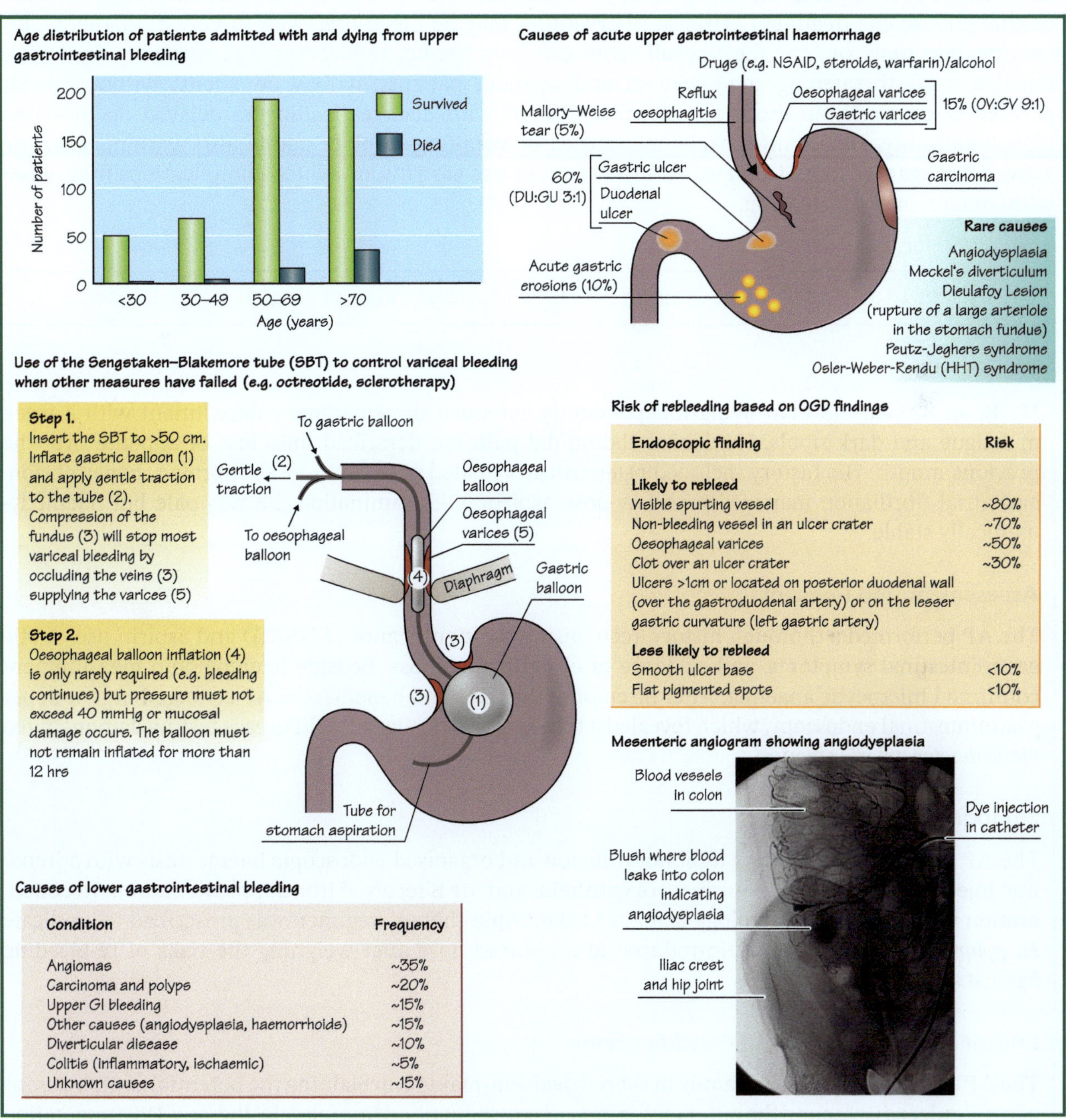

Risk of rebleeding based on OGD findings

Endoscopic finding	Risk
Likely to rebleed	
Visible spurting vessel	~80%
Non-bleeding vessel in an ulcer crater	~70%
Oesophageal varices	~50%
Clot over an ulcer crater	~30%
Ulcers >1cm or located on posterior duodenal wall (over the gastroduodenal artery) or on the lesser gastric curvature (left gastric artery)	
Less likely to rebleed	
Smooth ulcer base	<10%
Flat pigmented spots	<10%

Causes of lower gastrointestinal bleeding

Condition	Frequency
Angiomas	~35%
Carcinoma and polyps	~20%
Upper GI bleeding	~15%
Other causes (angiodysplasia, haemorrhoids)	~15%
Diverticular disease	~10%
Colitis (inflammatory, ischaemic)	~5%
Unknown causes	~15%

FIGURE 16.1   Upper and lower GI bleeding. *Source:* Leach (2014)/John Wiley & Sons.

considering temporary cessation of aspirin are crucial steps. Eradication therapy combining a proton pump inhibitor with two antibiotics is recommended when *H. pylori* is present, whereas acid suppression alone is sufficient if the bacterium is absent. Endoscopic follow-up, typically at six weeks, is essential to confirm healing, particularly of gastric or suspicious duodenal ulcers.

Acute upper gastrointestinal bleeding requires immediate resuscitation and urgent therapeutic endoscopy, for example, with adrenaline injection, thermal coagulation, or clip placement. High-dose intravenous proton pump inhibitor therapy reduces the risk of re-bleeding. If haemorrhage continues despite endoscopic treatment, surgical intervention may be life-saving even in very old patients. Risk stratification tools such as the Rockall score can help predict re-bleeding and mortality. Perforation remains a life-threatening complication, and in older patients, it may be 'silent', without obvious peritonitis, especially in those on corticosteroids or with diabetes leading to delayed diagnosis and higher mortality. Persistent unexplained nausea or vomiting in older adults also warrants early and active investigation, as gastrointestinal ulceration, severe gastritis, or related complications may present without pain or overt bleeding.

Case Study 16.2　The Role of AP and Management of Peptic Ulcer Disease

Presentation

Mr B, an 82-year-old man living independently, attended the emergency department with a week of fatigue and dark stools. He denied abdominal pain but described mild loss of appetite over the previous month. His history included osteoarthritis treated with high-dose ibuprofen, hypertension, and atrial fibrillation managed with low-dose aspirin. On examination, he was pale but haemodynamically stable.

Assessment and Reasoning

The AP performed a thorough history, recognising the significance of NSAID and aspirin use, subtle gastrointestinal symptoms, and evidence of chronic blood loss. Bedside haemoglobin measurement confirmed microcytic anaemia. After discussing the risks and benefits, the AP arranged urgent upper gastrointestinal endoscopy, which revealed a bleeding gastric ulcer. Rapid urease testing demonstrated *Helicobacter pylori* infection.

Management

The AP initiated proton pump inhibitor infusion and organised endoscopic haemostasis with adrenaline injection. NSAIDs and aspirin were withheld, and Mr B received iron supplementation. In collaboration with the gastroenterology team, a 14-day triple-therapy regimen was prescribed to eradicate *H. pylori*. Aspirin was later reintroduced at a reduced dose after weighing the risks of re-bleeding against stroke prevention.

Ethical and Person-centred Considerations

The AP engaged Mr B and his family in shared decision-making, explaining the potential complications of peptic ulcer disease and the rationale for staged reintroduction of antiplatelet therapy. Documentation reflected careful consideration of Mr B's autonomy, cardiovascular risk, and quality of life.

CONSTIPATION IN FRAILTY AND OLDER AGE

Constipation is highly prevalent in older people, affecting about one-third of community-dwelling adults older than 60 years and more than half of those living in care homes (Arco et al., 2022; Pilat, 2022). Besides discomfort, it can precipitate serious complications. In frail individuals, repeated straining may provoke vasovagal syncope or precipitate myocardial or cerebral ischaemia, while severe faecal loading can cause anorexia, nausea, abdominal pain, and, in rare cases, stercoral ulceration with life-threatening perforation (Gough et al., 2016). Chronic symptoms frequently diminish quality of life, impairing mobility, mental health, and social participation (De Giorgio et al., 2015).

PATHOPHYSIOLOGY AND RISK FACTORS

Constipation may result from primary motility disturbance (normal transit, slow transit, or disorders of defaecation) or secondary causes such as polypharmacy, metabolic disease, neurological disorders, or mechanical obstruction. Drugs commonly responsible include opioids, calcium channel blockers, anticholinergics, and iron supplements. Ageing reduced physical activity, low fibre intake, inadequate hydration, female sex, and poverty all contribute (Pilat, 2022). Histological changes in the ageing colon such as denser collagen and fewer myenteric neurons are reported but not thought to be dominant factors.

ASSESSMENT AND DIAGNOSIS

Comprehensive evaluation requires a detailed bowel, diet, and drug history; physical examination; and attention to red-flag signs of colorectal malignancy, such as rectal bleeding, weight loss, or change in stool calibre (NICE NG12, 2021). Abdominal and rectal examinations remain essential for detecting faecal loading, masses, or anorectal disease and should be performed with consent and a chaperone (Villanueva Herrero et al., 2024).

MANAGEMENT

Management is stepwise and multidisciplinary:

Non-pharmacological *measures* including optimising fluid and fibre intake, encouraging mobility, adjusting contributory drugs, and ensuring privacy and routine are the first step. Practical measures such as using a foot stool and forward-leaning posture can facilitate defaecation (Takano et al., 2018).

Pharmacological therapy begins with bulk-forming laxatives (e.g. ispaghula husk) if there is no impaction and hydration is inadequate. Osmotic agents such as macrogols are preferred when stool remains hard or evacuation unsatisfactory. Stimulant laxatives like bisacodyl can be added if required, and combination regimens are often necessary for opioid-induced constipation (British National Formulary, 2025).

Persistent or severe cases should prompt referral for gastroenterological assessment and consideration of anorectal manometry or endoscopy (Heidelbaugh et al., 2021).

For faecal impaction, escalating doses of macrogols are advised, with stimulant or rectal preparations if softening is incomplete. In rare, resistant cases, phosphate enemas or oil enemas may be required (Pilat, 2022). Early recognition and regular review are vital since delayed treatment can lead to overflow incontinence or perforation. Other key gastrointestinal disorders in older adults are summarised in Table 16.1.

TABLE 16.1   Key gastrointestinal disorders in older adults.

Condition	Pathophysiology/ key features	Typical presentation in older adults	Diagnostic considerations	Main management points
Irritable bowel syndrome (IBS)	Functional disorder causing abdominal pain, bloating, and altered bowel habit without structural abnormality. New onset in later life is rare.	Chronic fluctuating symptoms from youth may persist. Alarm features such as weight loss, bleeding, or nocturnal pain argue against IBS.	Diagnosis of exclusion after careful investigation to rule out malignancy, diverticulitis, or inflammatory bowel disease.	Dietary adjustment (low fibre for bloating; high fibre for constipation), antispasmodics such as mebeverine, bulking agents, and cautious use of loperamide or codeine for diarrhoea.
Angiodysplasia	Fragile, dilated submucosal vessels prone to bleeding; prevalence increases with age.	Recurrent or occult gastrointestinal bleeding leading to iron deficiency anaemia; rarely brisk haemorrhage.	Often a diagnosis of exclusion after repeated negative investigations. Colonoscopy may reveal lesions; mesenteric angiography identifies active bleeding.	Endoscopic diathermy for visible lesions, iron replacement, and in persistent bleeding, medical therapy such as tranexamic acid or oestrogen.
Microscopic colitis (collagenous or lymphocytic)	Idiopathic inflammation with microscopic mucosal changes but normal macroscopic appearance.	Chronic or intermittent watery, non-bloody diarrhoea without systemic toxicity.	Colonoscopy with multiple biopsies confirms diagnosis.	Dietary measures, anti-diarrhoeal agents, mesalamine, or oral steroids (e.g. budesonide) if needed.
Intestinal ischaemia	Compromised mesenteric blood supply; may be acute (embolism or thrombosis) or chronic (arterial stenosis).	Severe abdominal pain disproportionate to examination findings; intestinal angina causes postprandial pain, while acute small-bowel ischaemia presents with sudden pain and rectal bleeding.	Elevated lactate and metabolic acidosis raise suspicion. Angiography or urgent imaging helps confirm diagnosis.	Prompt fluid resuscitation and antiplatelet therapy for chronic mesenteric ischaemia; emergency revascularisation or laparotomy for acute infarction.

TABLE 16.1 (Continued)

Condition	Pathophysiology/ key features	Typical presentation in older adults	Diagnostic considerations	Main management points
Ischaemic colitis	Transient colonic hypoperfusion, often precipitated by hypotension or vascular disease.	Sudden lower abdominal pain with bloody diarrhoea; may follow dehydration or shock.	Colonoscopy or CT to exclude alternative pathology.	Bowel rest, fluid replacement, and correction of precipitating factors. Monitor for strictures requiring later intervention.
Inflammatory bowel disease (IBD)	Immune-mediated chronic inflammation (ulcerative colitis or Crohn's disease) with a second incidence peak in older age.	Diarrhoea with or without blood, abdominal pain, weight loss, and extra-intestinal manifestations (arthritis, eye or skin disease).	Stool cultures to exclude infection, blood tests for anaemia and inflammation, colonoscopy and biopsy.	Stepwise therapy with 5-aminosalicylates, corticosteroids, and immunomodulators; surgery for complications or refractory disease.
Diverticular disease	Herniation of mucosa through the muscular wall, usually in the sigmoid colon.	Mostly asymptomatic. Symptomatic disease causes left-sided pain or constipation. Diverticulitis presents with pain, fever, and diarrhoea; can lead to abscess, perforation, haemorrhage, or fistula.	CT colonography or colonoscopy to confirm diagnosis and rule out malignancy.	High-fibre diet for uncomplicated disease; antibiotics and supportive care for diverticulitis; surgery for complications.
Chronic liver disease (including cirrhosis and non-alcoholic fatty liver disease)	Progressive fibrosis from alcohol, viral hepatitis, or metabolic causes such as obesity and diabetes.	Non-specific symptoms such as fatigue, anorexia, confusion, or falls; signs of portal hypertension or hepatic failure may emerge late.	Liver function tests, viral serology, autoantibody panels, iron studies, and ultrasound with Doppler.	Treat underlying cause, manage complications (ascites, varices), and support nutrition; consider hepatology referral.
Gallbladder disease (gallstones, cholecystitis)	Biliary stones and inflammation of the gallbladder wall.	Often silent. When symptomatic, may mimic reflux or diverticular disease. Acute cholecystitis can present atypically without pain and carries a high mortality if untreated.	Ultrasound for diagnosis.	Conservative management for asymptomatic stones; intravenous antibiotics for acute cholecystitis; early surgical review if no improvement.

(Continued)

TABLE 16.1   (Continued)

Condition	Pathophysiology/ key features	Typical presentation in older adults	Diagnostic considerations	Main management points
Bowel obstruction	Mechanical blockage from causes such as severe constipation, colonic tumour, sigmoid volvulus, strangulated hernia, adhesions, or diverticular stricture.	Abdominal distension, pain or colic, vomiting, and cessation of stool or flatus. Signs can be subtle; obstruction may present with only bloating or nausea.	Abdominal X-ray (supine usually adequate), CT to localise and identify cause, and careful groin examination for hernia.	Early surgical assessment; bowel rest (nil by mouth, nasogastric tube), intravenous fluids, correction of electrolytes, and prophylactic low-molecular-weight heparin. Surgery or endoscopic decompression if conservative treatment fails.
Intestinal pseudo-obstruction (Ogilvie's syndrome)	Functional paralysis of the colon, often precipitated by severe illness, electrolyte imbalance (especially hypokalaemia), immobility, or drugs such as opiates and anticholinergics.	Abdominal distension, vomiting, and radiological evidence of large-bowel dilatation but with reduced or absent bowel sounds.	Abdominal X-ray or CT to exclude mechanical obstruction.	Supportive care with hydration, correction of electrolytes and precipitating factors, and bowel rest; decompression or surgery if conservative measures fail.

CONCLUSION

Gastrointestinal disease in later life is common, multifactorial, and frequently atypical. Outcomes improve when clinicians pair systematic assessment (including nutrition and hydration) with timely investigation, early complication prevention, and clear shared decision-making grounded in capacity and values. A multidisciplinary approach anchored in CGA delivers safer, more person-centred care.

Take-Home Messages

1. Treat nutrition and hydration as core clinical issues; screen routinely and act early.
2. Always consider serious pathology when new symptoms arise in older adults, especially dysphagia, weight loss, bleeding, or persistent vomiting.
3. Choose investigations that answer a focused question and minimise harm; endoscopy is often safe and informative in frailty.

4. Manage constipation proactively with lifestyle measures plus staged pharmacotherapy; address drugs that impair motility.

5. Decisions on assisted feeding must follow capacity assessment; best interest reasoning; and documented, compassionate dialogue with patients and families.

REFERENCES

Arco, S., Saldaña, E., Serra-Prat, M. et al. (2022). Functional constipation in older adults: prevalence, clinical symptoms and subtypes, association with frailty, and impact on quality of life. *Gerontology* 68 (4): 397–406.

Bowker, L., Price, J., and Smith, A. (2012). *Oxford Handbook of Geriatric Medicine*, 2e. Oxford: Oxford University Press.

British Geriatrics Society, Burrows, K., Romano, V. and Smith, A. (2025) *Comprehensive Geriatric Assessment: Nutrition and Hydration*. Available at: `https://www.bgs.org.uk/cga-nutrition-and-hydration` (accessed 2 February 2026).

British National Formulary (2025). Constipation: treatment summaries [Online]. `https://bnfc.nice.org.uk/treatment-summaries/constipation/` (accessed 20 September 2025).

Chen, Y.C., Malfertheiner, P., Yu, H.T. et al. (2024). Global prevalence of *Helicobacter pylori* infection and incidence of gastric cancer between 1980 and 2022. *Gastroenterology* 166 (4): 605–619.

De Giorgio, R., Ruggeri, E., Stanghellini, V. et al. (2015). Chronic constipation in the elderly: a primer. *BMC Gastroenterology* 15: 130.

Gough, A.E., Donovan, M.N., Grotts, J., and Greaney, G.C. (2016). Perforated stercoral ulcer: a 10-year experience. *Journal of the American Geriatrics Society* 64 (4): 880–884.

Heidelbaugh, J., Martinez de Andino, N., de Andino, N.M. et al. (2021). Diagnosing constipation spectrum disorders in primary care. *Journal of Clinical Medicine* 10 (5): 1092.

Kang, D.W., Lee, J.W., Park, M.Y. et al. (2025). Impact of *Helicobacter pylori* eradication on age-specific risk of incident dementia in patients with peptic ulcer disease: a nationwide population-based cohort study. *GeroScience* 47 (1): 1161–1174.

Khor, P.Y., Vearing, R.M., and Charlton, K.E. (2022). The effectiveness of nutrition interventions in improving frailty and its associated constructs related to malnutrition and functional decline among community-dwelling older adults: a systematic review. *Journal of Human Nutrition and Dietetics* 35 (3): 566–582.

Laur, C.V., McNicholl, T., Valaitis, R., and Keller, H.H. (2017). Malnutrition or frailty? Overlap and evidence gaps in the diagnosis and treatment of frailty and malnutrition. *Applied Physiology, Nutrition, and Metabolism* 42 (5): 449–458.

Leach, R. (2014). *Critical care medicine at a glance*, Thirde. Chichester, West Sussex: Wiley.

National Institute for Health and Care Excellence (NICE) (2021). *NG12: Suspected Cancer—Recognition and Referral*. London: NICE.

Pilat, D. (2022). Constipation in the elderly. RCGP Learning Blog, 20 September.

Takano, S., Nakashima, M., Tsuchino, M. et al. (2018). Influence of foot stool on defecation: a prospective study. *Pelviperineology* 37 (3): 101–103.

Thomson, K.H., Rice, S., Arisa, O. et al. (2022). Effectiveness and cost-effectiveness of oral nutritional supplements in frail older people who are malnourished or at risk of malnutrition: a systematic review and meta-analysis. *The Lancet Healthy Longevity* 3 (10): e654–e666.

UK Biobank (2025). *Helicobacter pylori* infection, its treatment and colorectal cancer risk: a two-phase study using treatment data from the UK Clinical Practice Database and serology information from the UK Biobank [Online]. `https://www.ukbiobank.ac.uk/projects/helicobacter-pylori-infection-its-treatment-and-colorectal-cancer-risk-a-two-phase-study-using-treatment-data-from-the-uk-clinical-practice-database-and-serology-information-from-the-uk-biobank/` (accessed 20 September 2025).

Villanueva Herrero, J.A., Abdussalam, A., and Kasi, A. (2024). Rectal exam. In: *StatPearls*. Treasure Island, FL: *StatPearls Publishing*.

CHAPTER 17

Genitourinary System

Aim

The aim of this chapter is to strengthen advanced practitioners' knowledge and critical understanding of age-related changes in the genitourinary system, with particular emphasis on prostate disorders, urinary incontinence, and sexual health, so that assessment, diagnosis, and management are evidence based, holistic, and person centred.

LEARNING OUTCOMES

On completion of this chapter, readers will be able to:

1. Critically appraise the effects of ageing on the male and female genitourinary systems, including hormonal and structural changes.
2. Evaluate the clinical presentation, investigation, and management of benign prostatic hyperplasia, prostate cancer, urinary incontinence, and related conditions using current NICE and British Geriatrics Society guidance.
3. Integrate frailty assessment, multimorbidity, and patient preference into decisions on pharmacological, surgical, and palliative care.
4. Address sexual health issues in later life with sensitivity, recognising the influence of illness, medication, and psychosocial factors.
5. Apply a comprehensive, person-centred approach to the prevention, early detection, and treatment of complications such as urinary retention, infection, and sexual dysfunction.

SELF-ASSESSMENT QUESTIONS

1. In a frail older man with lower urinary tract symptoms, how would you distinguish benign prostatic hyperplasia from alternative causes (e.g. malignancy, infection, and medication effects), and how would this distinction alter investigation and first-line management?
2. A care-home resident with vascular dementia develops distressing urge incontinence and sexual disinhibition after a recent dopamine-agonist dose increase. Outline your stepwise assessment and management plan, integrating frailty assessment, medicine optimisation, safeguarding, and the Mental Capacity Act best interest framework.

INTRODUCTION

Ageing affects the genitourinary system in both sexes. In women, dropping oestrogen levels after menopause leads to thinning and loss of elasticity of the vaginal mucosa, reduced lubrication, and increased risk of urinary and genital infection; the uterus and ovaries also atrophy. In men, testicular volume, sperm production, and semen quality gradually decline; erectile recovery slows; and benign prostatic enlargement may cause urinary symptoms. A minority develop symptomatic testosterone deficiency. Across both sexes, reduced sexual activity often reflects illness, medication, or social factors rather than ageing alone. Hormone replacement or testosterone therapy can help selected patients but require careful monitoring. For further physiological changes, refer to Chapter 10.

BENIGN PROSTATIC HYPERPLASIA

Benign prostatic hyperplasia (BPH) is a non-cancerous enlargement of the prostate gland accompanied by increased smooth muscle tone (Prostate Cancer UK, 2025). The resulting narrowing of the bladder outlet produces lower urinary tract symptoms (LUTSs) collectively referred to as prostatism. Histological evidence of BPH is almost universal in men older than 70 years, and around one-quarter to one-half of those older than 65 years' experience symptoms. The clinical course varies: Some men remain stable, others gradually worsen, and a minority improve spontaneously.

CLINICAL FEATURES AND ASSESSMENT

LUTSs are often grouped into (NICE, 2025a):

- Obstructive symptoms: slow urinary stream, hesitancy, straining, nocturia, and acute retention or chronic retention with overflow incontinence.
- Irritative symptoms: frequency, urgency, dysuria, and urge incontinence.

Macroscopic haematuria, urinary infection, or obstructive renal failure may also occur. Symptoms can be aggravated by certain medicines such as sedating antihistamines, while some drugs (for example, tricyclic antidepressants) may lessen urgency but worsen retention.

Evaluation should include a thorough history; symptom scoring (for example, using the International Prostate Symptom Score); physical examination of the genitals, abdomen, and nervous system; and digital rectal examination. A smooth, symmetrically enlarged prostate is typical of BPH, whereas irregularities may suggest cancer or calculi. Investigations are selected to exclude alternative diagnoses and identify complications and may include urinalysis, renal function tests, prostate-specific antigen (PSA) measurement when appropriate, ultrasonography of the renal tract, urine flow studies, and cystoscopy if haematuria is present.

MANAGEMENT

Treatment is guided by symptom severity, patient preference, and the presence of complications. However, conservative care is usually indicated. Ongoing follow-up and monitoring is appropriate for mild-to-moderate LUTSs without complications (NICE, 2025). Advice may include reducing evening fluid intake, reviewing unnecessary diuretics, and arranging regular clinical and renal function review. The annual risk of acute urinary retention is about 1–2%.

PHARMACOLOGICAL THERAPY

- Alpha-adrenergic blockers (e.g. tamsulosin and doxazosin) relax prostatic and bladder neck smooth muscle, improving urine flow within days. Side effects include postural hypotension and dizziness, so slow-dose titration and caution in frail patients are essential (Sica, 2005).
- 5-Alpha reductase inhibitors (e.g. finasteride) shrink the prostate by inhibiting conversion of testosterone to dihydrotestosterone, with benefit usually apparent after several months. They are most effective when the gland is substantially enlarged. Adverse effects may include reduced libido or erectile dysfunction. Because PSA levels fall during therapy, measured values should be doubled to estimate underlying cancer risk. If a single class of drug is inadequate, switching or combining therapies can be considered.

SURGICAL AND MINIMALLY INVASIVE OPTIONS

Surgery is recommended when symptoms remain troublesome, complications develop (e.g. recurrent infection, persistent haematuria, or obstructive renal failure), or drug treatment fails. Transurethral resection of the prostate (TURP) is the established standard, offering symptom relief in over 90% of patients but carrying risks such as retrograde ejaculation, erectile dysfunction, or incontinence (Rassweiler et al., 2006). Less invasive procedures such as transurethral incision of the prostate, microwave thermotherapy, or needle ablation may suit selected patients with smaller glands or high surgical risk, although long-term data are more limited. Open prostatectomy is reserved for very large prostates or when concomitant bladder surgery is required (Cho et al., 2021). For men with acute or chronic retention who are unfit for or decline surgery, long-term catheterisation may be the most practical option (Spinos et al., 2023). Intermittent trials without a catheter can be undertaken but may not always succeed.

PROSTATE CANCER IN OLDER ADULTS

Prostate carcinoma is the most frequently diagnosed malignancy in men, with incidence rising sharply with age and a median age at diagnosis exceeding 70 years (NICE, 2021). Many men die with, rather than from, the disease and remain asymptomatic or present only with lower urinary tract obstruction.

Because many tumours remain indolent, the potential risks and burdens of curative treatments often outweigh benefits in those with limited life expectancy.

ASSESSMENT AND DIAGNOSIS

Prognosis depends largely on tumour stage and histological grade, commonly expressed as the Gleason score (Swanson et al., 2021). Localised disease is often identified incidentally during investigations for BPH or after a raised PSA level. Digital rectal examination can be normal in early disease. Locally advanced tumours have breached the prostatic capsule and carry a less favourable outlook. Up to half of men present with metastatic spread, which may remain asymptomatic or cause urinary symptoms, bone pain, anaemia, weight loss, or pathological fractures.

Investigations may include PSA testing, full blood count, renal and liver function tests, imaging such as bone scans or MRI for staging, and transrectal ultrasound-guided biopsy for histological confirmation (NICE, 2025b). PSA levels, although helpful for monitoring disease activity, are neither specific nor entirely sensitive and can be increased by benign conditions such as prostatitis, urinary infection, or recent instrumentation.

MANAGEMENT PRINCIPLES

Management should reflect tumour grade, disease stage, symptom burden, and the patient's overall health and life expectancy (NICE, 2025b). In men with low-grade, localised cancer and anticipated survival less than 10 years, active surveillance or 'watchful waiting' with regular PSA monitoring is often appropriate. Curative options include radical prostatectomy or radiotherapy, but both carry significant risks such as urinary incontinence and erectile dysfunction (NICE, 2025b).

Hormone manipulation, usually with luteinising hormone-releasing hormone (LHRH) agonists or antiandrogens, remains the cornerstone of therapy for metastatic disease, often providing symptom control for one to two years (Zhao et al., 2024). Eventually, resistance to hormonal treatment is common, leading to disease progression. Complications of advanced disease include bone pain, pathological fractures, urinary retention, renal impairment, and spinal cord compression, all requiring timely palliative measures (Table 17.1).

Case Study 17.1   Frail Older Man with Newly Diagnosed Prostate Cancer

Mr H is an 82-year-old widower living alone with support from his daughter. He has a Clinical Frailty Scale score of 6 (moderately frail) and a history of chronic obstructive pulmonary disease, hypertension, and mild cognitive impairment.

He presents to a same-day emergency care service with worsening lower urinary tract symptoms and new-onset nocturia. An AP conducts a comprehensive assessment, including targeted history, physical examination, and point-of-care investigations.

Rectal examination shows an asymmetrically enlarged, firm prostate. Blood tests show a PSA of 34 μg/L, with normal renal function. In line with NICE guidelines for prostate cancer (2025), the AP arranges an urgent urology referral, provides a bladder diary and discusses conservative measures for symptom relief. He also initiates shared decision-making about investigations and treatment, considering Mr H's frailty, comorbidities, and life expectancy.

Subsequent imaging confirms locally advanced prostate adenocarcinoma without distant metastases. After multidisciplinary discussion involving oncology, urology, and palliative care, the agreed management is hormone therapy with active surveillance, prioritising symptom control and quality of life over curative intervention.

The AP coordinates follow-up, reviews side effects, and liaises with community services to support continence and maintain independence.

TABLE 17.1 Common causes of postmenopausal vaginal bleeding and related vulval disorders.

Condition	Typical features	Key risk factors	Diagnostic approach	Main management
Atrophic vaginitis	Vaginal dryness, irritation, and light bleeding from fragile epithelium	Oestrogen deficiency after menopause	Pelvic examination; exclusion of infection and malignancy	Topical vaginal oestrogen; emollients and avoidance of irritants
Endometrial hyperplasia	Irregular or heavy bleeding	Unopposed oestrogen (obesity, oestrogen-only HRT, tamoxifen)	Transvaginal ultrasound for endometrial thickness; hysteroscopy and biopsy if ≥ 5 mm	Progestogen therapy or hysterectomy depending on severity and histology
Endometrial or cervical polyps	Intermittent painless bleeding	Increasing age, oestrogen exposure	Speculum examination, hysteroscopy	Polyp removal and histological assessment
Genital tract malignancy (endometrium, cervix, vulva, vagina, ovary)	Persistent or heavy bleeding, discharge, pelvic pain	Age, obesity, unopposed oestrogen, HPV (for cervical)	Pelvic examination, ultrasound, biopsy	Surgery ± radiotherapy or systemic therapy depending on site and stage
Vaginal or urinary infection	Bleeding with discharge, dysuria or odour	Diabetes, poor hygiene, instrumentation	Vaginal swabs, urine culture	Antimicrobial treatment according to culture
Spurious bleeding	Blood from urinary or rectal source misidentified as vaginal	Haematuria, haemorrhoids	Urinalysis, rectal examination	Treat primary urinary or bowel cause
Vaginal prolapse (cystocoele, rectocoele, uterine descent, enterocele)	Sensation of pelvic pressure, visible or palpable bulge, ulceration with bleeding in severe cases	Multiparity, obesity, chronic cough or constipation	Pelvic examination: imaging if needed	Pelvic floor exercises, topical oestrogen, pessary fitting or surgical repair

(Continued)

TABLE 17.1   (Continued)

Condition	Typical features	Key risk factors	Diagnostic approach	Main management
Vulvitis	Pruritus, burning, superficial bleeding from scratching	Candida infection, irritant dermatitis, occasionally STIs	Visual inspection, swabs if infection suspected	Antifungal or mild topical steroid therapy; remove irritants
Lichen sclerosus/ squamous hyperplasia	White atrophic or thickened plaques, pruritus, possible fissuring	Post menopause	Vulval inspection and biopsy to rule out malignancy	High-potency topical steroids; long-term follow-up
Vulval carcinoma	Painless lesion, sometimes pruritic or bleeding, may be ulcerated	Increasing age, chronic inflammatory dermatoses	Vulval biopsy	Wide local excision or vulvectomy ± radiotherapy

URINARY INCONTINENCE

Urinary incontinence is common in older adults, affecting about two in five women older than 60 years (British Geriatrics Society [BGS], 2019). It arises from diverse mechanisms including weakened urethral support (stress incontinence), detrusor overactivity leading to urgency (urge incontinence), a combination of these (mixed incontinence), bladder outlet obstruction causing overflow, abnormal fistulous connections, or functional factors such as immobility or cognitive impairment. Any consultation with an older person should include an appropriate question on continence, and a positive response should prompt a comprehensive evaluation. Key history explores storage symptom frequency, urgency, stress leakage, nocturia, and voiding problems such as hesitancy, intermittent stream, or incomplete emptying. Clinicians should also ask about pain, haematuria, bowel habits, childhood urinary issues, and coexisting illnesses including diabetes or heart disease and review any drugs that may worsen incontinence.

Examination covers the cardiovascular, abdominal, pelvic, and neurological systems, with cognitive screening when appropriate. Inspection may show atrophic changes or prolapse; pelvic floor muscle strength can be graded during a vaginal examination, and a cough or strain test may reproduce leakage. Digital rectal examination is recommended in all patients to assess anal tone, rectal pathology, and, in men, prostate size. Initial investigations include a bladder diary, urinalysis with culture if needed, blood tests (full blood count, renal profile, glucose, and calcium), and post-void residual bladder scanning. Imaging or specialist tests are reserved for specific concerns such as haematuria, pelvic masses, or refractory symptoms.

Management begins with correction of reversible causes such as urinary infection, constipation, medication side effects, delirium, or poorly controlled diabetes. Lifestyle interventions like weight optimisation, smoking cessation, reduction of caffeine and alcohol, and bowel regulation are first line for all types. Stress incontinence may respond to pelvic floor muscle training, vaginal cones, or continence advisory support, with mid-urethral sling surgery considered for suitable candidates (Sims et al., 2022). Urge incontinence is managed with bladder training and, if required, antimuscarinic drugs or β_3-adrenoceptor agonists such as mirabegron, with intravaginal oestrogen used when vaginal atrophy contributes (NICE, 2025c). Bladder outlet obstruction, including BPH, may require alpha-blockers, 5-alpha-reductase inhibitors, or surgical procedures such as transurethral prostatectomy, according to the underlying cause (Creta et al., 2024). Referral to specialist services is indicated for red-flag features such as haematuria, pelvic organ prolapses beyond the introitus, pain with micturition, suspected malignancy, or persistent symptoms despite appropriate therapy (BGS, 2019).

SEXUAL HEALTH AND AGEING

Many older adults continue to value sexual intimacy, yet the frequency of both penetrative and non-penetrative sexual activity typically diminishes with age (Grabovac and McDermott, 2023). This reduction is shaped by multiple influences: loss of a partner, age-related physiological changes such as reduced vaginal lubrication or less reliable erections, chronic illness and medication effects (notably β-blockers), psychological conditions such as depression or poor self-esteem, limited privacy in residential settings, and cultural or societal attitudes. Sensitive and holistic enquiry is needed to explore these factors and to support individuals who report sexual difficulties.

ERECTILE DYSFUNCTION

Normal erection depends on coordinated neurological, vascular, hormonal, and psychological mechanisms (Mirone et al., 2022). In later life, erectile dysfunction is common and usually multifactorial. Medications especially antihypertensives (e.g. β-blockers and some diuretics), certain antidepressants, alcohol, and hormone-suppressing agents are frequent contributors alongside vascular and neurological disease. Purely psychogenic impotence is rare.

Clinical assessment should document the onset, pattern, and any psychological stressors. Examination includes cardiovascular and neurological evaluation, genital inspection, and assessment of mood. Basic blood tests (full blood count and renal and glucose profile) are typically sufficient; hormonal testing is reserved for men with loss of libido suggesting hypogonadism (NICE, 2024).

Management focuses on correcting reversible causes, adjusting offending drugs, and treating coexisting physical or mental illness (NICE, 2024). Pharmacological options include phosphodiesterase-5 inhibitors such as sildenafil, which enhance penile blood flow and are generally safe except in men using nitrates, and alprostadil delivered intra-urethrally or by injection when oral agents are unsuitable. Mechanical aids like vacuum devices are effective but less often maintained long term (NICE, 2024).

HYPERSEXUALITY

Sexual disinhibition may arise in some people with dementia or frontal lobe lesions and in a minority of patients with Parkinson's disease treated with dopamine agonists (De Giorgi and Series, 2016). Careful evaluation of behavioural triggers and associated risks is vital. Management emphasises environmental adaptation and carer support, with psychotropic medication considered only when necessary.

Case Study 17.2   Hypersexuality in a Frail Older Adult with Learning Disability

Mr P is a 74-year-old man with moderate intellectual disability and vascular dementia following a frontal lobe stroke. He lives in a supported residential home and has a Clinical Frailty Scale score of 7 (severely frail). Staff report new episodes of sexual disinhibition: inappropriate touching of staff and residents and frequent explicit remarks. There is increasing concern about safeguarding the dignity of other residents and the distress caused to care staff.

An AP undertakes a comprehensive assessment. With support from a learning disability nurse and speech and language therapist, she uses simplified communication aids to involve Mr P in history-taking and consent discussions.

Physical examination rules out acute causes such as urinary tract infection, pain, or constipation. A careful review of medicines shows he is taking a dopamine agonist for parkinsonian symptoms, which is known to increase sexual drive. Collateral history from carers confirms a recent dose increase coinciding with the behaviour change.

Working with the multidisciplinary team (MDT) including neurology, psychiatry, learning disability services, and social care, the AP balances competing priorities: safeguarding other residents, respecting Mr P's rights and autonomy, and addressing the underlying neuropsychiatric drivers.

After shared decision-making with Mr P's family and best interest discussions under the Mental Capacity Act, the dopamine agonist is tapered and discontinued. Behavioural strategies are implemented: increased meaningful activity, structured daily routine, and supervised social contact. A low-dose antipsychotic is started cautiously after MDT agreement to help manage persistent disinhibition.

The AP provides ongoing review, adjusting care plans as Mr P's cognition and mobility change, and documents all decisions to demonstrate proportionality and adherence to legal and ethical standards. Staff receive training in de-escalation techniques and safeguarding procedures. Over the following weeks, the behaviours diminish, maintaining Mr P's dignity and the safety of others.

Key Learning for APs

- Hypersexuality in frail older adults with cognitive impairment or learning disability requires thorough assessment to exclude reversible causes, including medication effects.
- Complex decision-making should combine legal safeguards (e.g. Mental Capacity Act best interest framework), ethical reasoning, and close collaboration with neurology, psychiatry, and social care.
- Multidisciplinary and family engagement ensures that risk is balanced with the person's rights, supporting dignified and person-centred care.

CONCLUSION

Ageing brings structural and hormonal changes that influence urinary and sexual function in both sexes. Disorders such as BPH, prostate cancer, urinary incontinence, and sexual dysfunction are common, interrelated and frequently compounded by frailty, multimorbidity, and polypharmacy. Evidence-based assessment and management grounded in national guidance and supported by multidisciplinary collaboration are essential to optimise outcomes, relieve symptoms, and preserve quality of life. Sensitive exploration of sexual health and continence issues, together with shared decision-making, ensures care remains individualised and respectful.

> ### Take-Home Messages
>
> 1. Routinely enquire about urinary and sexual symptoms and correct reversible factors such as infection, medication effects, or constipation.
> 2. Base investigations and treatment on national guidance, integrating frailty assessment and the person's goals of care.
> 3. Involve MDTs to deliver focused pharmacological, surgical, and supportive interventions.
> 4. Promote dignity, autonomy, and quality of life through holistic, person-centred management of genitourinary disorders in older adults.

REFERENCES

British Geriatrics Society (2019). CGA in Primary Care Settings: patients presenting with urinary incontinence. In: *Good Practice Guide.* https://www.bgs.org.uk/16-cga-in-primary-care-settings-patients-presenting-with-urinary-incontinence (accessed 20 September 2025).

Cho, J.M., Moon, K.T., Lee, J.H. et al. (2021). Open simple prostatectomy and robotic simple prostatectomy for large benign prostatic hyperplasia: comparison of safety and efficacy. *Prostate International* 9 (2): 101–106.

Creta, M., Russo, G.I., Bhojani, N. et al. (2024). Bladder outlet obstruction relief and symptom improvement following medical and surgical therapies for lower urinary tract symptoms suggestive of benign prostatic hyperplasia: a systematic review. *European Urology* 86 (4): 315–326.

De Giorgi, R. and Series, H. (2016). Treatment of inappropriate sexual behavior in dementia. *Current Treatment Options in Neurology* 18 (9): 41.

Grabovac, I. and McDermott, D.T. (2023). Sexuality and sexual activity in older age: an age old issue? *The Lancet Regional Health – Western Pacific* 39: 100831.

Mirone, V., Fusco, F., Cirillo, L., and Napolitano, L. (2022). Erectile dysfunction: from pathophysiology to clinical assessment. In: *Practical Clinical Andrology* (ed. G. Cavallini, I. Goldstein, E.A. Jannini, et al.), 25–33. Cham: Springer International Publishing.

National Institute for Health and Care Excellence (NICE) (2021) *NICE.* Available at: nice.org.uk/guidance/ng131/evidence/full-guideline-pdf-6781033550 (accessed 2 February 2026).

National Institute for Health and Care Excellence (NICE) (2024). Erectile dysfunction. Clinical Knowledge Summaries. https://cks.nice.org.uk/topics/erectile-dysfunction/ (accessed 20 September 2025).

National Institute for Health and Care Excellence (NICE) (2025) *Urinary tract infection (lower) in women: management.* Available at: https://cks.nice.org.uk/topics/urinary-tract-infection-lower-women/ (accessed 2 February 2026).

National Institute for Health and Care Excellence (NICE) (2025a). *LUTS in Men.* London: National Institute for Health and Care Excellence https://cks.nice.org.uk/topics/luts-in-men/ (accessed 20 September 2025).

National Institute for Health and Care Excellence (NICE) (2025b). Prostate cancer: How should I assess a person with suspected prostate cancer? Clinical Knowledge Summaries. https://cks.nice.org.uk/topics/prostate-cancer/diagnosis/assessment/ (accessed 20 September 2025).

National Institute for Health and Care Excellence (NICE) (2025c). Incontinence – urinary, in women: antimuscarinic (anticholinergic) medicines. Clinical Knowledge Summaries. https://cks.nice.org.uk/topics/incontinence-urinary-in-women/prescribing-information/antimuscarinic-anticholinergic-medicines/ (accessed 20 September 2025).

Prostate Cancer UK (2025). *Other Prostate Problems: Enlarged Prostate.* Prostate Cancer UK https://prostatecanceruk.org/prostate-information-and-support/just-diagnosed/other-prostate-problems/enlarged-prostate (accessed 20 September 2025).

Rassweiler, J., Teber, D., Kuntz, R., and Hofmann, R. (2006). Complications of transurethral resection of the prostate (TURP)—incidence, management, and prevention. *European Urology* 50 (5): 969–980.

Sica, D.A. (2005). Alpha1-adrenergic blockers: current usage considerations. *The Journal of Clinical Hypertension* 7 (12): 757–762.

Sims, L., Hay-Smith, J., and Dean, S. (2022). Pelvic floor exercises and female stress urinary incontinence. *British Journal of General Practice* 72 (717): 185.

Spinos, T., Katafigiotis, I., Leotsakos, I. et al. (2023). Rezūm water vapor therapy for the treatment of patients with urinary retention and permanent catheter dependence secondary to benign prostate hyperplasia: a systematic review of the literature. *World Journal of Urology* 41 (2): 413–420.

Swanson, G.P., Trevathan, S., Hammonds, K.A. et al. (2021). Gleason score evolution and the effect on prostate cancer outcomes. *American Journal of Clinical Pathology* 155 (5): 711–717.

Zhao, J., Chen, J., Sun, G. et al. (2024). Luteinizing hormone-releasing hormone receptor agonists and antagonists in prostate cancer: effects on long-term survival and combined therapy with next-generation hormonal agents. *Cancer Biology & Medicine* 21 (11): 1012–1032.

CHAPTER 18

Renal System

Aim

This chapter aims to provide advanced practitioners (APs) and clinicians with an evidence-based overview of renal system changes in ageing and frailty, focusing on the recognition and management of acute kidney injury (AKI), chronic kidney disease (CKD), and key renal pathologies. It highlights the implications of these conditions for complex decision-making, medicines optimisation, and person-centred care in frail older adults.

LEARNING OUTCOMES

After engaging with this chapter, readers will be able to:

1. Critically explain age-related structural and physiological changes in the kidneys and how these changes increase vulnerability to AKI and CKD.
2. Evaluate the risk factors, pathophysiology, clinical presentation, and complications of AKI and CKD in frail older adults, applying current evidence and NICE guidance.
3. Analyse and apply assessment, investigation, and management strategies for AKI, CKD, and selected renal disorders (nephrotic syndrome, glomerulonephritis, and renal artery stenosis), including safe prescribing and fluid management.
4. Demonstrate advanced clinical reasoning and leadership in complex renal cases, integrating multidisciplinary care and shared decision-making in the context of frailty.

SELF-ASSESSMENT QUESTIONS

1. In a frail older adult with suspected AKI, how would you differentiate pre-renal, intrinsic, and post-renal causes, and how would this guide immediate management and decisions on nephrology referral?
2. An older patient with stage 3 CKD shows a steady decline in estimated glomerular filtration rate (eGFR) and recurrent hyperkalaemia. Outline your approach to medicines optimisation, cardiovascular risk management, and shared decision-making about renal replacement versus conservative care.

INTRODUCTION

Age-related Renal Changes Relevant to Frailty

With ageing, renal reserve declines even in the absence of overt disease. Glomerular filtration rate (GFR) typically falls after 40 years due to fewer functioning glomeruli, increased glomerulosclerosis, and reduced renal blood flow (around 10% per decade, especially in the cortex). Renal mass reduces by 20–30% by age 90 years, and distal nephron diverticula and benign retention cysts are common (Bowker et al., 2012). These structural and haemodynamic changes impair the kidney's ability to excrete solutes and drugs, raising susceptibility to nephrotoxins, ischaemia, and drug toxicity despite normal plasma urea and creatinine.

Homeostatic regulation of water and electrolytes is blunted: sodium equilibrium is reached more slowly, urine concentration and dilution fall about 5% per decade, renin and aldosterone levels drop by 30–50%, thirst sensation is reduced, and responsiveness to vasopressin declines (Bowker et al., 2012). Clinically, this predisposes older adults to hyponatraemia, hypernatremia, dehydration during illness, hypokalaemia from poor intake or diuretics, and hyperkalaemia where GFR is low or potassium-retaining drugs are used. Declining renal 1-hydroxylase activity lowers vitamin D and can mildly raise parathyroid hormone, while loss of circadian sodium handling leads to nocturia. For further physiological changes with the renal system, refer to Chapter 10.

Acute Kidney Injury (AKI) in Frailty

AKI is a rapid decline in kidney function, developing within seven days or less, that results in retention of nitrogenous waste and disruption of fluid, electrolyte and acid–base balance. Diagnosis relies on an acute rise in serum creatinine and/or reduced urine output, and the term encompasses structural damage and functional impairment beyond the older concept of acute renal failure (KDIGO, 2012; Think Kidneys, 2018; NICE, 2023). Figure 18.1 demonstrates the pathophysiology and clinical aspects of AKI.

Why Frail Older Adults Are Vulnerable

Frail patients have reduced haemodynamic reserve, polypharmacy (non-steroidal anti-inflammatory drugs [NSAIDs], angiotensin-converting enzyme [ACE] inhibitors/angiotensin II receptor blockers [ARBs], and diuretics), and higher sepsis and obstruction risk, all of which increase AKI incidence and adverse outcomes. Routine creatinine monitoring is recommended in acutely unwell adults, especially those ≥65 years or exposed to nephrotoxins, and urine output should be tracked (NICE, 2023).

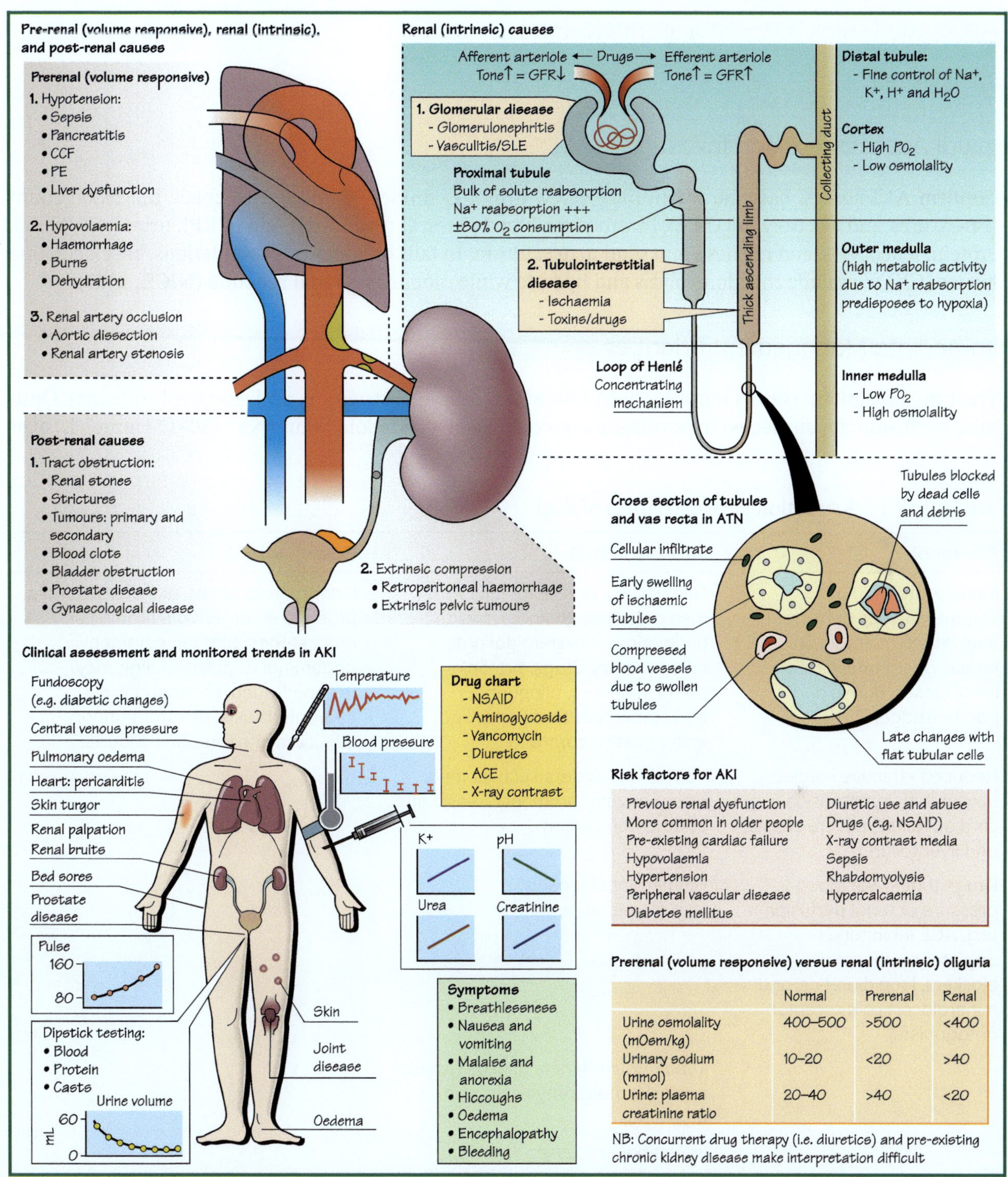

Prenatal (volume responsive) versus renal (intrinsic) oliguria

	Normal	Prerenal	Renal
Urine osmolality (mOsm/kg)	400–500	>500	<400
Urinary sodium (mmol)	10–20	<20	>40
Urine: plasma creatinine ratio	20–40	>40	<20

FIGURE 18.1 Pathophysiology of AKI and clinical aspects. *Source*: Leach (2014)/John Wiley & Sons.

Aetiology (Think 'Pre-renal–Intrinsic–Post-renal')

See Table 18.1.

Initial Assessment and Investigations

Confirm AKI against baseline creatinine; review drugs; examine volume status; check full blood count (FBC), urea and electrolytes (U&E), bicarbonate/blood gases, C-reactive protein (CRP), urinalysis (blood, protein, leucocytes, and nitrites), and send urine culture. In falls or 'long-lie' presentations, check creatine kinase (CK) to exclude rhabdomyolysis and hydrate while monitoring renal function (NICE, 2023).

Immediate Management Priorities

Treat the precipitant (sepsis bundle, control bleeding, relieve obstruction, and stop nephrotoxins). Optimise perfusion: for suspected hypovolaemia, give a 500 mL crystalloid bolus (Na^+ 130–154 mmol/L) over

TABLE 18.1   Key aetiological categories of AKI.

Pre-renal	Intrinsic (renal)	Post-renal
Inadequate circulating volume, such as dehydration (inability to maintain oral intake, gastrointestinal or renal losses, burns, and haemorrhage)	Nephrotoxic or tubular injury from medicines (e.g. aminoglycoside antibiotics, non-steroidal anti-inflammatory drugs, proton-pump inhibitors, allopurinol, chemotherapeutic agents, and iodine-based contrast)	Urinary tract obstruction, for example, prostate enlargement, ureteric or renal stones, blocked catheter, abdominal or pelvic malignancy, retroperitoneal fibrosis, chronic hydronephrosis, recurrent urinary infection, or neurogenic bladder
Reduced effective cardiac output with hypotension (e.g. cardiac failure, severe sepsis, and liver failure)	Vascular disorders such as renal artery or vein thrombosis, vasculitis, or atheroembolism	—
Drugs that lower blood pressure or renal perfusion (e.g. ACE inhibitors, angiotensin receptor blockers, loop diuretics, and mineralocorticoid receptor antagonists)	Glomerular diseases (e.g. glomerulonephritis)	—
—	Tubular disorders (e.g. acute tubular necrosis, rhabdomyolysis, and myeloma)	—
—	Interstitial processes (e.g. drug-induced or autoimmune interstitial nephritis and lymphomatous infiltration)	—

Source: Adapted from NICE (2023), Makris and Spanou (2016), Levey and James (2017), and Think Kidneys (2018).

<15 minutes, then reassess; in patients at high risk of fluid overload (e.g. heart failure), titrate cautiously with close clinical review. Monitor: strict input–output (consider a catheter for accurate urine output), serial creatinine/electrolytes, and weight (NICE, 2023).

Managing Complications

Hyperkalaemia: protect myocardium with intravenous (IV) calcium when indicated; shift potassium intracellularly (insulin–glucose; consider nebulised salbutamol; IV bicarbonate if acidotic), and remove potassium (diuretics if appropriate, potassium binders, dialysis when refractory). Metabolic acidosis, fluid overload, pulmonary oedema, or uraemic complications (pericarditis and encephalopathy): involve nephrology/critical care early and consider renal replacement therapy (RRT). Decisions should be based on overall clinical status, not a single laboratory value.

When to Refer Urgently

Referral to nephrology is indicated in cases of stage 3 AKI, suspected nephritis, vasculitis, interstitial nephritis or myeloma, an uncertain cause, inadequate response to treatment, complications, or CKD stages 4–5. Obstructive uropathy requires rapid urological intervention (nephrostomy or stent, ideally within 12 hours once diagnosed).

Contrast and Procedures

For adults having iodine-based contrast, apply the 2024 NICE update: encourage oral hydration; consider IV volume expansion in very high-risk inpatients; weigh the risk–benefit in emergencies, do not delay necessary imaging (NICE, 2024). Frailty independently raises AKI risk and worsens outcomes; incorporate early medicines review, cautious fluid strategies, delirium prevention, and rapid mobilisation, and ensure post-AKI follow-up because of the heightened risk of CKD and readmission (Jiesisibieke et al., 2019).

Case Study 18.1   Complex Decision-Making by an AP in Frailty with AKI

Mr H, an 86-year-old man with known frailty (Clinical Frailty Scale 6), stage 3 chronic kidney disease, heart failure with preserved ejection fraction, mild cognitive impairment, and osteoarthritis, was admitted from a care home with acute confusion, poor oral intake and a two-day history of vomiting. Regular medication included furosemide, lisinopril, and ibuprofen as needed.

Initial Assessment

On arrival, he was hypotensive (blood pressure [BP] 92/58 mmHg), tachycardic, and afebrile, with dry mucous membranes and reduced urine output (<150 mL in the past 12 hours). Capillary refill was delayed. Blood tests revealed creatinine 210 µmol/L (baseline 115 µmol/L), urea 18 mmol/L, potassium 5.8 mmol/L, and C-reactive protein 82 mg/L. Urinalysis showed leucocytes and nitrites. Chest X-ray was clear, and renal ultrasound excluded obstruction.

Decision-making Process

The AP led the initial management. Using NICE (2024) AKI guidance, she rapidly identified stage 2 AKI superimposed on chronic kidney disease, likely pre-renal and septic in origin. Key decisions included:

Immediate stabilisation: with input from a critical care outreach nurse, she commenced cautious IV isotonic crystalloid (500 mL over 15 minutes, then reassessment) given the risk of fluid overload due to heart failure.

Medication review: she suspended lisinopril, furosemide, and PRN NSAIDs to avoid further renal hypoperfusion and hyperkalaemia.

Diagnostics and treatment: urine and blood cultures were obtained before starting empirical intravenous antibiotics for suspected urinary sepsis.

Electrolyte management: hyperkalaemia was treated promptly with IV calcium gluconate, insulin–glucose infusion, and nebulised salbutamol.

Advanced care planning: recognising the patient's frailty and fluctuating cognition, she discussed goals of care with family and the care-home general practitioner (GP), confirming that hospital-based escalation, including temporary renal replacement therapy, was appropriate if required.

Ongoing Management and Outcome

The AP arranged hourly urine output monitoring, daily weights, and serial blood tests. After 48 hours of careful fluid titration and antibiotic therapy, renal function improved (creatinine 140 μmol/L) and urine output normalised. The patient returned to his care home on day 5 with clear instructions for medicines re-initiation and a follow-up renal review.

This case highlights the complexity of AP decision-making: rapid recognition of AKI, balancing aggressive treatment against frailty-related risks, coordinating multi-professional care, and integrating shared decision-making. It illustrates how advanced practitioners can apply national guidance (NICE NG148 2024) with clinical judgement to optimise outcomes for frail adults.

Chronic Kidney Disease (CKD) in Older and Frail Adults

CKD is a persistent and usually progressive reduction in kidney function that is not reversible (NICE, 2025). It is frequent in later life, and its prevalence is rising as populations age and diabetes and hypertension become more common. Globally, around 9% of adults are affected, with diabetes contributing to up to half of cases (Webster et al., 2017; KDIGO, 2024). In the United Kingdom, more than 1.9 million adults carry a CKD diagnosis, though many remain undetected, and approximately 6% have moderate-to-severe impairment (G3–G5) (Molokhia et al., 2020). Rates are particularly high in older people, with studies showing several-fold greater prevalence in those over 75 years compared with younger adults (Fraser and Roderick, 2016; Hirst et al., 2020; BMJ Best Practice, 2022; NICE, 2025).

Identifying and Assessment

Impaired renal function is frequently detected incidentally through elevated urea or creatinine. The eGFR is now routinely reported and helps reveal early impairment. Even small creatinine rises are significant in frail or low-weight older adults because serum creatinine reflects muscle mass as well as filtration rate. Creatinine clearance calculated using equations such as Cockcroft–Gault (Cockcroft and Gault, 1976) or eGFR provide a more accurate guide for drug dosing and disease staging.

Aetiology

Common causes are long-standing hypertension, diabetes mellitus, chronic urinary obstruction (often prostate-related), glomerulonephritis, and renovascular disease. In a considerable number of late presentations, the cause remains unclear.

Management Principles

1. Confirm persistence: repeat renal function tests when the patient is clinically stable and correct reversible factors such as hypovolaemia or medication effects.
2. Slow disease progression: optimise blood pressure and glycaemic control, and consider ACE inhibitors or angiotensin receptor blockers if not contraindicated.
3. Prevent complications: review medicines, avoid nephrotoxic drugs and unnecessary contrast, adjust doses of renally excreted agents, and monitor for anaemia, mineral and bone disorders, acidosis, and hyperkalaemia.
4. Address cardiovascular risk: manage dyslipidaemia and atherosclerotic risk factors.
5. Plan ahead: estimate the rate of decline from serial eGFR values, arrange early nephrology input when impairment is moderate to severe, and discuss renal replacement or conservative care in the context of frailty and life expectancy.

Common Complications

Hypertension and hyperlipidaemia are both causes and consequences of CKD and require active treatment (NICE, 2025). Salt and water retention may lead to oedema, while secondary hyperparathyroidism, renal osteodystrophy, anaemia, peripheral or autonomic neuropathy, metabolic acidosis, and hyperkalaemia become more prominent as GFR falls (NICE, 2025). Table 18.2 shows the other renal conditions that affect elderly people.

TABLE 18.2 Other renal diseases that affect elderly people.

Condition	Pathophysiology	Typical presentation in later life	Common causes	Core investigations	Main management principles
Nephrotic syndrome	Increased glomerular permeability with heavy proteinuria (>3 g/day), hypoalbuminemia, oedema, and secondary hyperlipidaemia	Generalised oedema (often mistaken for cardiac failure), frothy urine, malaise, muscle wasting, and variable blood pressure; heightened risk of infection, thrombosis, and renal impairment	Membranous and minimal-change nephropathy, primary glomerulonephritis, and amyloidosis; secondary to diabetes, chronic infection, autoimmune disease, and malignancy; sometimes triggered by NSAIDs	Urinalysis and 24-h urinary protein, U&E, liver and thyroid tests, autoantibodies (antinuclear antibodies [ANA] and antineutrophil cytoplasmic antibodies [ANCA]), complement, hepatitis serology, serum and urine electrophoresis, renal ultrasound, and usually renal biopsy	Salt and fluid restriction, careful diuretic use, prophylactic anticoagulation if immobile, prompt infection surveillance, and disease-specific immunosuppression under nephrology supervision
Glomerulonephritis	Immune-mediated inflammation of glomeruli, causing haematuria and proteinuria with reduced filtration	Non-specific systemic illness (nausea, malaise, arthralgia, pulmonary infiltrates); may also present with hypertension, oedema, haematuria, red cell casts, or acute renal failure	Post-infectious (streptococcal and staphylococcal), autoimmune vasculitides (e.g. ANCA-associated), lupus nephritis, IgA nephropathy, and Goodpasture's disease; sometimes idiopathic	Same baseline tests as for nephrotic syndrome, plus disease-specific antibodies (e.g. anti-glomerular basement membrane [anti-GBM]), and renal biopsy for definitive diagnosis	Supportive therapy, blood pressure control, and early nephrology input; immunosuppressive treatment except in post-infectious cases; dialysis if severe
Renal artery stenosis	Atherosclerotic narrowing of the renal artery, reducing renal perfusion and activating renin–angiotensin system	Often asymptomatic; may present with resistant hypertension, unexplained rise in creatinine after ACE inhibitor, renal bruit, asymmetric kidney size, flash pulmonary oedema, or hypokalaemia	Predominantly atheromatous disease; rarely fibromuscular dysplasia in younger adults	Duplex Doppler, CT, or magnetic resonance imaging (MR) angiography if renal function allows, or digital subtraction angiography (gold standard)	Optimise cardiovascular risk management and blood pressure (avoiding ACE inhibitors if bilateral disease); revascularisation with angioplasty or stent if renal function deteriorates or hypertension remains uncontrolled

Source: Bowker et al. (2012)/with permission of Oxford University Press.

Case Study 18.2   AP Management of Renal Artery Stenosis in a Frail Older Adult

Patient Background

Mr H, an 82-year-old man with severe frailty (Clinical Frailty Scale 7), long-standing hypertension, and peripheral vascular disease, was referred to the same day emergency care (SDEC) service following a sudden rise in serum creatinine from 125 to 210 µmol/L over three weeks. He reported no urinary symptoms. His blood pressure remained persistently elevated (>180/95 mmHg) despite three antihypertensive agents, including an ACE inhibitor.

Assessment

An AP performed a comprehensive review. Physical examination revealed a right-sided abdominal bruit. There was no evidence of urinary tract obstruction on point-of-care ultrasound. The AP suspected renal artery stenosis precipitating acute kidney injury on chronic kidney disease.

Decision-making and Management

- Medication adjustment: The ACE inhibitor was withheld immediately in line with NICE NG203 guidance, recognising the risk of further renal perfusion compromise.
- Diagnostic strategy: The AP arranged computed tomography (CT) angiography after confirming eGFR was above the safety threshold for contrast, and discussed pre-hydration with the renal consultant to mitigate contrast-induced injury.
- Multidisciplinary coordination: Vascular surgery and nephrology teams were involved early to plan revascularisation if significant stenosis was confirmed.
- Risk communication and planning: The AP facilitated a discussion with the patient and family about the benefits and risks of angioplasty and stent placement versus conservative management, taking into account frailty and life expectancy.

Outcome

Imaging confirmed significant unilateral renal artery stenosis. After shared decision-making, the patient underwent successful percutaneous angioplasty with stent insertion. Post-procedure, blood pressure stabilised, and creatinine fell to 150 µmol/L.

Reflection on the AP Role

This case demonstrates how an AP integrates advanced assessment, interpretation of imaging, medicines optimisation, and shared decision-making to manage complex renal-vascular disease in a frail patient. The AP applied NICE CKD guidance (NG203) and evidence on renovascular hypertension to guide timely intervention and prevent further renal decline.

CONCLUSION

Renal ageing reduces reserve and blunts homeostatic responses, making frail older adults particularly susceptible to AKI, CKD, and related complications. Prompt recognition, evidence-based treatment, and careful medicines and fluid management can prevent irreversible damage and improve outcomes.

Advanced practitioners are central to early identification, coordination of multidisciplinary input and tailoring of interventions to each patient's comorbidities, preferences, and life expectancy.

Take-Home Messages

1. Renal ageing leads to reduced glomerular filtration rate, diminished renal blood flow, and impaired water–electrolyte homeostasis, increasing frailty-related vulnerability to AKI and CKD.

2. Even small rises in serum creatinine can indicate significant impairment in older or low-muscle-mass individuals.

3. Early recognition and treatment of AKI, including careful fluid management and medicines review, can prevent irreversible renal injury.

4. CKD prevalence increases sharply with age; proactive blood pressure, glycaemic, and cardio-vascular risk control can slow progression and reduce complications.

5. APs play a key role in integrating assessment, diagnostics, multidisciplinary input, and shared decision-making to deliver safe, person-centred renal care in frail older adults.

REFERENCES

BMJ Best Practice (2022). *Chronic Kidney Disease*. BMJ Best Practice https://bestpractice.bmj.com/topics/en-gb/65 (accessed 20 September 2025).

Bowker, L., Price, J., and Nicol, M. (2012). *Oxford Handbook of Geriatric Medicine*, 2e, 361–375. Oxford: Oxford University Press.

Cockcroft, D.W. and Gault, H. (1976). Prediction of creatinine clearance from serum creatinine. *Nephron* 16 (1): 31–41.

Fraser, S.D.S. and Roderick, P.J. (2016). Epidemiology of chronic kidney disease in the UK: trends, risk factors and outcomes. *Clinical Medicine* 16 (6): 614–618. https://doi.org/10.7861/clinmedicine.16-6-614.

Hirst, J.A., Hill, N.R., O'Callaghan, C.A., and Hobbs, F.D.R. (2020). Prevalence of chronic kidney disease in older people: systematic review. *Age and Ageing* 49 (6): 970–978. https://doi.org/10.1093/ageing/afaa145.

Jiesisibieke, Z.L., Tung, T.H., Xu, Q.Y. et al. (2019). Association of acute kidney injury with frailty in elderly population: a systematic review and meta-analysis. *Renal Failure* 41 (1): 1021–1027.

KDIGO (2012). KDIGO clinical practice guideline for acute kidney injury. *Kidney International. Supplement* 2 (1): 1–138.

Kidney Disease: Improving Global Outcomes (KDIGO) (2024). KDIGO clinical practice guideline for the evaluation and management of chronic kidney disease. *Kidney International. Supplement* 14 (1): 1–150.

Leach, R. (2014). *Critical Care Medicine at a Glance*, 3e. Chichester: Wiley-Blackwell.

Levey, A.S. and James, M.T. (2017). Acute kidney injury. *Annals of Internal Medicine* 167 (9): ITC66–ITC80.

Makris, K. and Spanou, L. (2016). Acute kidney injury: definition, pathophysiology and clinical phenotypes. *The Clinical Biochemist Reviews* 37 (2): 85.

Molokhia, M., Curcin, V., Majeed, A., and Saxena, S. (2020). Chronic kidney disease in primary care: prevalence and impact. *British Journal of General Practice* 70 (692): e278–e285. https://doi.org/10.3399/bjgp20X708125.

National Institute for Health and Care Excellence (NICE) (2023). *Acute Kidney Injury: AKI*. London: NICE https://cks.nice.org.uk/topics/acute-kidney-injury/background-information/definition/.

National Institute for Health and Care Excellence (NICE) (2024). Acute kidney injury: prevention, detection and management (Guideline NG148). Published 18 December 2019, last updated 16 October 2024. London: NICE. https://www.nice.org.uk/guidance/ng148

National Institute for Health and Care Excellence (NICE) (2025). Chronic kidney disease: background information – prevalence. Clinical Knowledge Summaries. https://cks.nice.org.uk/topics/chronic-kidney-disease/background-information/prevalence/ (accessed 21 September 2025).

Think Kidneys (2018). *Acute Kidney Injury: Guidance and Resources for Health and Social Care Staff*. UK Renal Registry.

Webster, A.C., Nagler, E.V., Morton, R.L., and Masson, P. (2017). Chronic kidney disease. *The Lancet* 389 (10075): 1238–1252. https://doi.org/10.1016/S0140-6736(16)32064-5.

CHAPTER 19

Endocrinology System

Aim

This chapter explores key endocrine disorders encountered in later life, highlighting how physiological ageing, frailty, and multimorbidity influence presentation, investigation, and management. It integrates current UK and European guidance to support advanced clinical practitioners in providing safe, individualised care that balances metabolic control with quality of life.

LEARNING OUTCOMES

By the end of this chapter, readers will be able to:

1. Explain the main age-related changes in endocrine physiology and their clinical relevance in frailty.
2. Critically appraise how ageing modifies the presentation and treatment goals for diabetes, thyroid disease, menopause, and adrenal disorders.
3. Apply evidence-based approaches to diagnosis and management, including the use of national guidelines and dynamic testing.
4. Demonstrate advanced clinical reasoning, ethical decision-making, and multidisciplinary collaboration when caring for frail older adults with endocrine disease.
5. Formulate patient-centred care plans that integrate symptom control, safety-netting, and end-of-life considerations.

SELF-ASSESSMENT QUESTIONS

1. In a frail older adult with type 2 diabetes, how would you individualise glycaemic targets and select therapies to minimise hypoglycaemia while addressing cardiovascular risk and polypharmacy?

2. An 82-year-old with new weight loss, fast atrial fibrillation, suppressed thyroid-stimulating hormone (TSH), and elevated FT4 is taking warfarin. Outline your immediate management, medicines-safety considerations (including anticoagulation), and longer-term options (antithyroid drugs versus radioiodine) tailored to frailty.

DIABETES AND FRAILTY

Diabetes mellitus becomes increasingly prevalent with advancing age and is a major endocrine concern in frailty. Recent data indicate that in England, the prevalence of both diagnosed and undiagnosed diabetes in people aged 65 years and over is approximately 21% (NHS Digital, 2022). Prevalence in the general adult population is lower (around 7–8%), but is considerably elevated in certain ethnic minority groups, especially Asian and Black communities. Both type 1 and type 2 diabetes may present in later life, although type 2 diabetes is by far the most common. Type 2 disease in older adults is usually driven by insulin resistance in peripheral tissues, whereas a minority of lean older adults develop a phenotype marked by impaired insulin secretion and islet autoimmunity, leading to poor response to oral hypoglycaemic agents and a clinical picture closer to type 1 diabetes. Increasing numbers of people with long-standing type 1 diabetes are now reaching older age, often after decades of insulin therapy with relatively few complications (Joint British Diabetes Societies Inpatient Care, 2023).

Older adults with type 2 diabetes frequently require escalation to insulin to maintain glycaemic stability, yet it is essential to distinguish between those who are insulin-dependent (type 1, requiring continuous insulin to avoid ketoacidosis) and those who are insulin-requiring (type 2, who can safely have insulin withheld for short periods). Secondary diabetes is also more frequent in later life, commonly triggered by corticosteroids, high-dose thiazide diuretics, chronic pancreatitis, or endocrine disorders such as Cushing's syndrome and hyperthyroidism (NICE, 2022).

Clinical presentation in frail older adults is often subtle. Classical symptoms such as polyuria, polydipsia, and weight loss may be absent or delayed because of age-related physiological changes, including reduced renal glucose excretion thresholds and diminished thirst perception. Consequently, many individuals remain undiagnosed until detected by opportunistic blood testing or during intercurrent illness (NICE, 2022). Presenting features may include delirium, falls, recurrent infections such as candidiasis or cellulitis, unexplained weight loss, or cardiovascular events.

Diagnosis follows standard biochemical thresholds for random, fasting, or post-prandial plasma glucose, confirmed by repeat measurement unless acute metabolic decompensation is evident. In some lean older patients, fasting glucose may be normal and post-prandial testing or oral glucose tolerance testing is required. HbA1c is valuable for monitoring but is insufficient alone for diagnosis (Joint British Diabetes Societies Inpatient Care, 2023).

Management in frailty prioritises symptom relief and quality of life over strict glycaemic normalisation. Tight glucose targets may confer short-term benefits such as improved mood or cognition but carry increased risks of hypoglycaemia, falls, and fractures. Reasonable targets for HbA1c are often 7.5–8.5%, with fasting glucose of 7–10 mmol/L. Guideline-based recommendations for frail older adults often favour higher HbA_1c targets (7.5–8.5%) and fasting glucose levels in the region of 7–10 mmol/L, balancing the potential cognitive or mood benefits of tighter control against elevated risks of hypoglycaemia, falls, and fractures (Leung et al., 2018; Joint British Diabetes Societies Inpatient Care, 2023). Lifestyle interventions, balanced nutrition, modest weight reduction, and light endurance exercise remain fundamental but must be tailored to cognitive and functional capacity. Education of patients, families, and care-home staff is crucial to ensure safe and consistent care.

Pharmacological therapy usually begins with oral agents. Metformin is preferred for overweight individuals with preserved renal function, while sulphonylureas are often chosen for lean patients with impaired insulin release, provided that there is careful monitoring for hypoglycaemia. Other options include pioglitazone and α-glucosidase inhibitors where appropriate. Insulin is indicated when oral agents are inadequate or contraindicated, when hyperglycaemia is severe, or in absolute insulin deficiency. Long-acting once-daily insulin regimens, supported by community or specialist diabetes nurses, often suit frail older adults. In advanced age, insulin requirements may fall as appetite, body mass, and renal function decline, allowing simplification or withdrawal of therapy (NICE, 2022).

Comprehensive surveillance remains essential. Annual review should include assessment of glycaemic control, weight, cardiovascular risk factors, renal function (including microalbuminuria), retinal health, oral health, and foot care. Early recognition and management of complications such as neuropathy, nephropathy, retinopathy, and vascular disease help preserve function and quality of life. Blood pressure control is particularly important for cardiovascular risk reduction, and statins and low-dose aspirin may be appropriate unless contraindicated (Joint British Diabetes Societies Inpatient Care, 2023).

Diabetic emergencies in older adults present unique challenges. Hyperosmolar hyperglycaemic state (previously called hyperosmolar non-ketotic state) carries high mortality and typically results from infection and severe dehydration (Alsararatee, 2024). Hypoglycaemia is more frequent with age because of attenuated counter-regulatory responses and blunted autonomic warning signs; it may mimic cerebrovascular events or contribute to cognitive decline and falls (NICE, 2022).

End-of-life care focuses on comfort (Alsararatee et al., 2025). Medication doses are gradually reduced as oral intake diminishes and renal clearance falls. In many people with type 2 diabetes, therapy can be simplified or discontinued, while those with type 1 diabetes require minimal basal insulin until the very final stage. Blood glucose monitoring is reduced to situations where symptoms of hypo- or hyperglycaemia occur, and rigid dietary restrictions are inappropriate. Diabetes within frailty demands an approach that balances metabolic control with the overarching aim of preserving well-being and dignity (Muszalik et al., 2022). Individualised goals, regular review, and close collaboration between primary care, specialist teams, and carers are key to safe and effective management in this vulnerable population.

HYPOTHYROIDISM IN OLDER ADULTS

Hypothyroidism is an endocrine disorder characterised by insufficient production or action of the thyroid hormones thyroxine (T4) and triiodothyronine (T3), leading to reduced metabolic activity in multiple organs (Chaker et al., 2022). Regulation involves a hypothalamic–pituitary–thyroid axis in which thyrotropin-releasing hormone stimulates pituitary secretion of thyroid-stimulating hormone, which in turn promotes thyroidal release of T4 and T3; much of the circulating T4 is subsequently converted to the biologically active T3 within peripheral tissues (Monteiro-Martins et al., 2024). Abnormal thyroid function tests (TFTs) may arise from non-thyroidal illness or from medicines that interfere with thyroid hormone production, metabolism, or assay accuracy; consultation of the British National Formulary (BNF) is advised when prescribing or interpreting results.

The prevalence of hypothyroidism rises steadily with age and is consistently higher in women. In iodine-sufficient settings such as the United Kingdom, spontaneous primary hypothyroidism affects about 1–2% of the general population, but the prevalence is up to ten times higher in women and increases with age (Mendes et al., 2019; Gottwald-Hostalek, 2022). A meta-analysis of 17 European studies reported a total prevalence of 3%, with subclinical hypothyroidism affecting 5.9% of women and 3.4% of men, and overt hypothyroidism affecting 0.8% of women and 0.3% of men (Garmendia Madariaga et al., 2014). A broader European review estimated overt hypothyroidism to range from 0.2–5.3% depending on diagnostic criteria

(BMJ Best Practice., 2024). UK-specific data also confirm age-related trends. Analysis of a large primary care dataset ($n = 66{,}843$) from North-East England found a point prevalence of treated hypothyroidism of 4.5% in 2016, with prevalence increasing in older age groups (Ingoe et al., 2017). National prescribing data show an increase in treated hypothyroidism from 2.3% to 3.5% of the United Kingdom population between 2005 and 2014, again with higher rates in women and older adults (Razvi et al., 2019).

Subclinical hypothyroidism, defined by raised serum TSH with normal free thyroxine, affects 5–10% of adults, with the highest frequencies in older women (Okosieme et al., 2016; Biondi, 2019). In a UK primary care screening study of people aged over 65 years, about 5% were found to have subclinical hypothyroidism (Chaker et al., 2022). However, physiological increases in TSH that occur with ageing may lead to overestimation of disease prevalence in the very old.

CLINICAL PRESENTATION

Onset is typically insidious over months or years, and manifestations are often subtle in older adults, becoming evident only during acute illness (NICE, 2024a,b). Possible features include cold intolerance, dry skin, thinning hair, weight change, constipation, malaise, reduced mobility, proximal muscle weakness, myalgia or arthralgia with raised creatine kinase, bradycardia, heart failure, pericardial or pleural effusion, and non-pitting oedema (myxoedema) (Figure 19.1). Neuropsychiatric changes such as low mood, slowed cognition, or rarely frank dementia may occur. Other findings can include delayed tendon reflex relaxation, gait disturbance, anaemia of various types, hyponatraemia, and lipid abnormalities. In many cases, only the response to treatment confirms that symptoms were thyroid-related (NICE, 2024a,b).

INVESTIGATION

Because clinical assessment is insensitive and treatment is straightforward, clinicians should maintain a low threshold for TFTs in older people. Opportunistic screening in primary or secondary care is reasonable, while recognising that severe systemic illness can transiently lower thyroid hormones (non-thyroidal illness or 'sick euthyroid' syndrome) (Bowker et al., 2012).

- Overt primary hypothyroidism is diagnosed when serum TSH is raised, and free thyroxine (FT4) is low.
- Subclinical (or compensated) hypothyroidism is defined by elevated TSH with normal FT4 and may carry an increased risk of atherosclerotic disease.
- Anti-thyroid peroxidase antibodies can support an autoimmune aetiology and guide management in subclinical disease. Any discrete thyroid nodule warrants ultrasound and, if indicated, radionuclide imaging or fine-needle aspiration to exclude malignancy (Table 19.1) (NICE, 2024a,b).

MANAGEMENT

All patients with overt hypothyroidism should receive replacement therapy even if they feel well, as treatment usually improves energy and metabolic function. In subclinical disease, levothyroxine is recommended when there are symptoms, markedly raised TSH, borderline FT4, positive thyroid autoantibodies, or associated autoimmune disorders. Others can be monitored at six- to twelve-month intervals, starting therapy if progression occurs.

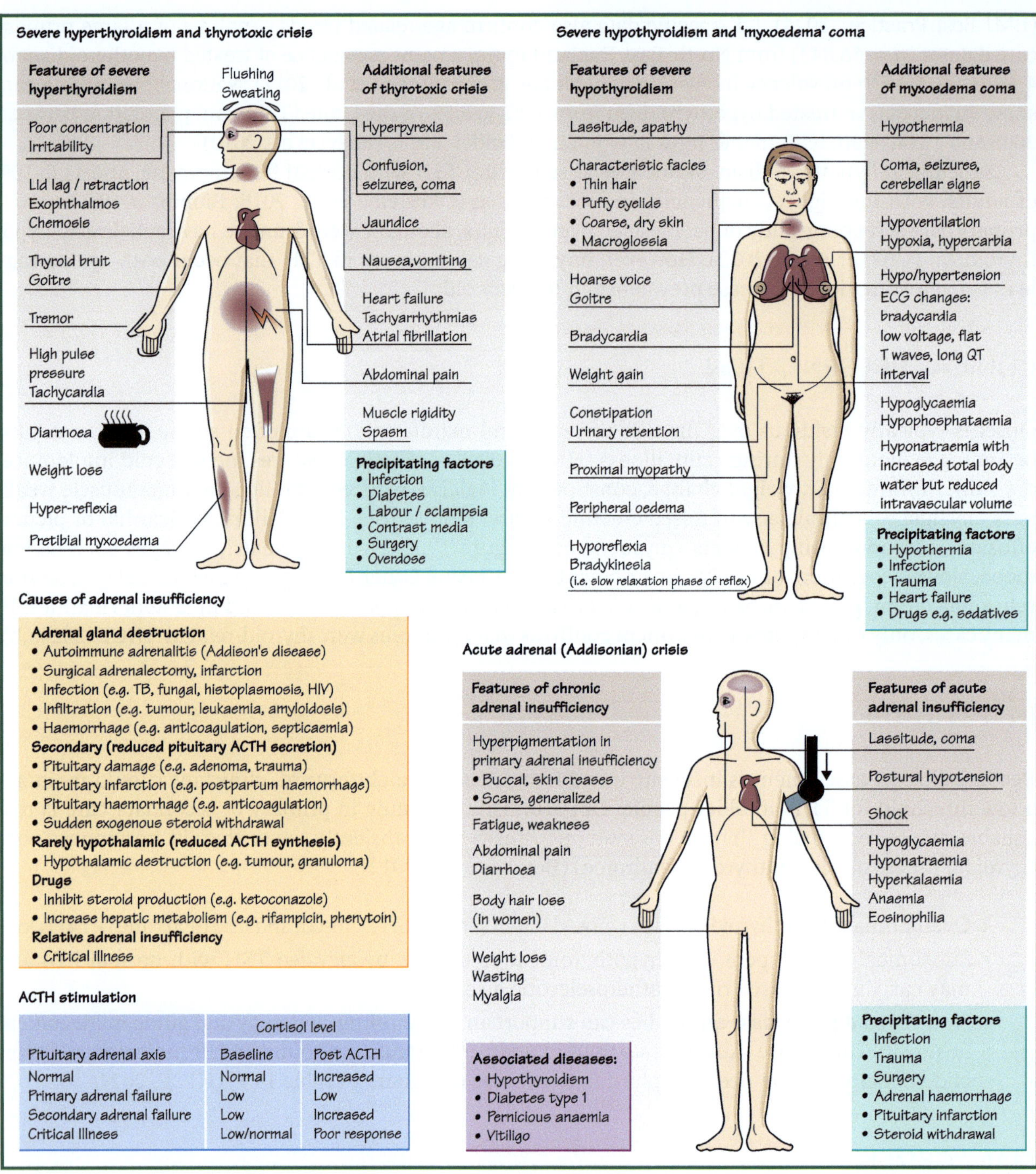

ACTH stimulation

Pituitary adrenal axis	Cortisol level	
	Baseline	Post ACTH
Normal	Normal	Increased
Primary adrenal failure	Low	Low
Secondary adrenal failure	Low	Increased
Critical illness	Low/normal	Poor response

FIGURE 19.1   Endocrine emergencies. *Source*: Leach (2014)/John Wiley & Sons.

TABLE 19.1 Interpretation of thyroid function test patterns.

TSH result	Free T4/free T3 pattern	Most consistent diagnosis	Other possible explanations
Low	Raised	Thyrotoxicosis, e.g. toxic solitary nodule	Graves' disease; thyroid inflammation; excess thyroid hormone therapy; post-radioiodine therapy; accidental or deliberate over-replacement
Low	Reduced	Non-thyroidal illness (sick euthyroid syndrome)	Secondary or pituitary-related hypothyroidism
High	Reduced	Primary hypothyroidism	Post-operative or post-radioiodine ablation; after external neck irradiation
High	Normal	Subclinical hypothyroidism	Recovery phase after systemic illness; inconsistent use of levothyroxine; medication effects
High	Raised	Rare, usually a TSH-secreting pituitary tumour	Laboratory error; inconsistent levothyroxine use
Normal	Reduced	Central (pituitary or hypothalamic) hypothyroidism	Drug-related assay interference

Adapted from Bowker et al. (2012) and NICE (2024a).

Levothyroxine is introduced cautiously, often at 25 µg daily, with dose titration every four to six weeks guided by TSH levels. The aim is to maintain TSH within the mid-normal range (around 1–3 mU/L). Over-replacement risks atrial fibrillation and osteoporosis, whereas under-treatment may result in persistent lethargy and cognitive impairment. Most older adults require 50–125 µg daily, adjusted for body weight (NICE, 2024a,b).

Long-term, thyroid status and dosage should be reviewed annually (British Thyroid Foundation, 2025). Because absorption is impaired by food, the tablet is best taken on an empty stomach. Missed doses can be taken when remembered, and occasional twice-weekly or weekly dosing with higher amounts can be used where adherence is difficult.

DRUG INTERACTIONS

Numerous medicines can affect thyroxine absorption or metabolism. Enzyme-inducing antiepileptics (e.g. phenytoin, carbamazepine, and primidone), barbiturates, and rifampicin accelerate hormone breakdown (Centanni et al., 2025). Iron salts, calcium supplements, colestyramine, and aluminium-containing antacids reduce absorption and should be separated from thyroxine by at least two hours. Amiodarone has complex, often biphasic effects, and β-blockers may inhibit the conversion of T4 to triiodothyronine (T3). As thyroid function normalises, dosage adjustments of insulin, oral hypoglycaemic agents, digoxin, warfarin, theophylline, and corticosteroids may be necessary.

HYPERTHYROIDISM IN OLDER ADULTS

Hyperthyroidism refers to excessive synthesis and release of thyroid hormones from the thyroid gland itself, resulting in raised circulating levels of thyroxine and triiodothyronine (Shahid et al., 2023). Thyrotoxicosis describes the clinical state of thyroid hormone excess in the bloodstream, whatever its origin, and therefore includes but is not limited to hyperthyroidism (NICE, 2025). Hyperthyroidism becomes more common with increasing age and is an important consideration in frailty, where subtle or atypical manifestations can delay diagnosis. A European meta-analysis of 17 population studies reported an overall prevalence of 0.75% for hyperthyroidism (diagnosed and undiagnosed) and an incidence of 51 per 100,000 person-years, with higher rates in women (82 per 100,000) than men (16 per 100,000) (Garmendia Madariaga et al., 2014).

Subclinical disease is particularly relevant in frailty. The prevalence of subclinical hyperthyroidism rises with age and may reach around 2% in people aged over 65 years, as shown in an English community survey of 5,950 older adults (Franklyn and Boelaert, 2012). A recent review places the overall prevalence of subclinical hyperthyroidism at 0.7–1.4% in general adult populations but emphasises the higher frequencies in elderly cohorts (Lee and Pearce, 2023). Earlier UK studies support these trends. The Whickham community survey reported hyperthyroidism in 2.7% of women and 0.23% of men, with incidence estimates of 100–200 cases per 100,000 per year, findings largely attributed to middle-aged and older groups (Tunbridge et al., 1977). A subsequent UK follow-up confirmed prevalence of 0.5–2% in women, again with strong age and sex effects (NICE, 2025).

AETIOLOGY

The most frequent cause in older people is toxic multinodular goitre, which typically evolves slowly from a previously euthyroid multinodular gland to autonomous hormone secretion. Graves' disease remains an important autoimmune cause but often presents without classical goitre or ophthalmopathy (NICE, 2025). Other recognised aetiologies include inadvertent over-replacement with levothyroxine, iodine excess (for example, from amiodarone or contrast media), transient thyroiditis (including subacute or Hashimoto's thyroiditis in its destructive phase), and less commonly solitary autonomous nodules, thyroid carcinoma secreting T4, or TSH-producing pituitary tumours.

CLINICAL PRESENTATION

Older adults frequently show non-specific or atypical manifestations. Weight loss, fatigue, anorexia, mood change, or depression, muscle weakness and functional decline may predominate ('apathetic hyperthyroidism') (Figure 19.1). Classical adrenergic features, such as tremor, palpitations, heat intolerance, and sweating, are often absent or muted, especially if the person is taking β-blockers. Cardiovascular complications, notably atrial fibrillation, heart failure, and angina, are relatively common. Increased bone turnover may cause osteoporosis or hypercalcaemia (NICE, 2025).

INVESTIGATION

A low threshold for thyroid function testing is recommended in older patients, particularly those with cardiovascular disease or unexplained weight loss.

- Overt hyperthyroidism is characterised by suppressed or undetectable TSH with raised FT4 and/or FT3.
- Subclinical hyperthyroidism shows persistently low TSH with normal FT4 and FT3.

If TSH is only mildly suppressed (0.1–0.5 mU/L), drugs or intercurrent illness should be excluded. Measurement of thyroid autoantibodies supports a diagnosis of Graves' disease. Radioisotope scanning can distinguish between diffuse uptake (Graves'), multiple autonomous nodules (toxic nodular goitre), or low uptake (thyroiditis).

MANAGEMENT

Treatment aims to prevent complications such as atrial fibrillation and bone loss and to alleviate symptoms (NICE, 2025).

* Thionamides (carbimazole or propylthiouracil) are used for initial control and, in Graves' disease, may achieve long-term remission.
* β-blockers provide rapid relief of adrenergic symptoms and are particularly useful in coexisting cardiac disease.
* Radioiodine therapy offers definitive treatment and is well tolerated in older adults; most patients eventually require lifelong levothyroxine replacement.
* Surgery is rarely needed and is reserved for selected cases, such as a very large goitre or intolerance of other therapies.

Subclinical hyperthyroidism warrants treatment if TSH is persistently <0.1 mU/L or if the person has risk factors such as osteoporosis or cardiovascular disease; otherwise, careful three- to six-monthly review is appropriate (Bowker et al., 2012).

Learning Event: Advanced Practice Decision-Making for Hyperthyroidism in a Frail Older Adult

Presentation

Mrs P, 82, lives alone with four daily care visits. Background: hypertension, paroxysmal atrial fibrillation (on warfarin), osteoporosis, and mild cognitive impairment. She presents to same day emergency care with six-week weight loss, fatigue, and new exertional breathlessness. Pulse 106 bpm irregular; blood pressure (BP) 148/74 mmHg; hand tremor minimal; no eye signs. Electrocardiogram (ECG) confirms fast AF. Thyroid function: TSH <0.01 mU/L, FT4 29 pmol/L, FT3 7.2 pmol/L.

As the advanced practitioner (AP) leading the front-door assessment, you consider aetiology, risk, and feasibility of therapies in the context of frailty and polypharmacy. You explain that hyperthyroidism can precipitate atrial fibrillation (AF) and bone loss in older adults and that rapid symptom control with a β-blocker plus disease-modifying therapy is standard (NICE NG145).

Diagnostic Reasoning

Absence of ophthalmopathy and a nodular thyroid on examination raises suspicion of toxic multinodular goitre, common in later life. You arrange thyroid receptor antibody testing and a radionuclide uptake scan as an outpatient to confirm the pattern (diffuse versus nodular) (NICE, 2025).

Immediate Management and Medicines Safety

You begin low-dose bisoprolol for symptomatic control and initiate carbimazole with written 'stop and seek help' advice about fever, sore throat, or mouth ulcers given the risk of agranulocytosis; you order baseline full blood count (FBC) and liver function tests (LFTs) (NICE, 2025). You also alert the anti-coagulation clinic because hyperthyroidism heightens sensitivity to warfarin, and dose requirements may change as the thyroid state is corrected (Howard-Thompson et al., 2014).

Legal and Ethical Aspect

Capacity is decision-specific. Mrs P understands the nature, benefits, material risks, and alternatives to treatment when information is presented with written prompts and involve-a-relative consent aids. She can weigh options and communicate a choice; she therefore has the capacity for this decision as per the Mental Capacity Act 2005 Code of Practice (UK Government, 2007). You document this using the General Medical Council (GMC) framework for shared decision-making and consent, ensuring discussion of material risks and reasonable alternatives in line with the GMC Guidance (2024).

As an AP, you anchor practice in the Nursing and Midwifery Council (NMC) Code: prioritise people, practise effectively, preserve safety, and promote professionalism and trust, particularly important when discussing risk, uncertainty, and follow-up (NMC, 2024).

The Shared Decision

Three options are set out in plain language with written summaries:

1. Antithyroid drugs (ATDs) long-term
2. Likely to control biochemistry; remission is less certain in nodular autonomy; requires monitoring; agranulocytosis is rare but serious. Suitable when radioiodine is impractical or declined (NICE, 2025).
3. Radioiodine (I-131)
4. High probability of durable control in nodular autonomy; often results in hypothyroidism needing replacement; requires radiation-safety precautions after dosing that can be challenging when carers and grandchildren visit frequently (NICE, 2025).
5. Surgery
6. Rarely first-line in frailty; considered for very large goitre or when other modalities are unsuitable; requires optimisation to euthyroid state first (NICE, 2025).

Mrs P initially leans towards radioiodine 'to be done with it' but is anxious about temporary separation from family carers and her great-grandchildren. You explore what matters to her—remaining at home with minimal disruption—using the GMC 'what matters to the patient' prompts and provide local nuclear medicine written advice so she can visualise practical restrictions (GMC, 2024).

MDT Collaboration

You convene a same-day virtual multidisciplinary team (MDT) involving endocrinology, cardiology, nuclear medicine, community pharmacy, and the frailty team.

- Endocrinology: confirms likely nodular autonomy; either ATD or radioiodine acceptable; suggests 'titration' regimen with carbimazole and reassessment at six to eight weeks (NICE, 2025).

- Cardiology/anticoagulation advises tighter international normalised ratio (INR) surveillance during thyrotoxicosis and after biochemical control because warfarin dose often needs reduction then escalation as euthyroidism returns (Howard-Thompson et al., 2014).

- Nuclear medicine: outlines home-precaution requirements post-I-131 and the need to limit close contact with children; provides written materials.

- Frailty team: reviews falls risk and bone health; recommends expedited dual-energy X-ray absorptiometry (DXA) review and fracture prevention plan given the catabolic state of thyrotoxicosis (NICE, 2025).

- All strands and rationales are documented in the consent note (GMC, 2024; NMC, 2024).

Outcome and Review

A shared plan is agreed: start carbimazole plus bisoprolol, weekly INR for four weeks, and community nursing checks. You book radionuclide scanning and a six-week review to revisit radioiodine once symptoms have settled. You provide blood-test schedules, red-flag advice for possible agranulocytosis, and a single point of contact. At review, TSH remains suppressed, but FT4 normalises; AF is rate-controlled; weight stabilises. Mrs P now prefers radioiodine and, having read the materials and arranged respite support, gives informed consent. She receives I-131 as an outpatient, follows exposure-reduction advice at home, and converts to hypothyroidism at three months, starting levothyroxine with annual monitoring thereafter (NICE NG145; UK radiation-safety guidance) (NICE, 2025).

Reflective Analysis

- Reasoning under uncertainty: initial therapy chosen to reduce immediate cardiovascular risk and allow time for values-based deliberation.

- Legal–ethical rigour: capacity assessed and recorded; material risks and alternatives discussed per Montgomery; dialogue structured by GMC consent guidance; practice aligned with the NMC Code.

- Communication: written and verbal information tailored to mild cognitive impairment; daughter included with the patient's permission; safety-netting explicit.

- System leadership: the AP coordinated an MDT across acute, community, and nuclear medicine services, aligning with NICE guidance and local policies.

MENOPAUSE AND (HORMONE REPLACEMENT THERAPY) HRT

Menopause is usually diagnosed clinically (typical age 45–55 years) (Monteleone et al., 2018). For burdensome vasomotor or genitourinary symptoms, HRT is first-line after individualised, informed discussion of benefits and risks; combined HRT increases breast cancer risk in a duration-dependent manner, and this risk diminishes after cessation, whereas HRT is not recommended solely for osteoporosis prevention in older age (British Menopause Society, 2023). Use local non-systemic oestrogens for isolated vulvovaginal atrophy when appropriate. Decisions in frailty should balance symptom relief against comorbidity, polypharmacy, and falls/fracture risk.

Case Study 19.1   Advanced Practice and Menopause/HRT in Frailty

Mrs T, a 72-year-old woman living in a supported housing complex, presents with severe vulvovaginal atrophy causing pain, recurrent urinary infections and sleep disturbance. She is known to the community services for long-term management of hypertension, atrial fibrillation, and osteoporosis. Despite her age, she reports that quality of life is dominated by urogenital discomfort.

The AP conducts a comprehensive assessment, reviewing falls risk, cognitive status and current medication, and liaises with the pharmacist to check for drug interactions. In multidisciplinary discussion with the patient's general practitioner (GP), gynaecology specialist nurse and continence physiotherapist, local vaginal oestrogen is agreed as first-line. The AP leads an in-depth, shared decision-making consultation, explaining that systemic HRT is not indicated for osteoporosis prevention at her age but that topical therapy carries minimal systemic absorption.

During follow-up, the AP monitors symptom relief, blood pressure, and endometrial safety, while coordinating with the pharmacist and district nurse to ensure correct application and adherence. This case illustrates advanced clinical reasoning balancing symptom control and safety in frailty, integrating national guidance (British Menopause Society, 2023), and demonstrating inter-professional leadership and patient-centred communication.

PRIMARY ADRENAL INSUFFICIENCY (ADDISON'S DISEASE)

Primary adrenal insufficiency (Addison's disease) remains uncommon but carries particular significance in frailty because even mild hormonal deficiency can precipitate acute decompensation during intercurrent illness. In the United Kingdom, autoimmune Addison's disease is estimated to affect roughly 1 in 14,000 people, with around 9,000 diagnosed cases and about 320 new cases annually (Addison's Disease Clinical Advisory Panel, 2020). Although the onset typically occurs between 30 and 50 years, late diagnosis or survival into older age means that a substantial proportion of patients are now living into frailty. Older adults are more likely to present atypically and to experience adrenal crisis during physical or psychological stress, highlighting the need for vigilance in frailty care. Female sex is a recognised risk factor (Betterle, 2019; Thomsen, 2020).

PRESENTATION

Onset is typically gradual and non-specific in later life. Common features include fatigue, unintentional weight loss, anorexia, abdominal discomfort, nausea or constipation, orthostatic and resting hypotension, low mood or delirium, and functional decline; hypoglycaemia and mild anaemia may occur. Generalised or patchy hyperpigmentation of skin and mucosa can develop, but may be absent early. Biochemistry often shows hyponatraemia, hyperkalaemia, and a mild metabolic acidosis. Intercurrent illness, trauma, or psychological stress can precipitate adrenal crisis with shock; this is a medical emergency (NICE, 2024b).

CAUSES

Autoimmune adrenalitis is most frequent (often alongside other autoimmune diseases). In older adults, past tuberculosis remains a consideration; less common causes include metastatic infiltration, lymphoma, haemorrhage/infarction, and drug-induced suppression (e.g. ketoconazole) (NICE, 2024b).

DIAGNOSIS

Use a low threshold for testing in frailty. A single random cortisol is unreliable because secretion is pulsatile; an 08:00 serum cortisol >400 nmol/L makes adrenal insufficiency unlikely, whereas <100 nmol/L strongly suggests the diagnosis (values between these ranges require dynamic testing) (NICE, 2024b). The short adrenocorticotropic hormone (ACTH) (Synacthen®) stimulation test is the preferred confirmatory test. Check adrenal autoantibodies and consider chest imaging if tuberculosis is suspected; adrenal computed tomography/magnetic resonance imaging (CT/MRI) can help distinguish autoimmune atrophy (small glands) from infection or tumour (enlarged glands). Always differentiate primary from secondary insufficiency (pituitary disease): ACTH is high in primary and low/normal in secondary (NICE, 2024b).

MANAGEMENT

Emergency (suspected crisis): do not delay. Give intravenous (IV) normal saline, correct electrolytes, and administer hydrocortisone 100 mg IV/IM (intramuscular) immediately, then regularly (e.g. six-hourly) with ongoing fluids; improvement is usually prompt. Issue and document a Steroid Emergency Card and provide sick-day rules (Bornstein et al., 2016; NICE, 2024b).

Long-term: physiological glucocorticoid replacement (usually hydrocortisone split dose; typical total 15–25 mg/day) plus fludrocortisone for mineralocorticoid deficiency with monitoring of blood pressure, electrolytes, and symptoms (salt craving and postural dizziness). In older adults, hypertension may emerge and require fludrocortisone dose reduction and non-diuretic antihypertensives. Educate patients/carers on stress-dosing and parenteral rescue (NICE, 2024b).

Adrenal Incidentalomas

Incidentally discovered adrenal masses are increasingly found on imaging in older people. The key questions are 'Is it malignant?' and 'Is it functional?'. Current European guidance recommends: (1) early determination of benignity/malignancy with high-quality imaging (homogeneous, lipid-rich lesions are usually benign adenomas), (2) structured hormonal assessment for cortisol autonomy, catecholamine excess, and in hypertensive or hypokalaemic patients aldosterone excess, and (3) MDT review for indeterminate or suspicious lesions and for those with clinically significant hormone excess. Large tumours or radiologically concerning features warrant surgical referral.
(Adapted from Fassnacht et al., 2023).

CONCLUSION

Endocrine disorders in older adults present unique diagnostic and therapeutic challenges. Normal ageing alters hormone secretion and tissue responsiveness, while frailty amplifies vulnerability to metabolic instability, drug side effects, and acute decompensation. Conditions such as diabetes, hypo- and hyperthyroidism, menopausal symptoms, and adrenal insufficiency require nuanced targets that prioritise well-being and dignity. APs are pivotal in delivering comprehensive assessment, shared decision-making, and coordinated care across acute, primary, and community settings.

Take-Home Messages

1. Physiological changes of ageing, including subtle shifts in thyroid and glucose homeostasis, can mask or mimic disease.
2. Diabetes and thyroid disorders often present atypically in frailty; treatment goals should emphasise comfort and prevention of complications rather than tight biochemical control.
3. Menopausal symptoms can remain clinically significant in older women; local oestrogen is preferred, and systemic HRT requires careful risk–benefit appraisal.
4. Addison's disease and adrenal crisis, though rare, carry high mortality; rapid recognition and immediate steroid replacement are life-saving.
5. Incidental adrenal masses demand structured imaging, hormonal assessment, and multidisciplinary team review to identify malignancy or hormone excess.
6. Advanced clinical practitioners must integrate diagnostic acumen with ethical reasoning, clear communication, and leadership of multidisciplinary care to optimise endocrine health in later life.

REFERENCES

Addison's Disease Clinical Advisory Panel (2020). Addison's disease: current UK epidemiology and clinical management.

Alsararatee, H.H. (2024). The role of ACPs in recognising and treating diabetic ketoacidosis and hyperosmolar hyperglycaemic state. *British Journal of Nursing* 33 (18): 868–875.

Alsararatee, H.H., Mukhtar, M., and Musawar, A. (2025). Ethical principles and challenges in end-of-life care for frail older adults. *British Journal of Nursing* 34 (11): 547–553.

Betterle, C. (2019). Epidemiology of Addison's disease. *Endocrinology and Metabolism Clinics* 48 (4): 731–746.

Biondi, B. (2019). Natural history, diagnosis and management of subclinical hypothyroidism in elderly people. *Endocrine* 66 (1): 63–71.

BMJ Best Practice (2024). *Hypothyroidism.* London: BMJ Publishing Group.

Bornstein, S.R., Allolio, B., Arlt, W. et al. (2016). Diagnosis and treatment of primary adrenal insufficiency: an endocrine society clinical practice guideline. *The Journal of Clinical Endocrinology & Metabolism* 101 (2): 364–389.

Bowker, L., Price, J., and Smith, S. (2012). *Oxford Handbook of Geriatric Medicine,* 2e. Oxford: Oxford University Press.

British Menopause Society (BMS) (2023). *What Is The Menopause?* London: British Menopause Society. August 2023. `https://thebms.org.uk/wp-content/uploads/2023/08/17-BMS-TfC-What-is-the-menopause-AUGUST2023-A.pdf` (accessed 21 September 2025).

British Thyroid Foundation (BTF) (2025). Levothyroxine (T4). `https://www.btf-thyroid.org/new-levothyroxine-prescribing-guidance` (accessed 21 September 2025).

Centanni, M., Duntas, L., Feldt-Rasmussen, U. et al. (2025). ETA guidelines for the use of levothyroxine sodium preparations in monotherapy to optimise the treatment of hypothyroidism. *European Thyroid Journal* 14 (4): e250123.

Chaker, L., Razvi, S., Bensenor, I.M. et al. (2022). Publisher correction: hypothyroidism. *Nature Reviews Disease Primers* 8 (1): 39.

Fassnacht, M., Tsagarakis, S., Terzolo, M. et al. (2023). European Society of Endocrinology clinical practice guidelines on the management of adrenal incidentalomas, in collaboration with the European Network for the Study of Adrenal Tumors. *European Journal of Endocrinology* 189 (1): G1–G42.

Franklyn, J.A. and Boelaert, K. (2012). Thyrotoxicosis. *The Lancet* 379 (9821): 1155–1166.

Garmendia Madariaga, A., Santos Palacios, S., Guillén-Grima, F., and Galofré, J.C. (2014). The incidence and prevalence of thyroid dysfunction in Europe: a meta-analysis. *The Journal of Clinical Endocrinology & Metabolism* 99 (3): 923–931.

General Medical Council (2024). *Decision Making and Consent.* London: GMC `https://www.gmc-uk.org/professional-standards/the-professional-standards/decision-making-and-consent` (accessed 21 September 2025).

Gottwald-Hostalek, U. (2022). Hypothyroidism in the elderly: challenges in diagnosis and treatment. *Drugs & Aging* 39 (1): 1–12.

Howard-Thompson, A., Luckey, A., George, C. et al. (2014). 'Graves' disease and treatment effects on warfarin anticoagulation. *Case Reports in Medicine* 1: 292468.

Ingoe, L., Phipps, N., Armstrong, G. et al. (2017). Prevalence of treated hypothyroidism in the community: analysis from general practices in North-East England with implications for the United Kingdom. *Clinical Endocrinology* 87 (6): 860–864.

Joint British Diabetes Societies Inpatient Care (2023). *JBDS 15: Inpatient care of the frail older adult with diabetes.* London: Association of British Clinical Diabetologists Available at: `https://abcd.care/sites/default/files/site_uploads/JBDS_Guidelines_Current/JBDS_15_Inpatient_Care_of_the%20Frail_Older_Adult_with_Diabetes_with_QR_code_February_2023.pdf`.

Leach, R.M. (2014). *Critical Care Medicine at a Glance*, 3e. Wiley Blackwell.

Lee, S.Y. and Pearce, E.N. (2023). Hyperthyroidism: a review. *JAMA* 330 (15): 1472–1483.

Leung, E., Wongrakpanich, S., and Munshi, M.N. (2018). Diabetes management in the elderly. *Diabetes Spectrum: A Publication of the American Diabetes Association* 31 (3): 245.

Mendes, D., Alves, C., Silverio, N., and Marques, F.B. (2019). Prevalence of undiagnosed hypothyroidism in Europe: a systematic review and meta-analysis. *European Thyroid Journal* 8 (3): 130–143.

Monteiro-Martins, S., Sterenborg, R.B., Borisov, O. et al. (2024). New insights into the hypothalamic–pituitary–thyroid axis: a transcriptome- and proteome-wide association study. *European Thyroid Journal* 13 (3): e240067.

Monteleone, P., Mascagni, G., Giannini, A. et al. (2018). Symptoms of menopause—global prevalence, physiology and implications. *Nature Reviews Endocrinology* 14 (4): 199–215.

Muszalik, M., Stępień, H., Puto, G. et al. (2022). Implications of the metabolic control of diabetes in patients with frailty syndrome. *International Journal of Environmental Research and Public Health* 19 (16): 10327.

National Institute for Health and Care Excellence (NICE) (2022). *Type 2 Diabetes in Adults: Management (NICE Guideline NG28)*. London: NICE https://www.nice.org.uk/guidance/ng28 (accessed 21 September 2025).

National Institute for Health and Care Excellence (NICE) (2024a). Clinical knowledge summaries: hypothyroidism. https://cks.nice.org.uk/topics/hypothyroidism/ (accessed 21 September 2025).

National Institute for Health and Care Excellence (NICE) (2024b). *Clinical Knowledge Summaries: Addison's Disease – Prevalence*. London: NICE https://cks.nice.org.uk/topics/addisons-disease/background-information/prevalence/ (accessed 21 September 2025).

National Institute for Health and Care Excellence (NICE) (2025) *Clinical Knowledge Summaries: Hyperthyroidism*. https://cks.nice.org.uk/topics/hyperthyroidism/ (accessed 21 September 2025).

NHS Digital (2022). *Health Survey for England, 2021: Adults' Health – Diabetes*. London: NHS Digital https://digital.nhs.uk/data-and-information/publications/statistical/health-survey-for-england/2021-part-2/adult-health-diabetes (accessed 21 September 2025).

Nursing and Midwifery Council (2024). *The Code: Professional Standards of Practice and Behaviour for Nurses, Midwives and Nursing Associates*. London: NMC https://www.nmc.org.uk/standards/code/ (accessed 21 September 2025).

Okosieme, O., Gilbert, J., Abraham, P. et al. (2016). Management of primary hypothyroidism: statement by the British Thyroid Association Executive Committee. *Clinical Endocrinology* 84 (6): 799–808.

Razvi, S., Korevaar, T.I., and Taylor, P. (2019). Trends, determinants, and associations of treated hypothyroidism in the United Kingdom, 2005–2014. *Thyroid* 29 (2): 174–182.

Shahid, M.A., Ashraf, M.A., and Sharma, S. (2023). *Physiology, Thyroid Hormone*. Treasure Island, FL: StatPearls Publishing.

Thomsen, A.F. (2020). Gender differences in autoimmune Addison's disease. *European Journal of Endocrinology* 182 (2): R27–R38.

Tunbridge, W.M.G., Evered, D.C., Hall, R. et al. (1977). The spectrum of thyroid disease in a community: the Whickham survey. *Clinical Endocrinology* 7 (6): 481–493.

UK Government (Department for Constitutional Affairs) (2007). *Mental Capacity Act 2005: Code of Practice*. London: TSO (current online version). https://www.gov.uk/government/publications/mental-capacity-act-code-of-practice (accessed 21 September 2025).

CHAPTER 20

Skin

Aim

To provide advanced practitioners (APs) with an in-depth understanding of common dermatological conditions affecting older adults, with a particular focus on cellulitis, chronic venous insufficiency, and leg ulceration, in order to enhance diagnostic accuracy, evidence-based management, and holistic care within frailty and end-of-life contexts.

LEARNING OUTCOMES

By the end of this chapter, readers should be able to:

1. Critically appraise the pathophysiological and clinical features of cellulitis, chronic venous insufficiency, and leg ulceration in frail older adults.
2. Evaluate diagnostic strategies, including microbiological, vascular, and histological assessments, in differentiating skin pathologies.
3. Formulate safe, evidence-based management plans that incorporate antimicrobial stewardship, wound care, compression therapy, and person-centred decision-making.
4. Reflect on the ethical, functional, and quality-of-life implications of skin disease in end-of-life care, integrating holistic and multidisciplinary perspectives.

SELF-ASSESSMENT QUESTIONS

1. What clinical indicators help to distinguish venous, arterial, and neuropathic ulcers in older adults, and how do these differences influence management?
2. How might frailty, polypharmacy, and multimorbidity alter the clinical presentation and therapeutic approach to cellulitis in older adults?

CELLULITIS IN OLDER ADULTS

Cellulitis is a deep bacterial infection of the skin and subcutaneous tissues that commonly affects the lower leg (NICE, 2025). Its incidence rises with advancing age, diabetes, immune compromise, and the presence of local skin breaches such as chronic ulcers, pressure injuries, lymphoedema, interdigital fungal infection, or minor trauma (Kumar et al., 2020). The usual pathogens are β-haemolytic streptococci, particularly *Streptococcus pyogenes*, and *Staphylococcus aureus*. In the context of open wounds or chronic lymphoedema, colonisation is often polymicrobial and may involve resistant organisms, including meticillin-resistant *S. aureus* (MRSA). The reported incidence of cellulitis varies widely, from 0.2 to 24.6 cases per 1,000 person-years, depending on the population studied (Dalal et al., 2017). Recurrence is frequent, and risk increases with each episode. In a large cohort of 36,276 adults with an initial episode of lower-limb cellulitis, 4,598 experienced at least one recurrence; cumulative incidences of first, second, and third recurrences were 6.3%, 17.2%, and 29.4% at 12 months, and 13.9%, 35.9%, and 52.9% at 5 years, respectively (Cannon et al., 2018).

Clinical Characteristics

The affected area is typically erythematous, warm, tender, and slightly raised with indistinct borders, and a cutaneous portal of bacterial entry is often identifiable (NICE, 2025). Systemic disturbance, fever, malaise, or rigors may develop. In some frail or cognitively impaired individuals, the presentation is non-specific, so a complete skin examination is important. Upward spread can result in lymphangitis and painful regional lymphadenopathy. Bacteraemia is not uncommon in nursing-home residents with pressure injuries and carries a mortality of up to 50% if inadequately treated (Bowker et al., 2012).

Assessment and Investigations

A full blood count may show leucocytosis, and blood cultures, ideally obtained before antimicrobial therapy, are positive in approximately one-quarter of cases. Local microbiological sampling, such as wound swabs, saline injection–aspiration or skin biopsy, is seldom required when empirical treatment is appropriate (NICE, 2025).

Management

For mild, uncomplicated disease in clinically stable individuals, oral therapy is suitable. Common first-line regimens are phenoxymethylpenicillin combined with flucloxacillin, erythromycin, or co-amoxiclav. The affected margin should be outlined with a waterproof marker to monitor progression, with review at 24–48 hours. Elevation of the limb limits oedema and blistering, reducing the risk of ulceration. Hospital admission and intravenous treatment with benzylpenicillin plus flucloxacillin or co-amoxiclav are indicated if there is systemic illness, lymphangitic spread, or failure of oral therapy. Intravenous therapy is continued until the erythema begins to recede, after which oral antibiotics complete a total course of up to two weeks, tailored to the clinical response. Broader-spectrum regimens should be initiated when cellulitis overlies ulcers, pressure injuries or chronic lymphoedema. Pain control, treatment of interdigital fungal infection, hydration assessment, and intravenous fluids when needed are integral components of care.

Condition	Typical features	Common sites/ organisms	Investigations	First-line management	When to escalate	Older adults
Erysipelas	Acute febrile illness; well-demarcated, bright erythema with oedema and pain; may follow a short flu-like prodrome; vesicles can rupture and crust	Face most often (bridge of nose and cheeks); also legs/arms/trunk; usually *Streptococcus pyogenes*	Clinical diagnosis; blood cultures if systemic illness	Parenteral benzylpenicillin for about 48 hours, then oral phenoxymethylpenicillin to complete about 10–14 days if not very mild	Admit if systemic toxicity, facial involvement with sepsis features, rapid progression, or poor oral intake	Bacteraemia is reported frequently; untreated mortality is substantial; recurrence over the life-course is common
Necrotising fasciitis	Severe, rapidly progressive pain and swelling; skin discolouration (violaceous), haemorrhagic bullae, and cutaneous anaesthesia; patient toxic with high fever	Limbs>trunk; Group A *Streptococcus* common; polymicrobial mixes may include *Staphylococci*, *Pseudomonas*, *Bacteroides*, diphtheroids, and coliforms	Urgent surgical review; bedside labs and blood cultures; imaging must not delay theatre	Immediate broad-spectrum IV antibiotics plus early surgical debridement	Any suspicion warrants emergency surgical assessment; haemodynamic instability or gas in tissues mandates immediate action	Early recognition is critical; review any 'cellulitis' that worsens over hours
Intertrigo	Superficial inflammation in opposing skin surfaces; soreness, maceration, fissuring; often pruritic	Flexures (groin, axillae, submammary, and inner thighs); friction and moisture predispose; secondary yeast infection is common	Clinical; consider skin scrapings if refractory	Meticulous hygiene; gentle cleansing and thorough drying; moisture control (absorbent powders/barrier preparations); topical imidazole ± 1% hydrocortisone; separate skin surfaces	Recalcitrant cases, recurrent secondary infection, or suspicion of alternative dermatoses for dermatology review	Incontinence, immobility and obesity increase risk; carer education is key

(*Continued*)

Condition	Typical features	Common sites/ organisms	Investigations	First-line management	When to escalate	Older adults
Dermatophyte infection (tinea)	Annular or sharply edged scaly lesions; pruritus; nail thickening/ discolouration if onychomycosis	Feet, groin, body, hands, nails, and scalp; Tinea spp.	Skin/nail scrapings for microscopy/ culture, where diagnosis is uncertain or before systemic therapy	Topical imidazole (e.g. clotrimazole) or topical terbinafine; consider oral terbinafine for resistant or nail/scalp disease once confirmed	Extensive disease, scalp involvement, or failure of topical therapy → consider systemic agents and specialist input	Check footwear, interdigital maceration; review liver function if considering systemic therapy
Candida (yeast) infection	Erythematous, sore, and macerated plaques in moist folds; satellite pustules; oral thrush with white plaques	Genital areas, flexures, peri-ungual skin, and oral cavity; risk with diabetes, poor denture fit, and broad-spectrum antibiotics	Clinical; swabs rarely needed unless refractory or recurrent	Topical imidazole for skin; combined steroid-antifungal short-term to settle inflammation; oral nystatin/miconazole/ amphotericin for thrush	Systemic symptoms or oesophageal disease → oral fluconazole; recurrent disease → review predisposing factors	Address moisture, glycaemic control, denture care and hygiene; consider drug interactions with azoles
Seborrhoeic dermatitis	Chronic erythematous and greasy scale; pruritus variable; may cause otitis externa or blepharitis	Scalp (dandruff), eyebrows/eyelids, nasolabial folds, post-auricular, beard, and central chest/ back; associated with Malassezia overgrowth	Clinical	Scalp: ketoconazole shampoo; skin folds/ face: ketoconazole wash and miconazole + 1% hydrocortisone cream; eyelids: warm compresses, lid hygiene, and short steroid course if needed	Severe, extensive, or refractory disease; suspected HIV or Parkinsonism warrants broader assessment	Relapsing course is usual; aim for control rather than cure; reinforce skin-care routines

CHRONIC VENOUS INSUFFICIENCY

Chronic venous insufficiency (CVI) is a frequent cause of leg discomfort, skin change, and ulceration in later life. It ranges from mild cosmetic concerns to persistent, painful ulceration that impairs mobility and independence. Prevalence increases with advancing age, obesity, prior leg trauma, superficial thrombophlebitis, and deep vein thrombosis (DVT). Long-term follow-up studies indicate that roughly one quarter of people with a history of DVT will develop venous insufficiency within two decades, and about 4% will eventually experience venous ulceration (Bowker et al., 2012). Although more cases are seen in women, this partly reflects female longevity.

Pathophysiology

CVI reflects failure of the calf-muscle venous pump and impaired venous return. Common mechanisms include post-thrombotic obstruction of the deep veins, incompetence of venous valves leading to reflux, and progressive microvascular changes with pericapillary fibrin deposition. These processes elevate venous pressure, damage the microcirculation, and set the stage for oedema, skin breakdown, and ulceration.

Clinical Manifestations

Varicose Veins

Early disease may present solely as superficial venous dilatation, often beginning with small submalleolar venous flares before progressing to tortuous, palpable varicosities. Symptoms can include aching, pruritus, superficial thrombophlebitis, or occasional bleeding. Support hosiery may relieve discomfort, and surgical ablation or endovenous procedures can be considered for symptomatic veins, but not when significant deep venous obstruction is present.

Oedema

Swelling typically worsens as the day progresses and improves with leg elevation. Patients may describe heaviness or fatigue in the legs. Low-dose thiazide diuretics can occasionally provide symptomatic relief but require careful monitoring because intravascular depletion is a risk in those who are not fluid overloaded.

Skin Changes

Persistent venous hypertension causes:

- Brown haemosiderin pigmentation from erythrocyte leakage.
- Telangiectasia and atrophic white scarring (atrophie blanche).
- Eczematous dermatitis with pruritic, weeping lesions that may respond to short courses of topical corticosteroids.
- Lipodermatosclerosis, in which fibrosis leads to circumferential induration and the characteristic 'inverted champagne bottle' lower-leg contour.

Venous Ulcers

Minor trauma to chronically inflamed skin can precipitate ulcer formation, typically in the gaiter region around the medial malleolus. Healing is slow, and recurrence is common without sustained compression therapy and management of underlying venous disease.

Leg Ulcers in Older Adults

Leg ulceration is a prevalent and costly condition, affecting about 1% of adults at any one time. Roughly half are purely venous in origin, about a tenth are arterial, a quarter have mixed venous–arterial aetiology, and the remainder arise from other causes such as diabetes, infection, vasculitis, haematological disorders, or malignancy (Bowker et al., 2012). Ulcers are often chronic, causing significant pain, immobility and psychosocial distress.

TYPICAL ULCER TYPES

Venous (Varicose) Ulcers

- Usually located around the medial malleolus along the line of the long saphenous vein.
- Shallow and tender, with irregular but non-undermined edges and a red or sloughy base.
- Accompanied by features of chronic venous insufficiency such as oedema, pigmentation, and lipodermatosclerosis.

Arterial (Ischaemic) Ulcers

- Appear on pressure or trauma sites, including the toes, heels, malleoli, and metatarsal heads.
- Deep, painful, and well-demarcated with a 'punched-out' appearance.
- Surrounding skin is pale, cool, and hairless, and peripheral pulses are diminished or absent.

Diabetic (Neuropathic) Ulcers

- Occur at weight-bearing areas of the foot.
- Typically, painless due to sensory neuropathy.
- Prone to infection and have undermined, irregular edges.

Malignant Ulcers

- Characteristically painless with raised or rolled edges.
- Suspect malignancy if an ulcer is non-healing or has an unusual appearance.

Principles of Assessment

Accurate identification of the underlying cause directs management. Clinical examination is supported by:

- Doppler ultrasound to detect venous obstruction or valve incompetence.
- Ankle–brachial pressure index (ABPI) to exclude or confirm arterial disease.

- Biopsy for suspected malignancy or for tissue culture when deep infection is a concern.
- Blood tests such as full blood count, glucose, erythrocyte sedimentation rate, and C-reactive protein, where systemic disease is possible.

General Management

- Encourage mobility and regular ankle exercises to enhance calf-muscle pump activity.
- Support smoking cessation.
- Provide adequate analgesia and simple, non-irritant dressings.
- Cleanse the ulcer with saline; routine antiseptic solutions are not recommended.
- Use systemic antibiotics only when there is clinical evidence of spreading infection.
- Reassess the diagnosis and care plan regularly if healing is delayed.

Venous Leg Ulcer Care

Venous ulcers are often chronic—median duration is around nine months—and recur frequently. Nevertheless, with appropriate treatment, around 70% will heal within three months.

Compression Therapy

Graduated, multilayer compression bandaging is the mainstay, applied only when ABPI is above 0.8. Compression reduces venous hypertension and enhances venous return. Bandages must be fitted by trained clinicians and adjusted for those with mixed arterial and venous disease. Intermittent pneumatic compression may be used when standard stockings are ineffective or poorly tolerated.

Elevation

Elevating the legs above heart level helps venous drainage and reduces oedema, though many older patients find this difficult to sustain. Elevating the foot of the bed during sleep is a practical alternative. Avoid elevation if significant arterial insufficiency is present.

Wound Care

Maintain a moist wound environment while avoiding maceration. Low-adherent dressings suffice in most cases; more complex impregnated products add cost and risk of contact dermatitis without proven benefit. Debridement of necrotic tissue, using gentle surgical techniques or larval therapy, may promote healing when appropriate.

Adjunctive Treatments

Low-dose aspirin and short courses of diuretics can be considered to aid healing or manage oedema. Pentoxifylline may have some benefit, but evidence is limited. Skin grafting or surgical correction of incompetent veins is an option when standard measures fail.

Condition	Key clinical features	Common triggers/risk factors	Essential investigations	First-line management	Points specific to frailty and older age
Malignant melanoma	Rapidly enlarging or colour-changing pigmented lesion; irregular outline; may bleed or itch; early metastasis	Sun exposure, fair skin, and family history	Dermoscopic assessment and excision biopsy	Wide surgical excision; oncology referral for advanced disease	Often detected late in older men; prognosis worsens with lesion thickness
Squamous cell carcinoma	Firm, indurated or hyperkeratotic nodule that may ulcerate; occasionally painful	Cumulative UV light, chronic scars or ulcers, and smoking	Biopsy for histology and margin planning	Surgical excision with ~5 mm margin; radiotherapy if surgery is unsuitable	May arise at ulcer edges; lymph node spread in 5–10%
Basal cell carcinoma	Pearly papule with rolled edge and surface telangiectasia ('rodent ulcer'); locally invasive but rarely metastatic	Sun damage, chronic scarring, and ionising radiation	Excision biopsy	Surgical excision or Mohs micrographic surgery; radiotherapy for recurrence or frail patients	Excellent survival, but local tissue destruction if ignored
Bullous pemphigoid	Chronic autoimmune blistering with tense bullae on erythematous or normal skin; pruritic, but the patient is usually well	Age >70 years; may follow trauma or drugs	Skin biopsy (linear IgG at basement membrane) and autoantibody assay	Potent topical or oral corticosteroids; consider steroid-sparing agents	Relapsing course; monitor for steroid adverse effects (osteoporosis and diabetes)
Severe blistering infections (e.g. cellulitis with bullae, impetigo and eczema herpeticum)	Rapid onset, painful erythema with vesicles or bullae; systemic upset possible	Streptococcal or staphylococcal infection, chronic ulcers, and eczema	Swabs and blood cultures if febrile	Prompt systemic antibiotics; wound care	Sepsis risk is higher in frail, immobile, or diabetic patients
Pruritus of systemic origin	Generalised itch often without rash; may disturb sleep and mood	Chronic kidney or liver disease, iron deficiency, haematological malignancy, thyroid disease, diabetes, and some drugs	FBC, ferritin, renal, and liver profiles, thyroid function, and glucose	Treat underlying cause; liberal emollients; antihistamines or menthol/urea creams for symptom relief	Persistent scratching can lead to infection or lichenification
Scabies (including Norwegian/crusted type)	Intense nocturnal itch; burrows on fingers, wrists, axillae, umbilicus, nipples, or groin	Close person-to-person contact and care-home outbreaks	Clinical; dermoscopy or skin scraping if uncertain	Whole-body permethrin or malathion for patient and close contacts; repeat in 7 days	Immunocompromised or frail patients may develop heavy mite loads requiring oral ivermectin and barrier nursing
Lichen simplex chronicus	Localised, thickened, lichenified plaque caused by repetitive scratching	Emotional stress and chronic pruritus	Clinical	Potent topical or intralesional steroids; capsaicin cream; occlusive dressings to break itch–scratch cycle	Behavioural support is vital when cognitive impairment contributes to scratching

Condition	Features	Causes/associations	Investigations	Management	Notes
Pruritus ani	Persistent perianal itching, sometimes with excoriation or secondary infection	Faecal soiling, loose stools, threadworm, and contact dermatitis	Consider swabs and stool tests for parasites	Improve hygiene (gentle cleansing and barrier creams); short course of topical steroid ± antifungal	Limited mobility and arthritis can hinder personal hygiene and prolong symptoms
Dermatophyte (tinea) infection	Scaly, annular, and itchy lesions; thickened nails (onychomycosis)	Warm and moist skin folds; occlusive footwear	Skin/nail scrapings for microscopy/culture	Topical imidazole or terbinafine; oral therapy if resistant or nail/scalp involvement	Monitor liver function if systemic antifungals are required
Candida (cutaneous or oral)	Erythematous, sore plaques with satellite pustules in flexures or oral mucosa	Diabetes, antibiotics, poor denture fit, and high moisture	Clinical; swab if recurrent	Topical imidazole ± mild steroid; oral nystatin or fluconazole if extensive	Rigorous moisture control and denture care reduce recurrence
Seborrhoeic dermatitis	Greasy, erythematous scaling on scalp, face (eyebrows and nasolabial folds), and chest	Overgrowth of *Malassezia* yeast; Parkinson's disease; HIV	Clinical	Ketoconazole shampoo or wash; miconazole + mild topical steroid for inflamed areas	Chronic relapsing course; regular maintenance treatment is often needed
Asteatotic (xerotic) eczema	Dry, cracked, and itchy skin, especially on shins and forearms	Reduced skin lipids in ageing, over-washing, and cold weather	Clinical	Liberal emollients (paraffin-based for severe dryness); avoid hot baths and harsh soaps	Prevent excoriation and secondary infection by keeping nails short
Actinic keratoses	Rough, scaly patches on sun-exposed skin; premalignant	Chronic ultraviolet exposure	Clinical; confirm with biopsy if doubtful	Cryotherapy, topical 5-fluorouracil, or diclofenac	Monitor for progression to squamous cell carcinoma
Bowen's disease	Well-demarcated, erythematous scaly plaques (intraepidermal carcinoma)	Sun damage, arsenic, and HPV	Skin biopsy	Cryotherapy, curettage, topical 5-fluorouracil, or surgical excision	Small risk of invasive squamous carcinoma—ensure follow-up
Lentigo maligna	Slowly enlarging irregular pigmented macule on sun-exposed skin	Chronic UV exposure	Dermoscopy and biopsy	Surgical excision or careful monitoring if frail	May transform into invasive melanoma if untreated
Benign lesions (seborrhoeic warts, skin tags, and Campbell de Morgan spots)	Seborrhoeic warts: 'stuck-on' brown plaques; skin tags: soft pedunculated growths; Campbell de Morgan spots: bright red papules	Ageing skin and friction	Clinical	Removal for cosmetic reasons (cryotherapy, curettage, or simple excision)	Reassure regarding benign nature; treat only if symptomatic or for appearance

CONCLUSION

Dermatological conditions such as cellulitis, chronic venous insufficiency, and leg ulcers are common in frail populations, often reflecting broader physiological decline and impaired tissue repair. Accurate assessment, early recognition of complications, and integrated multidisciplinary care are essential to improving comfort, preventing sepsis, and preserving dignity at the end of life.

Take-Home Messages

1. Skin disorders in frailty often present atypically and require a comprehensive clinical assessment.
2. Cellulitis in older adults carries significant morbidity and mortality; early treatment and prevention of recurrence are paramount.
3. Chronic venous insufficiency and leg ulcers demand long-term management strategies centred on compression, mobility, and wound optimisation.
4. Ethical considerations, including comfort, autonomy, and proportionality of interventions, are integral in end-of-life dermatological care.
5. Multidisciplinary collaboration between nurses, physicians, tissue viability specialists, and palliative care teams optimises outcomes and quality of life.

REFERENCES

Cannon, J., Dyer, J., Carapetis, J., and Manning, L. (2018). Epidemiology and risk factors for recurrent severe lower limb cellulitis: a longitudinal cohort study. *Clinical Microbiology and Infection* 24 (10): 1084–1088.

Dalal, A., Eskin-Schwartz, M., Mimouni, D. et al. (2017). Interventions for the prevention of recurrent erysipelas and cellulitis. *Cochrane Database of Systematic Reviews* 6 (6): CD009758.

Kumar, M., Ngian, V.J.J., Yeong, C. et al. (2020). Cellulitis in older people over 75 years–are there differences? *Annals of Medicine and Surgery* 49: 37–40.

National Institute for Health and Care Excellence (NICE) (2025). Cellulitis – acute: background information – prevalence. NICE Clinical Knowledge Summaries. https://cks.nice.org.uk/topics/cellulitis-acute/background-information/prevalence/ (accessed 21 September 2025)

CHAPTER 21

Musculoskeletal System

Aim

This chapter explores the principal musculoskeletal disorders encountered in later life, including osteoporosis, osteoarthritis, giant cell arteritis with polymyalgia rheumatica, cervical spondylosis with myelopathy, bone and joint infection, foot disorders, hand and peripheral nerve conditions, hip and shoulder disorders, crystal arthropathies, Paget's disease, contractures, and muscle weakness. It integrates current evidence and national guidance to support advanced practitioners (APs) in recognising key clinical features, applying diagnostic strategies, and delivering evidence-based, person-centred management with attention to frailty.

LEARNING OUTCOMES

After engaging with this chapter, readers will be able to:

1. Analyse the pathophysiology, risk factors, and typical presentations of common musculoskeletal conditions in older adults.
2. Apply recommended diagnostic investigations and differentiate between similar musculoskeletal disorders.
3. Formulate safe, evidence-based management plans incorporating pharmacological, non-pharmacological, and surgical options.
4. Evaluate how frailty modifies disease expression, treatment choice, and outcomes, and incorporate this into holistic care planning.
5. Reflect on the role of advanced clinical practitioners in multidisciplinary management, secondary prevention, and patient education.

SELF-ASSESSMENT QUESTIONS

1. An 80-year-old with frailty presents with new shoulder and hip girdle pain, morning stiffness, headache, and transient visual blurring. Outline your immediate investigations and management, including steroid, bone-protection, and referral plans.
2. A 78-year-old man with recurrent falls and a recent vertebral fracture needs secondary fracture prevention. How would you assess risk (including tool choice), start treatment, and integrate falls prevention and medicines optimisation?

OSTEOPOROSIS IN LATER LIFE

Osteoporosis is characterised by reduced bone mass and deterioration of micro-architecture, producing skeletal fragility and a high risk of low-energy fractures (NICE, 2025). The condition reflects a chronic imbalance in bone remodelling in which osteoclastic resorption outpaces osteoblastic formation (Figure 21.1). Osteoporosis is widespread yet frequently under-diagnosed and under-treated. In the United Kingdom, around one-third of women over 70 years have sustained a vertebral fracture, and nearly one-third of those over 90 years have experienced a hip fracture (Bowker et al., 2012). Fragility fractures impose a major health and economic burden, with hip fractures alone estimated to cost £1.9 billion annually in England (Rapp et al., 2012). Men sustain fewer fractures but experience higher mortality after hip fracture than women (Kannegaard et al., 2010; Smith et al., 2014).

Pathophysiology

Peak bone mass is achieved by the third decade of life, after which a gradual loss of approximately 0.5% per year is normal (Drahota et al., 2013). Post-menopause, bone resorption can accelerate to 5% annually. Smoking, high alcohol intake, low body weight, endocrine disorders such as hypepost-menopause hypogonadism, chronic kidney disease, and prolonged immobility further intensify bone loss. Medications, including glucocorticoids, anticonvulsants, and long-term heparin, also increased the risk. Genetic factors, adequate calcium and vitamin D intake in youth, and regular weight-bearing exercise influence the level of peak bone mass and later vulnerability.

Clinical Features and Diagnosis

Osteoporosis itself is asymptomatic until a fragility fracture occurs, typically involving the vertebrae, hip, or distal radius. Vertebral fractures can present as sudden pain, gradual height loss, or progressive kyphosis, which may impair respiratory mechanics and balance. Blood tests are usually normal; elevated calcium or alkaline phosphatase should prompt investigation for alternative diagnoses such as malignancy or Paget's disease. Dual-energy X-ray absorptiometry (DEXA) is the diagnostic standard, with a T-score $\leq$–2.5 defining osteoporosis and –1 to –2.5 indicating osteopenia (National Osteoporosis Guideline Group, 2024; NICE, 2025).

Prevention and Management

Lifestyle interventions, such as adequate dietary calcium and vitamin D, regular weight-bearing exercise, smoking cessation, and moderation of alcohol, are essential throughout life but particularly critical before peak bone mass is achieved. In older adults, vitamin D and calcium supplementation

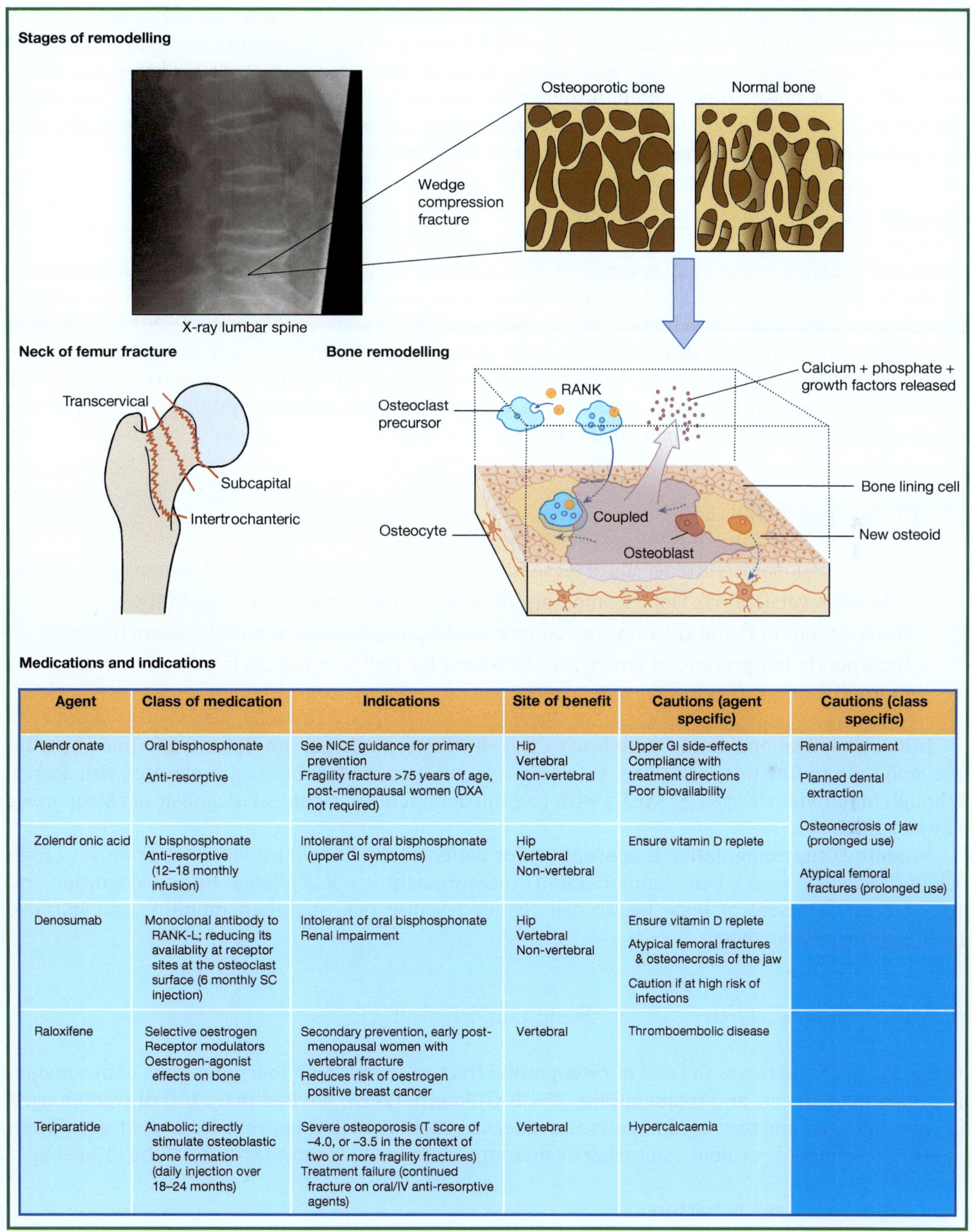

Agent	Class of medication	Indications	Site of benefit	Cautions (agent specific)	Cautions (class specific)
Alendronate	Oral bisphosphonate Anti-resorptive	See NICE guidance for primary prevention Fragility fracture >75 years of age, post-menopausal women (DXA not required)	Hip Vertebral Non-vertebral	Upper GI side-effects Compliance with treatment directions Poor biovailability	Renal impairment Planned dental extraction Osteonecrosis of jaw (prolonged use) Atypical femoral fractures (prolonged use)
Zolendronic acid	IV bisphosphonate Anti-resorptive (12–18 monthly infusion)	Intolerant of oral bisphosphonate (upper GI symptoms)	Hip Vertebral Non-vertebral	Ensure vitamin D replete	
Denosumab	Monoclonal antibody to RANK-L; reducing its availablity at receptor sites at the osteoclast surface (6 monthly SC injection)	Intolerant of oral bisphosphonate Renal impairment	Hip Vertebral Non-vertebral	Ensure vitamin D replete Atypical femoral fractures & osteonecrosis of the jaw Caution if at high risk of infections	
Raloxifene	Selective oestrogen Receptor modulators Oestrogen-agonist effects on bone	Secondary prevention, early post-menopausal women with vertebral fracture Reduces risk of oestrogen positive breast cancer	Vertebral	Thromboembolic disease	
Teriparatide	Anabolic; directly stimulate osteoblastic bone formation (daily injection over 18–24 months)	Severe osteoporosis (T score of −4.0, or −3.5 in the context of two or more fragility fractures) Treatment failure (continued fracture on oral/IV anti-resorptive agents)	Vertebral	Hypercalcaemia	

Geriatric Medicine at a Glance, First Edition. Adrian Blundell and Adam Gordon. © 2015 by John Wiley & Sons, Ltd. Published 2015 by John Wiley & Sons, Ltd.

FIGURE 21.1 Osteoporosis. *Source*: Blundell and Gordon (2015)/John Wiley & Sons.

remain beneficial, especially for those who are frail or housebound. Bisphosphonates are first-line pharmacological agents for secondary prevention following a fragility fracture and may be initiated empirically in women over 75 years without the need for bone densitometry (Bowker et al., 2012). Alternatives for those intolerant of bisphosphonates include denosumab, raloxifene, strontium ranelate or, in selected cases, teriparatide. Vertebroplasty can be considered for persistent pain after vertebral compression fractures when conservative measures fail.

Broader Perspectives on Bone Health

Evidence from large cohort studies shows that fracture risk is shaped not only by bone mineral density but also by frailty, sarcopenia, and lifestyle. Reduced muscle strength, slow gait speed, and low vitamin D levels are all associated with higher fracture rates and poorer recovery (Tajar et al., 2013; Rosengren et al., 2012). Environmental factors such as floor surface in residential care can also influence injury severity after falls (Simpson et al., 2004). Men who experience hip fractures face a particularly high risk of mortality within 12 months, underlining the importance of early case-finding and comprehensive geriatric assessment (Smith et al., 2014).

KEY PRACTICE POINTS

- Assume osteoporosis in older adults presenting with low-trauma fractures unless proved otherwise.
- Address reversible risk factors: smoking, alcohol, poor nutrition, and immobility.
- Initiate vitamin D and calcium, and commence bisphosphonates promptly where indicated.
- Incorporate fall-prevention strategies and assess for frailty to reduce fracture recurrence and mortality.

Initial investigations should include urea and electrolytes, calcium, phosphate, alkaline phosphatase, and thyroid function tests. DXA scanning is recommended for those with elevated risk scores, although in individuals aged ≥75 years with low-impact fractures, a clinical diagnosis of osteoporosis may be sufficient.

Vitamin D supplementation is appropriate for patients with known osteoporosis or those at high risk of deficiency, even when serum 25(OH)D measurement is not available. Early recognition and proactive management of bone health can reduce fracture risk, maintain mobility, and improve quality of life in later years.

FRAGILITY-FRACTURE RISK IN FRAIL OLDER ADULTS

Frailty markedly increases the risk of osteoporotic fracture, combining low bone mass with sarcopenia, impaired balance, and frequent falls. NICE Guidance (2025) advises that all frail women aged 65 years and older and men aged 75 years and older should have their fracture risk assessed, even when no other risk factor is evident. An earlier evaluation is warranted if they have any of the following:

- A previous fragility fracture.
- Current or repeated oral corticosteroid therapy.

- Recurrent falls, very low body mass index ($<18.5\,\text{kg/m}^2$), smoking, or alcohol intake above 14 units per week.
- Secondary causes of osteoporosis such as hypogonadism, untreated premature menopause, endocrine disease (e.g. diabetes and hyperthyroidism), chronic inflammatory or malabsorptive disorders, chronic kidney or liver disease, or prolonged immobility.

For frail patients, the QFracture® tool is preferred to FRAX® as it incorporates comorbidities and falls. A 10-year risk of around 10% or higher generally triggers dual-energy X-ray absorptiometry (DXA) to measure bone mineral density, although very high-risk individuals (for example, those with a recent vertebral fracture) may start bisphosphonate therapy without delay. Alongside pharmacological prevention, attention to vitamin D and calcium sufficiency and a structured falls-prevention programme is essential.

OSTEOARTHRITIS IN LATER LIFE

Osteoarthritis (OA) is the most prevalent degenerative joint disease in older adults and a major cause of pain, disability, and loss of independence (NICE, 2025). Although incidence increases with age, OA represents a failure of the joint's normal repair mechanisms rather than an inevitable feature of ageing. OA is diagnosed in about half of people aged over 65, placing it among the most common long-term conditions alongside hypertension (Kingston et al., 2018). Despite this, it is under-recognised in primary care records and is not included in the UK Quality and Outcomes Framework for routine review. Yet mortality is higher in those affected: a population study showed an all-cause standardised mortality ratio of 1.5 (Nüesch et al., 2011). This highlights the need to view OA as a chronic disease requiring proactive surveillance, early identification, and systematic follow-up (NICE, 2023).

Pathophysiology

OA reflects whole-joint failure. There is progressive loss and fissuring of articular cartilage with narrowing of the joint space, subchondral bone remodelling, and osteophyte formation. Synovial and capsular inflammation, vascular congestion, and reduced ligament elasticity contribute to pain and instability. Genetic susceptibility, advancing age, female sex, and high bone density increase risk, while obesity, previous trauma, and repetitive mechanical loading are modifiable factors. Secondary OA may develop after inflammatory arthritis, neuropathic joint disease, or congenital abnormalities such as hip dysplasia (NICE, 2023).

Clinical Manifestations

Pain is typically insidious, aggravated by movement and eased by rest, and can disturb sleep and mood. Morning stiffness is brief, and only one or a few joints are usually affected initially. Limitations of function, such as difficulty rising from a chair, dressing, or walking is common, and severe disease can precipitate falls and musculoskeletal frailty through sarcopenia and osteoporosis. Examination may reveal Heberden's nodes, bony deformity of knees or hips, fixed flexion deformities (detectable with Thomas' test), crepitus, effusion, and muscle wasting.

Diagnostic Approach

OA remains a clinical diagnosis because symptoms often correlate poorly with radiological change. Plain radiographs help assess structural severity, revealing joint-space narrowing, osteophytes, subchondral sclerosis and cysts, and guide surgical planning (NICE, 2023). Blood tests are normal; abnormal inflammatory markers warrant reassessment.

COMPREHENSIVE MANAGEMENT

Non-pharmacological Strategies

A holistic approach, recommended by NICE (2023), starts with education, self-management, and regular exercise to maintain strength and balance. Even individuals with established frailty benefit from targeted physical activity, which can improve gait speed and reduce falls (Fairhall et al., 2014). Weight optimisation, supportive footwear, heat or cold application, and appropriate walking aids enhance function and safety.

Pharmacological Treatments

Regular paracetamol remains first line, with escalation to weak opioids for persistent pain, acknowledging the risks of sedation and constipation. NSAIDs, preferably topical or in short oral courses with gastroprotection, can relieve acute flares. Capsaicin cream and intra-articular corticosteroid injections provide localised relief when indicated.

Surgical Interventions

Joint replacement is highly cost-effective in well-selected patients, yielding substantial gains in quality-adjusted life years (Jenkins et al., 2013). In 2018, more than 215,000 hip and knee replacements were performed in the United Kingdom, with most recipients classified as ASA 1–2 and recovering after an average hospital stay of three days (British Geriatrics Society, 2019). For older adults with frailty, surgery is primarily directed at alleviating severe pain and supporting mobility, with careful pre-operative optimisation and realistic goal setting.

Towards Proactive Care

Failure to manage OA proactively permits progressive functional decline and musculoskeletal frailty. Early recognition, annual review, and timely referral for surgical assessment are key to maintaining independence and reducing the wider consequences of chronic pain and inactivity.

FRAILTY AND GIANT CELL ARTERITIS

Giant cell arteritis is an inflammatory disease of medium- and large-calibre arteries in which granulomatous inflammation damages the vessel wall, most often involving branches of the carotid artery and, in some cases, the aorta and its major branches (NICE, 2024a,b). The precise trigger remains uncertain, but the disorder is thought to result from an aberrant immune response in genetically susceptible older adults. Frailty and GCA frequently intersect because the disease predominantly affects older adults, the group in whom frailty is most prevalent. UK data show that GCA is rare before 50 years, with the highest incidence of 7.4 per 10,000 person-years occurring in women aged 70–79 years (NICE, 2024a). More than twice as many women as men are affected (NICE, 2024a). These demographics overlap strongly with the population at risk of frailty, where multimorbidity, sarcopenia, and polypharmacy are common.

Frailty compounds the clinical challenge of GCA. Older patients often present with reduced physiological reserve, which can mask classic symptoms such as headache, increase the likelihood of steroid-related adverse effects (osteoporosis, myopathy, and diabetes), and complicate long-term glucocorticoid tapering. Careful risk–benefit assessment, vigilant monitoring for treatment toxicity, and proactive falls and bone-protection strategies are therefore essential when managing GCA in frail individuals.

Pathogenesis

The disease is characterised by chronic vascular inflammation with infiltration of giant cells and T lymphocytes, leading to intimal hyperplasia, luminal narrowing, and ischaemia. Although an autoimmune mechanism is suspected, no specific antigen or autoantibody has been identified. GCA shares certain pathogenetic pathways with polymyalgia rheumatica (PMR), but the vascular distribution differs.

Clinical Manifestations

Symptoms may be systemic or local:

1. Constitutional features: fever, fatigue, weight loss, and malaise.
2. Musculoskeletal: proximal muscle pain and morning stiffness reminiscent of PMR.
3. Cranial arteritis: scalp tenderness, new-onset temporal headache, and jaw claudication are typical. Patients often report pain when brushing hair or wearing a hat.
4. Visual complications: transient monocular visual loss (amaurosis fugax) or sudden permanent blindness can result from occlusion of the posterior ciliary arteries supplying the optic nerve.
5. Neurological sequelae: ischaemic stroke may occur if carotid branches are involved.
6. Large-vessel involvement: subclavian, vertebral, or aortic inflammation can cause limb claudication, aneurysm, or dissection.

GCA should always be considered in anyone over 50 years presenting with a new headache, scalp tenderness, or unexplained visual disturbance.

Investigations

Laboratory markers show marked systemic inflammation, with erythrocyte sedimentation rate often exceeding 100 mm/h and C-reactive protein markedly elevated (Bowker et al., 2012). Mild normochromic anaemia or renal impairment may be present. Temporal artery biopsy remains the diagnostic gold standard but has limited sensitivity because of skip lesions and rapidly declining histological changes once treatment begins. Imaging of large vessels with ultrasound, MRI, or PET-CT is increasingly used where clinical suspicion is high (NICE, 2024a).

Management

Immediate high-dose glucocorticoids are mandatory to prevent irreversible visual loss. Oral prednisolone 40–60 mg daily is standard for uncomplicated cases, while intravenous methylprednisolone may be required if visual symptoms are present (NICE, 2024a). Therapy is tapered gradually over many months, guided by symptoms and inflammatory markers, and relapse is common. Osteoporosis prophylaxis with calcium, vitamin D, and a bisphosphonate should start with steroid initiation. Steroid-sparing immunosuppressants such as methotrexate or azathioprine can be considered for patients with recurrent relapse or unacceptable steroid toxicity (Kobza et al., 2021).

POLYMYALGIA RHEUMATICA

PMR is an inflammatory condition of later life that produces bilateral pain and pronounced morning stiffness in the shoulder and pelvic girdles (NICE, 2024b). It is almost never seen before the age of 50 years. Onset is typically rapid, developing over days, and can be accompanied by systemic symptoms such as low-grade fever, fatigue, weight loss, and low mood. Despite the disabling pain, physical examination often reveals little abnormality.

PMR is predominantly a disorder of later life and therefore overlaps closely with the population most affected by frailty. Incidence and prevalence rise sharply with age, and the disease is rare before 50 years (Matteson, 2017; Lundberg et al., 2022). In the United Kingdom, population-based data show an incidence of about 96 per 100,000 among people over 40 years, with prevalence approaching 1% in those aged 55 years and above (Partington et al., 2018; Yates et al., 2016). Rates are consistently higher in women and in the oldest age groups (Lundberg et al., 2022; Espígol-Frigolé et al., 2023).

Because frailty is strongly age related, many individuals with PMR present with reduced physiological reserve, multimorbidity, and polypharmacy. Long-term corticosteroid therapy required in around one-fifth of cases for symptom control can worsen sarcopenia, precipitate osteoporosis, and impair glucose regulation, thereby reinforcing frailty trajectories (Dasgupta et al., 2007; Ameer and McNeil, 2014; Mahmood et al., 2020). These observations highlight the need for integrated management that addresses musculoskeletal health, fall prevention, and metabolic monitoring in frail older adults with PMR.

Pathophysiology

PMR shares immunopathological features with giant cell arteritis, suggesting a spectrum of disease. The primary source of pain and stiffness is thought to be synovial and bursal inflammation rather than direct muscle pathology (NICE, 2024b).

Diagnostic Features

Diagnosis is clinical and demands careful exclusion of mimicking conditions. Key features include:

- Age over 50 years.
- Persistent bilateral aching and morning stiffness of at least 30 minutes affecting the shoulders, hips, or the cervical region for at least one month.

- Elevated markers of inflammation, typically erythrocyte sedimentation rate (ESR) above 40 mm/h or raised C-reactive protein (CRP).

Supportive findings may include normocytic anaemia and mild disturbances in liver or renal function. Muscle enzymes and electromyography are normal, and temporal artery biopsy is positive only if concurrent giant cell arteritis is present. Failure to respond promptly to glucocorticoids should prompt reconsideration of the diagnosis.

Management

Oral prednisolone, usually 15 mg daily, often achieves relief within 24–48 hours. Once symptoms and inflammatory markers resolve, the dose is tapered, first more quickly and then in smaller decrements below 10 mg, guided by clinical response and serial ESR or CRP (NICE, 2024b). Relapse is treated by stepping back to the previous effective dose before re-titration. Many patients can discontinue therapy within 6–12 months, though treatment for 2–3 years is common. Long-term corticosteroids require bone protection with calcium, vitamin D, and a bisphosphonate from the outset. Steroid-sparing agents such as methotrexate or azathioprine may be considered in relapsing or steroid-intolerant cases.

Avoiding Diagnostic and Treatment Pitfalls

Conditions such as OA, chronic infection, or malignancy may mimic PMR and can transiently improve with steroids. Thorough baseline documentation and early review of treatment response are therefore essential. Steroid withdrawal can itself produce aches that resemble relapse; concurrent inflammatory marker testing helps to distinguish these scenarios. Shared decision-making about diagnosis, monitoring, and steroid tapering is crucial to prevent unnecessary long-term therapy and its complications (NICE, 2024b).

Case Study 21.1   Coexisting GCA and PMR

Presentation

Mr B, a 74-year-old retired teacher with a background of controlled hypertension and mild frailty (Clinical Frailty Scale 4), attended a same day emergency care (SDEC) clinic with a five-day history of severe new headache over the right temple, scalp tenderness when combing his hair, and transient blurred vision. He also described three weeks of aching shoulders and hips with pronounced morning stiffness, lethargy, and unintentional weight loss.

Initial Observations

- Temperature: 37.8 °C
- Blood pressure: 168/90 mmHg
- Pulse: 78 bpm, regular
- Respiratory rate: 18 breaths/min
- Oxygen saturation: 97% on air

Assessment

A systematic history explored vascular risk factors, visual changes, and constitutional symptoms. Examination showed:

- Tender, thickened right temporal artery with reduced pulsation.
- Limited shoulder abduction due to pain, but no true muscle weakness.
- No focal neurological deficits.

Clinical Reasoning

The combination of cranial artery tenderness, new-onset headache, jaw claudication, and transient visual loss strongly suggested giant cell arteritis. The history of bilateral shoulder and hip stiffness with raised inflammatory markers pointed to coexisting PMR. Recognising the risk of sudden, irreversible blindness, the AP initiated high-dose oral prednisolone 60 mg immediately, in line with NICE and British Society for Rheumatology (BSR) guidance, and arranged urgent ophthalmology input.

Investigations

- ESR 104 mm/h and CRP 98 mg/L.
- Normocytic anaemia on full blood count.
- Temporal artery ultrasound followed by biopsy (within five days) confirmed arteritis.
- Baseline DEXA scan and vitamin D level to support bone protection.
- Screening for diabetes and blood pressure monitoring to anticipate steroid side effects.

Management and Follow-Up

- Added calcium, vitamin D, and a bisphosphonate at the outset of steroid therapy.
- Planned tapering of glucocorticoids, with a slower schedule once the dose reached 10 mg to prevent relapse of PMR symptoms.
- Provided written education on recognising visual symptoms and the need for immediate review if they recur.
- Arranged a combined follow-up with rheumatology, ophthalmology, and a frailty team to address falls prevention and nutrition.

Outcome

The patient's headache and jaw pain resolved within 48 hours, and shoulder stiffness improved over the first week. He remained under multidisciplinary review for gradual steroid tapering and ongoing frailty management.

Key Learning Points

- Integrated presentation: PMR and GCA may coexist, requiring vigilance for overlapping symptoms.
- Advanced clinical reasoning: rapid assessment of headache, visual disturbance, and musculo-skeletal pain allows life-saving early treatment.

Holistic management: frailty assessment, bone protection, and close monitoring of steroid-related complications are as important as controlling vascular inflammation.

CERVICAL SPONDYLOSIS AND MYELOPATHY

Age-related degeneration of the cervical spine can compress both the exiting nerve roots and the spinal cord. This combination of radiculopathy and myelopathy produces a mixture of lower- and upper-motor-neurone deficits, leading to pain, sensory change, and weakness. Although degenerative changes of the cervical spine are common in older adults, clinically significant cord compression usually develops after the age of 50. Progression is often insidious but can occasionally be abrupt, particularly after trauma.

Clinical Presentation

Symptoms

- Neck pain and stiffness are frequent but do not reliably indicate neural involvement. Pain may radiate to the shoulder, chest, or arm in a dermatomal pattern.
- Hand and arm dysfunction is an early feature, with clumsiness during fine tasks, numbness, paraesthesia, and weakness.
- Lower-limb signs appear later, with spastic weakness, gait imbalance, or ataxia, and a tendency to fall.
- Bladder disturbance is uncommon and typically late.

Examination

- Upper limbs display lower-motor-neurone changes: weakness, wasting, and loss of segmental reflexes. A classic finding is that the inverted supinator reflex tapping the wrist fails to elicit the normal brachioradialis response but provokes finger flexion.
- Lower limbs show upper-motor-neurone features such as hyperreflexia, increased tone, clonus, and extensor plantar responses. Severe disease may cause spastic paraparesis with a defined sensory level.

DIFFERENTIAL DIAGNOSIS

Conditions that may mimic cervical myelopathy include syringomyelia, motor neurone disease (typically without sensory loss), peripheral neuropathy, vitamin B12 deficiency, and other spastic paraparesis syndromes.

INVESTIGATIONS

- Magnetic resonance imaging (MRI) is the investigation of choice, clearly defining bony changes, soft-tissue encroachment, and cord compression.
- Plain radiographs are useful mainly to exclude instability or other structural lesions, as degenerative changes are common and often asymptomatic.

- Computed tomography (CT) assists in surgical planning, and nerve conduction studies can help distinguish peripheral nerve disease.

MANAGEMENT

Conservative measures such as analgesia or a cervical collar may relieve radicular pain but do not halt progression. Surgical decompression, usually a laminectomy with fusion, is the definitive treatment and should be considered when there is:

- Progressive or rapidly evolving neurological deficit (short-term corticosteroids may be used while surgery is arranged).
- Intractable pain unresponsive to non-operative care.
- Established myelopathy rather than isolated radiculopathy.

Surgery can reduce further deterioration and alleviate pain, but recovery of lost neurological function is often incomplete. A thorough discussion of risks, benefits, and realistic outcomes is essential, especially in older patients with comorbidities or frailty. Table 21.1 demonstrates the other MKS presentations.

CONCLUSION

Musculoskeletal disorders in later life are heterogeneous but share key themes of chronicity, multimorbidity, and interaction with frailty. Early recognition, comprehensive assessment, and tailored interventions covering lifestyle, pharmacotherapy, surgery, and rehabilitation are essential to preserve function, reduce pain, and maintain independence.

Take-Home Messages

1. Frailty amplifies the impact of musculoskeletal disease and should be assessed routinely.
2. Prompt diagnosis and early intervention, especially in conditions such as giant cell arteritis, prevent irreversible complications.
3. Bone protection with calcium, vitamin D, and bisphosphonates is a cornerstone of care when long-term corticosteroids or fragility fractures are present.
4. Regular exercise, weight optimisation, and fall-prevention strategies remain central to sustaining musculoskeletal health at any age.
5. Advanced clinical practitioners play a pivotal role in integrating medical, surgical, and rehabilitative care to optimise outcomes for older adults.

TABLE 21.1 Other MSK presentations.

Spine

Condition	Typical presentation	Key examination	First-line investigations	Immediate/first-line management	When to refer/operate	Frailty considerations
Cervical spondylotic myelopathy	Insidious neck ± arm pain; hand clumsiness; later gait imbalance/falls; uncommon urinary symptoms	ULs: LMN signs (wasting and segmental reflex loss; inverted supinator). LLs: UMN signs (hyperreflexia, spasticity, and upgoing plantars)	MRI cervical spine (modality of choice). Plain films for alignment/instability; CT for bony detail; NCS/EMG if diagnostic doubt	Analgesia; short-term collar only for radicular pain; falls risk reduction	Progressive neurology, intractable pain, and established myelopathy → spinal surgery (decompression ± fusion)	Prehabilitation, delirium prevention, and VTE prophylaxis; set realistic goals—pain relief and halting decline are more likely than neurological recovery

Bone and joint infection

Condition	Typical presentation	Key examination	First-line investigations	Immediate/first-line management	When to refer	Frailty considerations
Vertebral osteomyelitis/discitis	Weeks of back pain and malaise; often thoracolumbar; fever may be absent; source often urinary/catheters/IVs	Localised vertebral tenderness; ± paravertebral spasm; screen neurology	Blood cultures; FBC/CRP/ESR; MRI spine (early diagnostic changes); CT-guided biopsy for organism	Analgesia, immobilisation as needed; targeted IV antibiotics once cultures obtained (empirical cover if septic)	Spinal/ID teams; urgent if neural compromise, abscess, and failure to respond	Early nutrition and pressure-area care; monitor for deconditioning and opioid sensitivity
Osteomyelitis (foot/other bones)	Non-healing ulcer or post-op wound; diabetic foot pain may be blunted by neuropathy	Probe-to-bone test; local warmth and swelling; vascular and neuropathy assessment	Blood cultures; inflammatory markers; X-ray (late); MRI foot; bone biopsy for culture/histology	Debridement of necrotic tissue; targeted prolonged antibiotics; off-loading	Ortho/vascular/podiatry MDT for debridement, revascularisation, or amputation decisions	Off-loading devices, safe footwear, and glucose control; community nursing support

(Continued)

TABLE 21.1 (Continued)

Foot (older adults)

Problem	Typical presentation	Key examination	Management essentials	Refer when	Frailty considerations
Onychogryphosis/ onychomycosis/ ingrown nails	Thick, painful, or discoloured nails; recurrent infection	Nail deformity; surrounding cellulitis	Podiatry care; footwear optimisation; nail care; antifungals when indicated (monitor LFTs if oral)	Refractory infection and severe deformity	Facilitate access to foot care; carers taught inspection
Callus/corns/fissures	Localised plantar pain; breaks in skin	Hyperkeratosis and focal tenderness	Debridement, pressure relief, and emollients; footwear review	Recurrent breakdown or ulceration	Falls risk from painful gait; pressure-ulcer prevention
Neuropathic (Charcot) foot	Swollen, warm, deforming, painless foot in neuropathy	Collapsed arch ('rocker-bottom') and instability	Weight-bearing X-ray; MRI if doubt	Immediate off-loading; specialist podiatry/ orthopaedics	Charcot suspected or progressive deformity
Peripheral arterial disease	Claudication, rest pain, and tissue loss	Pulses and ABPI	ABPI/toe pressures; vascular imaging	Risk factor control; wound care	Critical ischaemia → urgent vascular

Hand and peripheral nerve

Condition	Presentation	Examination	Investigations	Management	Referral trigger	Frailty considerations
Heberden/ Bouchard nodes (hand OA)	Bony enlargement; functional nuisance > pain	DIP/PIP bony swellings; crepitus	X-ray only if diagnostic doubt	Splints, hand therapy, topical NSAIDs, and pacing	Severe pain/ function loss	Adaptive aids; falls risk if grip is poor
Trigger finger	Locking/catching and worse mornings	Palpable A1 pulley nodule; triggering	Clinical	Splinting and NSAIDs; corticosteroid injection; release if refractory	Persistent locking or functional loss	Day-case under LA is feasible in frail pts
Carpal tunnel syndrome	Nocturnal paraesthesia and median distribution; thenar weakness late	Positive Tinel/ Phalen; sensory change; weak abduction	NCS if atypical/ pre-op	Night splints; steroid injection; surgical release usually curative	Thenar wasting, refractory symptoms	Local anaesthesia surgery; post-op hand therapy

Repetitive strain injury	Overuse pain; normal neuro exam	Local tendon tenderness	Clinical	Load modification, ergonomics, analgesia, and physio	Persistent disability	Education prevents recurrence
Complex regional pain syndrome	Disproportionate limb pain, swelling, colour/temperature change, and limited ROM	Allodynia and trophic change	Clinical ± triple-phase bone scan (early)	Early mobilisation and desensitisation; analgesia; consider steroids, short course; bisphosphonates for pain	Specialist pain/rehab if refractory	Early recognition prevents chronicity

Hip

Condition	Presentation	Examination	Investigations	Management	Key 'red flags'/referral	Frailty considerations
Hip fracture	Acute hip/groin pain ± fall; some can still walk	Pain on rotation; shortened/external rotation (not universal)	Pelvis and hip AP + lateral; MRI if X-ray negative and high suspicion	Almost all require surgery; comprehensive geriatric assessment; secondary fracture prevention	Urgent ortho admission; early surgery	High 30-day mortality; delirium prevention; osteoporosis Rx
Hip OA	Activity-related deep ache; stiffness after rest	↓ROM all planes; antalgic gait	X-ray if persistent symptoms	Exercise, weight management, simple analgesia, and aids; consider injection	Refer if pain/disability despite conservative care	THR outcomes can be excellent in robust older adults
Other hip pain causes	Paget disease, radicular pain, metastasis, septic arthritis, knee-referred, and psoas abscess	Specific signs (fever, cachexia, and spinal signs)	Targeted labs/imaging; joint aspiration if septic arthritis suspected	Aetiology-specific	Septic arthritis = urgent aspiration/IV antibiotics	Early imaging when red flags present

(Continued)

TABLE 21.1   (Continued)

Back pain in older adults

Domain	What to look for	Investigations	Management priorities
Assessment	Pain character/radiation; neuro/bowel/bladder; fever/weight loss; vertebral tenderness; gait	FBC, ESR/CRP (myeloma screen if ESR↑), Ca/ALP, and PSA; MRI for cancer/infection/compression; bone scan for multifocal	Diagnose cause first; WHO analgesia ladder; physio; weight reduction; TENS; consider targeted injections
Red flags	Acute neuro deficit, sphincter disturbance, fever, weight loss, new severe pain, and known cancer	MRI urgent	High-dose IV steroids if cord compression suspected; urgent oncology/ortho referral
Common causes	Facet OA (common with age); osteoporotic crush fractures; malignancy; infection (vertebral OM/discitis)	As above	Bisphosphonates/calcitonin for painful vertebral collapse; radiotherapy for metastases; urgent decompression if compression

Shoulder

Condition	Presentation	Examination	First-line management	Imaging	Escalation
Frozen shoulder	Painful stiffness → stiff phase months	Loss of external/internal rotation and abduction	Physio/exercise; intra-articular steroid for pain	Clinical ± US	Refractory stiffness → hydrodilatation/arthroscopic release
Bicipital tendinitis	Anterior shoulder pain; worse with supination	Local bicipital groove tenderness	Rest and NSAIDs; steroid injection; stretches	US if doubt	Persistent symptoms → ortho
Rotator cuff tendinitis	Dull ache; 'painful arc' 60°–120°	Impingement signs; preserved passive ROM	Rest, physio, and NSAIDs; subacromial injection	US useful	Ongoing pain → arthroscopic decompression
Rotator cuff tear	Post-trauma or attritional; weakness	↓Active ROM > passive	Analgesia and physio; injections	US/MRI	Consider repair depending on function/comorbidity
Dislocation	Fall (anterior) or seizure (posterior)	Deformity; neurovascular check	Analgesia/sedation; reduction; sling; rehab	X-ray pre/post	Recurrent instability → ortho
Glenohumeral OA	Post-traumatic commoner	Crepitus; ↓external rotation/abduction	Analgesia; mobilisation; injections	X-ray	Consider shoulder arthroplasty if refractory

Crystal arthropathies

Condition	Presentation	Diagnostic pointer	Management (acute)	Long-term/prevention	Frailty considerations
Gout	Hot, red, and exquisitely tender joint (often foot/ankle); fever possible	Joint aspirate: needle-shaped, negatively birefringent urate crystals	NSAID (with PPI) **or** colchicine protocol **or** short oral steroids; joint injection if sepsis excluded	Address drugs/alcohol; weight; consider allopurinol after recurrent attacks (cover with low-dose colchicine/NSAID)	NSAIDs often limited—prefer steroids/intra-articular routes; monitor renal function
Pseudogout (CPPD)	Acute large-joint synovitis (knee, wrist, and shoulder)	Aspirate: rhomboid, **positively** birefringent CPPD; chondrocalcinosis on X-ray	Intra-articular steroids; NSAIDs; short oral steroids; colchicine	Rarely needs chronic prophylaxis	Exclude sepsis; treat precipitating illness (e.g. intercurrent illness/trauma)

Systemic bone disease

Condition	Presentation	Key tests	Management	When to refer	Frailty considerations
Paget's disease of bone	Often asymptomatic ↑ALP; bone pain; deformity; skull changes; hearing loss; pathological fracture	ALP (bone isoenzyme); X-ray: mixed lysis/sclerosis; bone scan 'hot spots'	IV bisphosphonates (pain, pre-op vascularity, fracture healing, and neuro compression); analgesia; surgery for deformity/fracture	Symptomatic disease; neuro compression; complex deformity	Assess falls/hearing; plan surgery with bone turnover suppression pre-op

Contractures

Aspect	Key points	Management
Aetiology	Immobilisation (stroke, dementia, and fractures) and spasticity; connective tissue shortening	Prevent with early mobilisation/positioning; passive stretch programmes; seating
Complications	Pain, hygiene problems, pressure injury, and functional loss	Physio, serial casting (selected), and botulinum toxin for spasticity; selected tendon release
Frailty	High prevalence in care homes; often multi-factorial	MDT approach; carer education; pressure care; realistic functional goals

(Continued)

TABLE 21.1   (Continued)

Muscle Symptoms and Weakness			
Category	**Clinical clue**	**Core tests**	**Management**
True myopathy/NMJ/ neuropathy	Objective weakness; fatigability; fasciculations (MND); sensory loss (neuropathy)	CK, electrolytes, TFTs, B12/folate/ Vit D, and myeloma screen; NCS/ EMG; MRI/CT if CNS signs; biopsy selected	Treat cause; review drugs (statins and steroids); targeted rehab
Joint disease 'pseudo-weakness'	Pain-limited power around arthritic joints	X-ray/US as needed	Analgesia and joint-directed therapy
Asthenia	'Tired/weak' without objective deficit	Screen for systemic disease, depression, and deconditioning	Exercise, nutrition, and address mood/comorbidity

REFERENCES

Ameer, F. and McNeil, J. (2014). Polymyalgia rheumatica: clinical update. *Australian Family Physician* 43 (6): 373–376.

Blundell, A. and Gordon, A. (2015). *Geriatric Medicine at a Glance*, 1e. Chichester: Wiley Blackwell.

Bowker, L., Price, J., Smith, S., and Kinnaird, M. (2012). *Oxford Handbook of Geriatric Medicine*, 2e. Oxford: Oxford University Press.

British Geriatrics Society (2019). *Osteoarthritis – Are We Managing This Chronic Disease as Proactively as We Should?* British Geriatrics Society, 21 October https://www.bgs.org.uk/blog/osteoarthritis-are-we-managing-this-chronic-disease-as-proactively-as-we-should (accessed 21 September 2025).

Dasgupta, B., Matteson, E.L., and Maradit-Kremers, H. (2007). Management guidelines and outcome measures in polymyalgia rheumatica (PMR). *Clinical and Experimental Rheumatology* 25 (6): S130.

Drahota, A.K., Ward, D., Udell, J.E. et al. (2013). Pilot cluster randomised controlled trial of flooring to reduce injuries from falls in wards for older people. *Age and Ageing* 42 (5): 633–640.

Espígol-Frigolé, G., Dejaco, C., Mackie, S.L. et al. (2023). Polymyalgia rheumatica. *The Lancet* 402 (10411): 1459–1472.

Fairhall, N., Sherrington, C., Lord, S.R. et al. (2014). Effect of a multifactorial, interdisciplinary intervention on risk factors for falls and fall rate in frail older people: a randomised controlled trial. *Age and Ageing* 43 (5): 616–622.

Jenkins, P.J., Clement, N.D., Hamilton, D.F. et al. (2013). Total HIP and knee replacement: a cost-utility analysis. In: *Orthopaedic Proceedings*, vol. 95 February, Supp_5, 8–8. Bone & Joint.

Kannegaard, P.N., van der Mark, S., Eiken, P., and Abrahamsen, B. (2010). Excess mortality in men compared with women following a hip fracture. *Osteoporosis International* 21 (9): 1743–1748.

Kingston, A., Robinson, L., Booth, H. et al. (2018). Projections of multi-morbidity in the older population in England to 2035: estimates from the Population Ageing and Care Simulation (PACSim) model. *Age and Ageing* 47 (3): 374–380.

Kobza, A.O., Herman, D., Papaioannou, A. et al. (2021). Understanding and managing corticosteroid-induced osteoporosis. *Open Access Rheumatology: Research and Reviews* 13: 177–190.

Lundberg, I.E., Sharma, A., Turesson, C., and Mohammad, A.J. (2022). An update on polymyalgia rheumatica. *Journal of Internal Medicine* 292 (5): 717–732.

Mahmood, S.B., Nelson, E., Padniewski, J., and Nasr, R. (2020). Polymyalgia rheumatica: an updated review. *Cleveland Clinic Journal of Medicine* 87 (9): 549–556.

Matteson, E.L. (2017). Polymyalgia rheumatica: clinical features and diagnosis. *Rheumatic Disease Clinics of North America* 43 (1): 73–92.

National Institute for Health and Care Excellence (NICE) (2023). Clinical knowledge summaries: osteoarthritis. https://cks.nice.org.uk/topics/osteoarthritis/ (accessed 21 September 2025).

National Institute for Health and Care Excellence (NICE). Clinical knowledge summaries: giant cell arteritis–definition.2024a.https://cks.nice.org.uk/topics/giant-cell-arteritis/background-information/definition/ (accessed 21 September 2025).

National Institute for Health and Care Excellence (NICE) (2024b). Clinical knowledge summaries: polymyalgia rheumatica – prevalence. https://cks.nice.org.uk/topics/polymyalgia-rheumatica/background-information/prevalence/ (accessed 21 September 2025).

National Osteoporosis Guideline Group (NOGG) (2024). Clinical guideline for the prevention and treatment of osteoporosis. Updated December 2024. `https://www.nogg.org.uk/full-guideline` (accessed 21 September 2025).

NICE (2025). Osteoporosis: prevention of fragility fractures – Clinical Knowledge Summaries (CKS). `https://cks.nice.org.uk/topics/osteoporosis-prevention-of-fragility-fractures/` (accessed 21 September 2025).

Nüesch, E., Dieppe, P., Reichenbach, S. et al. (2011). All cause and disease specific mortality in patients with knee or hip osteoarthritis: population based cohort study. *BMJ* 342.

Partington, R.J., Muller, S., Helliwell, T. et al. (2018). Incidence, prevalence and treatment burden of polymyalgia rheumatica in the UK over two decades: a population-based study. *Annals of the Rheumatic Diseases* 77 (12): 1750–1756.

Rapp, K., Becker, C., Cameron, I.D. et al. (2012). Femoral fracture rates in people with and without disability. *Age and Ageing* 41 (5): 653–658.

Rosengren, B.E., Ribom, E.L., Nilsson, J.Å. et al. (2012). Inferior physical performance test results of 10,998 men in the MrOS Study is associated with high fracture risk. *Age and Ageing* 41 (3): 339–344.

Simpson, A.H.R.W., Lamb, S., Roberts, P.J. et al. (2004). Does the type of flooring affect the risk of hip fracture? *Age and Ageing* 33 (3): 242–246.

Smith, T., Pelpola, K., Ball, M. et al. (2014). Pre-operative indicators for mortality following hip fracture surgery: a systematic review and meta-analysis. *Age and Ageing* 43 (4): 464–471.

Tajar, A., Lee, D.M., Pye, S.R. et al. (2013). The association of frailty with serum 25-hydroxyvitamin D and parathyroid hormone levels in older European men. *Age and Ageing* 42 (3): 352–359.

Yates, M., Graham, K., Watts, R.A., and MacGregor, A.J. (2016). The prevalence of giant cell arteritis and polymyalgia rheumatica in a UK primary care population. *BMC Musculoskeletal Disorders* 17 (1): 285.

END-OF-LIFE MEDICINE AND ETHICAL DIMENSIONS

CHAPTER 22

Advance Care Planning and Difficult Conversations

Aim

The aim of this chapter is to provide advanced practitioners (APs) with the knowledge, skills, and professional confidence to initiate and lead advance care planning and end-of-life discussions, including treatment escalation and resuscitation decisions, in a manner that is evidence based, person centred, and aligned with national policy and professional standards.

LEARNING OUTCOMES

By the end of this chapter, readers will be able to:

1. Differentiate between palliative care, end of life, dying, death, and died and explain the clinical and communicative significance of these terms.
2. Identify triggers for advance care planning, including frailty, prognostic indicators, and the surprise question, and integrate relevant assessment tools such as the OACC suite.
3. Apply advanced communication strategies, including the SPIKES framework, to share serious news sensitively and explore patient values, goals, and preferences.
4. Plan, record, and review treatment escalation plans and DNACPR decisions in line with national guidance and organisational governance requirements.

SELF-ASSESSMENT QUESTIONS

1. Describe how you would use the SPIKES framework to communicate a new diagnosis of an incurable illness.
2. How would you ensure that a treatment escalation plan or DNACPR decision is both clinically appropriate and accessible across care settings?

> To speak openly about the future is not to diminish hope, but to redefine it, shaping care that preserves meaning, comfort, and humanity.

INTRODUCTION

End-of-life (EOL) care involves more than relieving physical symptoms; it also supports patients and families through emotionally complex experiences. Central to this care is open, honest, and compassionate communication about values, preferences, and treatment escalation and resuscitation decisions to ensure care remains person centred. Advanced care planning (ACP) provides a framework for these discussions, enabling patients to articulate priorities such as comfort, independence, or family presence and to document their wishes for future treatment in anticipation of a time when they may be unable to decide for themselves. The National Institute for Health and Care Excellence (NICE, 2019) and the General Medical Council (GMC, 2024) identify ACP as a basis of good palliative care.

Patients are considered to be approaching the end of life when they are likely to die within the next twelve months, a definition that includes those with advanced, progressive, incurable conditions; general frailty with co-existing illness; or those at risk of sudden deterioration from an acute event such as stroke or sepsis (NHS England, 2022). Recognising this stage is critical, as it allows anticipatory care planning before crisis occurs. Tools such as the surprise question 'Would I be surprised if this patient were to die in the next year?' together with general and disease-specific indicators of decline help clinicians identify when to begin these discussions and ensure that treatment plans, care preferences, and supportive measures remain aligned with individual values.

Multi-Professional Framework (MPF) for Advanced Practitioners

(Adapted from NHS England, 2025)

This chapter maps to the following statement within the MPF:

1. Clinical practice: 1.1, 1.2, 1.3, 1.5, 1.7, 1.9
2. Leadership and management: 2.1, 2.2, 2.5
3. Education: 3.1, 3.3, 3.5
4. Research: 4.1, 4.2

Accreditation Consideration

This chapter maps to the statement with the following national accretional document:

Curriculum framework for advanced practice in the care of older people (NHS England, 2022)

1. Core Capabilities CiPs: 1–5
2. Generic Clinical CiPs: 1–5
3. Specialty Clinical CiPs (older People): 1–4

Curriculum framework for advanced practitioners in the case of the palliative and end-of-life care (NHS England, 2023a)

1. Clinical pillar: 1.1, 1.2, 1.3, 1.4
2. Leadership and management: 2.1, 2.2
3. Education: 3.1, 3.3, 3.4
4. Research: 4.1

Curriculum for advanced practitioners in acute medicine (NHS England, 2023b)

1. Core CiPs: 1–4
2. Generic Clinical CiPs: 1–6
3. Specialty Clinical CiPs (Acute Medicine): 1–5 and acute conditions

Are We Using the 'D' Words?

- **Dying** describes the process of life ending, usually over hours or days, when the body shows signs of irreversible decline such as loss of appetite, reduced consciousness, and altered breathing.
- **Death** refers to the moment when all vital functions, including the heart and breathing, have ceased and life is no longer sustainable.
- **Died** is the factual term used after death has occurred, important for documentation, certification, and sensitive communication with families. Using these words accurately and without rewording helps professionals convey information clearly; support decision-making; and provide compassionate, honest dialogue at a critical time.

Are We Using the Same Language?

- **Dying** refers to the final stage of life when death is imminent and irreversible, typically measured in hours or days.
- **Palliative care** is a broader approach aimed at relieving suffering and improving quality of life for people with life-limiting conditions, regardless of prognosis. Palliative care may begin early in an illness and continue for months or years, encompassing symptom control, psychosocial support, and advanced care planning.
- **End of life** specifically focuses on the physical, emotional, and spiritual needs present in the last days of life.

WHY IS IT IMPORTANT TO RECOGNISE DYING?

Recognising when a person is entering the dying phase is essential not only for clinical decision-making but also for supporting patients and families to prepare practically, emotionally, and spiritually. Early acknowledgement of dying creates opportunities for patients to put their affairs in order, make a will, or arrange visits from loved ones, including those living abroad. It also allows space to meet spiritual or religious needs, whether through chaplaincy involvement, prayer, or other faith-based practices. For families, clear communication about what to expect reduces uncertainty and helps them to cope with the transition from active treatment to a focus on comfort. For APs, openly addressing the reality of dying demonstrates professional integrity, fosters trust, and ensures that care remains centred on dignity and quality of life.

> 'I've learned that people will forget what you said, people will forget what you did, but people will never forget how you made them feel' (Angelou, 2004).

INDICATOR TOOLS

Prognostication tools, including the Outcome Assessment and Complexity Collaborative (OACC) suite, support the timely assessment of people with life-limiting illness (Bausewein et al., 2018). The OACC measures such as the Australia-modified Karnofsky Performance Status (AKPS) (Abernethy et al., 2005) and Phase of Illness and Integrated Palliative Care Outcome Scale (IPOS) provide structured ways to monitor functional status, symptom burden, and psychosocial concerns (Nakajima, 2022). In addition, the ePrognosis platform (`https://eprognosis.ucsf.edu/`) (developed by the University of California, San Francisco) provides validated prognostic calculators that estimate life expectancy based on clinical indicators and functional status. These tools can help clinicians discuss prognosis, guide treatment intensity, and plan advanced care, particularly for frail or older adults. Incorporating ePrognosis as an evidence-based resource strengthens the use of objective indicators when considering EOL care and shared decision-making. By capturing these dimensions, they enable APs to plan care, evaluate outcomes, and ensure that the patient's priorities and holistic needs are recognised and addressed (Figure 22.1).

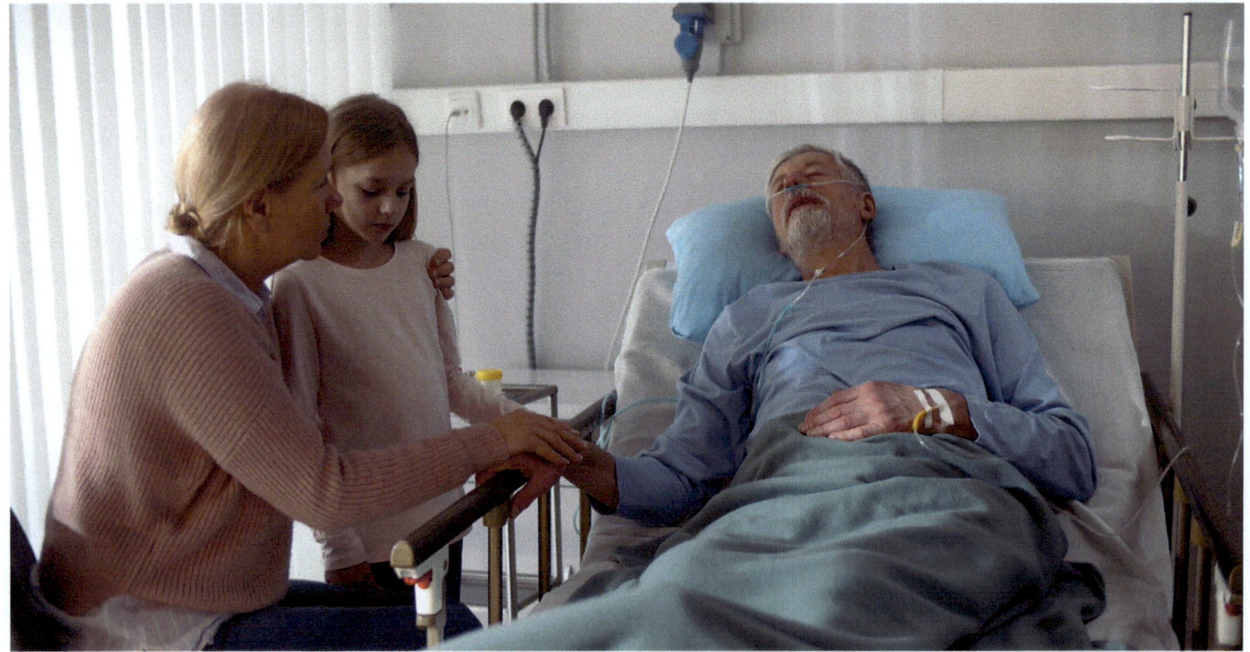

FIGURE 22.1   Supporting the dying person. *Source*: nimito/Adobe Stock Photos.

ADVANCED CARE PLANNING (ACP)

'Advance care planning is a process that supports adults at any age or stage of health in understanding and sharing their personal values, life goals, and preferences regarding future medical care. The goal of advance care planning is to help ensure that people receive medical care that is consistent with their values, goals and preferences during serious and chronic illness' (Sudore et al., 2017). ACP can and should begin even when the future course of illness is uncertain. Early conversations allow preferences to be revisited as health or circumstances change and help people focus on what matters most to them. Everyday changes such as increased frailty, a significant fall, or bereavement provide natural opportunities to open these discussions. By starting sensitively and honestly, practitioners enable individuals to retain control and make meaningful choices despite the unpredictability of their condition (British Geriatrics Society, 2020). Individuals can only make informed decisions about their future care when they understand both the possible prognosis of their illness and the limits of medical treatment. A narrow question such as whether to attempt cardiopulmonary resuscitation (CPR) does not give enough context for a genuine choice. APs who lead ACP need to recognise frailty, explain how it shapes illness and recovery, and describe the likely advantages and burdens of intensive interventions. Presenting information in this way supports thoughtful planning and helps patients and families prepare for recovery or further decline.

ACP has been shown to improve outcomes for patients, families, and healthcare systems. Evidence indicates that patients who participate in ACP are more likely to receive care aligned with their values and less likely to undergo burdensome interventions at the EOL (Houben et al., 2014). Families report greater confidence in decision-making and experience fewer feelings of guilt and conflict (Brighton and Bristowe, 2016).

National and international frameworks highlight ACP as a priority. NICE (2019) guidance on EoL care states that discussions about future preferences should be a routine part of care for people with progressive illness. Similarly, the GMC (2024) stresses the ethical duty to involve patients in decisions about their care and to document outcomes clearly.

BENEFITS OF ACP

- Respecting autonomy: Patients' values shape care.
- Reducing unwanted interventions: Avoids escalation to treatments unlikely to benefit.
- Improving coordination: Ensures continuity across primary, secondary, and community care.
- Supporting families: Provides clarity and reassurance during crises.
- Professional confidence: Staff feel more supported when decisions are documented.

PRINCIPLES OF COMMUNICATION IN ACP

Skilled communication is the foundation of ACP. Without it, even the most detailed documentation becomes meaningless. Effective ACP discussions share several key features:

1. **Shared responsibility:** ACP is everyone's role, not just senior consultants. All clinicians should create opportunities for discussion.

2. **Timely initiation:** Conversations should start early, ideally soon after diagnosis of a life-limiting condition, and be revisited regularly.
3. **Person-centredness:** The style and content must be adapted to the individual's cultural background, health literacy, and readiness.
4. **Clarity and honesty:** Avoiding euphemisms helps build trust, even when prognosis is uncertain.
5. **Iterative process:** ACP is dynamic; plans should evolve with changes in health and preferences.

Starting ACP conversations can feel frightening. Patients often expect clinicians to take the lead, but professionals may hesitate for fear of taking away hope or causing distress. However, those patients generally appreciate openness when approached sensitively.

Strategies for Initiating Conversations Include

- Using clinical triggers: Look for signs that indicate the patient may be approaching the final phase of life, such as repeated unplanned hospital admissions, a noticeable decline in physical function, progressive frailty, or worsening disease despite optimal therapy. These events provide natural opportunities to introduce planning discussions, framed around ensuring care matches the patient's needs as their health changes.
- Asking open questions: Rather than beginning with medical options, start with values-based questions such as, 'What matters most to you in the time ahead?' or 'What are you hoping for, and what are you worried about?' Such open approaches invite the patient to set the agenda, ensure their perspective is central, and help practitioners to understand priorities beyond purely clinical outcomes.
- Normalising ACP: It is important to present ACP as a routine and positive element of holistic care, not as an indication that healthcare professionals are 'giving up'. For example, explaining that 'we have these conversations with all of our patients to make sure care is consistent with their wishes' helps reduce stigma and builds trust.
- Acknowledging uncertainty: Prognostication is often difficult, and clinicians should be transparent about this. Acknowledging that the future may not be entirely predictable but emphasising that planning can reduce distress and ensure appropriate care reassures patients and families. For instance, you might say, 'We cannot be certain about exactly what will happen, but making plans now can help ensure you remain comfortable, and your wishes are respected.'

DIFFICULT CONVERSATIONS

Breaking bad news is a core but demanding element of EOL care that requires a structured approach. Effective conversations begin with thoughtful preparation; choosing a quiet, private setting; and allowing enough time. It is essential to explore what the patient and family already know and what they wish to discuss, to identify who they would like present, and to respect cultural and spiritual preferences. Using simple, clear, and honest language, free of euphemism, helps ensure understanding. Silence and pauses give space for emotional processing, while approaches such as the SPIKES framework (Setting, Perception, Invite, Knowledge, Empathy, Summary) support a logical and sensitive flow (Baile et al., 2000).

Checking comprehension; responding with empathy; and offering written information, follow-up contacts, and opportunities for further discussion reinforce trust. Accurate documentation and communication with the wider multidisciplinary team ensure that agreed plans and care priorities are shared, providing continuity and dignity at the end of life.

Difficult conversations with patients are routine in frailty and palliative care settings. In the wake of the COVID-19 pandemic, the Care Quality Commission (CQC) raised concerns about Do Not Attempt Cardiopulmonary Resuscitation (DNACPR) decisions and related discussions, emphasising its recommendations for the need for clear and appropriate communication (CQC, 2021).

Role of APS and the Spikes Framework

An AP can use the SPIKES (Setting, Perception, Invitation, Knowledge, Empathy, Strategy and Summary) framework to guide the delivery of difficult conversations in a structured and compassionate way.

Setting begins with arranging a quiet, private room and ensuring that adequate time is available, inviting the patient and any chosen relatives or carers.

During **Perception**, the AP explores the patient's understanding of their illness and what they suspect about its progression.

At the **Invite** stage, the AP seeks permission to share further details, gauging how much information the patient wishes to receive.

In **Knowledge**, the AP explains the clinical situation clearly and honestly, avoiding euphemisms, and allowing pauses for questions and emotional responses.

Moving to **Empathy**, the AP acknowledges and validates feelings, offering emotional support, and, if appropriate, access to chaplaincy or psychological services.

Finally, in **Summary**, the AP recaps key points, discusses next steps such as advance care planning or symptom control, and ensures that follow-up contact details are provided. By following these steps, the AP maintains dignity, promotes shared decision-making, and aligns care with the patient's values and preferences.

Case Study: Newly Diagnosed with Cancer and the Role of AP

The AP arranges a quiet consultation room, ensures there are no interruptions and invites the patient to have their partner present (**Setting**).

Sitting at the eye level, she begins, 'Before we look at the results, could you tell me what you already understand about the tests you had?' (**Perception**).

The patient explains that they know a mass was found but are unsure of its significance. The AP asks gently, 'Would you like me to explain what the biopsy has shown and what it could mean for your health?' (**Invite**).

When the patient agrees, she continues in clear, simple language, 'The biopsy shows that the lump in your bowel is a cancer. This means some of the cells are growing in an uncontrolled way. The good news is that treatments are available, and we can plan these with you.' She stops, allowing silence while the patient absorbs the news (**Knowledge**). Seeing visible distress, she says softly: 'I can see this is a shock. It is natural to feel overwhelmed and frightened. We are here to support you' (**Empathy**).

After the patient's questions, the AP summarises: 'Today we have discussed the diagnosis. The next steps will include further scans to check whether the cancer has spread and a meeting with the specialist team to talk through treatment choices. I will give you written information and contact details so that you can reach us at any time' (**Summary**).

THE RECOMMENDED SUMMARY PLAN FOR EMERGENCY CARE AND TREATMENT (ReSPECT) FORM

It is developed by the Resuscitation Council UK, providing a structured way for patients, families, and healthcare professionals to record personalised recommendations for emergency care (Resuscitation Council UK, 2025a). Its aim is to ensure that if a person is unable to communicate in a crisis, clinicians can make decisions that reflect the individual's own values and priorities. Unlike a single decision about CPR, the ReSPECT process supports broader planning: It considers treatments the person would want to receive, those that may be limited, and situations where natural death would be preferred.

Completion of the form is ideally part of ACP, initiated during routine care or at key points such as a new diagnosis of a life-limiting condition. The conversation should include exploration of what matters most to the person such as comfort, prolonging life, or remaining at home balanced with realistic clinical options. The form is then signed and dated, and it travels with the patient across care settings so that ambulance staff, hospital teams, and community services can see and respect the documented recommendations (Resuscitation Council UK, 2025a).

ReSPECT is not a legally binding document, but it carries significant professional weight and should be reviewed whenever circumstances change (Resuscitation Council UK, 2025b). It complements but does not replace other documents such as DNACPR orders or advance decisions to refuse treatment. By encouraging early, honest dialogue and making preferences visible in emergencies, the ReSPECT process supports person-centred, safe, and ethically sound care.

TREATMENT ESCALATION PLANS AND DNACPR

Treatment Escalation Plans (TEPs) provide a structured record of which treatments should or should not be offered if a patient's condition deteriorates. TEPs clarify decisions about hospital admission, intravenous therapy, non-invasive ventilation, or transfer to critical care, ensuring that interventions remain proportionate to clinical need and consistent with the person's goals. These plans help avoid crisis decision-making and give all members of the multidisciplinary team clear guidance on the ceiling of treatment, thereby promoting timely, coordinated care.

DNACPR decisions are a specific element of treatment escalation planning. They record that CPR will not be attempted if the heart or breathing stops, because it would be clinically futile or inconsistent with the patient's wishes. DNACPR does not mean withdrawal of care; active symptom control, comfort measures, and appropriate treatments continue. Sensitive communication is essential: Clinicians should explain the rationale, explore patient and family understanding, and document discussions carefully. Decisions must be reviewed regularly, as preferences and clinical circumstances may change.

Healthcare professionals are not obliged to provide treatment they consider clinically ineffective or inappropriate, and DNACPR decisions fall within this scope. Where CPR might be successful, or if there is doubt about its effectiveness, the patient must be consulted and may accept or decline CPR. If the patient lacks decision-making capacity, family members should be consulted; where a valid Lasting Power of Attorney (LPA) for health and welfare exists, that attorney may decline CPR on the patient's behalf.

If the clinical team concludes that CPR would be ineffective, they must inform the patient or their family. No patient or relative can compel clinicians to provide CPR. However, courts have found breaches of Article 8 of the Human Rights Act (the right to respect for private and family life) when adequate information was not provided. Where disagreement persists, seeking an independent second opinion is good practice.

In some cases, clinicians may delay implementing a DNACPR decision if immediate application would compromise care or if more time is needed for the patient and family to adjust to the prognosis.

DOCUMENTATION AND GOVERNANCE

Documentation is fundamental to safe and effective palliative care. APs should record discussions contemporaneously, noting all attendees and the decisions reached. ReSPECT and DNACPR forms must be signed, dated, and stored so that they are readily accessible across all care settings, including hospitals, primary care, and ambulance services. Electronic health records should be updated without delay and relevant community and specialist teams informed to ensure continuity of care. Organisational governance should mandate staff training and regular audit of ACP practice, providing assurance that documentation is accurate, current, and aligned with professional and legal standards.

CONCLUSION

ACP and treatment escalation discussions are central to high-quality EOL care. By recognising the signs of approaching death, using clear and consistent language, and applying structured approaches such as SPIKES and ReSPECT, APs can ensure that care decisions respect patient values, avoid futile interventions, and maintain dignity. Consistent documentation, regular review, and inter-professional collaboration safeguard these preferences across care settings and uphold ethical and legal standards.

Take-Home Messages

1. Early, honest, and well-documented conversations support person-centred care and reduce unnecessary interventions at the end of life.
2. Using precise terms such as palliative care, end of life, dying, death, and died enhances clarity and trust.
3. Structured frameworks such as SPIKES, ReSPECT, and treatment escalation plans help align clinical decisions with individual goals.
4. DNACPR decisions must be communicated sensitively, reviewed regularly, and clearly recorded to remain valid and accessible.
5. Advanced practitioners have a key leadership role in coordinating multidisciplinary input, ensuring legal compliance and sustaining dignity for patients and families.

REFERENCES

Abernethy, A.P., Shelby-James, T., Fazekas, B.S. et al. (2005). The Australia-modified Karnofsky Performance Status (AKPS) scale: a revised scale for contemporary palliative care clinical practice [ISRCTN81117481]. *BMC Palliative Care* 4 (1): 7.

Angelou, M. (2004). *The collected autobiographies of Maya Angelou*. New York: Random House.

Baile, W.F., Buckman, R., Lenzi, R. et al. (2000). SPIKES—a six-step protocol for delivering bad news: application to the patient with cancer. *The Oncologist* 5 (4): 302–311.

Bausewein, C., Schildmann, E., Rosenbruch, J., Haberland, B., Tänzler, S. and Ramsenthaler, C. (2018) Starting from scratch: implementing outcome measurement in clinical practice.

Brighton, L.J. and Bristowe, K. (2016). Communication in palliative care: talking about the end of life, before the end of life. *Postgraduate Medical Journal* 92 (1090): 466–470.

British Geriatrics Society (2020). End of life care in frailty: advance care planning. https://www.bgs.org.uk/end-of-life-care-in-frailty-advance-care-planning (accessed 17 September 2025).

Care Quality Commission (2021). *Protect, Respect, Connect – Decisions About Living and Dying Well During COVID-19: CQC's Review of 'Do Not Attempt Cardiopulmonary Resuscitation' Decisions During the COVID-19 Pandemic.* London: Care Quality Commission.

General Medical Council (GMC) (2024). Treatment and Care Towards the End of Life: Good Practice in Decision Making. https://www.gmc-uk.org/ethical-guidance/ethical-guidance-for-doctors/treatment-and-care-towards-the-end-of-life (accessed 17 September 2025).

Houben, C.H., Spruit, M.A., Groenen, M.T. et al. (2014). Efficacy of advance care planning: a systematic review and meta-analysis. *Journal of the American Medical Directors Association* 15 (7): 477–489.

Nakajima, N. (2022). Palliative Care Outcome Scale assessment for cancer patients eligible for palliative care: perspectives on the relationship between patient-reported outcome and objective assessments. *Current Oncology* 29 (10): 7140–7147.

National Institute for Health and Care Excellence (NICE) (2019). End of life care for adults: service delivery. NICE guideline [NG142]. https://www.nice.org.uk/guidance/ng142 (accessed 17 September 2025).

NHS England (2022). Ambitions for palliative and end of life care: a national framework for local action 2021-2026. https://www.england.nhs.uk/publication/ambitions-for-palliative-and-end-of-life-care-a-national-framework-for-local-action-2021-2026/ (accessed 17 September 2025).

NHS England (2023a). *Palliative and end of life care advanced practice area specific capability and curriculum framework.* NHS England. Available at: https://advanced-practice.hee.nhs.uk/wp-content/uploads/sites/28/2025/01/Palliative-and-end-of-life-care-advanced-practice-area-specific-capability-and-curriculum-framework-NHSE.pdf (accessed 30 January 2026).

NHS England (2023b). *Acute medicine advanced practice area specific capability and curriculum framework.* NHS England. Available at: https://advanced-practice.hee.nhs.uk/wp-content/uploads/sites/28/2025/03/Acute-medicine-advanced-practice-area-specific-capability-and-curriculum-framework-NHSE.pdf (accessed 30 January 2026).

NHS England (2025). *Multi-professional framework for advanced practice in England – Edition 2025.* NHS England. Available at: https://advanced-practice.hee.nhs.uk/wp-content/uploads/sites/28/2025/05/Multi-professional-framework-for-advanced-practice-in-England---Edition-2025.pdf (accessed 29 January 2026).

Resuscitation Council UK (2025a). *ReSPECT for healthcare professionals.* https://www.resus.org.uk/respect/respect-healthcare-professionals (accessed 17 September 2025).

Resuscitation Council UK. (2025b) *CPR recommendations, DNACPR and ReSPECT.* https://www.resus.org.uk/public-resource/cpr-decisions-and-dnacpr (accessed 17 September 2025).

Sudore, R.L., Lum, H.D., You, J.J. et al. (2017). Defining advance care planning for adults: a consensus definition from a multidisciplinary Delphi panel. *Journal of Pain and Symptom Management* 53 (5): 821–832.

CHAPTER 23

Managing the Most Common Symptoms in End-of-Life Medicine

Aim

The aim of this chapter is to equip advanced practitioners (APs) with the knowledge and clinical competence to assess and manage the most common symptoms encountered in end-of-life care including pain, breathlessness, nausea and vomiting, agitation and delirium, and respiratory tract secretions using evidence-based pharmacological and non-pharmacological strategies that prioritise comfort, dignity, and patient preferences.

LEARNING OUTCOMES

By the end of this chapter, readers will be able to:

1. Critically appraise the pathophysiology and clinical impact of key end-of-life symptoms, including pain, dyspnoea, nausea, delirium, and secretions.
2. Select and safely titrate first-line and adjunctive medications for these symptoms, applying national guidance and adjusting for frailty or renal or hepatic impairment.
3. Integrate non-pharmacological interventions with pharmacological care to optimise comfort and reduce distress for patients and families.
4. Demonstrate person-centred decision-making that incorporates patient goals, anticipatory prescribing, and timely review within a multidisciplinary framework.
5. Reflect on ethical, professional, and communication skills needed to deliver compassionate symptom management in complex or rapidly changing end of life.

SELF-ASSESSMENT QUESTIONS

1. What pharmacological and non-pharmacological interventions are recommended for managing pain, breathlessness, nausea, agitation, and respiratory tract secretions in end-of-life care?
2. How should medicines and doses be adjusted for frail older adults or those with renal or hepatic impairment to ensure safe and effective symptom control?

> To manage symptoms well is to listen beyond the body,
> to hear the language of suffering and respond with
> compassion, precision, and presence.

INTRODUCTION

End-of-life (EoL) care is an essential aspect of healthcare that focuses on the management of patients who are nearing the end of their lives (Akdeniz et al., 2021). Effective prescribing is central to this care, aiming to alleviate suffering and improve quality of life in patients facing advanced illness (Kastbom, 2021). The prescription of medications must be based on comprehensive clinical judgement, patient preferences, and current best practices. This review aims to explore the prescribing guidance for EoL care, focusing on common symptoms experienced at this stage of life and the medications used to manage them. Effective symptom management in EoL care requires a multifaceted approach, addressing physical, psychological, and social aspects of care. Among the key symptoms to be managed are pain, breathlessness, nausea, delirium, and agitation, with each requiring focused prescribing strategies. This chapter specifically addresses the essential management of key symptoms commonly encountered in EoL, including pain, breathlessness, nausea and vomiting, agitation, and respiratory tract secretions. It draws on the National Institute for Health and Care Excellence (NICE) guidelines, alongside other national and international frameworks, to provide evidence-based prescribing guidance for effective symptom relief.

Multi-Professional Framework (MPF) for Advanced Practitioners

(Adapted from NHS England, 2025)

This chapter maps to the following statement within the MPF:

1. Clinical practice: 1.1–1.11
2. Leadership and management: 2.1, 2.2, 2.3, 2.5, 2.6
3. Education: 3.1, 3.2, 3.3, 3.5
4. Research: 4.1, 4.2, 4.3

Accreditation Consideration

This chapter maps to the statement with the following national accretional documents:

Curriculum framework for advanced practice in the care of older people (NHS England, 2022)

1. Core CiPs: 1–5
2. Generic Clinical CiPs: 1–6
3. Specialty Clinical CiPs (Older People): 1–4

Curriculum framework for advanced practitioners in the case of the palliative and end-of-life care (NHS England, 2023a)

1. Clinical pillar: 1, 2, 3, 4
2. Leadership and management: 2.1, 2.2, 2.3
3. Education: 3.1, 3.2, 3.3, 3.4
4. Research: 4.1, 4.2

Curriculum for advanced practitioners in acute medicine (NHS England, 2023b)

1. Core CiPs: 1, 2, 3, 4
2. Generic Clinical CiPs: 1–5
3. Specialty Clinical CiPs (acute medicine): 1–5 and acute conditions

BREATHLESSNESS

Breathlessness, or dyspnoea, is a common and distressing symptom in EoL care, significantly impairing quality of life (Campbell et al., 2021). It is particularly associated with advanced conditions such as cancer, heart failure, and chronic obstructive pulmonary disease (COPD). A recent systematic review and meta-analysis of 67 studies involving 78,409 patients with advanced cancer reported a prevalence of dyspnoea of 43% (Hou et al., 2025). The symptom is highly subjective, often described as 'air hunger', and does not always correlate with objective markers such as oxygen saturation or respiratory rate. For patients, the sensation provokes fear and anxiety, while families may view worsening breathlessness as a sign of imminent death. For advanced practitioners (APs), careful assessment and timely intervention are therefore essential. Tools such as the Modified Borg Dyspnoea Scale (Doherty et al., 2006) and the Edmonton Symptom Assessment System (Hui and Bruera, 2017) can aid evaluation, although the patient's own description remains central.

Non-pharmacological strategies should be considered first line. Simple interventions, such as repositioning patients upright or laterally with head elevation, can reduce diaphragmatic load (Dickman, 2010). Opening windows or using a handheld fan directed at the face provides relief through trigeminal nerve stimulation (Saunders, 2022). Breathing techniques, including pursed-lip breathing and activity pacing, promote control, while reassurance and calm communication help reduce associated anxiety (Zemel, 2022; Saunders, 2022). Occupational therapy input can support energy conservation, and maintaining a calm, uncluttered environment reduces sensory burden.

Pharmacological management is indicated where symptoms persist despite basic interventions. Morphine sulphate is considered the first-line agent, reducing the central perception of breathlessness and associated anxiety (Obarzanek et al., 2023). Initial dosing is typically 2.5–5 mg subcutaneously, with repeat doses every 30 minutes if needed (Dickman, 2010). If three or more as-required doses are required in 24 hours, conversion to a continuous subcutaneous infusion using a T34 syringe pump is recommended, with the daily dose calculated as 50% of the patient's usual oral morphine and titrated by 30% if necessary (Northampton General Hospital End of Life Care Policy, 2025). Where anxiety or panic exacerbates symptoms, midazolam (2.5 mg subcutaneously as required or 5–10 mg by infusion) may be added (St Nicholas Hospice Care, 2012; García-López et al., 2023). For frail or elderly patients, or those with renal or hepatic impairment, starting doses should be reduced (e.g. 2.5 mg morphine PRN) to minimise the risk of sedation and overdose. In opioid-naïve patients, an antiemetic such as haloperidol (0.5–1 mg subcutaneously PRN) may be required to prevent nausea.

PAIN MANAGEMENT

Pain is one of the most distressing symptoms for patients at the EoL, often requiring careful assessment and management to ensure comfort (Gerber et al., 2022). Opioids, such as morphine, are the essential of pain management in EoL care, with their use based on evidence supporting their effectiveness in controlling moderate-to-severe pain (NICE, 2025). Oral morphine is typically the first-line option for pain management. However, in patients who are unable to take oral medications, subcutaneous morphine via a syringe pump may be necessary (Franklin and Lovell, 2025). Subcutaneous administration provides continuous infusion of medication, ensuring steady pain relief without the need for frequent administration. This approach is particularly useful for patients with advanced cancer or end-stage organ failure, where pain control is paramount (Gawande, 2014). Effective pain management requires regular monitoring to assess both the efficacy of pain relief and the potential for side effects, such as sedation, constipation, and respiratory depression. Dose adjustments should be made based on these factors, with consideration given to the patient's renal function and existing comorbidities (Franklin and Lovell, 2025). For example, patients with renal impairment may require reduced doses of opioids due to slower clearance, which increases the risk of opioid toxicity (Smith et al., 2022). For these patients, it is essential to consult with specialists such as palliative care teams or a nephrologist for appropriate dose titration and to ensure that potential side effects are mitigated.

In addition to opioids, adjuvant medications such as steroids and bisphosphonates may be prescribed to manage bone pain or neuropathic pain (Pickering et al., 2024). Medications such as gabapentin or amitriptyline can be used for neuropathic pain, while dexamethasone is often used in cancer patients to alleviate inflammatory pain and swelling. These adjuvants enhance the analgesic effect and can be particularly useful in patients with complex pain syndromes. For patients on oral morphine who require continuous pain relief, it may be necessary to convert their oral doses to a subcutaneous infusion (Biesiada et al., 2023). The EoL medication guidance of Buckinghamshire Healthcare NHS Trust and Buckinghamshire Clinical Commissioning Group (2021) suggests dividing the total oral morphine dose by 2 (50%) to determine the appropriate subcutaneous dose. For instance, a patient on 60 mg oral morphine daily would require 30 mg subcutaneously, administered via a syringe pump over 24 hours. This ensures that pain relief is maintained consistently, avoiding the peaks and troughs that can occur with intermittent oral dosing.

In addition, PRN doses of morphine are often prescribed at one-sixth of the total daily dose to manage breakthrough pain (Greater Manchester and Eastern Cheshire Strategic Clinical Networks, 2019). For example, a patient receiving 30 mg of morphine over 24 hours via subcutaneous infusion may require

5 mg PRN. These doses should be adjusted based on the patient's pain level, with careful monitoring for efficacy and potential side effects. If PRN doses are required frequently, the total daily dose may need to be increased to ensure that adequate pain relief is maintained. It is important to note that lower starting doses should be used in certain vulnerable populations, such as elderly, frail, cachectic, or patients with renal or liver failure, as they may be more susceptible to the sedative effects and toxicity of opioids (Gawande, 2014). In these cases, starting with morphine sulphate 2.5 mg PRN subcutaneously is recommended. Regular reviews of the patient's pain levels and side effects, as well as any adjustments to the dose, are essential to maintain optimal care (Franklin and Lovell, 2025).

NAUSEA AND VOMITING

Nausea and vomiting are common and often distressing symptoms in EoL care, frequently caused by disease progression, medication side effects, or metabolic disturbances (Ijaopo et al., 2023). Other contributors include bowel obstruction, central nervous system involvement, and psychological distress. Because multiple neurochemical pathways may be implicated, assessment should aim to identify the most likely mechanism, as this informs treatment selection. Management is generally practical, starting with a single antiemetic targeted at the suspected pathway and escalating to combination therapy if symptoms persist. Once stability is achieved, rationalising medication helps to minimise side effects and polypharmacy. For APs, it is important to understand the cause of nausea and vomiting in order to determine the pathway so that appropriate antiemetics can be prescribed (Table 23.1).

Furthermore, APs should be careful when selecting antiemetics, as certain medications may be contraindicated or require cautious use in specific patient groups. For instance, cyclizine can exacerbate congestive heart failure and should be avoided in such cases, while haloperidol may be a safer option for patients with chronic renal impairment (Dickman, 2010). Non-pharmacological approaches such as reassurance, avoidance of known triggers, and complementary therapies may also support symptom control.

The approach to management should always be individualised, taking into account the patient's overall condition, previous response to therapy, and tolerance of medications. For those already benefiting

TABLE 23.1   Nausea and vomiting pathways.

Pathway/site	Mechanism	Main receptor targets	Medication options
Chemoreceptor trigger zone (CTZ)	Detects circulating toxins, drugs, and metabolites	Dopamine (D2), serotonin (5-HT3), NK1	Haloperidol, prochlorperazine, olanzapine, ondansetron, granisetron, aprepitant
Cortex	Sensory input (smells, sights), anxiety, ↑ ICP	Higher cortical pathways	Benzodiazepines (e.g. lorazepam, midazolam), corticosteroids (for raised ICP), acupuncture
Peripheral (GI tract)	Mechanical stretch, mucosal injury, local toxins	Dopamine (D2), serotonin (5-HT3)	Metoclopramide, ondansetron, granisetron, mirtazapine
Vestibular system	Motion sickness, labyrinth disorders	Histamine (H1), acetylcholine (M1)	Antihistamines (diphenhydramine, hydroxyzine), anticholinergics (hyoscine hydrobromide, scopolamine patch)

from an antiemetic, continuation via continuous subcutaneous infusion, such as a T34 syringe pump, can provide consistent relief (Gawande, 2022). In patients not previously established on treatment, haloperidol is commonly initiated at low subcutaneous doses (0.5–1 mg as required), with a maximum daily dose of 10 mg. If two or more breakthrough doses are required within 24 hours, conversion to a continuous infusion, such as haloperidol 3 mg over 24 hours, offers a more stable option. Where haloperidol is ineffective or poorly tolerated, levomepromazine may be considered, either as a subcutaneous bolus or a continuous infusion at 6.25–12.5 mg over 24 hours (Northampton General Hospital End of Life Care Policy, 2025). Special caution is required in vulnerable groups, including frail older adults and those with renal or hepatic impairment. In such cases, lower starting doses (e.g. haloperidol 0.5 mg PRN) and careful monitoring for sedation or extrapyramidal symptoms are recommended. Regular reassessment is essential to ensure that therapy remains effective, side effects are minimised, and treatment continues to align with the patient's comfort and dignity.

DELIRIUM AND AGITATION

Restlessness and agitation often result from uncontrolled pain, anxiety, breathlessness, or delirium (Chin et al., 2023). These symptoms significantly impact the patient's comfort and quality of life, making their effective management essential. The first step in managing restlessness or agitation is identifying any underlying causes such as uncontrolled pain, anxiety, or physical discomfort (e.g. a full bladder or rectum). Addressing these causes promptly is essential before initiating pharmacological treatment. Midazolam is typically the first-line treatment for agitation, prescribed as a 2.5–5 mg subcutaneous PRN injection (Dickman, 2010), with repeat doses every 30 minutes as needed (Lock and Law, (2021). If two or more doses are required within 24 hours, a subcutaneous infusion of 10 mg midazolam via a T34 McKinley syringe pump is recommended, with the option to increase the dose gradually up to 30 mg per 24 hours for ongoing symptom management. For patients with delirium or psychotic features such as hallucinations, haloperidol can be used, with 0.5–1 mg PRN subcutaneously, increasing to a 3 mg subcutaneous infusion with 10 mg midazolam if required (Northampton General Hospital End of Life Care Policy, 2025). If haloperidol is ineffective, levomepromazine can be introduced at 12.5–25 mg PRN subcutaneously every 2 hours or via subcutaneous infusion at 50 mg over 24 hours. Again, special consideration must be given to vulnerable patients, including the elderly, cachectic, or those with renal or liver failure, who may need lower starting doses of sedatives to avoid potential side effects. The use of midazolam, haloperidol, and levomepromazine ensures that restlessness and agitation are effectively managed in a compassionate, patient-centred manner, improving the patient's comfort and quality of life in their final stages (St Nicholas Hospice Care, 2012).

MANAGEMENT OF RESPIRATORY TRACT SECRETIONS

Noisy secretions can often occur in patients nearing the EoL. These secretions are often a natural part of dying and may not necessarily require treatment unless they become troublesome for the patient or their loved ones (NICE, 2021). The first step in managing these symptoms is adjusting the patient's position, which may help alleviate the accumulation of secretions (Dickman, 2010). In cases where the patient experiences troublesome secretions, glycopyrronium (a muscarinic receptor antagonist) is commonly prescribed to manage these symptoms (Parker-Smith and Corbett, 2023). Initially, a subcutaneous injection of 200 µg of PRN (as needed) may be given every four hours. If symptoms persist, the dose can be increased to 400 µg subcutaneously, followed by 200 µg every four hours, with a maximum of 1.2 mg per 24 hours. In patients who require more continuous relief, glycopyrronium may be administered via a syringe pump, delivering a subcutaneous infusion of 800 µg over 24 hours (Parker and Aslett, 2024). Supportive care is also important. In a small number of cases, gentle suction may be helpful, but medications may not always be effective. In addition, it is essential to reassure family and friends, emphasising that this symptom, while distressing, is common and expected in the dying process (Etland, 2021).

MULTIDISCIPLINARY APPROACH

EoL care is best delivered through a multidisciplinary approach (Harasym et al., 2021), with input from doctors, nurses, pharmacists, social workers, and palliative care teams. This collaborative model ensures that symptom management is optimal, patient needs are comprehensively addressed, and ethical considerations are respected. Involving patients and families in discussions about treatment goals, preferences, and potential side effects of medications is a key component of person-centred care (Ellis-Smith et al., 2021). The focus should always be on improving the quality of life and providing comfort, rather than aggressive interventions aimed at prolonging life.

CHALLENGES IN MENTAL HEALTH PRESCRIBING

Patients with severe mental illness, such as schizophrenia or major depression, often present unique challenges at the end of life, including impaired communication, fluctuating capacity, and limited insight into physical deterioration (Edwards et al., 2021). These factors complicate prescribing decisions, particularly when balancing psychotropic medications with palliative treatments and managing risks associated with polypharmacy. The MENLOC systematic review (Edwards et al., 2021) emphasised that diagnostic overshadowing, fragmented care pathways, and enduring stigma frequently lead to the under-recognition of symptoms and delays in the initiation of appropriate EoL prescribing. These patient-level complexities are compounded by broader systemic issues within the mental health workforce.

The Royal College of Nursing (RCN, 2024) has reported persistent underinvestment in mental health nursing, leading to critical vacancy rates and a reliance on temporary staff unfamiliar with patients' complex needs, factors that may compromise safe prescribing. Furthermore, a 2023 RCN survey revealed that 63% of mental health nurses believe their professional role is being diluted, citing concerns over generic job titles, limited role recognition, and constrained career progression (RCN, 2023). These conditions contribute to professional demoralisation, erode prescribing confidence, and restrict autonomous practice. In addition, the forthcoming Mental Health Bill 2025 introduces legislative reforms intended to modernise mental health care (UK Parliament, 2025); however, these changes may create uncertainty around scope of practice and introduce additional educational requirements for nurse prescribers. While primary research specifically focused on advanced nurse prescribers in mental health remains limited, the 2025 Health and Social Care Report on inpatient mental health services highlights key structural challenges, including non-therapeutic environments, workforce instability, and fragmented interprofessional collaboration (Health and Social Care Safety Investigation Branch, 2024). Such conditions directly impact the quality and safety of prescribing decisions, limiting the capacity of advanced practitioners to deliver consistent, empathetic, person-centred, evidence-based care. These clinical and systemic challenges highlight the need for targeted research and policy reform to support and retain advanced mental health nurse prescribers within a sustainable, well-resourced framework.

CONCLUSION

Prescribing for EoL care is a complex process that requires careful attention to the individual's symptoms, clinical condition, and overall prognosis. Medications must be tailored to alleviate common symptoms such as pain, breathlessness, nausea, and delirium, while maintaining patient comfort and dignity. Evidence-based guidelines, such as those provided by NICE and the EoL medication guidance, provide valuable frameworks for effective prescribing in this context. However, clinical judgement and regular assessment are essential in ensuring that the approach remains flexible and responsive to the patient's changing needs. Ongoing education, training, and multidisciplinary teamwork are crucial for ensuring that healthcare providers can deliver high-quality, compassionate care during this critical stage of life. The ultimate goal of prescribing at the EoL should always be to alleviate suffering; enhance comfort; and provide a dignified, peaceful death for the patient.

Case Study 23.1   I Can't Catch My Breath

Mr J, 78, GOLD IV COPD and HFpEF, bedbound, on long-term oxygen at home. Now in hospice with escalating dyspnoea at rest, RR 28, SpO_2 92% on 2 L/min, anxious, using accessory muscles. On regular tiotropium/indacaterol, PRN salbutamol neb, sertraline 50 mg. No opioids currently.

Tasks for the AP

1. Perform a focused assessment and identify reversible versus non-reversible causes.
2. Initiate immediate non-pharmacological measures.
3. Prescribe first-line pharmacological management and plan rescue medication.
4. Decide when to convert to a continuous SC infusion and calculate a starting dose.
5. Safety: what will you do differently if he becomes drowsy or if eGFR is 28 mL/min?

Key Discussion Points

- Assessment: pattern, triggers, orthopnoea, secretions, wheeze, anxiety; exam incl. work of breathing; ESAS/Borg; consider infection/PE unlikely in last days if no red flags.
- Non-pharmacological: upright/forward-lean, fan to face, breathing coaching, calm reassurance, minimize stimuli; brief family explanation to reduce fear.
- Pharmacology: morphine SC 2.5 mg PRN q30–60 min (opioid-naïve), consider midazolam 2.5 mg SC PRN if panic prominent; oxygen not routinely escalated as $SpO_2 \geq$ 90%.
- Conversion: if $\geq$3 PRNs in 24 hours, start CSCI morphine via T34. If total PRN used = 10 mg/24 h, start ~10 mg/24 h (or 50% of any established oral dose where relevant) and prescribe PRN morphine = 1/6 of 24 hours dose.
- Renal impairment/frailty: start at lower end (morphine 1–2 mg SC PRN), extend PRN interval; monitor sedation; consider oxycodone SC if morphine intolerance/accumulation locally permitted.

Case Study 23.2   Constant Nausea and No Bowel Movements

Ms L, 64, metastatic ovarian cancer, 3 days of nausea/vomiting, colicky pain, minimal stool/flatus, tinkling bowel sounds. eGFR 75, LFTs normal. On cyclizine 50 mg TDS PO from GP without benefit. History of HFpEF.

Tasks

1. What is the likely mechanism(s) of nausea and vomiting?
2. Choose a single first-line antiemetic and justify based on pathway.
3. What will you avoid and why?
4. If two or more PRNs are needed in 24 hours, what CSCI will you start? Include dose.
5. Add two non-pharmacological measures and a communication point for family.

Key Points

- Mechanism: suspected malignant bowel obstruction → GI/peripheral + CTZ.
- First-line: haloperidol 0.5–1 mg SC PRN for CTZ; add metoclopramide only if no complete obstruction and no colic; consider levomepromazine if refractory.
- Avoid: cyclizine in heart failure (can worsen CHF) (Dickman, 2010).
- CSCI: haloperidol 3 mg/24 h via T34 if multiple PRNs needed; alternative levomepromazine 6.25–12.5 mg/24 h if haloperidol not tolerated.
- Non-pharmacological: small sips, oral care, trigger avoidance; communicate mechanism-based plan and expectations; review constipation/NG decompression if appropriate/goals concordant.

Learning Points

1. Opioids such as morphine are essential to manage moderate-to-severe pain in EoL care, with careful dose adjustments based on the patient's response and comorbidities, particularly renal function.
2. The management of breathlessness involves both pharmacological treatments (e.g. morphine) and non-pharmacological interventions (e.g. repositioning and reassurance) to address both the physical and emotional aspects of the symptom.
3. Haloperidol is often the first-line medication for managing nausea and vomiting in EoL care, but if ineffective, alternative options such as levomepromazine or midazolam can be considered.
4. Agitation and restlessness in EoL care require careful assessment for underlying causes, with midazolam and haloperidol commonly used for symptom relief, often in combination for comprehensive management.

Take-Home Messages

1. Timely recognition and proactive management of common EoL symptoms—pain, breathlessness, nausea and vomiting, agitation, and respiratory secretions—are essential to patient comfort and dignity.

2. Management should combine evidence-based pharmacological treatments with non-pharmacological approaches and clear, compassionate communication.

3. Regular review and dose adjustment are vital, particularly in frail older adults or those with renal or hepatic impairment.

4. Anticipatory prescribing and multidisciplinary collaboration help prevent crises and ensure that care remains consistent with patient preferences and national guidance.

5. Ongoing education and reflective practice strengthen clinical confidence and maintain high standards of palliative and EoL care.

REFERENCES

Akdeniz, M., Yardımcı, B., and Kavukcu, E. (2021). Ethical considerations at the end-of-life care. *SAGE Open Medicine* 9: 20503121211000918.

Biesiada, A., Ciałkowska-Rysz, A., and Mastalerz-Migas, A. (2023). Subcutaneous drug supply in the practice of a primary care physician—a literature review. *Family Medicine & Primary Care Review* 25 (4): 449–454.

Buckinghamshire Healthcare NHS Trust and Buckinghamshire Clinical Commissioning Group (2021). Conversion of opioid medicines dosages: guideline 699FM.3. `https://www.bucksformulary.nhs.uk/docs/Guideline_699FM.pdf` (accessed 28 April 2025).

Campbell, M.L., Donesky, D., Sarkozy, A., and Reinke, L.F. (2021). Treatment of dyspnea in advanced disease and at the end of life. *Journal of Hospice & Palliative Nursing* 23 (5): 406–420.

Chin, M.S., Roth, A.J., and Matsoukas, K. (2023). Anxiety in palliative care. In: *Handbook of Psychiatry in Palliative Medicine: Psychosocial Care of the Terminally Ill*, 3rde (ed. W. Breitbart and H.M. Chochinov), 62. Oxford: Oxford University Press.

Dickman, A. (2010). *Drugs in Palliative Care*, 1e. Oxford: Oxford University Press.

Doherty, D.E., Belfer, M.H., Brunton, S.A. et al. (2006). Chronic obstructive pulmonary disease: consensus recommendations for early diagnosis and treatment. *Journal of Family Practice* 55 (11): S1–S1.

Edwards, C., Hannigan, B., Coffey, M. et al. (2021). *End-of-life care for people with severe mental illness: mixed methods systematic review and thematic synthesis. Palliative Medicine* 35 (10): 1778–1793. `https://doi.org/10.1177/02692163211037480`.

Ellis-Smith, C., Tunnard, I., Dawkins, M. et al. (2021). Managing clinical uncertainty in older people towards the end of life: a systematic review of person-centred tools. *BMC Palliative Care* 20: 1–41.

Etland, C. (2021). Palliative and end-of-life care. In: *Critical care nursing: diagnosis and management*, 9the (ed. L.D. Urden, K.M. Stacy, and M.E. Lough), 150. London: Elsevier.

Franklin, A.E. and Lovell, M.R. (2025). Pain and pain management in palliative care. In: *Textbook of Palliative Care* (ed. R.D. MacLeod and L. Van den Block), 163–189. Springer Nature Switzerland AG: Cham, Switzerland.

García-López, I., Chocarro-González, L., Martín-Romero, I. et al. (2023). Pediatric palliative care at home: a prospective study on subcutaneous drug administration. *Journal of Pain and Symptom Management* 66 (3): e319–e326.

Gawande, A. (2014). *Being mortal: Medicine and what matters in the end.* Metropolitan Books.

Gawande, A. (2022). Medications in end-of-life care. In: *Palliative Touch: Massage for People at the End of Life*, 145.

Gerber, K., Willmott, L., White, B. et al. (2022). Barriers to adequate pain and symptom relief at the end of life: a qualitative study capturing nurses' perspectives. *Collegian* 29 (1): 1–8.

Greater Manchester and Eastern Cheshire Strategic Clinical Networks (2019). *Palliative Care Pain and Symptom Control Guidelines for Adults: For Staff Providing Generalist Palliative Care*, 5e. `https://www.england.nhs.uk/north-west/wp-content/uploads/sites/48/2020/01/Palliative-Care-Pain-and-Symptom-Control-Guidelines.pdf` (accessed 28 April 2025).

Harasym, P.M., Afzaal, M., Brisbin, S. et al. (2021). Multi-disciplinary supportive end of life care in long-term care: an integrative approach to improving end of life. *BMC Geriatrics* 21 (1): 326.

Health and Social Care Safety Investigation Branch (2024). Mental health inpatient settings: patient safety investigation report, March. `https://www.hssib.org.uk/patient-safety-investigations/mental-health-inpatient-settings/` (accessed 3 July 2025).

Hou, T., Ho, M.H., Jia, S., and Lin, C.C. (2025). The prevalence and factors of dyspnoea among advanced cancer survivors: a systematic review and meta-analysis. *Cancer Nursing* 10–1097. `https://doi.org/10.1097/NCC.0000000000001490`.

Hui, D. and Bruera, E. (2017). The Edmonton Symptom Assessment System 25 years later: past, present, and future developments. *Journal of Pain and Symptom Management* 53 (3): 630–643.

Ijaopo, E.O., Zaw, K.M., Ijaopo, R.O., and Khawand-Azoulai, M. (2023). A review of clinical signs and symptoms of imminent end-of-life in individuals with advanced illness. *Gerontology and Geriatric Medicine* 9: 23337214231183243.

Kastbom, L. (2021). *A good death from the perspective of patients with severe illness and advance care planning (ACP) in patients near end-of-life.* Linköping: Linköping University Electronic Press 1769.

Lock, A. and Law, S. (2021). *Anticipatory Medication Clinical Guidelines. Sandwell and West Birmingham Hospitals NHS Trust.* Available at: `https://www.swbh.nhs.uk/wp-content/uploads/2021/01/Anticipatory-Medication-Clinical-Guidelines-Jan-2021.pdf` (accessed 3 February 2026).

National Institute for Health and Care Excellence (NICE) (2021). Palliative care – secretions. Clinical Knowledge Summaries. `https://cks.nice.org.uk/topics/palliative-care-secretions/` (accessed 28 April 2025).

National Institute for Health and Care Excellence (NICE) (2025). Prescribing in palliative care. `https://bnf.nice.org.uk/medicines-guidance/prescribing-in-palliative-care/` (accessed 28 April 2025).

NHS England (2022). *Older people advanced practice area specific capability and curriculum framework.* NHS England. Available at: `https://advanced-practice.hee.nhs.uk/wp-content/uploads/sites/28/2025/01/Older-people-advanced-practice-area-specific-capability-and-curriculum-framework-NHSE.pdf` (accessed 30 January 2026).

NHS England (2023a). *Palliative and end of life care advanced practice area specific capability and curriculum framework.* NHS England. Available at: `https://advanced-practice.hee.nhs.uk/wp-content/uploads/sites/28/2025/01/Palliative-and-end-of-life-care-advanced-practice-area-specific-capability-and-curriculum-framework-NHSE.pdf` (accessed 30 January 2026).

NHS England (2023b). *Acute medicine advanced practice area specific capability and curriculum framework*. NHS England. Available at: `https://advanced-practice.hee.nhs.uk/wp-content/uploads/sites/28/2025/03/Acute-medicine-advanced-practice-area-specific-capability-and-curriculum-framework-NHSE.pdf` (accessed 30 January 2026).

NHS England (2025). *Multi-professional framework for advanced practice in England – Edition 2025*. NHS England. Available at: `https://advanced-practice.hee.nhs.uk/wp-content/uploads/sites/28/2025/05/Multi-professional-framework-for-advanced-practice-in-England---Edition-2025.pdf` (accessed 29 January 2026).

Northampton General Hospital End of Life Care Policy (2025). *End of Life Care Policy*. Northampton: Northampton General Hospital NHS Trust.

Obarzanek, L., Wu, W., and Tutag-Lehr, V. (2023). Opioid management of dyspnea at end of life: a systematic review. *Journal of Palliative Medicine* 26 (5): 711–726.

Parker, K. and Aslett, M. (2024). Medicines management in palliative care including syringe pumps. In: *Handbook of Palliative Care* (ed. S. Russell, C. Faull, and W. Prentice), 306–327. Oxford: Wiley-Blackwell.

Parker-Smith, J. and Corbett, C. (2023). Approach to respiratory secretions at the end of life. In: *Beyond Evidence-Based Medicine: Clinical Pearls from Experienced Physicians* (ed. R. Junckerstorff, S. Brady, and A.K. Aung), 127–129. Springer Nature Singapore Pte Ltd: Singapore.

Pickering, M.E., Delay, M., and Morel, V. (2024). Chronic pain and bone-related pathologies: a narrative review. *Journal of Pain Research* 2937–2947.

Royal College of Nursing (2023). Is mental health nursing being diluted?, 27 July `https://www.rcn.org.uk/news-and-events/Blogs/is-mental-health-nursing-being-diluted-270723` (accessed 3 July 2025).

Royal College of Nursing (2024). Royal College of Nursing responds to HSSIB report on 'the delivery of safe and therapeutic care to adults in mental health inpatient settings', 24 October. `https://www.rcn.org.uk/news-and-events/Press-Releases/rcn-responds-to-hssib-mental-health-report-24102024` (accessed 3 July 2025).

Saunders, C. (2022). *Palliative Touch: Massage for People at the End of Life*. London: Jessica Kingsley Publishers.

Smith, K., Wang, M., Abdukalikov, R. et al. (2022). Pain management considerations in patients with opioid use disorder requiring critical care. *The Journal of Clinical Pharmacology* 62 (4): 449–462.

St Nicholas Hospice Care (2012). End of life medicines information pack. `https://stnicholashospice.org.uk/wp-content/uploads/2016/05/medicines-information-pack.pdf` (accessed 28 April 2025).

UK Parliament (2025). Mental health bill [HL]. Parliamentary bills, session 2024–25. `https://bills.parliament.uk/bills/3884` (accessed 3 July 2025).

Zemel, R.A. (2022). Pharmacologic and non-pharmacologic dyspnea management in advanced cancer patients. *American Journal of Hospice and Palliative Care* 39 (7): 847–855.

CHAPTER 24

Ethical Consideration in Frailty and End-of-Life Medicine

Aim

The aim of this chapter is to equip advanced practitioners (APs) with the legal knowledge, ethical reasoning, and practical skills required to lead complex decision-making in frailty and end-of-life care, ensuring that all interventions remain person centred, evidence based, and fully compliant with UK law and professional standards.

LEARNING OUTCOMES

By the end of this chapter, readers will be able to:

1. Conduct and document decision-specific capacity assessments in line with the Mental Capacity Act 2005; apply the best interests standard; and involve LPAs, advance decisions, and IMCAs appropriately.
2. Formulate proportionate end-of-life care plans that justify withholding or withdrawing treatment, decisions on ANH, and the use of palliative sedation and opioids under the doctrine of double effect, with safe anticipatory prescribing consistent with GMC and NICE guidance.
3. Apply confidentiality and data protection duties in family-involved care, preventing breaches while supporting shared decision-making and clear records of consent.
4. Implement lawful, least restrictive arrangements by recognising when Deprivation of Liberty Safeguards (DoLS) authorisation is required, leading multidisciplinary best interests processes for medical and social decisions, and engaging safeguarding and the Court of Protection when indicated.
5. Lead and justify ethical deliberation in contexts of frailty, multimorbidity, and resource constraint, challenging ageism and advocating for equitable, person-centred outcomes that uphold dignity.

SELF-ASSESSMENT QUESTIONS

1. How would you apply the Mental Capacity Act 2005 to assess and document decision-making capacity in a frail older adult whose cognition fluctuates, and what steps would you take if capacity is lacking?
2. In a scenario where a family requests life-prolonging treatment that offers minimal benefit, how would you use the principles of autonomy, beneficence, non-maleficence, and justice to guide ethically sound and legally defensible care planning?

> When medicine can no longer add days, ethics must ensure that those days still hold meaning, autonomy, and respect.

INTRODUCTION

The proportion of older adults in the United Kingdom is rising progressively, creating increasing demand for complex end-of-life (EoL) care. Current projections indicate that the population aged 65 years and older will grow from about 12.0 million in mid-2022 to 13.7 million by mid-2032, an increase of around 13.8%, while those aged 85 years and older are expected to almost double by mid-2047 (Office for National Statistics, 2025). Many of these older adults live with frailty and multiple long-term conditions, making their care needs distinct from those of people with a single terminal illness (National Institute for Health and Care Excellence [NICE], 2019; British Geriatrics Society, 2023a,b). Patterns of decline in advanced frailty vary widely, encompassing gradual deterioration as in late-stage dementia, sudden life-limiting events such as stroke or hip fracture, and unpredictable fluctuations triggered by acute episodes including delirium or functional crises (BGS, 2023a,b).

These diverse trajectories require health professionals to adopt flexible, ethically robust approaches that respect each person's values and circumstances (Van Den Noortgate and Van den Block, 2022a,b). Four established bioethical principles—autonomy, beneficence, non-maleficence, and justice—provide an essential foundation for such decision-making, guiding practitioners to honour patient preferences, promote well-being, avoid harm, and distribute resources fairly. Yet the realities of frailty and multimorbidity can challenge the application of these principles in isolation. An ethics of care perspective, which emphasises relationships, context and responsiveness, complements traditional bioethics by recognising the interdependence between frail individuals and their caregivers, thereby supporting a more holistic and patient-centred approach to care (Grealish, 1997a,b).

This chapter examines how these ethical principles, together with an ethics-of-care framework, inform clinical decision-making in EoL care for frail older adults. It highlights key challenges such as decisions about resuscitation, mental capacity assessments, and confidentiality and provides a structured foundation for practitioners seeking to deliver compassionate, ethically sound care that upholds dignity at the end of life.

Multi-Professional Framework (MPF) for Advanced Practitioners

Adapted from (NHS England, 2025)

This chapter maps to the following statement within the MPF:

1. Clinical practice: 1.1, 1.2, 1.3, 1.4
2. Leadership and management 2.0

3. Education: 3.0
4. Research: 4.0

Accreditation Consideration

This chapter maps to the statement with the following national accretional document:

Curriculum framework for advanced practice in the care of older people (NHS England, 2022):

1. Core CiPs: 1, 2, 3, 4, 5, 6
2. Generic Clinical CiPs 1, 3, 5, 6
3. Specialty Clinical CiPs (older People): 1, 2, 3, 4

Curriculum framework for advanced practitioners in the case of the palliative and end-of-life care (NHS England, 2023a)

1. Clinical pillar: 1.1, 1.2, 1.3, 1.4
2. Leadership and management: 2.0
3. Education: 3.0
4. Research: 4.0

Curriculum for advanced practitioners in acute medicine (NHS England, 2023b)

1. Core CiPs: 1, 2, 3, 4, 5, 6
2. Generic Clinical CiPs: 1, 2, 3, 4, 5, 6
3. Specialty Clinical CiPs 1–5 and acute medicine and acute conditions

ETHICAL PRINCIPLES IN END-OF-LIFE CARE

Providing EoL care to frail older adults is ethically demanding. Their illness trajectories are rarely linear, with periods of gradual deterioration, sudden acute events, and unpredictable fluctuations (BGS, 2023a,b; Van Den Noortgate and Van den Block, 2022a,b. Such complexity requires advanced clinical reasoning and a sound ethical framework. The classic bioethical principles: autonomy, beneficence, non-maleficence, and justice remain central (Beauchamp and Childress, 2013), yet frailty highlights the need for a relational, context-sensitive approach grounded in an ethics of care (Grealish, 1997a,b). Together these perspectives guide professionals in maintaining dignity, supporting choice, and ensuring fairness.

Autonomy

Autonomy concerns the individual's right to make informed and independent decisions about care (Yulianto and Awaludin, 2024). In EoL situations, decisions often focus on whether to continue life-prolonging interventions or prioritise comfort-centred palliative care (Alanazi et al., 2024). Respecting autonomy requires that patients understand the information, retain it long enough to weigh options, and can communicate their choices (Beauchamp and Childress, 2013). Frailty complicates this process. Cognitive fluctuation, communication barriers, and dependence on carers may impair decision-making. An ethics-of-care framework highlights relational autonomy, viewing decision-making as a shared and evolving process rather than a one-off act (Grealish, 1997a,b). Advanced care planning therefore needs to be iterative, revisiting preferences as the patient's condition changes.

The Mental Capacity Act (MCA) 2005 establishes a presumption of capacity unless proven otherwise and requires that all practicable steps be taken to support decision-making. When capacity is lost, advance statements, advance decisions, or lasting powers of attorney should guide care (Alzheimer's Society, 2024). Practitioners must ensure that these instruments are discussed and documented and must give primacy to the patient's expressed wishes even if these diverge from family expectations or clinical opinion (Kumar et al., 2024).

Beneficence and Non-maleficence: Balancing Benefit and Burden

Beneficence calls on clinicians to act in the patient's best interests, while non-maleficence requires avoidance of harm (Cheraghi et al., 2023). For frail individuals, treatments beneficial to fitter patients may offer little advantage and risk significant discomfort. Hospital admissions, invasive procedures, or aggressive therapies can exacerbate frailty or prolong the dying process without meaningful improvement in well-being (BGS, 2020; Crooms and Gelfman, 2020).

Good practice therefore emphasises palliative measures that relieve symptoms and support comfort. Non-maleficence requires careful weighing of risks and benefits before initiating or continuing any intervention (Akdeniz et al., 2021). When patients or families request treatments unlikely to provide benefit, professionals must explain likely outcomes and the ethical justification for a comfort-focused plan (Wiesen et al., 2021). Because clinical status can change quickly, continual reassessment is necessary to ensure treatment remains proportionate and appropriate.

Justice and Fairness

The Human Rights Act, (1998) provides a statutory basis for equitable and dignified healthcare. Key provisions include Article 2 (right to life), Article 3 (freedom from torture or inhuman or degrading treatment), Article 8 (respect for private and family life), and Article 14 (protection from discrimination). Justice requires that individuals receive equitable access to care and that scarce resources are distributed fairly. Frail patients are particularly vulnerable to implicit ageism and structural inequities (Koffman et al., 2023). Legal protections such as the Human Rights Act reinforce obligations to safeguard dignity, autonomy, and freedom from degrading treatment. Resource shortages, which become more acute during crises such as the COVID-19 pandemic, can heighten ethical dilemmas. Frameworks emphasise need-based allocation rather than judgements of social worth or chronological age (Berlinger et al., 2020; Satomi et al., 2020; Vergano et al., 2020). Clinicians, including APs should advocate to ensure that frail individuals receive equitable access to pain control, psychological support, and hospice services. An ethics-of-care perspective strengthens this commitment by attending to the patient's relationships and lived context (Grealish, 1997a,b). When conflict persists between clinicians and patients or their advocates, ACPs should seek a second opinion and, where available, input from a clinical ethics committee or mediator. If agreement remains unattainable, the Court of Protection provides the final legal determination.

Confidentiality and Privacy

Confidentiality is fundamental to trust and to the free expression of concerns and preferences (Akdeniz et al., 2021). In frailty, where family members are often closely involved, unintentional breaches of confidentiality are a recognised risk (Crotty et al., 2015). Protecting privacy is therefore both a professional and legal requirement under the Human Rights Act, 1998 and Data Protection Act 2018, which implement the UK General Data Protection Regulation. The MCA 2005 further stipulates that any sharing of personal information must reflect the patient's known wishes and best interests. Maintaining confidentiality requires explicit discussions with patients and families about how information will be shared. Clear documentation and careful communication reduce the chance of inadvertent disclosure and reinforce respect for autonomy and dignity.

SUBSTANTIVE ETHICS AND THE ETHICS OF CARE

Although the four principles provide a necessary foundation, frailty and multimorbidity often demand a broader ethical lens. Substantive ethics considers the patient's lived experience, social context, and interdependent relationships, going beyond abstract rules (Grealish, 1997a,b). This approach supports nuanced, situation-specific decisions. For example, autonomy becomes a continuing dialogue as capacity fluctuates; beneficence requires attention to psychological and spiritual well-being as well as physical comfort; justice calls for recognition of how poverty or isolation may limit access to services. By embedding these perspectives, APs can deliver EoL care that is both ethically rigorous and responsive to the realities of frailty.

LEGAL AND ETHICAL FRAMEWORKS FOR DECISION-MAKING IN END-OF-LIFE AND FRAILTY CARE

The Deprivation of Liberty Safeguards

The Deprivation of Liberty Safeguards (DoLS), introduced by the Mental Health Act 2007 as an amendment to the MCA 2005 and reinforced by the Care Act 2014, provide a legal framework to protect vulnerable adults who lack capacity from inappropriate restrictions on their freedom. They apply when continuous supervision or control and lack of freedom to leave amount to a deprivation of liberty, as clarified in case law such as *Cheshire West and Chester Council v P* (2014) (Supreme Court, 2014). Hospitals and care homes must always consider less restrictive alternatives and, if none are safe, obtain formal authorisation, appoint a representative, review the decision regularly, and allow appeal to the Court of Protection. In frailty and EoL care, DoLS are particularly relevant when advanced dementia or severe delirium necessitates measures such as locked wards or constant observation, ensuring that any deprivation of liberty remains lawful, proportionate, time limited, and centred on the person's best interests (BGS, 2015).

Lasting Power of Attorney

Making decisions about property and finances is an important consideration for frail individuals approaching the end of life. The MCA 2005 introduced the Lasting Power of Attorney (LPA) for property and financial affairs, allowing a competent adult to appoint a trusted person to manage financial matters such as paying bills, collecting benefits, or selling property, subject to any conditions set by the donor. Earlier Enduring Powers of Attorney (EPOA) remain valid if properly executed before October 2007. An LPA or EPOA cannot be made once the donor lacks the capacity to understand its implications, and where no such arrangement exists, the Court of Protection may appoint a deputy to manage finances. Testamentary capacity which is specific capacity to make a will that requires separate assessment and solicitors may seek a doctor's opinion where competence is uncertain. The law requires that the LPA is signed in the presence of an independent witness and supported by a certificate of capacity from a qualified third party, such as a solicitor or doctor, confirming that the person understands the authority being granted and is free from duress. Good practice recommends completing these arrangements when the individual is well, to avoid later disputes over capacity, and all discussions and assessments should be carefully documented to safeguard both the donor and the appointed attorney.

Decisions about medical treatment for adults who lack capacity are governed in the United Kingdom by the MCA 2005. This Act introduced the LPA for health and welfare, enabling a competent adult to appoint a trusted person to make future decisions about medical care and personal welfare, including consent to or refusal of treatment, provided this authority is explicitly stated and the LPA is registered with the Office of the Public Guardian. Such powers only come into effect when the donor loses capacity. In the absence of a valid LPA or advance directive, no individual including relatives who has an automatic right to decide on medical treatment for an adult without capacity. Clinicians are legally required to act in the person's best interests, taking into account any known wishes, values, or verbal statements, and should involve family members to help determine what the patient would have wanted. Where disagreements arise between relatives and the clinical team, a second opinion, consultation with an Independent Mental Capacity Advocate (IMCA), hospital legal advice, or recourse to the Court of Protection may be necessary. For patients whose capacity is uncertain, their views should be sought and carefully assessed, with the outcome and reasoning meticulously documented, recognising that a competent adult has the right to decline recommended treatment even when this may shorten life.

Social decisions for adults who lack capacity, such as determining where they should live, are subject to the same legal principles as medical decisions under the *Mental Capacity Act 2005*. Unless a valid LPA for health and welfare is in place, no one, including relatives, has automatic authority to decide on a person's accommodation or daily care arrangements. Clinicians must act in the individual's best interests, consulting family members and, where necessary, an IMCA, and ensuring that any plan is the least restrictive option in line with the DoLS. When a patient wishes to remain at home despite significant physical or cognitive risk, capacity must first be assessed. If the person has capacity, they may lawfully choose to accept those risks even against professional advice, although careful negotiation and practical safety measures may help reduce danger. Where capacity is lacking, a multidisciplinary best interests meeting and, in contentious cases, an application to the Court of Protection may be required to appoint a deputy to supervise welfare decisions. In every case, meticulous documentation of capacity assessments and the reasoning behind final decisions is essential for both ethical and legal accountability.

ADVANCE DIRECTIVES

Advance directives (ADs), also known as advance decisions or living wills, enable a competent adult to specify in advance which medical treatments they would refuse should they later lose capacity. Enshrined in the MCA 2005, a valid and applicable AD has the same legal force as a contemporaneous decision and can be verbal, although written forms are preferred for clarity. Typically used to decline life-sustaining treatments, an AD cannot demand interventions that are not clinically indicated or withdraw basic care such as nursing or analgesia. For an AD to be valid, healthcare professionals must confirm its authenticity and relevance to the current clinical situation; in emergencies or if doubt exists, appropriate treatment should proceed until clarification is obtained. Despite their value in supporting autonomy and reducing uncertainty for families and clinicians, ADs remain underused owing to limited public awareness, reluctance to initiate discussions, poor transfer of documentation between settings, and concerns that a person's preferences might change. They are most effective when developed within broader advance care planning, such as that promoted by the UK Gold Standards Framework, and when conditions follow a predictable trajectory, as in motor neuron disease, cancer, or advanced chronic obstructive pulmonary disease.

CHALLENGES IN END-OF-LIFE CARE

EoL care for frail individuals frequently involves family members who participate actively in decisions about treatment and future care (Pun et al., 2023). While their involvement can help ensure that the person's preferences are understood and honoured, it also raises risks of unintended breaches of confidentiality. For example, a clinician may disclose sensitive prognostic or treatment information to relatives without checking the patient's consent (Van den Block and MacLeod, 2019). Such breaches are ethically significant, especially when frail patients have diminished ability to express or enforce their privacy preferences because of cognitive decline or fluctuating communication capacity. These challenges underline the need for clinicians to maintain meticulous communication, ensuring that any exchange of information is aligned with the individual's stated wishes and with relevant legal safeguards, such as those provided by the Mental Capacity Act 2005.

CAPACITY ASSESSMENT IN END-OF-LIFE CARE

Assessing decision-making capacity is both a fundamental human right and a cornerstone of ethical and lawful medical practice (Beauchamp and Childress, 2013; HM Government, 2005). Capacity and competency are closely related concepts, but in the United Kingdom, the term *capacity* is the one established in statute. The law presumes that every adult has capacity unless proven otherwise, placing the burden of proof on the assessor. This presumption is crucial, because an incorrect finding of incapacity can unjustly deprive an individual of involvement in important decisions about health and lifestyle.

Capacity is decision specific and may fluctuate over time. Conditions such as dementia, delirium, or acute illness can temporarily impair mental function, and reversible factors should be addressed before assessment. Clinicians are expected to maximise the patient's ability to participate, for example, by ensuring optimal hearing and vision, treating intercurrent illness, and providing ample time for discussion and education (Jones and Morgan, 2024). Ignorance is not equivalent to incapacity: People should first receive information in a form they can understand, including repeated explanations, visual aids, or supported communication if needed.

The MCA 2005 specifies a functional test based on four abilities:

- Understanding—the person must comprehend the information relevant to the specific decision.
- Retaining—the person must retain that information long enough to make a choice.

- Weighing—the person must be able to use or weigh the information when deciding, which reflects the ethical principles of beneficence and non-maleficence.
- Communicating—the decision must be expressed, verbally or by any other reliable means.

Assessment should be tailored to each significant decision and carefully documented, including direct patient quotations where possible. In complex or borderline cases, a second professional opinion such as from a psychogeriatrician can add robustness (Schweitser et al., 2021). Importantly, individuals with capacity have the right to make decisions that others view as unwise or unconventional, and such choices must still be respected (Beauchamp and Childress, 2013).

When a person is found to lack capacity for a specific decision, practitioners must rely on valid advance directives or involve legally appointed decision-makers to ensure that care remains consistent with the individual's known values and previously expressed preferences (Jones and Morgan, 2024). This approach upholds autonomy and protects against well-intentioned but paternalistic decision-making.

DECISION-MAKING

The ability to make autonomous healthcare decisions depends on mental capacity—the competence to understand, retain, and weigh information relevant to a specific choice (Amaral et al., 2022). In the United Kingdom, the MCA 2005 provides the legal framework for assessing capacity and presumes that every adult can decide for themselves unless there is evidence to the contrary. Capacity is decision-specific: A person may be able to consent to one intervention but not another if the latter requires a more complex understanding. This feature is particularly significant in frailty, where cognition may fluctuate or gradually decline as the end of life approaches.

Progressive loss of capacity presents ethical and practical challenges. When advance directives are absent or ambiguous, clinicians must determine the patient's best interests by drawing on earlier statements of values or by consulting those close to the person. Advance statements such as preferences for place of care or for symptom management, though not legally binding, provide essential guidance for planning. If death is judged inevitable, decision-making should centre on dignity and comfort, avoiding any action intended to hasten death and ensuring that care accords with the patient's known wishes.

Balancing respect for autonomy with the duty to promote well-being therefore requires sensitive, ongoing dialogue. Health professionals must revisit decisions as capacity changes, document discussions carefully, and ensure that any intervention reflects both the individual's rights and the ethical standards of compassionate EoL care.

Palliative Sedation

Palliative sedation is employed to relieve severe, otherwise uncontrollable symptoms by deliberately lowering a patient's level of consciousness. Its use in frail individuals approaching the end of life raises significant ethical considerations (Galea, 2020). The practice seeks to uphold beneficence by alleviating intractable suffering, yet it can affect autonomy and non-maleficence because the person's ability to interact with loved ones and participate in decisions is inevitably reduced.

Although the aim of palliative sedation is comfort rather than hastening death, clinicians must ensure that treatment accords with the individual's own values and previously expressed preferences (Etland, 2021). Consent—obtained in advance wherever possible—and thorough documentation are essential. Ethical deliberation focuses on achieving effective symptom control while preserving dignity and avoiding any perception that life is being intentionally shortened, consistent with the principles articulated by Beauchamp and Childress (2013). Open, honest communication with families supports transparency and shared understanding throughout the process.

Withdrawing and Withholding Treatment

In EoL care, it is important to distinguish between withdrawing treatment stopping an intervention that has already begun and withholding treatment choosing not to start an intervention in the first place (Etland, 2021; American Medical Association, 2022). Both actions have significant ethical implications but are ethically and legally regarded as equivalent when the goal is to respect the patient's best interests rather than to hasten death.

For frail patients, whose potential to benefit from invasive or life-prolonging therapies may be limited, decisions about withholding or withdrawing life-sustaining measures are usually guided by a commitment to dignity, quality of life, and the avoidance of unnecessary suffering (Beil et al., 2023). Such decisions should begin with a clear understanding of the patient's own values and previously stated wishes, ideally documented in advance care plans, and involve open dialogue with family members or appointed proxies. Approached in this way, the process honours autonomy while fulfilling the principles of beneficence and non-maleficence, supporting a death that is both compassionate and ethically sound (Wong et al., 2024).

Anticipatory Prescribing

Effective symptom control in the last days of life often relies on anticipatory prescribing, whereby medicines are supplied in advance to manage predictable problems such as pain, agitation, breathlessness, nausea, and respiratory secretions. Both the British Medical Association and the National Institute for Health and Care Excellence highlight this proactive approach as a way to prevent avoidable distress and reduce the need for crisis interventions (British Medical Association, 2024; NICE, 2019).

Guidance from the General Medical Council (GMC) advises clinicians to assess likely symptom progression early and to prescribe appropriate medication in readiness, ensuring that frail patients receive timely relief while avoiding unnecessary pharmacological burden (GMC, 2024). Each prescription should be based on an individualised clinical assessment, with regular reviews so that dosages and drug choices can be adjusted as the patient's condition evolves (Ellershaw and Wilkinson, 2011; NICE, 2019).

Transparent communication is essential. The GMC stresses that prescribing plans should be discussed with the patient where possible, and with family members and the wider multidisciplinary team, to support understanding and prevent either under-treatment or inappropriate escalation (GMC, 2024). Clinicians must also remain alert to potential adverse effects such as opioid accumulation in renal impairment and the risk of respiratory depression. When symptom relief inadvertently shortens life, the doctrine of double effect provides the ethical justification for treatment aimed at comfort rather than hastening death (GMC, 2024).

ARTIFICIAL NUTRITION AND HYDRATION

Artificial nutrition and hydration (ANH) can prolong life but presents significant ethical challenges in the context of frailty and multimorbidity (Rochford, 2021). While it may prevent malnutrition or dehydration, ANH also carries risks including aspiration, infection, and discomfort from invasive procedures.

The GMC (2024) advises that each decision should be individualised, weighing potential benefits against burdens and considering the person's prognosis, symptom burden, and clearly expressed wishes. When frailty is advanced or illness is terminal, discontinuing ANH may represent an approach focused on comfort and dignity rather than life prolongation, provided that decisions are consistent with the patient's values and best interests.

DOCTRINE OF DOUBLE EFFECT

The doctrine of double effect is particularly relevant when managing distressing symptoms with opioid-based medicines in the last days of life. In older adults with renal impairment, opioids may accumulate, heightening the risk of toxicity, while in those with respiratory insufficiency opioids can both relieve breathlessness and depress respiratory drive (Faris et al., 2021). The GMC (2024) emphasises that when medication is carefully titrated and the intention is genuine symptom relief, any unintended life-shortening effect is ethically permissible. This principle provides important reassurance to clinicians who might otherwise fear that effective symptom control could be misconstrued as euthanasia.

ASSISTED DYING

Assisted dying remains illegal in the United Kingdom, yet public and professional debate continues over its potential legalisation (Mallion and Murphy, 2023). Proponents argue that it supports autonomy and may relieve intolerable suffering, while opponents highlight risks of coercion, diminished societal respect for life and potential impacts on vulnerable groups (Nuffield Council on Bioethics, 2023). These issues are particularly salient in frailty, where prolonged decline and complex symptoms can lead to profound distress. Health professionals must therefore balance respect for patient autonomy and compassion with their professional and legal obligations, ensuring that all care remains within the current legal framework (Alsararatee, 2024). The Terminally Ill Adults (End of Life) Bill seeks to permit assisted dying for mentally competent adults in England and Wales who have a terminal illness with a prognosis of six months or less. It sets out legal safeguards, including assessment by two independent doctors, confirmation of capacity, and oversight mechanisms to prevent coercion. At present, the Bill has passed all stages in the House of Commons including the first reading, second reading, committee and report stages, and third reading on 20 June 2025 and has entered the House of Lords, where it has had its first and second readings and awaits detailed committee scrutiny before further stages and possible Royal Assent (UK Parliament, 2025).

ORGAN DONATION

Organ donation is a recognised treatment for end-stage organ failure but is limited by the shortage of suitable organs. In the United Kingdom, it is considered when brain-stem death or circulatory death has been confirmed. Life-sustaining treatment should not be continued solely to allow donation. The decision must be voluntary and documented, and discussion with relatives should occur in a structured and unpressured way. If the person is on the Organ Donor Register, the process is more direct. After consent, blood is taken for tissue typing and for tests for HIV, hepatitis, and cytomegalovirus. A specialist nurse or transplant co-ordinator arranges retrieval and allocation. Before retrieval, organ perfusion and oxygenation are maintained through fluids, inotropes, and monitoring to support graft function.

Potential complications during retrieval are anticipated and managed. Emotional and practical support for relatives and staff continues throughout the process.

ELDER ABUSE

Elder abuse is any act or omission that harms or distresses an older person and remains widely under-reported. Community data suggest about 5% of older adults experience verbal abuse and around 2% physical abuse, with higher rates likely in care settings (Bowker and James, 2018). Forms include psychological abuse (intimidation and blaming), physical abuse (hitting, restraint, and inappropriate sedation), financial exploitation (misuse of money or property), sexual abuse, and neglect (failure to provide food, warmth, or basic care) (Figure 24.1). Perpetrators are often caregivers under stress, affected

"Example pictures"	Type	Examples	Indicators
	Physical "Infliction of physical force leading to body injury or pain"	Slapping/biting/punching Restraint Burning (cigarette) Being handled roughly	Unexplained bruises, falls, minor accidents
	Financial "Using funds without the authority of the owner"	Pushy sales persons Being paid as carer but not providing the care Selling items without consent (car, jewellery) Abuse of power of attorney for finances	Missing money, unpaid bills,lack of basic things, unexplained receipts
	Psychological "Use of mental cruelty or verbal threats to cause discomfort"	Name calling/shouting Being kept in isolation Being threatened Blaming	Fearful and nervous, harsh tones, strained relationship, low mood, confusion
	Neglect "Willful failure to assist someone to achieve activities of daily living"	Withholding food, medication, water and comfort Human needs not provided	Pressure sores, malnourished, dehydrated, dirty house, unkempt appearance, unused medication
	Sexual "Being involved directly or indirectly in sexual activity with no consent"	Sexual act Sexual comments Rape Being forced to watch pornography	Bruises in genital areas, fear of being touched
	Discrimination "Unjust treatment of people on the grounds of gender/ race/ age etc"	Ageism Racism	Treatment restriction on grounds of age Inequity with regards to levels of care
	Institutional "abuse within an institution such as care home or hospital"	Often used to refer to systematic abuse of more than one person, or one person on more than one ossasion at an institutional level– i.e. abuse is perpetrated by more than one person and is facilitated by policies and practices	Multiple admissions or safeguarding referrals from one institution due to health or social care issues Multiple complaints by relatives and care recipients High prevalence of indicators of neglect, e.g. pressure ulceration/malnutrition

FIGURE 24.1   Elderly abuse. *Source*: Blundell and Gordon (2015)/John Wiley & Sons.

by isolation, mental illness, or substance misuse. In the United Kingdom, the Care Act 2014 requires local authorities to safeguard adults at risk through multi-agency investigations and coordinated support. Prompt referral to adult safeguarding teams, careful documentation, and close monitoring are essential, and police or legal action may be necessary where serious harm is suspected.

RATIONING AND AGEISM IN HEALTH CARE

Decisions about how limited healthcare resources are allocated, often referred to as rationing, have been part of the National Health Service since its inception. Rising costs associated with complex technologies and advanced pharmacological treatments, together with increasing expectations of care, have made the process more explicit and frequently contested. Although no UK government has formally acknowledged rationing, policies described as efficiency savings or commissioning often involve choices about which interventions can be provided. Over time, responsibility for these decisions has shifted from individual clinicians, whose differing practices created inequity, to hospital managers and national bodies such as the NICE. NICE guidance is intended to standardise access to treatments across the country, yet variation persists, sometimes described as 'postcode prescribing', where the availability of drugs depends on local commissioning priorities.

One area of particular concern is ageism, where rationing occurs according to chronological age. The National Service Framework for Older People prohibits discrimination based solely on age, requiring care to be determined by clinical need (Department of Health, 2001). Nevertheless, older adults may still experience limited access to high-intensity treatments such as critical care. While some interventions may indeed confer less benefit in advanced age, biological ageing varies greatly and some therapies, such as thrombolysis for myocardial infarction, can yield significant gains in older populations because of higher baseline risk. Economic arguments that older adults consume disproportionate resources, especially in their final year of life, remain unconvincing because it is rarely possible to predict when that final year will begin.

Ethically, healthcare systems are challenged to reject assumptions that certain groups have less social worth or are politically less influential. Concepts such as the 'fair innings' argument, which proposes that younger people should have priority because older individuals have already had their share of life's opportunities, remain controversial. Such reasoning risks entrenching prejudice by suggesting that those who have used more healthcare, such as people living with chronic conditions, have already exhausted their entitlement to care. A fair and sustainable approach must therefore focus on clinical effectiveness and individual need, rather than age or perceived social value, ensuring that all patients receive equitable access to appropriate treatment throughout life (Oliver, 2013).

QUALITY-OF-LIFE CONSIDERATIONS

Quality of life is a central consideration in EoL decision-making. For frail individuals, aggressive interventions such as intensive care admission or invasive therapies may cause more harm than benefit, failing to improve and sometimes compromising overall well-being (Lapid et al., 2020). Emphasising comfort and dignity over mere prolongation of life reflects the ethical principle of beneficence, directing care towards what genuinely enhances the patient's final days. This perspective challenges traditional curative priorities; encouraging palliative approaches that address physical, emotional, and spiritual needs; and enabling individuals to live their remaining time with maximum comfort and respect.

Case Study 24.1 Complex End-of-Life Decision-Making in Advanced Practice

Patient Background

Mrs J, an 84-year-old woman with advanced frailty (Clinical Frailty Scale 7), severe heart failure, vascular dementia, and stage 4 chronic kidney disease, was admitted to the acute frailty unit following sudden worsening breathlessness and chest discomfort. Her general practitioner reported progressive weight loss and recurrent hospital admissions over the past year. She had no recorded advance decision or lasting power of attorney, but during previous reviews, she expressed a wish 'not to be kept alive on machines'.

Clinical Presentation and Assessment by the AP

On arrival, Mrs J was drowsy, with a blood pressure of 86/52 mmHg, heart rate of 118 bpm (irregular), respiratory rate of 30/min, and oxygen saturation of 82% on room air. Chest auscultation reveals widespread crackles. Point-of-care ultrasound shows biventricular failure with gross pleural effusions. Venous blood gases confirm metabolic acidosis.

The AP conducted a comprehensive advanced assessment, integrating cardiovascular, respiratory, and neurological examinations with bedside echocardiography and focused lung ultrasound. In consultation with cardiology, the AP determined that invasive ventilation or renal replacement therapy would offer minimal benefit and risk significant harm.

Ethical and Legal Complexity

Mrs J's fluctuating consciousness raised questions about decision-making capacity. Applying the Mental Capacity Act (2005), the AP evaluated her ability to understand, retain, weigh, and communicate information. At times, she could say she wanted 'comfort', but periods of confusion followed. Her only relative, a niece, believed 'everything possible' should be done.

The AP facilitated an urgent best-interests meeting, involving the niece, palliative care team, and senior consultant. The discussion considered Mrs J's previously stated preferences, current clinical condition, and likely outcomes. The AP explained that aggressive treatments, including intubation or dialysis, would not reverse her heart failure and could prolong discomfort.

Care Planning and Interventions

- Initiates oxygen therapy and low-dose intravenous diuretics for symptomatic relief.
- Implements anticipatory prescribing for pain, agitation and breathlessness, ensuring careful opioid titration consistent with the doctrine of double effect.
- Documents do not attempt cardiopulmonary resuscitation (DNACPR) order and detailed care plan, with agreement from the niece.
- Arranges for palliative care review and supports transfer to a side room for privacy and dignity.
- Considers the need for DoLS authorisation if continuous observation or gentle restraint is required to maintain comfort measures.

This case highlights the AP's pivotal role in synthesising advanced clinical assessment with complex ethical, legal, and family considerations. It illustrates leadership in urgent capacity assessment, end-of-life decision-making, and inter-professional communication, while ensuring that care remains patient-centred and consistent with statutory frameworks.

CONCLUSION

Ethical practice in frailty and EoL care requires more than the application of abstract principles: It depends on context-sensitive judgement, iterative capacity assessment, clear documentation, and honest communication that foregrounds the patient's values. The MCA provides the legal scaffolding for decision-specific capacity and best interests determinations; DoLS, LPA, and ADs translate preferences into lawful action; GMC and NICE guidance support safe symptom control, including anticipatory prescribing and proportionate analgesia. An ethics-of-care lens complements the four principles by recognising interdependence, relational autonomy, and the practical realities of multimorbidity. Against the backdrop of resource constraints and the risk of ageism, clinicians should advocate for equity, dignity, and comfort, ensuring decisions remain lawful, proportionate, and aligned with what matters most to the person.

Take-Home Messages

1. Capacity is decision-specific, can fluctuate, and must be supported before judged; respect for an unwise decision is a legal and ethical requirement when capacity is present.
2. Withholding and withdrawing treatment are ethically equivalent when guided by goals of care, proportionality, and the patient's values.
3. Anticipatory prescribing and careful opioid titration are central to comfort; intention matters under the doctrine of double effect.
4. DoLS, LPA, and ADs safeguard rights and make preferences actionable across medical and social decisions.
5. Vigilance for elder abuse and structured safeguarding responses are essential.
6. Equity requires resisting age-based rationing and focusing on need, effectiveness, and person-centred outcomes.

REFERENCES

Akdeniz, M., Yardımcı, B., and Kavukcu, E. (2021). Ethical considerations at the end-of-life care. *SAGE Open Medicine* 9: 20503121211000918.

Alanazi, M.A., Shaban, M.M., Ramadan, O.M.E. et al. (2024). Navigating end-of-life decision-making in nursing: a systematic review of ethical challenges and palliative care practices. *BMC Nursing* 23 (1): 467.

Alsararatee, H.H. (2024). The ethics of clinically assisted nutrition and hydration in adults and the role of the advanced clinical practitioner. *British Journal of Nursing* 33 (13): S14–S24.

Alzheimer's Society (2024) Advance Decisions and Lasting Power of Attorney. https://www.alzheimers.org.uk/get-support/legal-financial/advance-decisions-lasting-power-attorney-lpa (accessed 14 April 2025)

Amaral, A.S., Simões, M.R., Freitas, S. et al. (2022). Healthcare decision-making capacity in old age: a qualitative study. *Frontiers in Psychology* 13: 1024967.

American Medical Association (2022). Withholding or withdrawing life-sustaining treatment. https://code-medical-ethics.ama-assn.org/ethics-opinions/withholding-or-withdrawing-life-sustaining-treatment (accessed 23 September 2025).

Beauchamp, T.L. and Childress, J.F. (2013). *Principles of Biomedical Ethics*, 7e. Oxford: Oxford University Press.

Beil, M., van Heerden, P.V., Joynt, G.M. et al. (2023). Limiting life-sustaining treatment for very old ICU patients: cultural challenges and diverse practices. *Annals of Intensive Care* 13 (1): 107.

Berlinger, N., Wynia, M., Powell, T. et al. (2020). *Ethical Framework for Health Care Institutions Responding to Novel Coronavirus SARS-CoV-2 (COVID-19): Guidelines for Institutional Ethics Services Responding to COVID-19*. The Hastings Center `https://www.thehastingscenter.org/wp-content/uploads/HastingsCenterCovidFramework2020.pdf` (accessed 14 April 2025).

Blundell, A. and Gordon, A. (2015). *Geriatric Medicine at a Glance*, 1e. Chichester: Wiley Blackwell.

Bowker, L. and James, D. (2018). *Oxford Handbook of Geriatric Medicine*, 3e. Oxford: Oxford University Press.

British Geriatrics Society (2015). *Submission to the Law Commission in response to Consultation Paper 222: Mental Capacity and Deprivation of Liberty*. London. Available at: `https://www.bgs.org.uk/sites/default/files/content/attachment/2018-04-06/2015_bgs.on_dols%20%281%29.pdf`: British Geriatrics Society (accessed 3 February 2026).

British Geriatrics Society (2020). *End of life care in frailty: law and ethics*. `https://www.bgs.org.uk/resources/end-of-life-care-in-frailty-law-and-ethics` (accessed 14 April 2025).

British Geriatrics Society (2023a). *End of Life Care in Frailty: Guidance*. London: BGS.

British Geriatrics Society (2023b) Joining the dots: a blueprint for preventing and managing frailty in older people. `https://tinyurl.com/3wuuvtf3` (accessed 23 September 2025).

British Medical Association (2024). Anticipatory prescribing for end-of-life care. `https://www.bma.org.uk/advice-and-support/gp-practices/prescribing/anticipatory-prescribing-for-end-of-life-care` (accessed 23 September 2025).

Cheraghi, R., Valizadeh, L., Zamanzadeh, V. et al. (2023). Clarification of ethical principle of the beneficence in nursing care: an integrative review. *BMC Nursing* 22 (1): 89.

Crooms, R.C. and Gelfman, L.P. (2020). Palliative care and end-of-life considerations for the frail patient. *Anesthesia & Analgesia* 130 (6): 1504–1515.

Crotty, B.H., Walker, J., Dierks, M. et al. (2015). Information sharing preferences of older patients and their families. *JAMA Internal Medicine* 175 (9): 1492–1497.

Department of Health (2001). *National Service Framework for Older People*. London: Stationery Office `https://assets.publishing.service.gov.uk/media/5a7b4f16e5274a34770ead1c/National_Service_Framework_for_Older_People.pdf` (accessed 23 September 2025).

Ellershaw, J. and Wilkinson, S. (ed.) (2011). *Care of the Dying: A Pathway to Excellence*. Oxford: Oxford University Press ISBN: 9780191730177.

Etland, C. (2021). Palliative and end-of-life care. In: *Critical Care Nursing – E-Book* (ed. L.D. Urden, K.M. Stacy, and M.E. Lough), 150. Elsevier.

Faris, H., Dewar, B., Dyason, C. et al. (2021). Goods, causes and intentions: problems with applying the doctrine of double effect to palliative sedation. *BMC Medical Ethics* 22 (1): 141. `https://doi.org/10.1186/s12910-021-00709-0` (accessed 23 September 2025).

Galea L. (2020). Ethical analysis of the practice of sedation for end of life suffering. Master's thesis. University of Malta. `https://www.um.edu.mt/library/oar/handle/123456789/72407` (accessed 23 September 2025).

General Medical Council (2024). Treatment and care towards the end of life: good practice in decision making. `https://www.gmc-uk.org/professional-standards/the-professional-standards/treatment-and-care-towards-the-end-of-life` (accessed 23 September 2025).

Grealish, L. (1997a). Beyond Hippocrates: ethics in palliative care. *International Journal of Palliative Nursing* 3 (3): 151–155.

Grealish, L. (1997b). The ethics of care: a framework for examining ethical issues in palliative care. *Journal of Advanced Nursing* 26 (5): 948–953.

HM Government (2005). *Mental Capacity Act 2005*. London: The Stationery Office. Available at: https://www.legislation.gov.uk/ukpga/2005/9/contents (accessed 3 February 2026).

Human Rights Act 1998, c. 42. https://www.legislation.gov.uk/ukpga/1998/42/contents (accessed 25 September 2025).

Jones, J.R. and Morgan, J.D. (2024). Healthcare decision-making and advance care planning. In: *Evidence-Based Geriatric Nursing Protocols for Best Practice* (ed. M. Boltz, E.A. Capezuti, and T. Fulmer). Springer ISBN: 978-0-8261-5277-0.

Koffman, J., Shapiro, G.K., and Schulz-Quach, C. (2023). Enhancing equity and diversity in palliative care clinical practice, research and education. *BMC Palliative Care* 22 (1): 64.

Kumar, B.P., Paudel, P., Panja, A.K., and Sharma, S. (2024). Balancing paternalism and autonomy in healthcare: insights from Ayurveda. *International Journal of Ayurveda Research* 5 (3): 154–162.

Lapid, M.I., Koopmans, R., Sampson, E.L. et al. (2020). Providing quality end-of-life care to older people in the era of COVID-19: perspectives from five countries. *International Psychogeriatrics* 32 (11): 1345–1352. https://doi.org/10.1017/S10.1610220000836.

Mallion, J. and Murphy, L. (2023). *'Ending Death, Not Ending Life': Understanding Positive Attitudes Toward Assisted Dying in the UK*. LSBU School of Applied Sciences https://tinyurl.com/43yt4h8y (accessed 23 September 2025).

National Institute for Health and Care Excellence (NICE) (2019). End of life care for adults: service delivery. NICE guideline NG142. https://www.nice.org.uk/guidance/ng142/chapter/Recommendations#identifying-adults-who-may-be-approaching-the-end-of-their-life-their-carers-and-other-people (accessed 23 September 2025).

NHS England (2022). *Older people advanced practice area specific capability and curriculum framework*. NHS England. Available at: https://advanced-practice.hee.nhs.uk/wp-content/uploads/sites/28/2025/01/Older-people-advanced-practice-area-specific-capability-and-curriculum-framework-NHSE.pdf (accessed 30 January 2026).

NHS England (2023a). *Palliative and end of life care advanced practice area specific capability and curriculum framework*. NHS England. Available at: https://advanced-practice.hee.nhs.uk/wp-content/uploads/sites/28/2025/01/Palliative-and-end-of-life-care-advanced-practice-area-specific-capability-and-curriculum-framework-NHSE.pdf (accessed 30 January 2026).

NHS England (2023b) *Acute medicine advanced practice area specific capability and curriculum framework*. NHS England. Available at: https://advanced-practice.hee.nhs.uk/wp-content/uploads/sites/28/2025/03/Acute-medicine-advanced-practice-area-specific-capability-and-curriculum-framework-NHSE.pdf (accessed 30 January 2026).

NHS England (2025). *Multi-professional framework for advanced practice in England – Edition 2025*. NHS England. Available at: https://advanced-practice.hee.nhs.uk/wp-content/uploads/sites/28/2025/05/Multi-professional-framework-for-advanced-practice-in-England---Edition-2025.pdf (accessed 29 January 2026).

Nuffield Council on Bioethics (2023). Written evidence submitted by Nuffield Council on Bioethics (ADY0494). House of Commons Health and Social Care Committee inquiry into assisted dying/assisted suicide. https://committees.parliament.uk/writtenevidence/117234/pdf (accessed 23 September 2025).

Office for National Statistics (ONS) (2025). *National Population Projections: 2025-Based.* London: ONS.

Oliver, D. (2013). *We Must End Ageism and Age Discrimination in Health and Social Care.* The King's Fund https://www.kingsfund.org.uk/insight-and-analysis/blogs/end-ageism-age-discrimination-health-social-care (accessed 23 September 2025).

Pun, J., Chow, J.C.H., Fok, L., and Cheung, K.M. (2023). Role of patients' family members in end-of-life communication: an integrative review. *BMJ Open* 13 (2): e067304.

Rochford, A. (2021). Ethics of providing clinically assisted nutrition and hydration: current issues. *Frontline Gastroenterology* 12 (2): 128–132. https://doi.org/10.1136/flgastro-2019-101230 (accessed 23 September 2025).

Satomi, E., Souza, P.M.R., Thomé, B.C. et al. (2020). Fair allocation of scarce medical resources during COVID-19 pandemic: ethical considerations. *Einstein (Sao Paulo)* 18: eAE5775.

Schweitser, F., Stuy, J., Distelmans, W., and Rigo, A. (2021). Assessment of patient decision-making capacity in the context of voluntary euthanasia for psychic suffering caused by psychiatric disorders: a qualitative study of approaches among Belgian physicians. *Journal of Medical Ethics* 47 (12): e38.

Supreme Court (2014) Cheshire West and Chester Council v P; Surrey County Council v P [2014] UKSC 19. https://www.supremecourt.uk/cases/uksc-2013-0136.html (accessed 23 September 2025).

UK Parliament (2025). Terminally Ill Adults (End of Life) Bill [HL]: Bill stages. https://bills.parliament.uk/bills/3774 (accessed 28 September 2025).

Van den Block, L. and MacLeod, R.D. (ed.) (2019). *Textbook of Palliative Care.* Cham: Springer International Publishing ISBN 9783319777382.

Van Den Noortgate, N.J. and Van den Block, L. (2022a). End-of-life care for older people: the way forward. *Age and Ageing* 51 (7): afac078.

Van Den Noortgate, N. and Van den Block, L. (2022b). Palliative care for older people with frailty. *The Lancet Healthy Longevity* 3 (11): e744–e752.

Vergano, M., Bertolini, G., Giannini, A. et al. (2020). Clinical ethics recommendations for the allocation of intensive care treatments in exceptional, resource-limited circumstances: the Italian perspective during the COVID-19 epidemic. *Critical Care* 24 (1): 165.

Wiesen, J., Donatelli, C., Smith, M.L. et al. (2021). Medical, ethical, and legal aspects of end-of-life dilemmas in the intensive care unit. *Cleveland Clinic Journal of Medicine* 88 (9): 516–527.

Wong, V., Hassan, N., Wong, Y.P. et al. (2024). Nurses' adherence to ethical principles – a qualitative study. *Nursing Ethics* https://doi.org/10.1177/09697330241291159 Epub ahead of print (accessed 23 September 2025).

Yulianto, P. and Awaludin, S. (2024). Ethical principles of autonomy for patients receiving care in the Intensive Care Unit (ICU): a concept analysis. *Journal of Holistic Nursing Science* 11 (1): 28–36.

FUTURE DIRECTIONS

CHAPTER 25

The Future of Frailty and End-of-Life Medicine

Aim

The aim of this chapter is to explore how advanced practitioners (APs) can lead and transform frailty and end-of-life care in the context of rapid population ageing, complex multimorbidity, technological change, and evolving ethical and legal challenges.

LEARNING OUTCOMES

After studying this chapter, readers will be able to:

1. Demonstrate how APs apply advanced assessment, complex reasoning, and leadership to design and deliver integrated, person-centred services.
2. Evaluate ethical and legal considerations, including capacity law and equitable resource allocation, in complex clinical decision-making.
3. Formulate strategies for service innovation, workforce development, and policy influence within integrated care systems.

SELF-ASSESSMENT QUESTIONS

1. How can APs integrate predictive analytics and comprehensive geriatric assessment to anticipate deterioration in frail older adults?
2. In what ways can APs provide ethical leadership when a patient with dementia lacks capacity and no advance decision is in place?

> This chapter in frailty is written not in years lost,
> but in lives lived well where science, compassion,
> and resilience converge.

INTRODUCTION

According to the World Health Organization (WHO) (2024), by 2030, one in six people worldwide will be aged 60 years or older, with this group increasing from about 1 billion in 2020 to around 1.4 billion. By 2050, the global population aged 60 and older is projected to double to roughly 2.1 billion, while the number of people aged 80 years and older is expected to triple to about 426 million (WHO, 2024). England's population is ageing rapidly, with almost one in five people now aged 65 and older and nearly two in five aged 50 and older (Centre for Ageing Better, 2025). Projections indicate that by 2065, around one-quarter of the population will be older than 65 years and almost half will be older than 50 years, adding an estimated 6.5 million people to the older age group. Growth is most noticeable in rural and coastal areas, but pockets of high older-age density are found even in younger urban centres (Centre for Ageing Better, 2025). Furthermore, there is a projected 55% rise in England's over-85 population over the next 15 years, significantly intensifying pressure on services designed for frailty and end-of-life (EoL) care (NHS England, 2025). This demographic shift is expected to place substantial pressure on health and social care systems, with rising prevalence of frailty increasing demand for complex, long-term and end-of-life care services.

This chapter explores how APs can anticipate and influence future trajectories in frailty and EoL care. We examine demographic pressures, evolving care models, the future workforce, ethical and legal challenges, global perspectives, and strategic directions for advanced practice leadership. Our goal is to empower APs to lead adaptation in a rapidly ageing world.

Comorbidity, Complexity, and Health Use

Frailty rarely occurs in isolation: Multimorbidity is the norm. By 2037, two-thirds of older adults in England may have two or more health conditions and one-third will also have mental health needs (NHS England, 2023). In addition, the 10-Year Health Plan for England warns that demographic ageing and population growth will sharply increase the prevalence of long-term conditions and complex care needs, placing sustained pressure on health and care services (Department of Health and Social Care, 2025). The confluence of frailty and comorbidity challenges conventional, disease-specific medical models. Care utilization intensifies in later life, with frequent hospitalizations, polypharmacy, and transitions between care settings. These shifts escalate costs and strain systems already under workforce pressure.

INNOVATIONS IN MODELS OF CARE

Rapid population ageing demands not only more staff but also new ways of delivering care. Recent national guidance emphasises early recognition of frailty and proactive, person-centred management across the health and social care system (BGS, 2025). Systematic frailty identification at first contact whether in primary care, emergency department, or community services enables earlier advanced care planning and timely palliative input, reducing unplanned admissions and late crisis management.

A home-first philosophy is central, supporting older people to remain in familiar surroundings whenever safe and reducing hospital-acquired deconditioning. This requires integrated neighbourhood teams able to deliver urgent and routine care in the community at scale, coupled with early discharge planning when hospital admission is unavoidable. Such coordinated models also address unwarranted variation in service quality and ensure equitable access to high-value interventions, regardless of geography. Embedding these approaches aligns with the broader shift towards anticipatory, patient-centred EoL care. For advanced clinical practitioners, leadership in implementing frailty screening, orchestrating multidisciplinary responses, and initiating advanced care planning will be critical in ensuring that future services remain both ethically robust and sustainable.

Integrated and Community-based Care

One key transformation is the move from episodic hospital-centric treatment to integrated, community-based models. Virtual wards, hospital-at-home, and proactive home-based frailty services embed specialist expertise closer to patients, reducing hospital admissions. In the United Kingdom, integrated care systems (ICSs) have become the locus for coordinating these services. Kawashima and Evans (2023) highlighted that older people with non-cancer conditions are less likely to receive timely referral to palliative care services, in part, because their disease trajectories are less predictable. Proactive integration of geriatrics, palliative care, and community services can reduce avoidable crises, providing more person-centred, anticipatory EoL care.

Digital Health, AI, and Predictive Analytics

Emerging digital technologies, particularly artificial intelligence (AI), are expected to transform frailty assessment and EoL care. A recent bibliometric analysis shows rapid global growth in AI-frailty research, with leading contributions from the United Kingdom, United States, and Italy (Albarrati et al., 2025). Machine learning algorithms are being developed to predict frailty trajectories, anticipate dementia, and monitor sarcopenia, enabling earlier intervention and more personalised care planning. However, Albarrati and colleagues highlighted limited collaboration between research groups and a lack of validated tools for routine primary and community practice. To harness these advances, integrated health and social care systems will need to incorporate frailty-specific data into electronic records, invest in ethical governance of AI, and ensure that APs are trained to interpret and apply AI-derived insights. Implanting such technologies alongside established comprehensive geriatric assessment could enhance proactive, person-centred management of frailty in coming decades.

Strengthening Primary Care as the Front Line of Frailty Care

Primary care is uniquely placed to identify and manage frailty early, enabling timely interventions that may slow progression and avoid crises. Ludlow et al. (2023) highlighted opportunities to use electronic frailty indices and routinely collected data for systematic screening, supported by multi-component interventions such as tailored physical activity and nutrition programmes. Embedding frailty-specific items in primary care datasets and enhancing community capacity are key future priorities.

Advancing Assessment and Personalised Interventions

There is no single gold-standard frailty tool. More research is needed to clarify which components of the Comprehensive Geriatric Assessment (CGA) confer the greatest benefit in community settings. Evidence supports multi-component interventions, particularly those involving resistance training, and adapting disease-specific management (for example, diabetes or hypertension) to the degree of frailty. These innovations can help practitioners offer person-centred, cost-effective care. It is essential that elderly people are involved in research to explore and understand frailty and its consequences, as the complexity of their conditions means that some are often excluded from studies.

Building the Frailty-capable Workforce

Strengthening education and training in frailty is essential. Structured frailty training programmes can enhance clinicians' knowledge and confidence, while interdisciplinary collaboration across primary care, rehabilitation, mental health, and allied health supports holistic management. Future workforce planning must therefore embed frailty competence and interprofessional teamwork as core requirements.

THE FUTURE ADVANCED PRACTICE WORKFORCE

Meeting future health demands requires more than new models of care: It calls for a workforce equipped for complexity. Although NHS staffing has expanded since 2010, workforce growth has not kept pace with rising needs linked to population ageing. Vacancy rates remain high, particularly in community and services for older people, while the population older than 85 years is projected to grow by 55% over the next 15 years, amplifying pressure on frailty and EoL care (NHS England, 2023; NHS England, 2025). APs are well placed to address these gaps. Operating across primary, acute, and community settings, and bringing skills in prescribing, diagnostics, and leadership, they are critical to sustaining safe and effective care.

Strengthening frailty diagnosis and management will require coordinated national and international policy initiatives. Evidence from England and other European nations shows that making frailty screening a primary care performance measure encourages early recognition and structured management (Ruiz and Theou, 2024). Aligning health system incentives in this way would drive the integration of frailty teaching across undergraduate, postgraduate, and continuing professional development curricula. To embed lasting change, educational strategies must connect frailty identification with evidence-based interventions and remain centred on individual goals. The WHO highlights frailty and intrinsic capacity as core competencies for all professionals working with older adults and calls for standardised tools and validated interventions (WHO, 2017). International platforms such as the Global Frailty Network, the International Conference on Frailty and Sarcopenia Research, and the Johns Hopkins Older Americans Independence Center already disseminate research and best practice to advance these aims (Global Frailty Network, 2025; Johns Hopkins University Older Americans Independence Center, 2021).

APs are pivotal in operationalising these developments. Their advanced clinical and leadership capabilities enable them to integrate frailty screening and management within multidisciplinary teams, shape curricula, and lead interprofessional education programmes. Incorporating frailty-specific competencies into AP training and professional frameworks will help ensure that future clinical leaders can deliver coordinated, person-centred interventions. Broader collaboration is essential. Adoption of the

Institute for Healthcare Improvement's Age-Friendly Health Systems model, which emphasises Mentation, Mobility, Medications, and Matters Most, offers a unifying structure for frailty education and practice in diverse health systems (Mate et al., 2018). Developing global consensus on competencies and sharing adaptable educational models will further support APs and other clinicians to translate evidence into routine practice.

1. Looking ahead, the AP role should expand beyond direct clinical decision-making to encompass system design, education, service evaluation, and policy influence. Key future capabilities include:
   - Leading frailty and EoL pathways across care settings.
2. Applying digital tools, artificial intelligence, and remote monitoring.
3. Exercising competence in ethical deliberation, mental capacity law, and shared decision-making.
4. Mentoring multiprofessional teams and driving quality improvement.
5. Advocating for equitable access and evidence-informed resource planning.

Educational curricula should therefore evolve to promote lifelong learning in genomics, data science, bioethics, health policy, and strategic leadership. This comprehensive skill set will equip APs to guide the transformation of frailty and EoL care, ensuring resilience and quality in the face of demographic and clinical complexity.

Future Directions for Frailty and End-of-Life Care Under the NHS 2025 Plan

1. **Prevention and earlier intervention**

   The NHS Long-Term Plan 2025 emphasises preventive care and early detection of disease. For frailty and EoL care, this supports the expansion of screening and surveillance mechanisms in community and primary care settings to identify pre-frailty and early frailty. Proactive interventions such as exercise, nutrition, and polypharmacy review can delay frailty progression and reduce crisis admissions.

2. **Shift from hospital to community and home settings**

   The Plan promotes delivering more care outside hospital, reducing unnecessary admissions and length of stay. Frailty and EoL services should align: Models such as hospital-at-home, virtual wards, and mobile palliative teams will become central, enabling patients to remain in familiar surroundings whenever appropriate.

3. **Integrated care and neighbourhood teams**

   One of the Long-Term Plan's pillars is integrated care systems (ICSs) and neighbourhood models. Frailty/EoL care must be embedded in these networks, bridging primary care, community health, social care, and specialist palliative services. APs can lead the coordination among disciplines to ensure seamless transitions and continuity.

4. **Digital and data-driven care**

   The Plan expects greater use of digital tools, remote monitoring, AI, and predictive analytics. Frailty management can benefit predictive frailty scoring, alerting to deterioration, and supporting shared decision-making. However, APs must help ensure these tools are ethical, inclusive, and explainable to patients and families.

5. Workforce development and role expansion

   The Long-Term Plan calls for the growth of advanced clinicians across settings. Frailty and EoL care should become a core domain for AP roles not as a niche, but as integral to generalist practice. APs should develop skills in palliative care, complex decision-making, capacity assessments, and cross-disciplinary leadership.

6. Resource allocation, equity, and personalised care

   The Plan advocates outcome-based commissioning and reducing unwarranted variation. Frailty and EoL care must be included in outcome metrics. APs should advocate for equitable access across geographies, especially in underserved areas, and contribute to designing person-centred models that adjust resources based on individual needs rather than age or location.

7. Research, innovation, and evaluation

   The Long-Term Plan emphasises innovation and evaluation of new care models. Frailty and EoL initiatives should embed evaluation frameworks. APs can lead pragmatic trials, data collection, real-world evidence, and co-design with patients to refine care pathways and justify investment.

ETHICAL, LEGAL, AND RESOURCE CHALLENGES

Future Ageing and Shortage Bring Complex Ethical Dilemmas

Resource Allocation and Ageism

Scarcity of beds, ICU capacity, and workforce may bring pressure to ration care. Ageism—explicit or implicit—must be resisted. Allocation should be grounded in need, potential benefit and fairness, not chronological age. Ethical frameworks such as *fair innings* or social worth are deeply contestable. Instead, APs should lead equitable triage policies and ensure frail individuals retain access to palliative, hospice, and supportive care.

Autonomy, Capacity, and Algorithmic Decision Support

As decision support systems and predictive models become embedded, APs should safeguard autonomy. Algorithmic suggestions cannot override personalised judgement. Capacity assessment remains foundational. Legal tools such as advance decisions, LPAs, DoLS will grow in relevance as cognitive decline becomes more common. APs should be fluent in these mechanisms and lead multidisciplinary decision-making.

Technology and Equity

Digital innovations risk exacerbating disparities. Older adults in rural areas or of lower socioeconomic status may lack connectivity. APs should champion inclusive deployment of technology, ensure training, and monitor for inequitable outcomes.

Assisted Dying and End-of-Life Legislation

Global debates on assisted dying continue, and future legal reforms may reach jurisdictions where APs practise. In the United Kingdom, on 20 June 2025, the House of Commons passed the Terminally Ill Adults (End of Life) Bill by 314 votes to 291, advancing it for detailed scrutiny in the House of Lords

(UK Parliament, 2025). APs should stay up to date, contribute to debate, and prepare frameworks that preserve autonomy while protecting vulnerable people.

GLOBAL PERSPECTIVES AND HEALTH EQUITY

Frailty and EoL care are not UK concerns alone, high-income countries face severe pressure, but low- and middle-income countries will soon experience rapid ageing with limited resources. Frailty care in such settings must adapt to fewer healthcare resources, cultural differences in dying, and weaker legal infrastructure. Cross-national learning and adaptable models are essential. Even in resource-rich nations, disparities exist. Deprived regions, minority ethnic groups, rural populations, and those with lower digital access may suffer worse EoL care. APs should be advocates for equity, designing services to reach underserved groups.

Strategic Directions and Call to Action

To shape the future of frailty and EoL care, APs should consider these strategic moves:

1. Engage in policy and system design:

   Influence ICS strategies, frailty frameworks, and digital health policy to prioritise EoL care in older adults.

2. Lead service innovation:

   Pilot integrated frailty-palliative pathways, virtual wards, and predictive analytics at local scale and evaluate outcomes.

3. Strengthen education and research:

   Develop curricula that integrate bioethics, health informatics and leadership; promote practice-based research in frailty and EoL settings.

4. Build interdisciplinary leadership:

   Bring together palliative care, geriatrics, primary care, social services, and technology to co-produce sustainable care models.

5. Champion equity and dignity:

   Monitor for ageism, technology exclusion, and voice inequities in resource allocation; advocate for person-centred care across all demographic groups.

Case Study 25.1   AP Leadership in Complex Frailty and EoL Care

Background

Mrs J, an 84-year-old woman with advanced frailty (Clinical Frailty Scale 6), severe chronic obstructive pulmonary disease, type 2 diabetes, and progressing vascular dementia, lives alone in a rural village with limited transport. Over the previous year, she has had three unplanned admissions with delirium and pneumonia. She now shows marked weight loss and functional decline, signalling advanced frailty and approaching end of life.

Specialist Assessment and High-level Reasoning

An AP from the community frailty virtual ward conducted a comprehensive geriatric assessment in Mrs J's home, combining detailed physical examination, cognitive testing, and electronic frailty index data. The AP integrates laboratory results, remote monitoring trends, and predictive analytics to identify reversible factors, optimise symptom control, and anticipate potential deterioration. Recognising the interplay of multimorbidity, dementia, and social isolation, the AP judges that the main goals of care are comfort, safety, and avoidance of unnecessary hospitalisation.

Leadership in Complex Decision-making

When cognitive decline rendered Mrs J unable to make informed choices, the AP convened and chaired a formal best interests meeting with the GP, palliative care consultant, community nurses, social services, and family members. Drawing on the Mental Capacity Act 2005 and any available Lasting Power of Attorney, the AP framed the discussion around Mrs J's previously recorded preferences and current clinical evidence. Options such as future hospital transfer, antibiotics, non-invasive ventilation, and palliative sedation were critically appraised. Through skilled facilitation, the AP guided the team to consensus on a home-based, comfort-focused plan, documenting all decisions in the shared electronic record and ensuring legal compliance.

System Coordination and Service Design

The AP led the integrated neighbourhood team to operationalise the plan. Actions included proactive prescribing, rapid-response escalation pathways, and coordination of social care to maintain 24/7 cover. Recognising poor rural connectivity, the AP negotiated with the Integrated Care System for enhanced home visiting and alternative monitoring solutions, ensuring digital equity.

Outcome

Mrs J remained at home for the final eight months of life, experienced no further emergency admissions, and died peacefully with her family present. Post-bereavement evaluation confirmed that care was aligned with her wishes and avoided burdensome interventions.

CONCLUSION

The future of frailty and EoL care will be defined by demographic pressure, complexity of illness, resource constraints, and technological change. APs are well positioned to lead this evolution bridging domains of clinical expertise, system design, ethics, and leadership. By embracing integrated care models, advocating for equitable resource allocation, applying digital innovation thoughtfully, and elevating their role in shaping policy, APs can ensure that the next generation of frailty and EoL services remains humane, sustainable, and dignified.

Take-Home Messages

1. Demographic ageing demands proactive, integrated models of frailty and EoL care.
2. APs should combine expert clinical assessment with strategic leadership and ethical competence.

3. Digital innovation and AI should enhance, not replace, personalised care and human judgement.

4. Equitable access, respect for autonomy, and careful resource stewardship are central to future service design.

REFERENCES

Albarrati, A.M., Nazer, R., Abdelwahab, S.I., and Albratty, M. (2025). Artificial intelligence applications and aging (1995–2024): trends, challenges, and future directions in frailty research. *Archives of Gerontology and Geriatrics* 123: 105837.

British Geriatrics Society and Getting It Right First Time (2025). *Actions to Help Provide Effective Acute Care for Older People Living with Frailty*. London: BGS https://www.bgs.org.uk/resources/actions-to-help-provide-effective-acute-care-for-older-people-living-with-frailty (accessed 24 September 2025).

Centre for Ageing Better (2025). Our ageing population: the state of ageing 2025. https://ageing-better.org.uk/our-ageing-population-state-ageing-2025 (accessed 24 September 2025).

Department of Health and Social Care (2025). Fit for the future: 10 year health plan for england – executive summary. https://assets.publishing.service.gov.uk/media/6888a09964785256757383f3a/fit-for-the-future-10-year-health-plan-for-england-executive-summary.pdf (accessed 24 September 2025).

Global Frailty Network (2025). Global frailty network/frailty seminar series. https://frailtyscience.org/global-frailty-networkfrailty-seminar-series/ (accessed 26 September 2025).

Johns Hopkins University Older Americans Independence Center (2021). Frailty science: promoting resilience and healthy aging. 2021. https://frailtyscience.org/ (accessed 4 October 2023).

Kawashima, A. and Evans, C.J. (2023). Needs-based triggers for timely referral to palliative care for older adults severely affected by noncancer conditions: a systematic review and narrative synthesis. *BMC Palliative Care* 22 (1): 20.

Ludlow, K., Todd, O., Reid, N., and Yaman, H. (2023). Frailty in primary care: challenges, innovations, and future directions. *BMC Primary Care* 24: Article 129.

Mate, K.S., Berman, A., Laderman, M. et al. (2018). Creating age-friendly health systems—a vision for better care of older adults. *Healthcare* 6 (1): 4–6.

NHS England (2023). NHS long term workforce plan. https://www.england.nhs.uk/long-read/nhs-long-term-workforce-plan-2/ (accessed 24 September 2025).

NHS England (2025). Review of NHS performance and delivery. https://www.england.nhs.uk/long-read/review-of-nhs-performance-and-delivery/ (accessed 24 September 2025).

Ruiz, J.G. and Theou, O. (ed.) (2024). *Frailty: A multidisciplinary approach to assessment, management, and prevention*. Cham, Switzerland: Springer Nature Switzerland AG.

UK Parliament (2025). Terminally Ill adults (end of life) bill (Bill 3774). https://bills.parliament.uk/bills/3774 (accessed 25 September 2025).

World Health Organization (2017). WHO Clinical Consortium on Healthy Ageing: Topic focus – frailty and intrinsic capacity (report of consortium meeting, 1–2 December 2016, Geneva). WHO Report No. WHO/FWC/ALC/17.2. https://www.who.int/publications/i/item/WHO-FWC-ALC-17.2 (accessed 26 September 2025).

World Health Organization (2024). Ageing and health. https://www.who.int/news-room/fact-sheets/detail/ageing-and-health (accessed 24 September 2025).

Index

A

ablative procedures, 203
accessibility, comprehensive geriatric
    assessment, 118–119
acetylcholine, 178
achalasia, 269
ACP. *see* advanced care planning (ACP)
ACS. *see* acute coronary syndrome (ACS)
actinic keratoses, 323
action/intention tremor, 208
activities of daily living (ADLs), 62, 86, 102, 113
acute atrial fibrillation, 244
acute confusion with suspected dementia, 230
acute coronary syndrome (ACS)
    assessment in frail patients, 236
    complication, 239
    definition of, 235
    diagnosis, 236
    discharge and long-term care, 239
    frailty-specific considerations, 239
    management of, 236–238
    ongoing and secondary prevention, 238
    risk factors for, 235
    signs and symptoms, 235
acute kidney injury (AKI), 290
    aetiology, 292
    contrast and procedures, 293
    decision-making by AP, 293–294
    immediate management priorities, 292, 293
    initial assessment and investigations, 292
    managing complications, 293
    pathophysiology of, 291
    vulnerable frail older adults, 290
acute medicine, 199
acute sarcopenia, 166
acute seizures, 205
acute tracheobronchitis, 254–255
acute upper gastrointestinal bleeding, 272

Addison's disease, 310
    causes, 311
    diagnosis, 311
    management, 311
    presentation, 310
adjunctive therapies, for Parkinson's disease, 203
adjuvant medications, 360
ADLs. *see* activities of daily living (ADLs)
adrenal incidentalomas, 311
adrenocorticotropic hormone (ACTH), 311
ADs. *see* advance directives (ADs)
advance care planning (ACP), 11
advanced ageing, 187–188
advanced care planning (ACP), 348, 351
    benefits of, 351
    difficult conversations, 352–353
    principles of communication in, 351–352
advance decisions, 374–375
Advance Decision to Refuse Treatment (ADRT), 120
advance directives (ADs), 374–375
advanced practitioners (APs), 4, 16, 47, 57, 78, 133,
        218, 223, 226
    build and prove capability, 11
    clinical practice, 8, 10
    education, 8, 10
    engage with area-specific capability frameworks, 6
    leadership and management, 8, 10
    research, 8–9, 10
    role in frailty settings, 8, 10
    stability and assurance in, 5
AF. *see* atrial fibrillation (AF)
ageing, 110, 176, 204, 247, 280
    cardiovascular system, 179–181
    endocrine system, 184–186
    gastrointestinal system, 181–183
    genitourinary system, 183–184
    haematology and immune system, 186–188
    integumentary system, 186

nervous system, 178
    respiratory system, 179
age-related cardiovascular changes, 180–181
age-related renal changes, 290
agitation, 362
agnosia, 224
air hunger, 359
airway defence mechanisms, 179
AKI. *see* acute kidney injury (AKI)
alcohol consumption, 59
alcohol-related cognitive disorder, 229
alcohol use, 86
algorithmic decision support, 394
alpha-adrenergic blockers, 281
Alzheimer's disease, 223, 228
amantadine, for Parkinson's disease, 203
amiodarone, 305
anaemia, 186
angiodysplasia, 274
ANH. *see* artificial nutrition and hydration (ANH)
antibacterial therapy, 254–255
anticholinergic burden (ACB), 106, 153
Anticholinergic Cognitive Burden (ACB)
    Calculator, 153
anticipatory prescribing, EoL care, 377
anticoagulants, 154
anticoagulation, 261
antifungal agents, 270
anxiety, 58, 227
    management of, 227
    person-centred approaches, 227, 230
appetite, 268
appropriate polypharmacy, 150–151
apraxia, 224
area-specific capability frameworks, 6
    older people/frailty, 6–9
    palliative and end-of-life care, 9
arrhythmias, 239
    assessment and investigations, 240–241, 244
    causes and risk factors of, 243
    clinical presentation, 240–241, 244
    complications and prognosis, 241
    diagnosis, 240–241
    management, 241, 244–245
arterial blood gas analysis, 261
arterial (ischaemic) ulcers, 320

artificial intelligence (AI), 391
artificial nutrition and hydration (ANH), 377–378
aspiration, 270
aspiration pneumonia, 259
    diagnosis, 259
    management, 259
    risk factors, 259
assisted dying, 378, 394–395
assistive devices, 119
asteatotic (xerotic) eczema, 323
asterixis/metabolic tremor, 209
asthenia, 342
asthma, 262, 264
atrial fibrillation (AF)
    classification of, 243
    definition and clinical relevance, 241
atrophic vaginitis, 283
atypical parkinsonian disorders, 202
Australia-modified Karnofsky Performance Status
    (AKPS), 350
autoimmune adrenalitis, 311
autonomic impairment, 178
autonomy, end-of-life (EoL) care, 371–372

B
bacteraemia, 316
Bamford classification, stroke, 212
basal cell carcinoma, 322
beneficence, 372
benign lesions, 323
benign prostatic hyperplasia (BPH), 184, 280
    clinical features and assessment, 280–281
    management, 281
    pharmacological therapy, 281
    surgical and minimally invasive options, 281
benzodiazepines, 156, 205
benzylpenicillin, 316
β-hydroxy-β-methylbutyrate (HMB), 170
bicipital tendinitis, 340
biological plausibility and epidemiology, 23
bisphosphonates, 328
bladder capacity and compliance, 184
blood cultures, 256
blood glucose monitoring, 302
blood tests, 205
body mass index, 268

bone marrow stem cells, 186
bone resorption, 326
bowel and bladder health, 109–110
bowel obstruction, 276
Bowen's disease, 323
BPH. *see* benign prostatic hyperplasia (BPH)
bradyarrhythmias, 239, 241
breathing techniques, 359
breathlessness, 359–360
British Geriatrics Society (BGS), 102, 259, 260
British National Formulary (BNF), 302
bronchoscopy, 264
bullous pemphigoid, 322

C

calcium supplementation, 326
callus/corns/fissures, 338
candida (cutaneous or oral), 323
candida (yeast) infection, 317
capacity assessment
    in end-of-life care, 375–376
    frailty, 394
carbamazepine, 205
cardiac arrhythmias, 239
cardiac tamponade, 239
cardiology
    acute coronary syndrome, 235–239
    arrhythmias, 239–241
    atrial fibrillation, 241–245
    heart failure, 245–247
    hypertension, 247–249
cardiopulmonary resuscitation (CPR), 351
Cardiovascular Health Study (CHS), 21
cardiovascular system, 179–181
care plans, 113–114
Care Quality Commission (CQC), 353
carer education, 227
carer needs and burden, 117
carpal tunnel syndrome, 338
catechol-*O*-methyltransferase inhibitors, for
    Parkinson's disease, 203
cellulitis, 316
    assessment and investigations, 316
    clinical characteristics, 316
    management, 316
Centre for Advancing Practice, 6
cerebellar/brainstem signs, 214

cerebral hypoperfusion, 205
cervical spondylosis, 335
    clinical presentation, 335
    differential diagnosis, 335
    examination, 335
    investigations, 335–336
    management, 336
    symptoms, 335
cervical spondylotic myelopathy, 337
CFS. *see* Clinical Frailty Scale (CFS)
CGA. *see* comprehensive geriatric
    assessment (CGA)
chemical pneumonitis, 259
chemotherapy, 265
chest radiograph, 205, 254, 256, 259
cholinergic receptors, 178
chronic inflammation, 58
chronic kidney disease (CKD), 294
    aetiology, 295
    common complications, 295
    identifying and assessment, 295
    management principles, 295
chronic liver disease, 275
chronic obstructive pulmonary disease
    (COPD), 262–264
chronic or persistent atrial fibrillation, 244
chronic sarcopenia, 166
chronic venous insufficiency (CVI), 319
    clinical manifestations, 319
    pathophysiology, 319
    skin changes, 319
chronic wounds, 110
chronological age, 176
circadian rhythms, 185
cirrhosis, 275
CKD. *see* chronic kidney disease (CKD)
clarity and honesty, 352
Clinical Frailty Scale (CFS), 63, 134, 135, 259, 260
    in acute medicine, 141
clinical heterogeneity, 81
coagulation, 187
co-amoxiclav, 316
cognition, 113, 115
cognitive and psychosocial dimensions,
    exclusion of, 24–25
cognitive behavioural therapy for insomnia
    (CBT-I), 156

cognitive capacity, 38
cognitive decline, 63–64
cognitive frailty, 63
cognitive impairment, 58, 113, 115, 249
    assessment tools, 219, 220, 221
    clinical presentation, 218–219
    prevalence and impact, 218
combined exercise and nutrition, 168–169
communication, 120
communication challenges, 79–80
community-acquired pneumonia, 256
community and caregiver engagement, 41
community services and support, 119
comparable alternatives exist, 25
complexity of care, frailty, 64
complex regional pain syndrome, 339
comprehensive geriatric assessment (CGA), 11, 60,
        99, 104, 134, 195, 268, 392
    case study, 122–123
    in clinical practice, 103
    cognition, 115
    conduct, 101
    consider conducting, 101
    definition of, 100–101
    delirium, 115
    in end-of-life medicine, 123–124
    environmental domain of, 118–120
    in everyday care, 102
    functional domain of, 112–114
    future wishes domain, 120–121
    implementation, 122–124
    integration into primary care, 102
    perform, 101
    physical domain of, 103–112
    psychological domain of, 114–115
    sixth elements of, 103
    social domain of, 115–118
comprehensive person-centred assessment, 41
compression therapy, 321
computed tomographic pulmonary angiography
    (CTPA), 261
computed tomography (CT), 205, 225, 264
confidentiality, 373
Confusion Assessment Method (CAM), 222
confusion states and coma, causes of, 116
constipation, 273
    assessment and diagnosis, 273

in frail and end-of- life patients, 156
    management, 273–274
    pathophysiology and risk factors, 273
continence, 38, 113
continuity and care planning, 113–114
conversations, 352–353
    and communication, 120
COPD. see chronic obstructive pulmonary
        disease (COPD)
cough, 92–95
COVID-19 pandemic, 259, 353, 372
    evidence on outcomes, 260
    impact on sarcopenia, 167–168
    management and ongoing care, 260
    presentation and assessment, 260
    recovery and long-term impact, 260
cranial nerves and visual system, 213
C-reactive protein (CRP), 255
credentials, 6
CRP. see C-reactive protein (CRP)
CTPA. see computed tomographic pulmonary
        angiography (CTPA)
CVI. see chronic venous insufficiency (CVI)

D
D-dimer testing, 261
decision-making, EoL care, 376–377
decision support systems, 394
deep brain stimulation, 203
deep vein thrombosis (DVT), 319
deficit accumulation model, 16, 17, 25–26
dehydration, 112
delirium, 63–64, 115
    and agitation, 362
    assessment tools, 222
    definition and significance, 220
    identifying causes, 222–223
    mobility, 223
    nutritional support, 223
    prevalence of, 220
dementia, 115, 223–224
    case study, 230
    cognitive testing, 224
    communicating the diagnosis, 224
    investigations, 224–225
    physical and mental examination, 224
dementia with Lewy bodies (DLB), 228

demyelination, 178

dentition, 182

deprescribing, 151, 158
  embedding into multidisciplinary polypharmacy clinics, 156
  identifying and reversing prescribing cascades, 155
  individualising antihypertensive therapy, 153–154
  optimising anticoagulant use, 154
  polypharmacy and, 157–158
  practical guidance in, 153–154
  preventing hyponatraemia, 154
  reviewing ongoing indication for each medicine, 153
  and role of advanced practitioners, 149
  tools to support decision-making, 151–152

deprescription, 11

depression, 38, 58, 114–115, 229
  clinical features, 226
  clinical presentation, 225–227
  epidemiology and risk factors, 225
  management of, 226
  in older people, 225
  screening tools, 227

Deprivation of Liberty Safeguards (DoLS), 373

dermatophyte infection (tinea), 317

dermatophyte (tinea) infection, 323

diabetes mellitus
  clinical presentation, 301
  diagnosis, 301
  management, 301
  pharmacological therapy, 302
  prevalence of, 301

diabetes therapy in frail or end-of- life contexts, 154–155

diabetic (neuropathic) ulcers, 320

diarrhoea, 110

difficult conversations, 352–353

digital exclusion, 117

digital health, 171, 391

directory, 6

disability, 62

dislocation, 340

diverticular disease, 275

dizziness, classification of, 207

DNACPR. *see* Do Not Attempt Cardiopulmonary Resuscitation (DNACPR)

doctrine of double effect, 378

documentation, 355

Do Not Attempt Cardiopulmonary Resuscitation (DNACPR), 353, 354–355

dopamine agonists, for Parkinson's disease, 203

dopamine-producing neurons, 202

dopamine transporter imaging, Parkinson's disease, 203

doxycycline, 255

Dressler's syndrome, 239

Driver and Vehicle Licensing Agency (DVLA), 205

drug/alcohol withdrawal tremor, 209

drug history, 85

drug-induced parkinsonism, 202

drug-induced tremor, 209

dual-energy X-ray absorptiometry (DEXA), 326

dual sensory impairment, 38

DVT. *see* deep vein thrombosis (DVT)

dying, 349–350

dysphagia, 270

dyspnoea, 359

E

Earlier Enduring Powers of Attorney (EPOA), 374

early identification of progression, 23

echocardiography, 261

Edmonton Frail Scale (EFS), 139–140
  and TFI in community care, 144

effective management, 107

effective prescribing, 358

EFS. *see* Edmonton Frail Scale (EFS)

elder abuse, 121, 379–380

Elder Abuse Suspicion Index, 121

electrical conduction, 180

electrocardiography, 205

electroencephalography (EEG), 205, 225

electromyography, 206

electronic frailty index (eFI), 16, 27

electronic health records, 355

emergency and escalation planning, 121

emerging technological applications, 24

emotional well-being, 227

endocrine ageing, 185

endocrine disorders, 312

endocrine emergencies, 304
endocrine system, 184
   diabetes, 301–302
   energy balance and appetite regulation, 185–186
   glucose metabolism, 185
   gonadal hormones, 185
   hormone replacement therapy, 309–310
   hyperthyroidism, 305–309
   hypothalamic–pituitary axis, 185
   hypothyroidism, 302–305
   menopause, 309–310
   primary adrenal insufficiency, 310–311
   thyroid function, 185
end-of-life (EoL) care, 4, 348, 358, 390
   advance directives, 374–375
   AP leadership in, 395–396
   artificial nutrition and hydration, 377–378
   assisted dying, 378
   capacity assessment in, 375–376
   challenges in, 375
   decision-making, 376–377
   doctrine of double effect, 378
   elder abuse, 379–380
   ethical, legal, and resource challenges, 394–395
   ethical principles in, 371–373
   future advanced practice workforce, 392–394
   global perspectives and health equity, 395
   innovations in models of, 390–392
   legal and ethical frameworks for decision-making in, 373–374
   organ donation, 378–379
   quality-of-life considerations, 380
   rationing and ageism in health care, 380
end-of-life decision-making in advanced practice, 381
end-of-life legislation, 394–395
end-of-life medicine, 198
endometrial hyperplasia, 283
endometrial or cervical polyps, 283
energy balance and appetite regulation, 185–186
environmental domain of CGA, 118
   accessibility, 118–119
   community services and support, 119
   home safety, 118
   technology aids, 119–120
epilepsy, 204

   causes of, 205
   diagnosis, 205–206
   management, 205
   older adults with, 205
   primary (idiopathic) epilepsy, 204
   secondary, 204
ePrognosis, 350
equally important, 110, 118
eradication therapy, 272
erectile dysfunction, 285
   clinical assessment, 285
   management, 285
erysipelas, 317
erythrocyte sedimentation rate (ESR), 187
erythromycin, 316
ESR. *see* erythrocyte sedimentation rate (ESR)
essential tremor (ET), 208
European Society for Clinical Nutrition and Metabolism (ESPEN), 108
European Society of Cardiology (ESC), 241
European Working Group on Sarcopenia in Older People (EWGSOP), 165
exercise, 60, 168
exhaustion, 22

F
faecal incontinence, 110
fairness, 372
falls, 84
   fractures, and injury, 62
   history, 106–107
family history, 85
feasibility challenges in clinical settings, 24
feeling weaker, 78
fibrosis, 180
financial well-being, 117
5-alpha reductase inhibitors, 281
flucloxacillin, 316
flutter, 241
4AT tool, 222
fragility fractures, 326
   risk in frail older adults, 328–329
frail elderly, 17
frail older adults, vulnerable, 290
FRAIL scale, 136, 138–139
   in pre-operative assessment, 144

frailty, 4, 19, 47, 61–62, 78, 133, 235
   accurate identification and grading of, 133
   AP leadership in, 395–396
   assessment and clinical examination, 11
   beyond older age, 20
   biological and clinical factors, 58
   and chronic diseases, 59
   clinical and public health implications, 66
   comorbidity, complexity, and health use, 390
   complications of, 61–67
   comprehensive geriatric assessment, 60
   decline in quality of life and well-being, 65
   definition, 18
   development mechanism, 19
   economic and caregiver burden, 65–66
   epidemiology of, 47–51
   ethical, legal, and resource challenges, 394–395
   following critical illness, 29
   future advanced practice workforce, 392–394
   future directions, 61
   and giant cell arteritis, 330–331
   global perspectives and health equity, 395
   healthcare utilisation, 62–63
   healthy again, disability and multimorbidity, 19
   heart failure in, 245–246
   hospitalisation and readmission, 62–63
   identification and grading, 11
   implications for practice, 51–52
   infections and compromised immunity, 65
   innovations in models of care, 390–392
   institutionalisation and loss of autonomy, 63
   intrinsic capacity and, 38–39
   lifestyle factors, 59
   malnutrition and sarcopenia, 65
   measurement and setting, 64–65
   medication optimisation, 61
   mortality and prognosis, 63
   multicomponent interventions, 60
   multidomain management of, 67
   and multimorbidity, 249
   in older adults, 259
   in Parkinson's disease, 202
   psychological and cognitive factors, 58
   psychosocial approaches, 60–61
   recognising, 18
   risk factors, 58–59
   social and environmental determinants, 58
   special considerations in, 245
   status, 103, 105
frailty assessment tools, 133, 134–135
   Clinical Frailty Scale (CFS), 134, 135
   Edmonton Frail Scale (EFS), 139–140
   FRAIL scale, 136, 138–139
   Pictorial Fit-Frail Scale (PFFS), 135–136, 137–138
   Tilburg Frailty Indicator (TFI), 141–143
frailty-capable workforce, 392
frailty index (FI), 16, 26, 28–29, 61
frailty phenotype, 16, 22
   advantages of, 23–24
   criteria, 21
   disadvantages of, 24–27
   through the cardiovascular health study, 21
Fried frailty phenotype
   advantages of, 23–24
   disadvantages of, 24–27
frontotemporal dementia (FTD), 228
frozen shoulder, 340
functional assessment, 113
functional decline, 62
   and decompensation, 79
functional disorders, 270
functional domain of CGA, 112–113
   assessing ADLs and IADLs, 113
   cognition, nutrition, and continence, 113
   continuity and care planning, 113–114
   influences on function, 113
   interventions and reablement, 114
   structured functional assessment, 113
functional status, 86
future wishes domain of CGA, 120
   conversations and communication, 120
   emergency and escalation planning, 121
   legal tools, 120–121
   treatment preferences, 120

G

gait and function, 214
gait assessment, 90
gallbladder disease, 275
gastroenterology
   constipation, 273
   dysphagia, 270

nutrition, hydration, and weight loss, 268–269
  oesophageal disease, 269
  peptic ulcer disease, 270–272
gastrointestinal disease, 276
gastrointestinal disorders in older adults, 274–276
gastrointestinal system, 181–182
  ageing of, 182
  oesophagus and stomach, 182–183
  oral cavity and dentition, 182
  pancreas, liver, and gallbladder, 183
  small and large intestine, 183
gastro-oesophageal reflux disease (GORD), 269
GCA. *see* giant cell arteritis (GCA)
General Medical Council (GMC), 377
genital tract malignancy, 283
genitourinary system, 183
  benign prostatic hyperplasia, 280–281
  erectile dysfunction, 285
  hypersexuality, 285–286
  kidneys and renal function, 183
  lower urinary tract, 184
  prostate cancer, 281–284
  sex-specific changes, 184
  sexual health and ageing, 285
  sexual health in both sexes, 184
  urinary incontinence, 284–285
geriatric medicine, 12, 195
  MPF capabilities and, 197
GFR. *see* glomerular filtration rate (GFR)
giant cell arteritis (GCA), 330–331
  clinical manifestations, 331
  investigations, 331
  management, 332
  pathogenesis, 331
glenohumeral OA, 340
Global Leadership Initiative on Malnutrition
  (GLIM), 108
glomerular filtration rate (GFR), 183, 290
glomerulonephritis, 296
glucose metabolism, 185
gonadal hormones, 185
GORD. *see* gastro-oesophageal reflux disease (GORD)
gout, 341
governance, 6, 355
gram-negative bacilli, 257
Guillain–Barré syndrome (GBS), 210

H
haematology and immune system, 186
  clinical consequences, 187
  coagulation and inflammatory milieu, 187
  haematopoiesis and anaemia, 186
  immune ageing, 187
haematopoiesis, 186
Haemophilus influenzae, 255, 257
haloperidol, 223
healing outcomes, 112
healthcare systems, 120
health equity, 395
hearing loss, 38, 109
heart failure, 245–246
  definition, causes, and clinical features, 246
  frailty considerations, 246
  management, 246
  and pulmonary oedema management, 247
heart failure with preserved ejection fraction
  (HFpEF), 180
Heberden/Bouchard nodes (hand OA), 338
Helicobacter pylori, 270, 271, 272
hiatus hernia, 269
high-calorie foods, 223
hip fracture, 339
hip OA, 339
history of presenting complaints (HPCs), 81
history-taking
  communication challenges, 79–80
  functional decline and decompensation, 79
  key components of, 80–83
  multimorbidity and overlapping symptoms, 80
  in suspected stroke/TIA, 212–213
  under-reporting of symptoms, 80
HIV serology, 224
home safety, 118
hormone replacement therapy (HRT), 309–310
hospital-acquired pneumonia, 258
hospital-associated deconditioning, 114
hospitalisation and readmission, frailty, 62–63
hospitals and care homes, 373
HPCs. *see* history of presenting complaints (HPCs)
Human Rights Act (1998), 354, 372
hydration, 108, 112, 222, 268–269
hyperkalaemia, 293
hyperosmolar hyperglycaemic state, 302

hypersexuality, 285–286
hypertension, 247–248
  challenges in treating, 249
  diagnosis and assessment, 248
  management principles, 249
  treatment targets and evidence, 248
hyperthyroidism, 305
  advanced practice decision-making for, 307–309
  aetiology, 306
  clinical presentation, 306
  investigation, 306–307
  management, 307
hypnotics, 156
hypoglycaemia, 302
hyponatraemia, 154
hypothalamic–pituitary axis, 185
hypothyroidism, 302
  clinical presentation, 303, 304
  drug interactions, 305
  investigation, 303
  management, 303
  prevalence of, 302

I
IBD. *see* inflammatory bowel disease (IBD)
IBS. *see* irritable bowel syndrome (IBS)
IC. *see* intrinsic capacity (IC)
IGT. *see* impaired glucose tolerance (IGT)
immune ageing, 187
immunosenescence, 186, 187
impaired glucose tolerance (IGT), 185
incontinence, 112
Independent Mental Capacity Advocate (IMCA), 374
individualising antihypertensive therapy, 153–154
infections and compromised immunity, frailty, 65
inflammatory bowel disease (IBD), 275
inflammatory milieu, 187
influences on function, 113
influenza, 255
influenza-like illness, 255
insomnia
  in older adults, 210
  without long-term hypnotics, 156
institutionalisation and loss of autonomy, frailty, 63
instrumental activities of daily living (IADLs),
    62, 86, 113
integrated and community-based care, 391

Integrated Care for Older People (ICOPE), 35
Integrated Palliative Care Outcome Scale
    (IPOS), 350
integumentary system, 186
intertrigo, 317
interventions and reablement, 114
intestinal ischaemia, 274
intestinal pseudo-obstruction, 276
intravenous phenytoin, 205
intravenous therapy, 316
intrinsic capacity (IC), 35, 36–37, 66
  community and caregiver engagement, 41
  comparison between frailty and, 38–39
  comprehensive person-centred assessment, 41
  concept of, 36
  development of personalised care plan, 41
  ICOPE assessment pathway, 40–42
  initial screening, 41
  referral, monitoring, and review, 41
  six domains of, 37–39
iron supplementation, rationalising, 155
irritable bowel syndrome (IBS), 274
ischaemic colitis, 275
isolation, 116
iterative process, 352

J
joint disease 'pseudo-weakness, ' 342
joint problems, 107–108
justice, 372

K
Katz Index of Independence in Activities of Daily
    Living (Katz-ADL), 86, 87
kidneys and renal function, 183

L
lack of engagement, 119
lactulose, 156
lacunar stroke (LACS), 212
lamotrigine, 205
Lasting Power of Attorney (LPA), 120, 354, 373–374
late-life depression, 225
late-life psychosis, 229
left or right ventricular failure, 239
legal tools, 120–121
Legionella pneumophila, 257

leg ulcers, 320
lentigo maligna, 323
levetiracetam, 205
levodopa, for Parkinson's disease, 203
levomepromazine, 362
levothyroxine, 305
LHRH. *see* luteinising hormone-releasing
    hormone (LHRH)
lichen sclerosus/squamous hyperplasia, 284
lichen simplex chronicus, 322
lifestyle factors, frailty, 59
Lifestyle Interventions and Independence for
    Elders (LIFE), 62
living wills, 374–375
locomotor capacity, 37
loneliness, 116
long-term antiepileptic medication, 205
loop diuretics, 246
lorazepam, 223
low-dose thiazide diuretics, 319
lower urinary tract, 184
lower urinary tract symptoms (LUTSs), 280
low physical activity, 22, 59
lumbar puncture, 225
lung cancer, 264
    clinical presentation and assessment, 264
    management principles, 264
luteinising hormone-releasing hormone
    (LHRH), 282
LUTSs. *see* lower urinary tract symptoms (LUTSs)

M
macrogols, 156
macrolide antibiotics, 255
magnetic resonance imaging (MRI), 225
malignant melanoma, 322
malignant ulcers, 320
    general management, 321
    principles of assessment, 320–321
malnutrition, 59, 65, 108, 112, 268, 270
malnutrition-associated sarcopenia, 166
Malnutrition Universal Screening Tool
    (MUST), 108, 268
medication
    history and review, 105–106
    optimisation, 61
    side effects, 112

Medicines and Healthcare products Regulatory
    Agency (MHRA), 153
MENLOC systematic review, 363
menopause, 185, 309–310
Mental Capacity Act (MCA), 372, 374
mental health, 58, 63–64
mental health prescribing, 363
mental state examination, 224
microscopic colitis, 274
Mini-Cog, 224
Mini-Mental State Examination (MMSE), 224
mitochondrial dysfunction, 178
mobility and functional status, 112
moderate-to-severe depression, 226
Montreal Cognitive Assessment (MoCA), 224
morphine, 360
morphine sulphate, 360
mortality and prognosis, frailty, 63
motoric cognitive risk (MCR), 38
motor neurone disease (MND), 206
    diagnosis, 206
    management, 206
motor system, 214
multicomponent interventions, frailty, 60
multidisciplinary approach, 363
multidisciplinary integration, 12
multifactorial interventions, 107
multimorbidity, 58, 64, 105
    and overlapping symptoms, 80
multiple system atrophy, 202
multi-professional framework (MPF), 4, 5, 16,
    35, 99, 149
musculoskeletal system
    cervical spondylosis and myelopathy, 335–336
    osteoarthritis, 329–332
    osteoporosis, 326–329
    polymyalgia rheumatica, 332–335
Mycoplasma pneumoniae, 257
myelopathy, 335
myokine, 170

N
National Institute for Health and Care Excellence
    (NICE), 102, 106, 156, 259, 260, 264, 348, 358
natriuretic peptides, 246
nausea and vomiting, 361–362
necrotising fasciitis, 317

nephrotic syndrome, 296
nervous system, 178
neuroimaging, Parkinson's disease, 203
neuroleptic malignant syndrome (NMS), 210
neurological ageing, 215
neurology system
    epilepsy, 204–206
    motor neurone disease, 206–211
    Parkinson's disease, 202–204
    stroke, 212–215
neuropathic (charcot) foot, 338
new confusion, 92–95
noisy secretions, 362
non-alcoholic fatty liver disease, 275
non-maleficence, 372
non-pharmacological strategies, 359
non-resolving pneumonia, 257–258
non-small-cell lung cancer (NSCLC), 264
non-steroidal anti-inflammatory drugs
    (NSAIDs), 155, 270
non-valvular atrial fibrillation, 243
normal ageing, 115, 268
normal-pressure hydrocephalus (NPH), 229
NSCLC. *see* non-small-cell lung cancer (NSCLC)
nutrition, 37, 86, 108, 112, 113, 268–269
    combined exercise and, 168–169
    protein and, 169–170

O

OA. *see* osteoarthritis (OA)
occupational therapy, 359
oedema, 319
oesophageal disease, 269
oesophageal dysmotility, 270
oesophagus, 182–183
oestrogen deficiency, 185
Ogilvie's syndrome, 276
onychogryphosis/onychomycosis/ingrown nails, 338
operationalisation, variability in, 25
opioid-induced constipation (OIC), 156
opioids, 360
oral cavity, 182
oral morphine, 360
oral nutritional supplements (ONS), 108
organ donation, 378–379
organisational governance, 355

orthostatic blood pressure, 248
orthostatic hypotension, 249
orthostatic tremor, 209
osmotic agents, 156
osteoarthritis (OA), 329
    clinical manifestations, 329
    diagnostic approach, 330
    non-pharmacological strategies, 330
    pathophysiology, 329
    pharmacological treatments, 330
    surgical interventions, 330
    towards proactive care, 330
osteomyelitis (foot/other bones), 337
osteoporosis, 326, 327
    broader perspectives on bone health, 328
    clinical features and diagnosis, 326
    pathophysiology, 326
    prevention and management, 326, 328
Outcome Assessment and Complexity Collaborative
    (OACC), 350
Oxfordshire Community Stroke Project (OCSP), 212

P

PACS. *see* partial anterior circulation stroke (PACS)
Paget's disease of bone, 341
pain and joint problems, 107–108
Pain Assessment in Advanced Dementia (PAINAD)
    scale, 107
pain management, 360–361
palliative and end-of-life care framework, 9
palliative and supportive care, 265
palliative care, 198
palliative sedation, 376–377
pancreas, liver, and gallbladder, 183
paracetamol, 223
Parkinson's disease (PD), 202
    case study, 204
    clinical presentation, 202–203
    diagnosis, 202
    frailty in, 202
    investigations, 203
    management, 203
    non-motor symptoms, 203
    prevalence of, 202
    supportive and multidisciplinary care, 203
Parkinson's disease dementia (PDD), 228

paroxysmal atrial fibrillation, 244
partial anterior circulation stroke (PACS), 212
past medical and surgical history, 105
past medical history (PMH), 83–85
PC. *see* presenting complaint (PC)
PD. *see* Parkinson's disease (PD)
PE. *see* pulmonary embolism (PE)
peak bone mass, 326
pendant alarms, 119
peptic ulcer disease, 270–272
pericarditis, 239
peripheral and autonomic nerves, 178
peripheral arterial disease, 338
peripheral neuropathies, 209
persistent seizures, 205
personalised care plan, 41
personalised interventions, 392
person-centredness, 352
PFFS. *see* Pictorial Fit-Frail Scale (PFFS)
pharmacological management, 360
pharmacological therapy, 249, 273
pharmacotherapy, 227
phenoxymethylpenicillin, 316
PHN. *see* post-herpetic neuralgia (PHN)
physical examination in frail adult
    core elements of examination, 88–92
    general principles, 88
Pictorial Fit-Frail Scale (PFFS), 135–136, 137–138
    in culturally diverse primary care, 144
PINCH ME mnemonic, 222
PMH. *see* past medical history (PMH)
PMR. *see* polymyalgia rheumatica (PMR)
pneumonia, 255
    management and prognosis, 257–259
    presentation, assessment, and
        microbiology, 255–257
polymyalgia rheumatica (PMR), 332
    avoiding diagnostic and treatment pitfalls, 333
    case study, 333–334
    diagnostic features, 332–333
    management, 333
    pathophysiology, 332
polypharmacy, 11, 64, 85, 105, 106, 112, 149, 150
    appropriate polypharmacy, 150–151
    deprescribing and, 151, 157–158
    problematic polypharmacy, 151

polypharmacy clinics, 156
poor nutritional status, 108
positron emission tomography (PET), 225
posterior circulation stroke (POCS), 212
post-herpetic neuralgia (PHN), 209
postural and postprandial hypotension, 249
postural tremor, 208
PPIs. *see* proton pump inhibitors (PPIs)
predictive analytics, 391
predictive models, 394
predictive validity across populations, 23
prescribing cascades, 105
prescribing cascades, identifying and reversing, 155
prescription of medications, 358
presenting complaint (PC), 80–83
pressure ulcer, 111
primary adrenal insufficiency, 310
primary care, 391
primary (idiopathic) epilepsy, 204
primary sarcopenia, 165
privacy, 373
problematic polypharmacy, 151
prognostication tools, 350
progressive supranuclear palsy, 202
prostate cancer, 281–282
    assessment and diagnosis, 282
    case study, 282–283
    management principles, 282
prostate carcinoma, 281
protein and nutrition, 169–170
proton pump inhibitors (PPIs), 269
pruritus ani, 323
pruritus of systemic origin, 322
pseudogout, 341
psychiatry
    anxiety and emotional well-being, 227–230
    cognitive impairment, 218–220
    delirium, 220–223
    dementia, 223–225
    depression, 225–227
psychological capacity, 38
psychological domain of CGA, 114
    depression, 114–115
psychological health in older adults, 218
psychological well-being, 114
Public Health England (PHE), 241

pulmonary embolism (PE), 260
   management, 261–262
   presentation and assessment, 261
Pulmonary Embolism Severity Index (PESI), 261

Q

quality-adjusted life years (QALYs), 102
quality-of-life, 380

R

randomised controlled trials (RCT), 169
rationing and ageism in health care, 380
reablement, 114
Recommended Summary Plan for Emergency Care
   and Treatment (ReSPECT), 121
REFS. *see* Reported Edmonton Frail Scale (REFS)
renal ageing, 297
renal artery stenosis, 296, 297
renal function, 183
repetitive strain injury, 339
Reported Edmonton Frail Scale (REFS), 139
resilience, 18, 66
resource allocation and ageism, 394
ReSPECT process, 354
respiratory disorders, 265
respiratory system, 179
respiratory tract infections, 254
   acute tracheobronchitis, 254–255
   influenza and influenza-like illness, 255
   upper airways, 254
respiratory tract secretions, 362–363
restlessness, 362
rest tremor, 208
rhinorrhoea, 255
rigors, 208
riluzole, 206
Rockall score, 272
rotator cuff tear, 340
rotator cuff tendinitis, 340
routine screening, 115
Royal College of Emergency Medicine (RCEM), 102
Royal College of Nursing (RCN), 363
Royal College of Physicians (RCP), 102

S

safeguarding and modern risks, 117
salivary glands, 182

sarcopenia, 58, 65, 164
   aetiological factors and mechanisms of, 167
   barriers and challenges, 170
   consequences of, 166
   definition, 165
   diagnostic approaches, 168, 169
   epidemiology, 166
   and frailty, 165
   impact of COVID-19 on, 167–168
   interventions, 168–170
   pathophysiology, 167
   prevalence of, 166
   recent advances and emerging therapies, 170–171
   role of APs, 170
   types of, 165–166
sarcopenic obesity, 166
scabies, 322
SCLC. *see* small-cell lung cancer (SCLC)
Scottish 7-Step approach, 151
SDH. *see* subdural haematoma (SDH)
seborrhoeic dermatitis, 317, 323
secondary epilepsy, 204
secondary sarcopenia, 165
sedation, 223
seizures, 204
selective serotonin reuptake inhibitors (SSRIs), 154
sensory capacity (hearing and vision), 38
sensory dysfunction, 108
sensory impairment, 108–109
sensory system, 214
serotonin–noradrenaline reuptake inhibitors
   (SNRIs), 154
serotonin syndrome (SS), 210
severe blistering infections, 322
sex-specific changes, 184
sexual disinhibition, 285
sexual health, 87
   and ageing, 285
   in both sexes, 184
sexual history, 86–87
shared responsibility, 351
single drug to address multiple conditions safely, 155
single-photon emission computed tomography
   (SPECT), 225
skin
   cellulitis, 316–318
   chronic venous insufficiency, 319–320

integrity, 110–112

    typical ulcer, 320–323

sleep disorders, in older people, 211

sleep disturbance, 223

slowness, 22

small and large intestine, 183

small-bowel function, 183

small-cell lung cancer (SCLC), 265

smoking, 59, 86

social and environmental determinants, frailty, 58

social and functional history, 86

social decisions for adults, 374

social domain of CGA, 115–116

    carer needs and burden, 117

    financial concerns, 117

    protective factors, 117–118

    safeguarding and modern risks, 117

    social support, isolation, and loneliness, 116

    spiritual and cultural well-being, 117

social isolation, 58, 119

social support, 116

sodium valproate, 205

specialised outpatient care, barriers in, 24

sperm production, 184, 185

SPIKES framework, 353

spiritual and cultural well-being, 117

spurious bleeding, 283

squamous cell carcinoma (SCC), 322

standardisation, benefits of, 23–24

standardised and reproducible framework, 23

Staphylococcus aureus, 255, 257

stimulant laxatives, 156

stomach, 182–183

STOPP/START criteria, 151

Streptococcus pneumoniae, 255, 256

strict glycaemic targets, 154

stroke, 212

    bedside investigation priorities, 214

    classification, 212

    examination in, 213–214

    history taking in, 212–213

    prevention of early complications, 215

structural disorders, 270

structured functional assessment, 113

structured medication reviews (SMRs), 106

subclinical hyperthyroidism, 306

subclinical hypothyroidism, 303

subcutaneous morphine, 360

subdural haematoma (SDH), 210

substantive ethics and ethics of care, 373

supraventricular tachycardias, 241

surgical history, 83–85

swallowing problems, 270

syncope, 242

syphilis, 224

systematic enquiry, 88

systolic blood pressure (SBP), 153

T

tachyarrhythmia, 240

TACS. *see* total anterior circulation stroke (TACS)

technology aids, 119–120

technology and equity, 394

telecare devices, 119

telemedicine, 171

TEPs. *see* Treatment Escalation Plans (TEPs)

testicular mass, 184, 185

testosterone, 184, 185

TFI. *see* Tilburg Frailty Indicator (TFI)

TFTs. *see* thyroid function tests (TFTs)

thiazide diuretics, 154

thromboembolic events, 239

thrombolysis, 261

thyroid function tests (TFTs), 185, 302, 305

thyroid-stimulating hormone (TSH), 185

thyrotoxicosis, 305

thyrotoxic tremor, 208

TIA. *see* transient ischaemic attack (TIA)

Tilburg Frailty Indicator (TFI), 141–143

timely initiation, 352

'time-is-brain' principle, 212

tissue diagnosis, 264

total anterior circulation stroke (TACS), 212

transient ischaemic attack (TIA), 212

transparent communication, 377

Treatment Escalation Plans (TEPs), 354

treatment preferences, 120

Trial of ORG 10172 in Acute Stroke Treatment (TOAST), 212

trigeminal neuralgia (TN), 209

trigger finger, 338

true myopathy/NMJ/ neuropathy, 342

type 1 diabetes, 301

type 2 diabetes, 301

U

undernutrition, 268
under-reporting of symptoms, 80
unintentional weight loss, 22
unrecognised pain, 223
untreated arrhythmias, 241
upper and lower GI bleeding, 271
upper gastrointestinal endoscopy, 270, 271
upper respiratory tract, infections of, 254
urinary incontinence (UI), 38, 109, 284–285
urinary retention, 223
urinary tract infections (UTIs), 109, 184
UTIs. *see* urinary tract infection (UTIs)

V

vaginal or urinary infection, 283
vaginal prolapse, 283
valvular atrial fibrillation, 243
varicose veins, 319
vascular dementia, 228
vascular parkinsonism, 202
venous ulcers, 320
ventricular fibrillation, 241
ventricular tachycardia, 241
vertebral fractures, 326

vertebral osteomyelitis/discitis, 337
vision and hearing loss, 38
vision loss, 109
visual impairment, 109
vitality, 37
vitamin D deficiency, 169
vitamin D supplementation, 326, 328
vomiting, 361–362
vulval carcinoma, 284
vulvitis, 284

W

warfarin, 261
weakness, 22
weight loss, 268
withdrawing and withholding treatment,
    EoL care, 377
World Health Organization (WHO), 390

X

xerostomia, 182

Z

zopiclone, 156